D1270605

Musculoskeletal Tissue Regeneration

Orthopedic Biology and Medicine

Series Editors: *Yuehuei H. An and A. U. Daniels*

Orthopaedic Research Laboratory
Medical University of South Carolina, Charleston, SC

Musculoskeletal Tissue Regeneration: Biological Materials and Methods, edited by *William S. Pietrzak*, 2008

Repair and Regeneration of Ligaments, Tendons, and Joint Capsule, edited by *William R. Walsh*, 2005

Musculoskeletal Tissue Regeneration

Biological Materials and Methods

Edited by

William S. Pietrzak Ph.D.
Department of Bioengineering, University of Illinois at Chicago, Chicago, IL
and
Biomet, Inc., Warsaw, IN

Foreword by

Charles A. Vacanti, M.D.
Brigham and Women's Hospital, Boston, MA

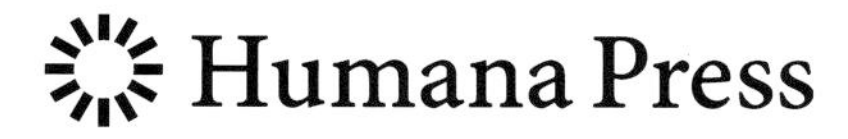

MT

William S. Pietrzak, Ph.D.
Department of Bioengineering
University of Illinois at Chicago
Chicago, IL
Biomet, Inc., Warsaw, IN
USA
billsp@uic.edu

Series Editors:

Yuehuei H. An and A. U. Daniels
Orthopaedic Research Laboratory
Medical University of South Carolina
Charleston, SC

ISBN: 978-1-58829-909-3 e-ISBN: 978-1-59745-239-7
DOI: 10.1007/978-1-59745-239-7

Library of Congress Control Number: 2008920308

Cover illustration: Prepared by Terry Armstrong, Warsaw, IN, representing cells, matrices, and signaling molecules - the three essential components of musculoskeletal tissue regeneration. Designed by William S. Pietrzak and Terry Armstrong.

Printed on acid-free paper

9 8 7 6 5 4 3 2 1

springer.com

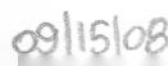

About the Editor

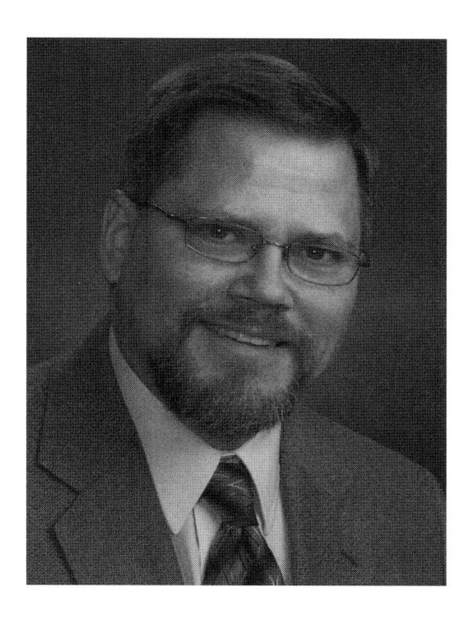

Originally from Chicago, Dr. William Pietrzak received his Bachelor of Science (1977) and Ph.D. (1988) bioengineering degrees from the University of Illinois at Chicago. His career has spanned several medical disciplines, including opthalmology, cardiovascular, and—for the past 16 years—orthopedics. He has published research on numerous technologies used for musculoskeletal tissue regeneration, including bioabsorbable fixation, bone graft substitutes, bone morphogenetic proteins, platelet rich plasma, and total knee and hip arthroplasty. Several of these publications have been centered around the foot, ankle, knee, hip, shoulder, and craniofacial skeleton. He is an inventor, with four patents in the fields of suture anchors and bioabsorbable fixation. In addition to his role as a reviewer for several biomedical journals, he serves on the Editorial Boards of the Journal of Craniofacial Surgery and the Journal of Applied Research in Clinical and Experimental Therapeutics. He is a member of the Society for Biomaterials and the Orthopaedic Research Society. Dr. Pietrzak is a Chief Research Scientist at Biomet, Inc., with a current emphasis on clinical research. He is also Adjunct Research Professor of Bioengineering at the University of Illinois at Chicago.

I dedicate this book to my wife, Karen, whose love and support helped make it happen; and my children, Brad and Becky, who inspire me to view the world through the eyes of a child—a world with limitless possibilities.

Foreword

Tissue engineering and regenerative medicine will ultimately have a more profound impact than most of us can fully appreciate. The combination of the principles of engineering with advances in the material sciences, and an increased understanding of developmental biology has the potential to influence developments in medicine and biotechnology more than any single advance in these fields during the last several decades.

I would first like to applaud the volume editor, Dr. Pietrzak, and the authors for their efforts in bringing together a group of interrelated topics to create a textbook emphasizing the Tissue Engineered generation of musculoskeletal tissue. The authors of this book are all established experts in their respective fields. The publication of a separate volume dedicated to musculoskeletal tissue regeneration as part of a series focusing on orthopedic biology and medicine is a reflection of the tremendous growth of knowledge and ongoing developments that have occurred in this field over the last decade.

Musculoskeletal Tissue Regeneration: *Biological Materials and Methods* is intended to cover the basic fundamentals and early treatment of musculoskeletal disease, tissue loss and wound healing, as well as provide a comprehensive summary of recent advances in regenerative medicine and tissue engineering as they relate to the musculoskeletal system, and should serve as a reference for researchers and graduate students in this discipline.

Since the initial descriptions of the field, the synthesis of new polymers and materials for use in the generation of engineered musculoskeletal tissue has increased dramatically. Cell/biomaterials and biomaterial/host interactions continue to be explored. The tremendous potential for the use of stem cells in tissue engineering and regenerative medicine is now widely appreciated, with some groups focusing on the use of fetal stem cells, and others employing adult stem or progenitor cells, to develop into various specialized tissues.

Practicing physicians in many disciplines are now starting to apply the techniques of musculoskeletal tissue engineering to patient care. This growing interest has resulted in expansion of the scope of regenerative medicine. The chapters presented in this text represent the multidisciplinary efforts of a multitude of scientists and clinicians. Various technologies described here may ultimately make a profound and lasting impact on the way that the healthcare industry functions in the treatment of many disease processes.

Any new developments in tissue and organ replacements have the potential to be controversial. Tissue engineering as a science and a medical discipline may be viewed by some as "unnatural." It is often difficult for society to reach an opinion on the relative merits and ethics of any new therapeutic. Both professionals and lay people are likely to examine the ethics of any new endeavor and weigh its relative merits, especially when that endeavor has the potential to employ other controversial techniques, such as stem cell manipulation. When one actually considers what physicians have done for centuries, the similarities between "conventional" treatment and tissue engineering become more obvious. If the basic premise of health care is that the body heals itself, then physicians do nothing more than optimize the environment most conducive to healing. Basically, physicians attempt to neutralize hostile factors at the same time that they enhance the supply of oxygen and nutrients that the body needs to heal itself. In Tissue Engineering, the same goal is achieved using a somewhat unique approach. Living cells that belong in the injured area are delivered using a scaffold that dictates the shape and function of the desired tissue. The physician then optimizes the local environment by maximizing the delivery of oxygen and the elimination of waste products. Under ideal conditions, this will then enable the body to heal itself. In this respect, the significant difference is that "tissue engineering" efforts are focused on the microenvironment, or the cellular level, as opposed to being focused on the macroenvironment, or the organ level, as is done in "traditional" medicine.

One hopeful outcome of this text is to demonstrate the skill and imagination that have been brought to bear to develop revolutionary new approaches to treat patients who are often desperately ill and have no alternative.

Finally, it is important to understand the current limitations of the field, and the need for developments in associated fields on which tissue engineering is predicated. Our expectations must be realistic as the field develops and knowledge is acquired. Initial applications may reflect the advantages of component therapy to replace lost function(s) of specific organs, rather than replacement of an entire organ. It is certainly possible that many tissue functions can be sufficiently recovered without the need to replace an entire organ. In this fashion, advances in human application can parallel advances in the science of the field, rather than generate hopes prematurely.

Although I believe that developments in this field will result in a tremendous advance in the treatment of many disease processes, the power of tissue engineering as a model to explore changes associated with developmental biology may equal its special applications to human health care.

Charles A. Vacanti, M.D.
Director of Tissue Engineering Laboratory and
Chair of the Department of Anesthesiology
Brigham and Women's Hospital
Boston, MA

Preface

The repair of musculoskeletal tissue is a vital concern of all surgical specialties, most notably orthopedics and related disciplines. While many of the surgical techniques in current use have their basis in methods that have been historically practiced, we now stand on the cusp of a revolution in musculoskeletal repair based on new tools that have recently become available or are about to emerge into clinical practice. These new tools include tissue engineering, gene therapy, stem cell applications, delivery of growth factors and many others. By their very nature, these tools require an interdisciplinary approach, utilizing teams comprised of surgeons, engineers, and scientists in collaboration between industry and academia. To function effectively as a team, each member must not only possess a core competency, but must also have a working knowledge of related fields.

Musculoskeletal Tissue Regeneration: *Biological Materials and Methods* aims to provide the reader with both basic and advanced knowledge of many of the newer methodologies being developed or introduced to the clinical arena. Collectively, the chapters, written by recognized experts in their field, provide an integration of the current state of knowledge about this important topic. It is hoped that this book will be a valuable resource for researchers, developers and clinicians, alike, and will help to provide a foundation to propel the technology through the 21st Century.

William S. Pietrzak, Ph.D.,
University of Illinois at Chicago, Chicago, IL
and
Biomet, Inc., Warsaw, IN

Contents

Section IV Generalized Approaches

Section V The Future

Contributors

Matthew Aleef, M.D., University of Pittsburgh Medical Center, Pittsburgh, PA

Fabrisia Ambrosio, Ph.D., M.P.T., Growth and Development Laboratory, Stem Cell Research Center, Department of Orthopaedic Surgery, Department of Physical Medicine and Rehabilitation, Children's Hospital of Pittsburgh, Pittsburgh, PA

Kyriacos A. Athanasiou, Ph.D., P.E., Department of Bioengineering, Rice University, Houston, TX

Stephen F. Badylak, D.V.M., Ph.D., M.D., Department of Surgery, McGowan Institute for Regenerative Medicine, Department of Surgery, University of Pittsburgh, Pittsburgh, PA

F. Alan Barber, M.D., F.A.C.S., Plano Orthopedic and Sports Medicine Center, Plano, TX

Thomas W. Bauer, M.D., Ph.D., Departments of Pathology and Orthopaedic Surgery, The Cleveland Clinic Foundation, Cleveland, OH

John G. Birch, M.D., Center for Excellence in Limb Lengthening & Reconstruction, Seay Center for Musculoskeletal Research, Texas Scottish Rite Hospital for Children, Dallas, TX

Michael L. Boninger, M.D., Department of Physical Medicine and Rehabilitation, University of Pittsburgh, Pittsburgh, PA

Michael H. Boothby, M.D., Southwest Orthopedic Associates, Fort Worth, TX

Barbara D. Boyan, Ph.D., Institute of Bioengineering and Bioscience, Georgia Institute of Technology, Atlanta, GA

Michael B. Boyd, D.O., Department of Orthopaedic Surgery, University of California at San Diego, La Jolla, CA

William D. Bugbee, M.D., Department of Orthopaedic Surgery, University of California at San Diego, La Jolla, CA

Pieter Buma, Ph.D., Department of Orthopaedics, University Medical Center Nijmegen, Nijmegen, the Netherlands

Alexander M. Cherkashin, M.D., Center for Excellence in Limb Lengthening & Reconstruction, Seay Center for Musculoskeletal Research, Texas Scottish Rite Hospital for Children, Dallas, TX

Yolanda Cillo, M.D., Medtronic, Inc., Memphis, TN

Anna V. Cuomo, M.D., Department of Orthopaedic Surgery, David Geffen School of Medicine at UCLA, Los Angeles, CA

Guy Daculsi, PhD, INSERM, Faculte de Chirurgie Dentaire, Universite de Nantes, Nantes, France

Bruce Doll, D.D.S., Ph.D., University of Pittsburgh, Pittsburgh, PA

Liisa M. Eisenlohr, Ph.D., M.B.A., LifeNet Health, Virginia Beach, VA

Benjamin D. Elder, M.S., Department of Bioengineering, Rice University, Houston, TX

Mario Ferretti, M.D., Department of Orthopedic Surgery, University of Pittsburgh Medical Center, Pittsburgh, PA

Renny T. Franceschi, University of Michigan School of Dentistry, Ann Arbor, MI

Abhi Freyer, B.A.S., Stone Research Foundation, San Francisco, CA

Freddie Fu, M.D., D.Sc. (Hon), D.Ps. (Hon), Department of Orthopedic Surgery, University of Pittsburgh Medical Center, Pittsburgh, PA

Takaaki Fujishiro, M.D., Ph.D., Department of Orthopaedic Surgery, Kobe University Graduate School of Medicine, Kobe, Japan

Victor M. Goldberg, M.D., Department of Orthopaedics, Case Medical Center, Cleveland, OH

Simon Görtz, M.D., Department of Orthopaedic Surgery, University of California at San Diego, La Jolla, CA

Jonathan N. Grauer, M.D., Department of Orthopaedics and Rehabilitation, Yale University School of Medicine, New Haven, CT

Robert J. Havlik, M.D., Division of Plastic Surgery, Indiana University School of Medicine, Indianapolis, IN

Jeffrey O. Hollinger, D.D.S., Ph.D., Bone Tissue Engineering Center, Carnegie Mellon University, Pittsburgh, PA

Stephen M. Howell, M.D., Department of Mechanical and Aeronautical Engineering, University of California at Davis, Davis, CA

Johnny Huard, Ph.D., Growth and Development Laboratory, Stem Cell Research Center, Department of Orthopaedic Surgery, Children's Hospital of Pittsburgh, Pittsburgh, PA

Douglas W. Jackson, M.D., Orthopaedic Research Institute at the Southern California Center for Sports Medicine and Long Beach Memorial Medical Center, Long Beach, CA

Ramsey C. Kinney, Ph.D., Institute of Bioengineering and Bioscience, Georgia Institute of Technology, Atlanta, GA

Hideo Kobayashi, M.D., Ph.D., Departments of Pathology and Orthopaedic Surgery, The Cleveland Clinic Foundation, Cleveland, OH

Keith W. Lawhorn, M.D., Advanced Orthopaedics and Sports Medicine Institute, Fairfax, VA

John P. LeGeros, Ph.D., Calcium Phosphate Research Laboratory, Department of Biomaterials & Biomimetics, New York University College of Dentistry, New York, NY

Racquel Z. LeGeros, Ph.D., Calcium Phosphate Research Laboratory, Department of Biomaterials & Biomimetics, New York University College of Dentistry, New York, NY

Yong Li, M.D., Ph.D., Growth and Development Laboratory, Stem Cell Research Center, Department of Orthopaedic Surgery, Children's Hospital of Pittsburgh, Pittsburgh, PA

Jay R. Lieberman, M.D., Director, New England Musculoskeletal Institute, Professor and Chairman, Department of Orthopaedic Surgery, University of Connecticut Health Center, Farmington, CT

Marina R. Makarov, M.D., Center for Excellence in Limb Lengthening & Reconstruction, Seay Center for Musculoskeletal Research, Texas Scottish Rite Hospital for Children, Dallas, TX

Theodore I. Malinin, M.S., M.D., Department of Orthopedics and Rehabilitation, Miller School of Medicine, University of Miami, Miami, FL

Mollie Manley, M.D., Department of Orthopaedic Surgery, University of Pittsburgh Medical Center, Pittsburgh, PA

Stefan Marlovits, M.D., M.B.A., Department of Traumatology, Medical University of Vienna, Vienna, Austria

William S. Pietrzak, Ph.D., Department of Bioengineering, University of Illinois at Chicago, Chicago, IL, Biomet, Inc., Warsaw, IN

Katrina Ruth, B.S., Smith and Nephew, Inc., Memphis, TN

Mikhail L. Samchukov, M.D., Center for Excellence in Limb Lengthening & Reconstruction, Seay Center for Musculoskeletal Research, Texas Scottish Rite Hospital for Children, Dallas, TX

Zvi Schwartz, D.M.D., M.D., Hebrew University Hadassah Faculty of Dental Medicine, Jerusalem, Israel

Wei Shen, M.D., Ph.D., Department of Orthopaedic Surgery, University of Pittsburgh Medical Center, Pittsburgh, PA

Bruce Simon, Ph.D., Biomet Osteobiologics, Parsippany, NJ

Josh Simon, Ph.D., Biomet Osteobiologics, Parsippany, NJ

Timothy M. Simon, Ph.D., Orthopaedic Research Institute at the Southern California Center for Sports Medicine and Long Beach Memorial Medical Center, Long Beach, CA

Andrew K. Simpson, M.D., Department of Orthopaedics and Rehabilitation, Yale University School of Medicine, New Haven, CT

Kimberly Singh, M.D., Institute of Bioengineering and Bioscience, Georgia Institute of Technology, Atlanta, GA

William D. Spotnitz, M.D., M.B.A., Surgical Therapeutic Advancement Center, Department of Surgery, University of Virginia Health System, Charlottesville, VA

Andreas Stavropoulos, D.D.S., Ph.D., Department of Periodontology and Oral Gerontology, School of Dentistry, University of Aarhus, Denmark

Kevin R. Stone, M.D., The Stone Clinic, San Francisco, CA

Arvydas Usas, M.D., Growth and Development Laboratory, Stem Cell Research Center, Department of Orthopaedic Surgery, Children's Hospital of Pittsburgh, Pittsburgh, PA

Marloes van Meel, Department of Orthopaedics, University Medical Center Nijmegen, Nijmegen, the Netherlands

Tony G. van Tienen, M.D., Ph.D., Department of Orthopaedics, University Medical Center Nijmegen, Nijmegen, the Netherlands

Rene P.H. Veth, M.D., Ph.D., Department of Orthopaedics, University Medical Center Nijmegen, Nijmegen, the Netherlands

Ann W. Walgenbach, RN, NP, MSN, The Stone Clinic, San Francisco, CA

Peter G. Whang, M.D., Department of Orthopaedics and Rehabilitation, Yale University School of Medicine, New Haven, CT

Joseph K. Williams, M.D., Craniofacial Plastic Surgery, Children's Healthcare of Atlanta, Atlanta, GA

Lloyd Wolfinbarger, Jr., Ph.D., LifeNet Health, Virginia Beach, VA

Jennifer E. Woodell-May, Ph.D., Biomet, Inc., Warsaw, IN

Color Plates

Color plates follow p. 288

Fig. 4.1 A vascularized fibular autograft used to treat osteonecrosis of the femoral head is shown. Most of the graft is viable one year after implantation, and it has provided an osteoconductive surface for a few areas of new bone formation. The (*) symbols mark the interface between cortical autograft and new bone that has formed in the femoral head
Fig. 4.2 The photomicrograph of histological sections through the center of a clinically failed intervertebral body fusion cage shows incorporated iliac crest autograft
Fig. 4.3 The lower-magnification photomicrograph shows unincorporated iliac crest autograft in a Harms cage that had been used for cervical fusion, but failed shortly after insertion. Although this case was not clinically successful, it illustrates an appropriate combination of cortical and cancellous bone fragments prepared from iliac crest
Fig. 4.4 The decalcified section of the shavings of one preparation of locally harvested autograft shows shavings of cancellous bone, almost completely devoid of cells. Fibrous tissue, hyaline cartilage and fibrocartilage were also present in this preparation
Fig. 7.3 Small/smaller (a) critical size defects subjected to regenerative treatment (e.g., covered with a membrane: dotted line) will heal with larger amounts of bone in terms of percent of defect fill than large/larger (b) critical size defects subjected to the same treatment during the same amount of time. Similarly, a 3-wall defect (b) subjected to regenerative treatment will present more bone fill than a 2- wall (c) or 1-wall (d) defect subjected to the same regenerative treatment during the same period of time
Fig. 7.4 The mandibular ramus is exposed (a) and four holes are drilled (b). A Teflon capsule is then placed and may be either left empty to serve as control (c) or be filled with biomaterial under testing (e.g., DBB) (d). The capsule is stabilized by means of sutures passing through the collar of the capsule and the holes in the ramus (e), and thus a tight adaptation of the capsule onto the bone surface can be achieved (f)
Fig. 7.5 In originally empty capsules bone formation (arrowheads) can be observed already after one month of healing (a), and increasing amounts of new bone are formed after two (b) and four months (c), until 12 months (d) where the capsules are almost entirely filled out with bone. The dotted line indicates the level of pristine bone
Fig. 7.6 Limited amounts of bone (arrowheads) confined in the vicinity of the pristine bone (dotted line) are observed inside capsules grafted with unsintered DBB after four (a) or 12months (b) of healing. The new bone grows in continuity with the host bone and in contact with the DBB particles (stars) (c), which occupy the major portion of the capsules. The amount of new bone remains basically stable for at least six months after capsule removal (d)
Fig. 7.7 Overview of a root with neighboring tissues removed six months after treatment with unsintered DBB+GTR (a). New cementum (arrows) with inserting collagen fibers and a new bone-like tissue (arrowheads) in direct contact with DBB particles (star) can be observed (b). A substantial portion of the defect was occupied by graft particles with empty osteocytic lacunae (arrowheads) embedded in a periodontal ligament-like connective tissue (c)

Section I

Background

1

Musculoskeletal and Wound Treatment Through the Ages: A Brief Historical Tour

William S. Pietrzak

Abstract: The healing of wounds and the treatment of musculoskeletal deficiencies are two of the most compelling matters that have occupied the attentions of physicians and surgeons throughout human history. At any given point in time, past or present, the state of the clinical art is the integration of all earlier failures and successes. Understanding and knowledge of the efforts of our forebears helps to not only maintain a continuity between our contemporary treatments and those of our ancient ancestors, but also, through extrapolation, may help us catch an early glimpse of what may yet come. The history of wound repair and treatment of musculoskeletal deficiencies may span, in a fashion, over 50,000 years of human existence, which may be up to half of the time that humans have walked the earth. Our ancient forebears were remarkably intelligent, insightful and creative, and one cannot help but be in awe of their accomplishments when presented with information from their written documents and/or unearthed artifacts and skeletal remains. This chapter presents an overview of the state of musculoskeletal treatment, wound healing and related surgery from prehistoric times through the eighteenth century.

Keywords: musculoskeletal, wound healing, history, ancient, surgery, treatment

1.1. Introduction

Virtually every surgical specialty is concerned with some aspect of musculoskeletal tissue repair. Many techniques have been developed for this purpose, based on mechanical, biological and electrical principles [1-11]. These methods were built upon the foundations laid by our predecessors, both recent and distant. Names that come to mind include Röntgen (pioneered radiography in the 1890s) [12]; Wolff (described the adaptive nature of bone architecture in 1892) [13]; Muller, et al. (founded the AO/ASIF in 1958) [14], and Urist (published landmark demineralized bone matrix paper in 1965) [15]. Relative

Department of Bioengineering, University of Illinois at Chicago, Chicago, IL, Biomet, Inc., Warsaw, IN

From: *Orthopedic Biology and Medicine: Musculoskeletal Tissue Regeneration, Biological Materials and Methods*
Edited by W. S. Pietrzak © Humana Press, Totowa, NJ

to the expanse of recorded history, however, these and other contemporaneous contributions can be considered to be recent.

Injury and disease have been around since before humans, and attempts at treatment have been recorded and/or preserved for many thousands of years. From our vantage point these early efforts, upon initial examination, may appear primitive. However, placed in the context of the period where there was little understanding of the natural world and technology was in its infancy, these ancient medical practices were truly marvels, with some concepts and methods described hundreds or even thousands of years ago, still relevant today. We owe a great deal to our ancient forbears, and a better understanding of their efforts and accomplishments will help us to better appreciate the current state of the art, and help prepare us for what lies ahead.

The story of the evolution of wound treatment is tied to the evolution of many other aspects of human existence, including that of medicine and surgery in general, material and fabrication technology, the understanding of biological and physiological concepts, as well as the evolution of social, political and religious matters. With regard to the last three, one only has to look at the current controversy regarding stem cell therapy to appreciate this [16]. There are several excellent historical texts that explain many of these interrelationships in detail [17-20]. The purpose of this chapter is to provide a brief overview of the progress made in musculoskeletal treatment, wound healing and related surgery over the ages through the 18th Century.

1.2. History of Wound Repair and Musculoskeletal Treatment

1.2.1. The Early Beginnings…50,000 B.C. to 1,000 B.C.

Modern *homo sapiens* are believed to have come into existence approximately 100,000 to 200,000 years ago in Africa [21]. One might speculate that with the ability to think, problem solve and make and use tools, it would only be a matter of time before man would become aware of his frailty and direct his intelligence to improve his physical condition when necessary. Some of the earliest evidence of this is eyed needles that were invented between 50,000 and 30,000 years ago before Christ [22, 23]. By 20,000 B.C. bone needles were developed to the point where they were not improved upon until the Renaissance. These needles may have been used for some type of wound closure, although the details are not certain.

Trephination, or the surgical creation of a hole in the cranium, is the oldest known surgical procedure and was practiced by Neolithic man in many regions of the world [17, 24]. The procedure was performed using sharpened flint instruments, with the removed fragments perforated and worn as amulets by the family or the patient, if he survived [17]. Insight into the motives of these early people may be gained by examining current procedures performed by native African communities, which include therapeutic treatment for head injuries such as fractures, and treatment for persistent headaches, epilepsy, intracranial tumors and mental disease [25]. What may be the earliest evidence of trephination came from the discovery, in 1996, of a well-preserved Neolithic male skeleton of an individual who died about 7,000 years ago at approximately 50 years of age that was found at the Stone Age burial site of Ensisheim in France [25]. In addition to the excellent state of preservation, this skeleton was remarkable in that the skull contained evidence of two trephinations.

It was clear that these holes were surgically induced while the individual was alive, as the anterior site showed complete bony healing while the posterior site showed partial healing.

Pre-Incan surgeons in Peru performed trephinations in great numbers as early as 3,000 B.C. [24] Six percent of 10,000 mummies from prehistoric Peru showed evidence of cranial trephination. There is strong evidence that cranioplasty, or defect repair, was performed in some of these cases. For instance, trephined Incan skulls have been discovered adjacent to shells, gourds and silver or gold plates, and there have been several reports of skulls found with these materials *in situ* [24]. In one case, a skull dating to 2,000 B.C. was found with the left frontal defect covered with a gold plate (Fig. 1.1). The choice of cranioplastic material may have been based on the social rank of the citizen undergoing trephination, with gourds being used for the common person, and precious metals reserved for nobility [24]. Cases in which the cranium healed tightly around the foreign body show that ancient South American cranioplasty was performed, at least in those cases, on the living cranium and were not postmortem procedures.

The earliest known Egyptian physician was Im-hotep, who lived in the reign of the Pharoh Zoser of the third dynasty (c. 2,980 B.C.) [21]. The *Edwin-Smith papyrus*, written in 1,600 B.C., was a transcript of a much older document written between 3,000 and 2,500 B.C., and deals primarily with surgery of the era [17]. This papyrus details 48 cases of clinical surgery, including injuries of the head, chest and spine, and describes the provisional diagnosis, examination, symptoms, diagnosis, treatment and prognosis of each. For example, case 47 was one in which there was a gaping wound in the soft tissues of the shoulder. Upon first examination, the wound was sutured. Upon second examination, the sutures were found to have loosened so adhesive strips were used to hold it together. Following this, the wound healed and recovered. For the most part, the described treatments were mechanical in nature and did not involve medicaments, early evidence of a distinction between surgery and medicine. Lacerations were drawn together

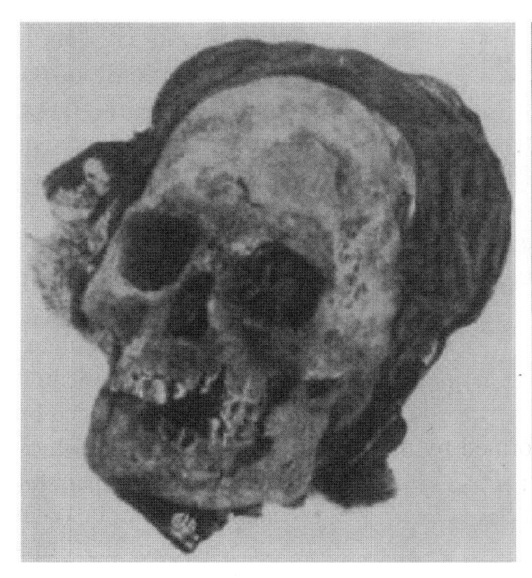

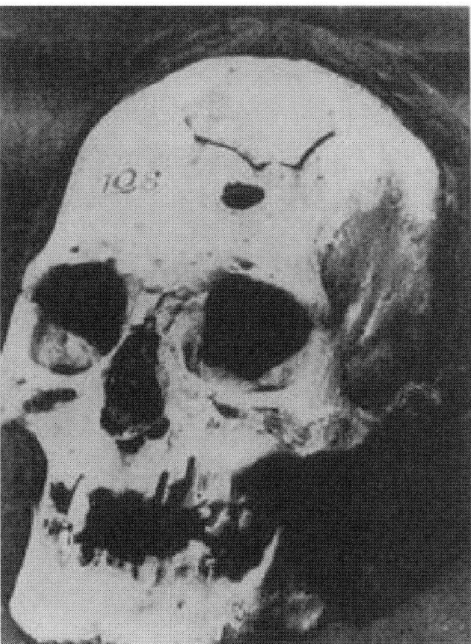

Fig. 1.1 Pre-Incan Skull (2,000 B.C.) with Trephination Left: hole covered with gold plate. Right, plate moved to expose hole Reproduced with permission. From: Sanan A, Haines SJ. Repairing holes in the head: a history of cranioplasty. Neurosurgery 1997;40:588-602

with linen strips, an early reference to sutures [22, 23]. Other references from this period describe linen strips coated with a sticky mixture of flour and honey, creating the earliest recorded skin closure strips.

It appears that as long ago as 4,000 years the Egyptians had the ability to treat forearm fractures with wooden splints. They also performed amputations [26]. Several investigators have reported prosthetic limb replacements in ancient Egyptian mummies, but it has been suggested that these devices were used to restore the integrity of the body in preparation for the afterlife [26]. Nerlich, et al. [26], however, reported on a 3,000-year-old mummy whose big toe of the right foot had been amputated during life, as evidenced by the intact layer of soft tissue and skin covering the site. A wooden toe replacement was attached to the forefoot using two wooden plates and leather strings (Fig. 1.2). Wear marks on the sole of the prosthetic toe indicated that it had been used.

In Babylon recurrent wars made surgery necessary, with the *Code of Hammurabi* – named after the king who reigned about 2,250 B.C. – setting a pay scale for surgeons based on the procedures and the social class upon which it was performed [17]. For setting a broken bone, the surgeon was to receive five shekels of silver. The Code also stated that, should the man lose his life or his eye, the surgeon should have his hands cut off [17].

Wagle [27] reported, in 1994, that a 3,000-year-old Egyptian female mummy had a two-component artificial toe attached directly to the first metatarsal of the right foot. The proximal, socket-like portion had a high radiographic

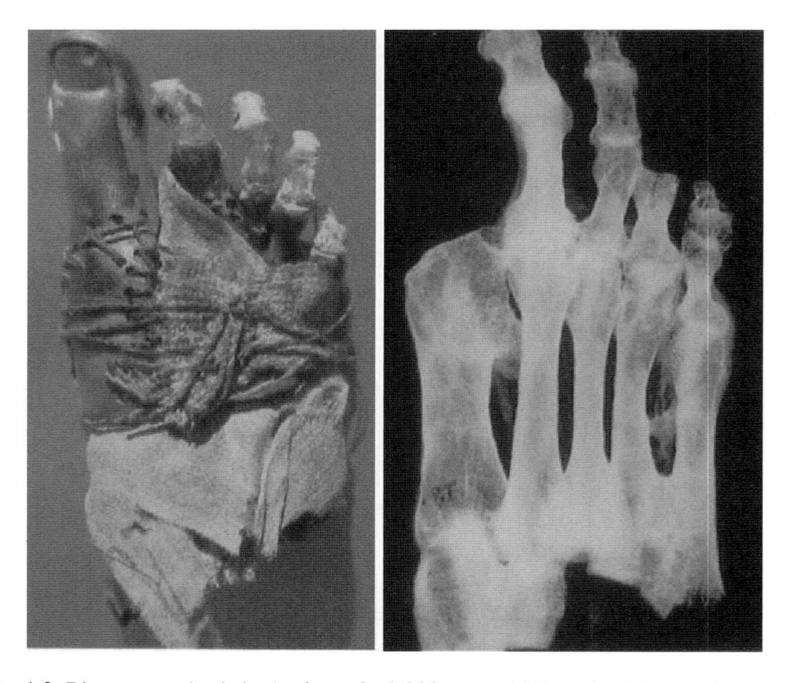

Fig. 1.2 Big toe prosthesis in the foot of a 3,000-year-old Egyptian Mummy Prosthesis was attached to the outside of the foot with two wooden plates and leather strings. Reprinted from The Lancet, vol 356, Nerlich AG, Zink A, Szeimies U, Hagedorn HG. Ancient Egyptian prosthesis of the big toe. 2176-2179, 2000, with permission from Elsevier

density on CT scan and was thought to be made of a high density ceramic, with the distal portion having a low radiographic density similar to air. As only CT analysis was performed, it was unclear whether the prosthesis was used during life or placed after death [26, 27]. There has also been debate about whether two dental prostheses found near Cairo were used intravitally, however, the absence of dental wear and dental calculus on the teeth suggest that they were not used in life [26].

1.2.2. 1,000 B.C. to 1000 A.D.

Homer's *Illiad*, an account of the siege of Troy by the Greeks, was written around 1,000 B.C. In it there are 147 records of war wounds. Of these, 106 were spear wounds with 80 percent mortality, 17 were sword thrusts with total mortality, 12 arrow wounds had 42 percent mortality and 12 wounds from slings had 66 percent mortality [17]. While Homer described the site and extent of the wounds in anatomical terms, he did not give much information about their treatment or the process of healing.

Shusruta of India is believed to have lived sometime between approximately 600 B.C to 600 A.D. and was a great physician and surgeon, although there is some question as to whether he was a historical figure or a legendary figure [17, 20]. In *Shusruta Samhita*, his collected work of medicine and surgery, a variety of blunt and sharp steel surgical instruments were described, including forceps, cannulae, knives, rasps, needles, probes, saws, razors, lancets, scissors, trocars, tubes, hooks and catheters [17, 19]. Sutures were made of cotton threads, hemp fibers, strips of leather, horse hair or animal sinews. Needles were straight, curved, two-edged and three-edged. Although sutures and needles were known, they were apparently not used for ligation. Rather, during amputations and other procedures, bleeding was controlled with boiling oil, hot metal cautery or pressure. Wounds were classified as incised, punctured or pierced, contused, crushed or lacerated and were to be thoroughly cleansed and all foreign bodies removed prior to suturing. An incised wound was to be sutured immediately, covered with cotton, or with the ashes of a burnt cloth, then bandaged. Shusruta believed in keeping wounds dry, stating that if a foreign body was left in the wound, pus would form. Thus, he understood the difference between primary and secondary wound healing. He was also a pioneer of anesthesia, using henbane (hyoscamus niger) and Indian hemp (cannabis indica) to deaden pain. A unique method of wound closure was practiced in at least one surgical procedure [22, 23]. Intestinal obstructions were surgically removed, with the bowel washed out with milk, lubricated with butter and closed with the heads of black ants. The ants, which had fierce jaws, were grasped by their bodies and directed to bite the bowel edges, at which time their bodies were twisted off—the first surgical clips!

Hippocrates, born on the island of Cos, (460 to 350 B.C.) is considered to be the "Father of Medicine" [20, 28]. More than 70 books bearing his name are collectively called the *Corpus Hippocraticum* and deal with both medicine and surgery. Three of the books deal with the skeletal system: "On Fractures", "On Articulations", and "Mochlicus (Instruments of Reduction)" [20]. These books indicate a systematic study of human anatomy. The recognition and management of disease and injuries was so complete that it remained standard for 2,000 years, and some of the methods are still in use today [20]. For fractures, reduction was accomplished by traction, plus manual manipulation. Bandages were applied initially as the extension was being maintained, but splints were not used during the first seven to 11 days to permit the swelling to subside. Both compound and simple fractures were dealt with, and complications of injuries, including sepsis, tetanus, osteomyelitis, gangrene and death, were described [20]. In the case of compound fractures and dislocations that could not be reduced, he advocated complete resection of the bones at the joints. Hippocrates was aware that dry wounds were known to heal well if the edges were kept closely approximated, achieving hemostasis with cautery [22]. In badly contused or infected wounds he attempted to promote suppuration using ointments to lessen inflammation and prevent complications. His was the first description of healing by first and second intention [17]. As far back as the time of Hippocrates it was recognized that fractures in children became stable in one month, while two to three months were required for adults [18]. Among his legacies is his advocacy for treatments based on rationality, rather than on tradition and wishful thinking [22].

The Roman medical journalist Aurelius Cornelius Celsus, who lived in the 1st Century A.D., wrote *De Re Medicina* and other books on medicine, providing ample evidence of medicine's advancement since Hippocrates [20, 23, 28]. His writings included descriptions of different organs, as well as used Greek names which are still in use today, including zygoma, vertebra, femur and cartilage [28]. As much of trauma in his day was due to arrows and other weapons, he gave instruction for the removal of such missiles from bone and soft tissue [28]. Celsus described the mode of repairing defects in the ears, lips and nose. In particular, he described the harelip operation: "...the edges having been pared, the margins are to be brought gently together, but, in cases where they cannot be coapted, semilunar incisions are to be made beyond the parts to be joined in order to aid their approach to each other" [28]. Stitches, and not pins, were to be used in such procedures. Teeth loosened by blows and falls were to be fastened to the firm teeth with gold, although he does not state whether gold wire or plate is to be used [28]. The following quote from Celsus is particularly noteworthy: "But, if at any time the bones have not united, in consequence of the dressings being frequently removed and the parts disturbed, the treatment to be adopted is obvious; for union may yet take place. If the fracture be of long standing, the limb is to be extended, in order to produce a fresh injury; the bones must be separated from each other by the hand, that their broken surfaces may be rendered uneven by the grating against each other; and if there be any fat substance, it must be abraded, and the whole reduced to a recent accident; yet great care must be employed, lest the ligaments or muscles be injured" [28]. Celsus also gave the first description of inflammation, i.e., redness, swelling, heat and pain [17]. His method of wound treatment was to cleanse the area of blood clots and foreign material, then suture. Ointments and drugs were used to hasten the formation of granulation tissue. He speaks of ligation of blood vessels, leaving the ligatures long so that they can be removed [17]. To distinguish a cranial fissure from a suture, Clesus quotes Hippocrates, advising to pour ink on the part, then scraping the bone, with the ink marking the presence of a fissure [19].

Galen of Pergamon (131 to 202 A.D.) treated and sutured the severed tendons of gladiators, hoping to restore mobility [23]. His method involved washing out the wounds with wine, then removing the clots and foreign bodies, followed by suturing. Many wounds healed without suppuration and the wounded were able to promptly return to their work. Unfortunately, Galen did not use this experience to promote primary wound healing and later advised the introduction of ointments and drugs that favored formation of "laudable pus" and healing by second intention. Due to his authority in medicine and surgery, the doctrine of healing by suppuration became the accepted doctrine for centuries, until the time of Lister [23]. He also employed traction and manipulation for injuries of the neck [28]. In *De Methodo Medendi* he espoused the virtues of silk sutures while suggesting that, if that is unavailable, gut sutures be used. He recognized the temporary nature of sutures derived from the intestines of herbivorous animals. Traditionally, such sutures have been termed "catgut," but have nothing to do with cats. This material was likely used as strings on early instruments such as the flute-like "Kit," hence, Kit-gut has likely been corrupted to catgut over the years [23]. Following trephination Galen and others described the placement of linen moistened in wine or the oil of roses over the dura mater and performed dressing changes until the wound granulated over [24].

Both Galen and Hippocrates recognized two types of wounds, one that was clean and dry and healed by first intention, and the other that was dirty and required drainage before healing [22]. In the 6th Century A.D. Aetius of Amida confused this, disregarding clean dry wounds and insisting that pus was a necessary process of healing.

Knowledge of Jewish surgery prior to 200 A.D. can be found in the Talmud [19]. Not only were the rabbis acquainted with the use of sutures, but they also freshened the edges of old wounds to obtain reunion and understood application of artificial body parts to replace loss, as applied to the trachea and cranium, and use of artificial teeth and wooden legs.

The Greek medical and surgical writer Paulos Æginta, who flourished at the end of the 6th and first half of the 7th Centuries A.D., described the fracture of the patella and its treatment as follows: "The symptoms are obvious, a solution of continuity, a hollow, and crepitation. The fracture is put in order by extending the leg, for thus the divided portions may be brought together with the fingers until the lips of the fracture mutually touch, and are united to one another, and the fractured pieces, when separated, are thus arranged together. For even if callus does not form, owing to the parts being drawn in different directions by the muscles and tendons from the thigh and leg, which are inserted into it, yet the separation is much diminished" [28]. Paulos described, in great detail, the many types of penetrating weapons of the day and their manner of extraction, noting that if the weapon lodged in any of the larger vessels, both sides should first be secured with ligatures [28].

Haly Abbas (930 to 994 A.D.) was born in Persia and collected a large number of observations from his extensive hospital experience [28]. Among these, he described treatment for fractures of the lower jaw, advising that the teeth be secured together with ligature before using compresses or bandages. He also discussed making wooden splints, avoiding their placement over processes of bone, and forbade their use in fractures in the presence of inflammation. Avicenna (Abu' Ali Ib n Sima, 980 to 1037 A.D.) of Bagdad practiced manipulation with traction for treating back ailments [18].

There is some controversy regarding the first endosseous alloplastic dental implant. One candidate is a black stone that was implanted in place of a lateral incisor, discovered in 1890 in Copan, Honduras, the ancient Mayan metropolis near the border of Guatamala [29]. Apparently, the stone had a great deal of tartar on it, signifying that it had probably been implanted during life. It was estimated that this implant was more than 1,000 years old. Another candidate is a mandible, likely from a woman about 20 years of age, found in 1931 in Honduras and believed to date to the 7th Century. Three missing incisors had been replaced by artificial teeth made from the shell of a bivalve mollusk (Fig. 1.3) [29]. The implants were triangular with the acute apical angle serving as the root. It is likely that the implants were placed during life as two of them were set firmly into the bone. The third implant was not firmly attached, and was also incorrectly placed, suggesting that it had fallen out and was carelessly placed in an incorrect position.

1.2.3. 1000 A.D. to 1500 A.D.

Albucasis of Spain (~1060 to 1122) prepared a treatise on the principles and practice of Arabian surgery, as taught by his predecessors [28]. In it he described his treatment of fractures of the femur with long splints, resecting sharp points of bone and spicula. He also spoke of four methods to reduce dislocations of the hip joint, the first of which rotated the limb in all directions.

During the 12th and 13th Centuries many universities were established in Italy, France and England, with Bologna becoming the medical center [17]. Hugo of Lucca (c. 1160 to 1257) was a lecturer in surgery at Bologna and, although left no known writings, his surgical teachings, especially regarding wound repair and healing, were quoted by his successor, Theodorice Borgnoni, better known as Theodoric [17]. He quoted Hugo as saying "In the first place, the sides of the wound should be debrided, or abraded, then the wound should be completely cleansed of fuzz, hair, or anything else, and lest it be wiped dry with lint moistened with warm wine; thus the sides of the wound

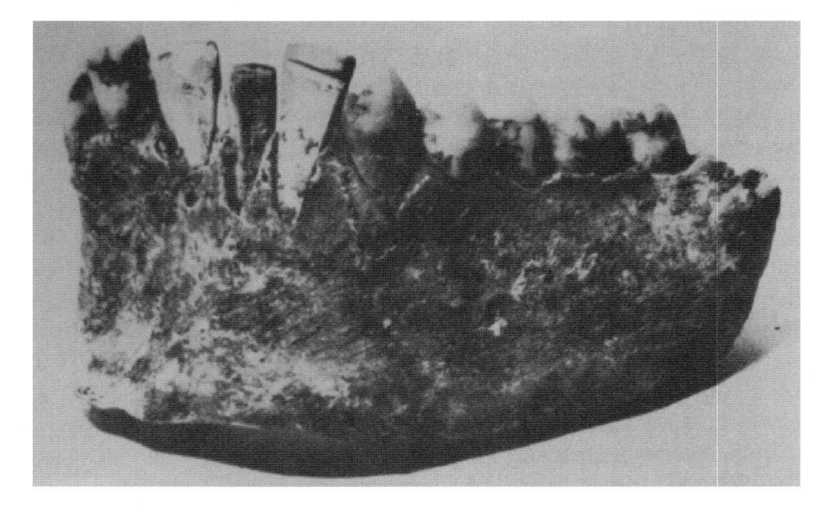

Fig. 1.3 Mayan Mandible Dating from 700 A.D. Contains three triangular incisors fabricated from the shells of bivalve mollusks [29] Reproduced by permission of the Journal of the History of Dentistry

may be united as well as possible in accordance with their original state; and let it bandaged in such a way that the re-approximation of the wound edges cannot be disturbed at all."

Bruno of Longoburgo of Padua University completed a surgical treatise called *Cyrurgia magna* in 1252 [17]. He made a clear distinction between primary wound healing and a "union which takes place through the intermediary of a flesh-like substance 'granulation tissue.' "

Theodoric completed his surgical textbook in 1266 which included many aspects of wound healing. He states "Indeed, above all else, a wound must be made clean" [17]. He also quotes Galen in the following passage "A suture must be made according to the size of the wound, for it ought to be done more deeply in a large wound than a small one. If a suture should be so tight that it produces pain, it will cause abscessing and swelling. But if it is at all slack, it will not hold the sides of the wound together" [17]. Theodoic also explains the misbelief that pus should be generated in wounds. "Such a practice is indeed to hinder Nature, to prolong the disease and to prevent conglutination and consolidation of the wound" [17]. Despite the efforts of Hugo, Theodoric and others to promote primary wound healing, other well-known surgeons of the time continued to advocate the production of "laudable pus" in their treatment of wounds.

Guy D. Chauliac (1300 to 1368) of France was surgeon to the French popes and, in 1363, wrote *Chirugia Magna*, which dealt with cataracts, hernias, fractures and dislocations [18]. Continuous traction with a weight and pulley was used to treat fractures of the femur. He stressed removal of foreign bodies and bits of bone from wounds and advised approximation of the damaged parts and preservation of the parts brought together, and the need to avoid damage to the involved organ. His philosophy of learning from medical history was "We are as children, standing on the shoulder of a giant, who sees all that he sees, and more beside." Nevertheless, Chauliac was a strict Galenist and insisted that laudible pus and suppuration were essential for wound healing. Due to his status as a great surgical authority, this set back the rational care of wounds for five centuries, until the discoveries of Lister in the role of bacteria in wound infection.

John of Arderne, born in 1307, is considered to be the "Father of English Surgery" [17]. He taught that wounds should heal without suppuration and should not be contaminated with salves and oils, but rather should be left to nature's powers to heal.

Two events occurred in the 15th Century that greatly contributed to the advancement and diffusion of medical and surgical knowledge throughout Europe [17, 28]: 1) the capture of Constantinople by the Turks, which resulted in the movement of Christians from that city into Italy, bringing with them rare and precise Greek medical manuscripts, and 2) the invention of the printing press.

1.2.4. 1500 to 1800, A.D.

Hans von Gersdorff of Germany published his book, *Feldtbuch der Wundtarzney*, in 1517 [19]. In it he described treatment for bullet wounds. To arrest bleeding, a styptic was applied: "Take of unslacked lime two ounces, vitriol, alum, each, once ounce, of aloes to be calcined, gallnuts, colophony each a quarter of an ounce; of the residuum in the retort when you made aquafortis two and a half ounces, and the white hair of the belly of a hare or deer chopped up, and mix all together thoroughly. When you use it, mix it with the white of eggs...But if an artery rages and will not be staunched then burn it with a cautery" [19].

Ambroise Paré (1509 to 1590) of France made several relevant contributions to surgery. Referring to his knowledge of Galen, he stated that: "...there was no speedier remedy for the staunching of blood than to bind the vessels ..." in the context that, at least in Europe, the principle means of staunching blood loss was with cautery [28]. During Paré's first attempt at ligature to arrest bleeding in a case requiring leg amputation, he had cautery available in case the ligature should fail. The operation using ligature was a success. He was the first to repair a laceration of the perineum with sutures and extract loose cartilage from the knee [28]. His written works describe drainage tubes to remove pus from deep-seated wounds and abscesses, a club-foot boot and models of artificial legs, hands, noses, ears and eyes. Until the middle of the 16th Century it was thought that gun powder was venomous and that the fired ball accumulated heat during flight and acted as a cautery when it penetrated tissue. It was common to treat wounds, particularly gunshot wounds, by pouring hot oil into them. In the battle before the Chateau de Villane, Paré and other surgeons were busy for many hours treating soldiers with gunshot wounds. When the supply of oil was exhausted, he began treating wounds with a mixture of egg yolks, oil of roses and turpentine [17, 28]. The day after treatment he wrote that those treated with the new method felt little pain and that there was little associated inflammation or tumor. In contrast, those treated with the "burning oil" were feverish, with great pain and tumor about the wound edges [28]. Following this observation he stated, "I determined never again to burn thus so cruelly the poor wounded with arquebuses (fire arms)" [17]. Like Guy de Chauliac, Paré advocated suppuration [17]. He advised use of an ointment or salve made from the boiling oil of lilies with earthworms that had been steeped in turpentine and a "just whelped" dog [17].

Hieronymus Fabricius d'Aquapendenta (1537 to 1619) was the most distinguished Italian surgeon at the start of the 17th Century [19]. His principal discoveries and writings relate to anatomy and embryology, but he was also a professor of surgery and his *Pentateuchos Chirugicum* (1582) and *Opera Chirugica* (1613) were important reference works for the next century. These contained many accounts of cases from other surgeons. With respect to intestinal wounds, he refers to animal sutures and the insertion of a piece of trachea from an animal to preserve the lumen of the gut [19].

The English surgeon William Clowes (1544 to 1604) wrote a treatise in 1591 entitled *A Proved Practice for All Yyoung Chirurgians, Concerning Burnings with Gun-powder, and Woundes made with Gun-shot, Sword, Halbard, Pike, Lance, or such other*, which was reprinted in 1596 and 1637, describing the treatment of weapons-induced wounds [28]. In it he details how amputations are to be performed. The skin and divided muscles were drawn over the cut end of the bone to form a letter X, covering the wound from every side. A "restrictive" mixture, which included a combination of various powders and hair from the belly of a hare, was then applied to stop bleeding [28].

Alexander Read, successor to Clowes, described three methods of keeping the edges of wounds together [17]. Extensive wounds were to be sutured with continuous or interrupted silk sutures. The least serious wounds were treated with snug bandaging. A third method involved gluing strips of adhesive plaster or cloth to the skin on either side of the wound, stitching the edges of the strips together with linen strands and drawing the edges together to approximate the wound. In this way the needle left no marks in the skin.

William Fabry of Hilden (1560 to 1624), also known as Fabricius Hildanus, has been called the "Father of German Surgery" [17, 19]. In his *Century of Surgical Cases* he presented a collection of his own cases. He believed in the efficacy of the "weapon salve," a concoction of human mummy, earthworms, pig's brain and moss taken from the skull of a man who had been killed or hanged and "gathered when the star Venus is predominant" [17]. The weapon causing the wound, with blood still on it, was smeared with the salve and carefully wrapped with clean linen. The dressing on the weapon was changed every three days. In reality, of course, this practice had nothing to do with wound healing. In fact the patient's wound was covered with a dressing and forgotten. Left to nature's healing powers, the wounds often healed uneventfully, but the weapon salve was given the credit. He advised amputation at an early stage of gangrene, specifying that the incision be made in the living and not the decayed flesh [19]. He also used cautery, rather than ligature, to treat arterial wounds [19].

There was controversy in the first half of the 17th Century on the sympathetic or magnetic cure of wounds using weapon salve [19]. Goclenius (1547 to 1628), professor of medicine at Marburg, thought the cure was a natural process. The priests thought it was magical with the aid of the devil. Van Helmont (1579 to 1644), a Belgian doctor, undertook to disprove both concepts, believing the effect due to what in later times was called "animal magnetism" [19].

John Woodall (1566 to 1643) was another prominent English surgeon who published several works including *The Surgeons Mate or Military & Domestique Surgery* (1617) and *Viaticum, Being the Path-Way to the Surgeons Chest* (1628) [19]. He espoused the tying of large vessels in cases of amputation, but if this fails, and also in the case of smaller vessels, recommended buttons of astringent and caustic powders. Interestingly, in gangrene, he urged amputation in the dead region instead of the living part, which was an old treatment that had, essentially, fallen into disuse. In cases of disease of the foot, he advocated amputating as low as the ankle instead of just below the knee, as was commonly done [19].

Thomas Gale, an English military surgeon, published a series of works in 1563 in which he corrected the errors concerning the presumed poisonous nature of bullet wounds and described the treatment of wounds, fractures and dislocations [28].

Another English surgeon, James Yonge (1646 to 1721) of Plymouth, published a small book entitled *Currus Triumphalis, é Terebinthô. Or an account of the many admirable Vertues of Oleum Terebinthinae. More particularly, of the good effects produced by its application to recent Wounds...And lastly, A new Way of Amputation, etc.* [19]. In it he took issue with Paré's method of ligature in amputation, calling it "tedious and often successless," but allowing for its use in other procedures. Significantly, the book may have been the first printed reference to the use of a tourniquet.

By the beginning of the 18th Century France was the leader in surgery in Europe, perhaps due, in part, to wars undertaken by Louis XIV [19]. By now surgeons knew that gunshot wounds were not poisonous and did not require cautery. As well, many surgeons knew that ordinary wounds that did not involve the bones required very little treatment. Nevertheless, the surgeons of the day prescribed and used oils, ointments, plasters, vulnerary drinks, etc., principally because surgeons were paid based upon the application of these remedies and not the visits [19]. Surgeons applied styptic powders, compression and cautery to check hemorrhage, and were generally reluctant to trust ligature for this purpose [19].

Micolas Andre de Boisregards (1658 to 1742) used the Greek terms "ortho" (straight) and "pais" (child) to produce the new word "orthopaedics," or straight child, publishing *L'Orthopedie* in 1741 [18]. This book helped to establish orthopaedics as a separate specialty. One of his illustrations for the principle of correcting deformities depicts a tree tethered to a post that has come to symbolize orthopaedics throughout the world. He taught ways of preventing and correcting deformities in children, as well as wrote on clubfeet, spinal curvature, bowed legs, congenital deformities and dislocations and other subjects.

Jean Louis Petit (1674 to 1750) of France was the most distinguished surgeon of the first half of the 18th Century [19]. In addition to inventing the screw tourniquet and improving the procedure of amputation, he demonstrated that clot formation is mainly responsible for the occlusion of arteries in wounds.

William Cheselden (1688 to 1752) of England was a surgeon-anatomist who published an atlas of anatomy in 1713 and an atlas of osteology in 1733 entitled *Osteographia or the Anatomy of the Bones* [18]. This work was of great value to both surgeons and lecturers.

Albrecht von Haller (1708 to 1777), a native of Bern, was one of the most influential German surgeons of the 18th Century [19]. His *Bibliotheca chirurgica* (1774 to 1775) is one of the most valuable published works on the history and literature of surgery, placing on firm foundation the use of the experimental method in dealing with surgical problems.

John Hunter (1728 to 1793) of Glasgow was an anatomist, experimenter and surgeon [18]. He was a pioneer in comparative anatomy and many of his mounted specimens, including those of a giant and a pigmy, were exhibited in the Hunterian Museum of the Royal College of Surgeons in London. Hunter conducted experiments on inflammation and tendon healing, as well as studies of diseases of the teeth, ligation of blood vessels and bone growth and structure.

John Abernathy (1764 to 1831) of England was a student of John Hunter [19]. In addition to his other accomplishments, Abernathy performed a neurectomy for neuralgia of the arm, beginning in the finger. He discovered that, following removal of one-half inch of nerve, reunion occurred along with the return of sensibility in the skin of the finger.

Jean Andre Venel (1740 to 1791) of Geneva, Switzerland can be considered the founder of modern orthopaedics [18]. In 1780 Venel acquired an old Abbey where he set up a multi-roomed hospital. In the basement was a workshop with technicians building devices and braces, as well as a large bath for patient therapy. The hospital primarily treated children with clubfeet, deformed lower limbs and scoliosis of the spine. The children would often remain at the hospital for months or years while receiving treatment, continuing their education with lessons from a school teacher. The children would wear their apparatus and be able to walk and play on the grounds of what was probably the first orthopaedic clinic in the world. Correction of lateral curvatures of the spine, performed with difficulty since the time of Hippocrates, was greatly improved by Venel. He used a mechanical apparatus to provide two methods of treatment. First, he stretched the spine using suspension and supported the spine with a corset-type device. Second, he used an apparatus with shoulder supports and applied side pressure on the convex side of the spinal curvature, allowing torsional corrections that had not been previously performed. For children under the age of 13 years, he used a special stretching bed at nighttime. This bed had straps which pulled the lower body toward the foot of the bed, as well as straps that ran under the shoulders and to the neck, forehead and temples that pulled the head and trunk upwards. The effect was to stretch the curved spine. During the day, a corset that rested on the pelvis as a distal support and on the shoulders and head as a proximal support was worn. Such continuous treatment – day and night – was a new concept.

1.3. Discussion

Volumes have been written about the early history of surgery and medicine and, due to space limitations, the above brief summary omits many other relevant individuals and contributions over the time interval considered. Nevertheless, sufficient detail has hopefully been provided to make the following points apparent. First, both progressive as well as regressive steps have occurred over the ages, as exemplified by the vacillation over primary vs. secondary wound healing, but, overall, progress has dominated resulting in advancement of technique over long periods of time. Second, the achievements during the beginning of civilization, when a basic understanding of biology was presumably lacking and technology was practically nonexistent, are amazing. In our era of sterile fields, anesthetic, antibiotics, bone grafts and substitutes, electrocautery and growth factor treatment, there remain complications of infection, bleeding and nonunion. That Neolithic man was able to successfully perform trephination is both a testament to his ability, as well as the robust tendency of the human body to heal. Third, while the history of medicine and surgery in general, and wound and musculoskeletal treatment in particular, are replete with dead-ends in methods and thinking, there remain a core of principles that are as relevant today as they were when they were discovered thousands of years ago. This is especially evident in the works of Hippocrates, as well as some of his predecessors and successors.

What does all of this tell us about where we are now and what the future holds? Although our lifestyle is arguably much different now than it was thousands, or even hundreds of years ago, to which, for better or worse, our physiology has adapted, there is no reason to believe that the basic regenerative capacity of the human body has changed over time. Thus, the fundamental healing response is the same today as it was in the time of Hippocrates, so what worked then continues to work today. Of course, current techniques may be more refined, but their basis is similar, if not identical, in many instances. As tremendous strides in genetics and molecular biology have been made in the 20th and early 21st Centuries, and the nature of the healing process, while not completely known, has been elucidated in some detail, different and improved healing interventions have become evident as indicated, for instance, by the burgeoning field of tissue engineering [30]. As for the future prediction is, and will remain, an inexact science unless, of course, technology changes this – an event that this author cannot predict! Nevertheless, three things appear to be relatively certain. First, new interventions will still be required to work within the context of the capabilities of the human body. To the extent that the human body continues to retain its heritage of the past, the same core principals that have withstood the test of time will continue to provide guidance. If, on the other hand, manipulation of the human genome changes the "playing field," this may be sufficient, in some instances, to obviate further intervention or may open new avenues for intervention in others. Second, new enabling technologies may be developed, whose existence cannot even be imagined now, which can open entirely new frontiers of musculoskeletal repair. Current leading technologies such as tissue engineering and nanotechnology hold much promise, but remain in their infancy [30, 31]. Third, and this is the most certain, future surgeons, physicians, scientists and bioengineers will look back upon our current era and, at first glance, say that our efforts were primitive, but then, upon closer inspection, say that we accomplished some truly marvelous things given our level of understanding and technology. But isn't that where this chapter began?

1.4. Conclusions

Treatment to enhance wound healing and effect musculoskeletal tissue repair has been an ongoing process, perhaps spanning as much as half of the collective existence of *homo sapiens*. While we have come a long way in producing effective treatments, we are "not there yet." Much work needs to be done before all wounds heal quickly and uneventfully with full restoration of form and function. While the task may seem daunting, we can move ahead confidently knowing that, indeed, "We are as children, standing on the shoulder of a giant..." – a giant that grows with each passing year.

References

1. Waris E, Konttinen YT, Ashammakhi N, Suuronen R, Santavirta S. Bioabsorbable fixation devices in trauma and bone surgery: current clinical standing. Expert Rev Med Devices 2004;1:229-240.
2. Uhthoff HK, Poitras P, Backman DS. Internal plate fixation of fractures: a short history and recent developments. J Orthop Sci 2006;11:118-126.
3. McFarland EG, Park HB, Keyurapan E, Gill HS, Selhi HS. Suture anchors and tacks for shoulder surgery, part I: biology and biomechanics. Am J Sports Med 2005;33:1918-1923.
4. Spotnitz WD. Surgical tissue adhesives: new additions to the surgical armamentarium. J Long Term Eff Med Implants 2003;13:385-387.
5. Bauer TW, Muschler GF. Bone graft materials. An overview of the basic science. Clin Orthop Rel Res 2000;371:10-27.
6. Sherman OH, Banffy MB. Anterior cruciate ligament reconstruction: which graft is best? Arthroscopy 2004;20:974-980.
7. Carlisle E, Fischgrund JS. Bone morphogenetic proteins for spinal fusion. Spine J 2005;5(6 Suppl):240S-249S.
8. Pietrzak WS, Eppley BL. Platelet rich plasma: biology and new technology. J Craniofac Surg 2005;16:1043-1054.
9. Ciombor DM, Aaron RK. The role of electrical stimulation in bone repair. Foot Ankle Clin 2005;10:579-593.

10. Nelson FR, Brighton CT, Ryaby J, Simon BJ, Nielson JH, Lorich DG, Bolander M, Seelig J. Use of physical forces in bone healing. J Am Acad Orthop Surg 2003;11:344-354.
11. Ge Z, Goh JC. Lee EH. Selection of cell source for ligament tissue engineering. Cell Transplant 2005;14:573-583.
12. Richardson RG. Surgery: Old and New Frontiers. New York: Charles Scribner's Sons, 1968.
13. Frost HM. A 2003 update of bone physiology and Wolff's Law for clinicians. Angle Orthod 2004;74:3-15.
14. Matter P. History of the AO and its global effect on operative fracture management. Clin Orthop Relat Res 1998;347:11-18.
15. Urist MR. Bone: formation by autoinduction. Science 1965;150:893-899.
16. Annas GJ, Caplan A, Elias S. Stem cell politics, ethics, and medical progress. Nat Med 1999;5:1339-1341.
17. Whipple AO. The story of wound healing and wound repair. Springfield, IL: Charles C. Thomas, 1961.
18. Mayba, MD. Bonesetters and others, pioneer orthopaedic surgeons. Henderson Books, Winnipeg, Manitoba, 1991.
19. Billings JS. The history and literature of surgery. New York: Argosy-Antiquarian, Ltd. 1970 (reprint) originally published 1895.
20. Zimmerman LM, Veith I. Great ideas in the history of surgery. Baltimore: The Williams & Wilkins Company, 1961.
21. Lieberman DE, McBratney BM, Krovitz G. The evolution and development of cranial form in Homo Sapiens. Proc Natl Acad Sci U S A. 2002;99:1134-9.
22. Mackenzie D. The history of sutures. Med Hist 1973;17:158-168.
23. Scott M. 32,000 years of suture. NATNEWS 1983;20:15-17.
24. Sanan A, Haines SJ. Repairing holes in the head: a history of cranioplasty. Neurosurgery 1997;40:588-602.
25. Alt KW, Jeunesse C, Buitrago-Téllez CH, Wächter R, Bos E, Pichler SL. Evidence for stone age cranial surgery. Nature 1997;387:768.
26. Nerlich AG, Zink A, Szeimies U, Hagedorn HG. Ancient Egyptian prosthesis of the big toe. Lancet 2000;356:2176-2179.
27. Wagle WA. Toe prosthesis in an Egyptian human mummy. AJR Am J Roentgenol 1994;162:999-1000.
28. Fisher GJ. A history of surgery. In: Ashhurst J, ed. International Encyclopedia of surgery. Vol. 6, 1886:1146-1202.
29. Bobbio A. The first endosseous alloplastic implant in the history of man. Bull Hist Dent 1972;20:1-6.
30. Atala A. Recent Developments in tissue engineering and regenerative medicine. Curr Opin Pediatr 2006;18:167-171.
31. Patel GM, Patel GC, Patel RB, Patel JK, Patel M. Nanorobot: a versatile tool in nanomedicine. J Drug Target 2006;14:63-67.

2

Musculoskeletal Fundamentals: Form, Function, and a Survey of Healing Strategies

Wei Shen, Mario Ferretti, Mollie Manley, and Freddie Fu

Abstract: During the last decade the basic research of orthopaedics has witnessed the revolution of cell biology, molecular biology and biomedical engineering. New concepts and technologies from these basic science fields have been quickly utilized in the research of orthopaedics, and will finally lead to the improvement of health care in the future. Among the new concepts and technologies, stem cells, gene therapy and tissue engineering showed their outstanding features and strong potential for future application in orthopaedics, just as they did in other medical fields. In this chapter we briefly summarize the basics of these topics and their application in orthopaedics. The advantages and drawbacks are discussed, as well as the current status of research. Additionally, although basic anatomy and histology of musculoskeletal tissue has been documented decades ago, we still briefly reviewed them in this chapter and wish to refresh the knowledge of the audience. The natural healing process of musculoskeletal tissues is also discussed in this chapter because no appropriate medical treatment can be applied without understanding the physiology and pathophysiology of the tissue.

Keywords: Stem cells, gene therapy, tissue engineering, musculoskeletal

2.1. Introduction

The musculoskeletal system is composed of many different tissues, which have different compositions, structures and physical properties. These tissues have unique natural healing processes when they sustain injures. In this chapter the basics of musculoskeletal tissues and their natural regenerative processes are briefly reviewed to serve as a cornerstone of this book. The concept and application of stem cells, gene therapy and tissue engineering are also reviewed here to update the knowledge of orthopaedic surgeons, scientists and bioengineers.

Department of Orthopaedic Surgery, University of Pittsburgh Medical Center, Pittsburg, PA

From: *Orthopedic Biology and Medicine: Musculoskeletal Tissue Regeneration, Biological Materials and Methods*
Edited by W. S. Pietrzak © Humana Press, Totowa, NJ

2.2. Musculoskeletal Tissues Basics and Their Natural Healing Processes

2.2.1. Bone

Bone is composed of bone cells and matrix. Osteoblasts produce Type I collagen to form bone, whereas osteoclasts break bone down. Osteocytes are resident cells in the matrix maintaining bone. The matrix is primarily composed of Type I collagen and associated inorganic compounds, the most prevalent of which is calcium hydroxyapatite, and organic compounds. The two general histological types of bone are cortical and cancellous. Cortical bones are composed of osteons and sustain most of the stress, while cancellous bones are composed of immature bone, known as trabeculae.

In general, bone injury is described as either a vascular etiology such as osteonecrosis, or a physical injury like a fracture. Osteonecrosis is caused by a mechanical disruption of the vascular supply of the bone which may eventually lead to infarction. Early changes include necrosis and death of the resident cells in the blood vessels, marrow and in the osseous matrix. Repair is usually initiated in the trabecular bone in the periphery of the lesion by increasing vascularity and osteoclastic migration. The osteoclasts reabsorb the necrotic trabeculae and new woven bone is deposited, giving the appearance of increased density on radiograph. This process of repair is termed creeping substitution. Due to the reabsorption of the trabeculae, the bone is fragile and failure of the matrix may lead to fractures and collapse in the beginning. This repair process may continue for up to two years, and the bone will become stronger.

The healing processes of bone fracture include inflammation, repair of the fracture and remodeling. These basic processes occur in the soft tissue, periosteum, cortex and bone marrow. Some of the factors that influence healing processes include disease state, nutrition, extent of injury, location and smoking cigarettes. After mechanical failure of the bone occurs, the blood supply is disrupted and bleeding occurs to create a local hematoma. Platelets release Platelet-Derived Growth Factor (PDGF) to recruit a source of inflammatory cells to the injury. Osteogenic precursor cells that are located in the surrounding periosteum differentiate into osteoblasts with the aid of growth factors such as Bone Morphogenic Protein (BMP). BMP-2 and BMP-7 have been shown in several clinical trials to accelerate fracture healing and decrease the rate of nonunion [1]. Bone formation begins only 24 hours after the initial injury, and has been described as primary and secondary. In order for primary healing to occur, the cortex of the fracture site must be realigned and stabilized. After reduction of the fracture site, minor cracks and breaks in the cortex remain, and angiogenesis occurs. Little or no callous is seen in primary healing. Secondary healing involves intramembranous and endochondral ossification and, contrary to primary healing, stabilization inhibits this process, while mobilization enhances it [2]. Soft callous forms between the two ends and are eventually replaced by a hard callous composed of woven bone. Transforming growth factor-beta (TGF-β) stimulates chondrogenic differentiation of periosteal mesenchymal cells during fracture healing at the callous [3]. After angiogenesis occurs and the cartilage has begun to form, it ossifies. In addition to TGF-β, Insulin-Like Growth Factor I (IGF-I) helps to stimulate bone formation. IGF-I has been shown to have a synergistic effect when combined with TGF-β [4]. Lastly, remodeling occurs and the calcified cartilage is reabsorbed and replaced by bone. This process is similar to the process at the physes during bone growth.

2.2.2. Articular Cartilage

Articular cartilage, composed of hyaline cartilage, can sustain years of use. However, once damage has occurred articular cartilage rarely recovers completely. Cartilage tissue can be damaged by direct trauma, inflammatory processes, infectious diseases or degenerative processes such as osteoarthritis. Interleukin-1 (IL-1) is a cytokine that acts in cartilage degradation by increasing Type I collagen synthesis, and repressing Type II collagen, the main collagen of healthy cartilage, from forming [5]. In contrast to vascularized tissues, articular cartilage does not have a good blood supply, and receives nutrients through diffusion in the synovial fluid. This affects the reparative process because a fibrin clot does not form at the injury site, therefore inflammatory cells cannot migrate into the tissue. Besides, articular cartilage contains mainly chondrocytes and lacks progenitor cells. Injuries to articular cartilage may be superficial or deep; the superficial lacerations do not heal because they do not cause hemorrhage. In this type of injury the chondrocyte has the potential to proliferate, but since the cells are unable to migrate it does not repair the defect. Deep injuries involve the bone as well, causing hemorrhage and migration of inflammatory cells and undifferentiated cells. The repair tissue in a chondral defect has a histological appearance of hybrid between hyaline and fibrocartilage, and does not completely restore pre-injury anatomy or mechanical function. Eventually this repair zone may degenerate further and results in densely packed collagen fibrils and loss of hyaline properties including elasticity and load bearing. The repair tissue has the ability to remain as it is or to remodel to more normal appearing articular cartilage.

2.2.3. Skeletal Muscle

Skeletal muscle is composed of units known as the sarcomere, which is the contractile element of the tissue. These are composed of myosin and actin, better known as the thick and thin filaments, respectively, and arranged in a parallel pattern. Myofibril is composed of sarcomeres separated by Z lines. Myofibrils make up a muscle fiber which makes up a muscle fascicle (Fig. 2.1).

Injury to the muscle can occur through ischemia and laceration, or genetic processes such as Duchenne (DMD) and Becker Muscular Dystrophy (BMD). Both diseases are X-linked and involve an abnormal gene for dystrophin resulting in total absence (DMD) or and an abnormally low amount of dystrophin (BMD). Dystrophin is important in the cell membrane of muscle for structural support and increasing membrane stiffness [6]. When children are born with these diseases they have normal appearing muscle. The muscle fibers go through a repetitive degenerative/regenerative process and are eventually replaced by fibrotic fatty tissue.

Muscle laceration does not regain the pre-injury properties after repair, but has been shown to recover 50 percent to 60 percent of ability to produce tension, and 80 percent to 100 percent of their ability to shorten, depending on the size of the injury [7]. Histologically the specimens showed variable size,

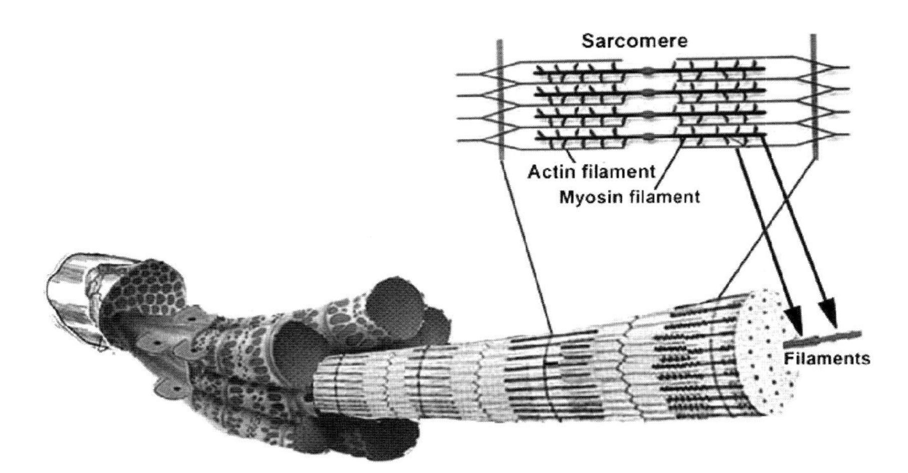

Fig. 2.1 The myofibrils, the major constituent of the muscle fibers, are made up of contractile units called sarcomeres. Two filamentary proteins called actin and myosin are the key components of a scaromere

fiber atrophy, increased fibrosis and centralization of the nucleus. Repair after a blunt trauma can be more complete, although it varies with age and morbidities of the patients. Unique to blunt trauma is myositis ossificans, which means bone formation within muscle. This typically occurs six to eight weeks after injury. Two studies of quadriceps contusions in West Point cadets showed formation of myositis ossificans in 20 percent and 9 percent of the study group, respectively [8, 9]. Surgery is contraindicated because it may intensify the heterotopic bone formation, and aggressive physiotherapy with passive stretching also increases the incidence of heterotopic bone formation [10]. Instead this is treated conservatively with the RICE principles of rest, ice, compression and elevation [11].

2.2.4. Tendon and Ligament

Tendons and ligaments have similar structures and properties. They are composed of Type I collagen arranged in uniform parallel rows, and fibroblasts that produce the collagen fibrils. Tendons attach muscle to bone and insert into bone through fibrocartilage. The fibrocartilage prevents the tendon from bending or compressing, protecting the fibers from wear and tear [12]. Sharpey's fibers are collagen fibers that extend into the bone at an angle to connect the tendon with the bone. Ligaments differ from tendons in that they are connections between bones, as opposed to bone to muscle, and they have more ground substance composed of glycosaminoglycans, mainly chondroitin sulfate and keratin sulfate, than tendons and a lower percentage of collagen.

There are two main types of tendons: sheathed tendons and paratenon-covered tendons. The difference between the two types is the vascular supply. The sheathed tendons' blood is supplied to part of the tendon and the avascular portion receives nutrients through diffusion. In the sheathed tendons cells from the epitenon and endotenon proliferate and migrate to the severed ends of the tendon, producing the majority of collagen [13]. A surgical repair is necessary in many cases to allow for early motion. This has been shown to decrease adhesions and restore the gliding surface of the sheath and tendon [14].

Paratenon-covered tendons heal better due to the higher vascularity of the tissue. After an injury the wound fills with inflammatory cells brought in by hematoma formation. Fibroblasts proliferate and produce granulation tissue, and VEGF is released to aid in capillary invasion into the gap in the tendon. The collagen fibrils are first oriented perpendicularly to the axis of the tendon, and begin to remodel due to stress placed on the tendon. Without stress added to the healing tissue, the tendon will not gain the tensile strength it originally had because of the alignment of collagen in the tendon [15].

The healing of ligaments has four basic phases: hemorrhage, inflammation, repair and remodeling [16]. The first phase is similar to other tissues with formation of a hematoma, fibrin clot, and release of inflammatory mediators such as bradykinins and histamine. During the next phase of repair phagocytosis continues and the clot is slowly transformed into granulation tissue. Eventually, at the end of the inflammatory stage, fibroblasts begin to form an immature extracellular matrix and Type III collagen. The third phase is a continuum of the inflammatory phase, and Type I collagen fibers are now the predominant in extracellular matrix produced. It is during the reparative phase that the collagen fibers align in a more parallel fashion, similar to pre-injury state.

2.2.5. Meniscus

The menisci are fibrocartilage rings attached to the tibial plateau. The medial ring is a semicircular shape and the lateral is circular. Once thought of as nonfunctional, the menisci are now considered as a vital component of the knee that functions to extend the articular surface contact area of the tibia and femur [17]. The menisci function mainly to distribute stress and provide shock absorption during weight bearing, stabilize the joint and provide lubrication to the joint [18, 19]. The menisci are composed mostly of Type I collagen arranged in three different layers: superficial, lamellar and central [20]. The tibial and femoral sides of the meniscus surface are covered by the superficial meshwork of thin fibrils. The lamellar layer is beneath the superficial network. The collagen fibril bundles in this layer intersect at various angles, although they are arranged in a radial direction in the area of the external circumference of the anterior and posterior segments. The central main layer is the primary portion of the meniscus collagen fibrils. The bundles of collagen fibrils in this layer are orientated in a circular manner (Fig. 2.2). Type I collagen is the most abundant type of collagen in the menisci, although Types II, III, V and VI have been identified. The menisci also have an abundant amount of water, as well as proteoglycans, elastin and cells [21]. Two types of cells are found within the meniscus, fusiform and ovoid cells that synthesize the extracellular matrix. There are three zones that are important in the healing process of the meniscus, going from the outside thick part to the inside thin part. The three zones of the meniscus are named red-red, red-white and white-white zones. These names are based on blood supply which is rich superficially and virtually does not exist deep within the meniscus. The red-red zone has excelling healing potential due to the rich vascular supply; the red-white zone still has a good prognosis, but the white-white zone has a bad prognosis with almost no potential for healing [22]. Chronic degeneration of the meniscus occurs with disruption of the normal anatomy of the knee, torn ACL and with 75 percent of primary osteoarthritis [23].

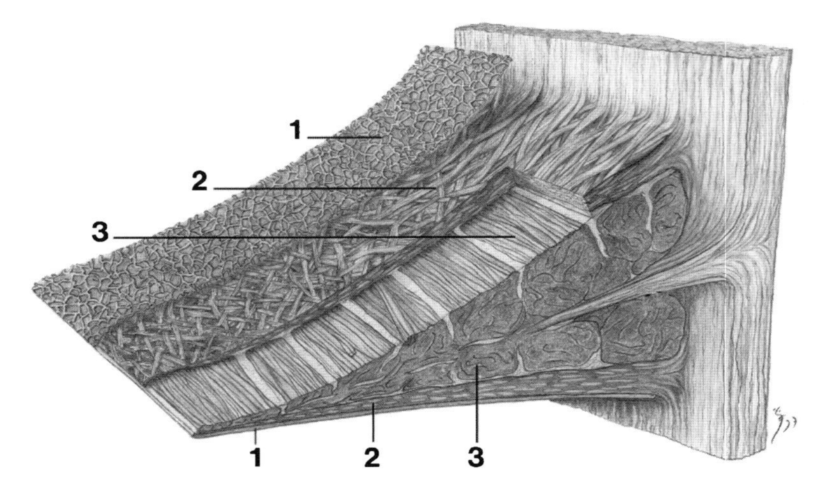

Fig. 2.2 Schematic drawing shows three distinct layers in the meniscus cross section: the superficial network (1), the lamellar layer (2) and the central layer (3)

2.2.6. Intervertebral Disc

The intervertebral disc is composed mainly of fibrocartilage. This fibrocartilage portion is known as the anulus fibrosus surrounding the nucleus pulposus. The collagen fibers are organized in rows of lamella in the anulus that become more complex and thick with age [24]. Collagen fibers anchor the anulus to the vertebral bodies. The disc is also composed of extracellular matrix and two different cell populations; the cells from the nucleus pulposus produce Type II collagen while the cells from the anulus fibrosus produce Types I and II [25]. It is important to note that the blood supply is located only in the outer few layers of the disc, and the number of vascular channels decreases early in life [26]. Many changes occur with aging, such as increased cell death, increased number and complexity of clefts and tears, neovascularization and the presence of granular material [27]. Two basic degenerative processes that occur in the intervertebral disc are degeneration and herniation. The characteristics of disc degeneration are similar to many normal, age-related changes; therefore it is difficult to differentiate between the two processes. The lamellar layers become more disorganized and may fissure more than aging alone. Also, it has been proposed that the disc height would not decrease during normal aging [28].

2.3. The Application of Stem Cells in Regeneration of Musculoskeletal Tissues

Stem cells have the ability to replicate themselves for the life of the organism. With certain stimulations stem cells are capable of differentiating into different cell types that make up the organism.

A fertilized egg is said to be totipotent, which means that it has the potential to generate all the cells and tissues that make up an organism. The fertilized egg replicates and differentiates until it produces a mature organism, which consists of more than 200 types of cells. The term pluripotent is used to describe embryonic stem cells that can give rise to cells derived from all three embryonic germ layers: mesoderm, endoderm and ectoderm. These three germ layers are the origin of all cells of the organism. The only difference between totipotent and pluripotent stem cells is that totipotent stem cells can also differentiate into cell types that are essential for embryonic development, but are not incorporated into the body of the embryo, including the extraembryonic tissues, placenta and umbilical cord.

Unipotent stem cells are capable of differentiating along only one lineage (a lineage may consist of different specific cell types). Adult stem cells in many tissues are typically unipotent and give rise to all the specialized cell types of the tissue from which it originated. They provide self-renewal capability to the tissue. Adult stem cells have been found in many tissues, including bone marrow, blood stream, cornea and retina of the eye, the dental pulp of the tooth, liver, skin, muscle, adipose tissue, gastrointestinal tract and pancreas. However, pluripotent stem cells may also exist in mature tissue and become activated after injury and tissue damage [29]. Under normal conditions adult stem cells are not pluripotent. However, it has been suggested that they may become pluripotent in certain circumstances [30].

From a therapeutic point of view, although embryonic stem cells may be versatile in repairing different tissues, they must be used as allografts unless therapeutic cloning techniques are utilized. Adult stem cells, however, can be used for autologous transplantation with reduced concern of immunogenecity. Remarkable progress has been achieved in assessing the characteristics of adult stem cells and their potential use in treating orthopaedic disorders. Since the application of stem cells in orthopaedics will also be covered in the topics of tissue engineering and gene therapy, here we will introduce the orthopaedic application of stem cells briefly.

2.3.1. Bone

The potential of mesenchymal stem cells (MSCs) in promoting bone healing has been demonstrated. Goel, et al. [31] evaluated the effect of bone marrow grafting in patients with a tibial nonunion, resulting in union in most patients. Siwach, et al. [32] treated 72 patients who had delayed or nonunion with a percutaneous injection of autogenous bone marrow. They achieved union in 68 of 72 patients. The application of scaffolds loaded with MSCs appears to be a more efficient technique capable of healing large defects. The outcome can be further enhanced by the addition of growth factors. Borden, et al. [33] combined BMP-7 with bone marrow MSCs and a polymeric microsphere matrix in an effort to treat large segmental defects in an animal model. The addition of BMP-7 seemed to up-regulate the osteogenic activity of MSCs and enhance the healing of the defect. Muscle-Derived Stem Cells (MDSCs) were studied as another source of adult stem cells that promote bone healing. MDSCs that were transfected to express BMP-4 and VEGF [34] were shown to significantly elicit bone healing [35]. However, it is worth noting that stem cells alone have limited ability in improving the healing of critical-sized bone defects without being genetically engineered to express specific growth factors.

2.3.2. Articular Cartilage

It has been demonstrated that MSCs are also capable of differentiating into chondrocytes and form cartilage tissue. Osteochondral defects could heal spontaneously because MSCs migrated from bone marrow may proliferate and differentiate into chondrocytes [36]. Stem cell-based cartilage repair has focused on discovering growth factors with the potential to promote chondrogenic differentiation, and the tissue engineering of cartilage. BMP2 and BMP9 have been shown to induce the activation of Sox-9 and lead to the chondrogenic differentiation of MSCs, as indicated by the expression of Type II collagen mRNA and the increased expression of aggrecan and other cartilage matrix proteins [37]. Tamai, et al. [38] studied the healing potential of full-thickness articular defects in an animal model by combining porous hydroxyapatite with recombinant human BMP-2 and a synthetic biodegradable polymer. It resulted in complete repair of the defect at six weeks. However, it's questionable whether tissue engineering construct could integrate with surrounding normal cartilage tissues and maintain its structure after being implanted into a defect.

2.3.3. Skeletal Muscle

Stem cell-based therapy could also be utilized in the treatment of Duchenne Muscular Dystrophy (DMD) patients, which are characterized by the lack of dystrophin protein. These patients are subjected to repeated injury and regeneration, and finally the depletion of MDSCs. Transplanted MDSCs successfully restored dystrophin expression upon implantation into MDX mice (an animal model of DMD) with a higher degree of efficiency than myoblast or satellite cell. This superior transplantation capability of MDSCs may be due to their immune privilege (less immune response), self-renewal ability and multipotential differentiation [39]. This group also reported that CD34-positive MDSCs have a better regeneration capacity than other subpopulations of MDSCs, and this superior regeneration capacity correlates with a better proliferation potential [40].

Using stem cells in other musculoskeletal tissues has recently been explored. Yamasaki, et al. [41] showed that when using a normal meniscus as scaffold and embedded with mesenchymal stromal cells derived from the bone marrow of GFP transgenic rats, the expression of extracellular matrices was detected histologically and expression of mRNA for aggrecan and Type X collagen was detected. Stiffness of the cultured tissue, assessed by the indentation stiffness test, had increased significantly after two weeks in culture, and approximated the stiffness of a normal meniscus. In the research of tendon and ligament tissue, gel-collagen sponge seeded with MSCs significantly improves patellar tendon repair, compared to the use of a gel-sponge composite alone in the range of *in vivo* loading [42]. Ge, et.al [43] showed that MSCs could promote synthesis of collagen Type I and collagen Type III in tissue-engineered anterior cruciate ligaments. However, both studies failed to improve the mechanical property of the construct to closely match those of the normal, native tissues. In the field of intervertebral disc, MSCs were transplanted to degenerative discs in rabbits [44]. They proliferated and differentiated into cells expressing some of the major phenotypic characteristics of nucleus pulposus cells, suggesting that these MSCs may have undergone site-dependent differentiation. However, their functional role needs to be evaluated in the future.

2.4. The Application of Gene Therapy in the Regeneration of Musculoskeletal Tissues

Gene therapy is defined as the insertion of functional genes into cells to replace the defective genes, and provide a specialized disease-fighting function. Genetic material can be delivered into the nucleus of cells by either virus-mediated or non–virus-mediated delivery methods. Although the non–virus-mediated delivery methods have their advantages – easy manipulation, low toxicity and less immune reaction – nowadays the use of viral vectors becomes more and more popular because it enables more efficient gene delivery rendered by the naturally evolved features of viruses. Genes that code for pathogenic protein products are modified or removed from the virus vector, and the genes of interest are inserted. The inserted genes may either integrate into host chromosomes or remain in a form of episome to produce the desired protein product. Various gene transfer strategies have been used to treat musculoskeletal diseases [45, 46]. In most orthopaedic applications, tissue-specific local delivery is a more desirable approach against systemic delivery, because local delivery requires less amount of vector, and it is safer by not disseminating the vector throughout the body. More importantly, musculoskeletal tissues usually lack blood supply and make them poor candidates for systemic delivery. Two basic strategies are used for the local gene delivery approach: *in vivo* and *ex vivo* [45, 46]. The *in vivo* technique involves direct injection of the vectors containing DNA into the targeted host tissue. In the *ex vivo* technique cells are genetically modified outside the body, and injected into the target site. Stem cells are now hot candidates in *ex vivo* technique, because under specific growth factor induction, stem cells can differentiate into desired cell types and regenerate musculoskeletal tissues. After all, the selection of appropriate strategy is based on various factors, like cell source, size of the insertion gene and the pathophysiology of diseased tissue.

2.4.1. Bone

The ability of gene therapy to repair bone defects has been examined by multiple independent laboratories using different gene transfer strategies. Using a non-viral delivery method, Bonadio and his colleagues [47] implanted a collagen sponge containing parathyroid hormone cDNA in a critical-sized canine tibial bone defect model. Although this study was not a total success, since bone production was insufficient at six weeks after implantation, it demonstrated the importance of identifying the optimal combination of matrix material and osteoinductive agent. Using *in vivo* technique, Baltzer and coworkers [48, 49] injected adenovirus Bone Morphogenic Protein-2 (Ad. BMP-2) into a rabbit femoral bone defect and reported osseous tissue formation. In another study of this group, the safety of using adenovirus was brought to light. Impressively, they [50] showed that 51 transgene expression was almost entirely restricted to the site of administration. Musgrave, et al. [51] also used Ad.BMP-2 in inducing ectopic bone formation in the thigh muscles of mice. Less bone was formed in immunocompetent animals than in immunocompromised animals. This may be due to the immune response elicited by the first generation adenovirus [52, 53]. Stem cells of different sources are commonly used as *ex vivo* delivery vehicles. The insertion of an osteoinductive protein gene into stem cells could further enhance bone repair responses because they would not only produce, but also respond to osteoinductive proteins. Lieberman, et Al. [54] transduced bone marrow mesenchymal stem cells with Ad.BMP-2 and observed a robust pattern of bone formation by injecting them into a critical-sized femoral bone defect. Peng, et al. [35] showed that muscle-derived stem cells genetically engineered to express human BMP-4 or VEGF could work synergistically to enhance bone formation.

2.4.2. Articular Cartilage

Many genes have been found useful in cartilage repair, including genes encoding growth factors like Transforming Growth Factor (TGF-β) superfamily, BMPs, Insulin-like Growth Factor-1 (IGF-1), Fibroblast Growth Factor (FGF) and Epidermal Growth Factor (EGF), transcription factors like Sox-9, L-Sox 5 and Sox-6, and signal transduction molecules like SMADs. In addition, proteins like Interleukin-1 Receptor a (IL-1Ra), soluble Tissue Necrosis Factor (TNF) receptors or inhibitors of MMPs (Matrix Metalloproteinases) may effectively reduce cartilage loss by blocking the increased level of IL-1 and TNF-α during cartilage degradation [55]. Several approaches to repair cartilage using gene transfer have been evaluated. Direct intra-articular injection of adenovirus containing IGF-1 cDNA increase matrix synthesis in both rabbit and horse models [56,57]. Kang, et Al. [58] have shown that *ex vivo* delivery of genetically modified chondrocytes to cartilage defects leads to transgene expression in full-thickness cartilage defects. Using an *ex vivo* approach, Ahrens and co-workers [59] reported that some BMP-2 or BMP-4 tranfected mesenchymal progenitor cells developed into chondrocytes, whereas some others also underwent osteogenic and adipocytic differentiation.

2.4.3. Tendon and Ligament

Tendon and ligament injures are common orthopaedic problems. Besides the common problems of gene therapy, scar tissue formation and adhesions are specific challenging problems for tendon and ligament [60]. Lou and co-workers [61] used Ad.BMP-12 to transfect tendon cells *in vitro* and tendons *in vivo* to investigate the effect BMP-12 on tendon repair. The *in vitro* experiment showed that tranduced tendon cells have a 30 percent increase in collagen Type I synthesis, whereas the *in vivo* experiment showed significantly higher ultimate failure force and lower stiffness in the treated animals four weeks after surgery. In ligament gene therapy MCL and ACL were used as models [60]. In a MCL rabbit model researchers created a 4-mm gap. Two weeks after surgery, hemagglutinating virus of Japan-conjugated liposomes containing antisense oligodeoxynucleotides to decorin was injected into the scar that filled the surgery gap [62-64]. Histology showed a more normal appearance and some return of the normal crimp pattern in the antisense group.

2.4.4. Skeletal Muscle

Severe muscle injuries can lead to functional impairment and may culminate in the formation of scar tissue. It was reported that the basal lamina surrounding mature myofibers acts as a barrier to direct gene transfer because it contains pores that are only about 40 nm in diameter [65]. Thus, the small adeno-associated virus (AAV) was rendered the advantage over other viruses in penetrating the basal lamina. Barton-Davis and his colleagues [66] showed that direct injection of AAV.IGF-1 into skeletal muscle can stimulate muscle regeneration. Duchenne muscle dystrophy is another major target of skeletal muscle gene therapy. The large size of the dystrophin gene is a challenge to gene therapy for Duchenne muscle dystrophy. The use of the high-capacity adenovirus has improved the effectiveness of gene transfer [67,68]. Recently, a minidystrophin and microdystrophin strategy has been developed [69, 70]. This approach is based on the fact that only a small part of this gene is responsible for its vital function [71]. Researchers have also evaluated gene transfer of utrophin as an alternative strategy to treat DMD [72] because the structure and function of utrophin and dystrophin are similar.

2.4.5. Meniscus

The research of gene therapy in meniscus repair is limited. However, its feasibility has been investigated in a rabbit model. LacZ, luciferase and green fluorescence protein were used as marker genes to investigate viral transduction in 50 lapine menisci for four weeks *in vitro*. Subsequently, 16 unilateral meniscus replacements were performed with *ex vivo* retrovirally transduced meniscal allografts. Gene expression was found in both superficial and deeper cell layers of the menisci. Marker gene expression was detectable for up to four weeks, although the level was declining over time. There was no evidence of cellular immune response in the transduced transplants [73].

2.4.6. Intervertebral Disc

Direct injection of recombinant adenovirus and AAV has been used to deliver cDNAs to the intervertebral disc. A dramatic increase in matrix synthesis was seen with the delivery of cDNAs encoding IGF-1, TGF-β, BMP-2, and the tissue inhibitor of metalloproteinases-1 (TIMP-1) [74, 75]. This seems to have a promising future in the prevention and treatment of degenerative disc disease. The duration of transgene expression in the intervertebral disc are usually prolonged, possibly due to the quiescent state of the cells, and lack of immune responses provided by the dense and avascular matrix structure of the intervertebral disc.

2.5. The Application of Tissue Engineering in the Regeneration of Musculoskeletal Tissues

Tissue engineering is an advanced therapy that aims at the repair, reconstruction and regeneration of specific tissues. Usually tissue engineering combines scaffold or matrix, living cells and/or biologically active molecules. The scaffold must be biocompatible and biodegradable. It should be able to provide a temporary structure, support cell colonization, migration, growth and differentiation, guide the tissue development and also act as a delivery vehicle of drugs or growth factors [76, 77]. The cells used are commonly pluripotent mesenchymal stem cells (MSCs) that can be isolated from various sites such as bone marrow, muscle and others. The MSCs are non-haematopoetic cells, exhibit a multilineage differentiation capacity and can develop into different cell types, including adipocytes, osteoblasts, chondrocytes, myocytes, tenocytes, neural cells and many others [78]. The MSCs may be only combined with scaffold [76]. However, they can be stimulated directly by biological molecules like growth factors [79] or modified genetically to produce a specific molecule continuously [80]. The biological factor is a key component of advancing tissue regeneration. It may be used to amplify cell expansion, strengthen phenotype, improve extracellular matrix production and, at the same time, reduce cell breakdown and catabolic degradation [81].

The existence of different techniques in tissue engineering demonstrates the experimental character of this approach. However, the experimental results are promising and some of these technologies already have been used in clinical trial [82, 83].

2.5.1. Bone

The treatment of large bony defects is a challenge to trauma and orthopaedic surgeons. Advances in tissue engineering have led to the development of new therapeutic options. The ideal therapy for bone healing and osteointegration must contain osteogenic, osteoinductive and osteoconductive elements. The osteogenic potential is represented by cells that can proliferate and differentiate in osteoblasts and, eventually, to osteocytes to produce bone tissue. Osteoinduction is the stimulation and activation of host mesenchymal stem cells from the surrounding tissue, which differentiate into bone-forming osteoblasts. Osteoconduction describes the facilitation and orientation of blood vessels and the creation of the new Haversian systems into the bone [84].

The cancelous bone autograft is the gold standard treatment for bone defects and contains good osteogenic element. The use of bone marrow aspirate also contains osteogenic elements [84]. Recently cell therapy using MSCs has been described for bone formation with an osteogenic potential [78, 82, 84].

The osteoinductive element is achieved by growth factors and BMPs. The FGF-2 and IGF-1 have been shown to increase callous size and strength [85, 86]. The addition of VEGF to osteoinductive factors (BMPs) improves bone healing [35]. Local injections of small amounts of Growth Hormone (GH) have a marked positive effect on rat fracture repair, without causing any systemic effects [87].

Since BMPs were first described by Urist in 1965 [88] numerous research projects have been developed to study their effect in bone healing. BMP-2 has been shown effective to better heal ulnar bone defect in rabbits [89], and it appears to enhance fracture healing in osteoporotic sheep [90]. In a prospective, randomized, controlled, single-blind study, 450 patients with an open tibial fracture were randomized to receive either the standard of care (intramedullary nail fixation), or the standard of care and an implant containing different dosages of rhBMP-2. The higher dosage of rhBMP-2 (1.50 mg/mL) group had a 44 percent reduction in the risk of failure, and significantly faster fracture healing than did the control patients [1]. BMP-4 and BMP-7 also demonstrated an enhancement in the bone healing in experimental model and clinical trials [91, 33].

Scaffolds provide a platform for bone ingrowth and satisfy the osteoconductive requirements. The demineralized bone matrix (DBM) is produced through decalcification of cortical bone. It provides osteoconductive and some osteoinductive properties. It can be supplied as a gel, malleable putty, flexible strips or injectable bone paste. However, clinical results are not uniformly good; consequently DBM is used as a "bone graft extender" rather than as a bone graft substitute [84]. Considerable advances have been made with synthetic bone substitutes. However, most of them allow osteointegration and osteoconduction, but not osteoinduction and osteogenesis. Ceramics are synthetic scaffold made from calcium phosphate, so as tricalcium phosphate (TCP) - ceramic and hydroxyapatite (HA). When attached to healthy bone osteoid is produced on the surfaces of the ceramic and results in new bone remodeling. A ceramic with higher porosity and lower density construct provides greater surface area for vascularization, and bony ingrowth. The osteoconductive scaffold provides an appropriate environment for bone cells and BMPs [84]. Injectable calcium phosphate is a ceramic composite. It can work as a void-filler and the osteointegration is followed by incorporation. Ultraporous beta tricalcium phosphate (β-TCP) is a highly porous void-filler that is composed of 90 percent interconnected void space with a broad range of porous size. The β-TCP architecture encourages vascularization and bone formation. Poly (lactic acid) (PLA), poly (glycolic acid) (PGA) and poly (lactic-co-glycolide) (PLGA) are saturated aliphatic polyesters that can be processed easily, and their degradation rates, physical and mechanical properties are adjustable over a wide range by using various molecular weights and copolymers. However, these polymers undergo a bulk erosion process that can cause failure of the scaffold. In addition, abrupt release of these acidic degradation products can cause a strong inflammatory response [92]. Biologic/synthetic composite grafts that contain osteogenic cells, osteoinductive growth factors and osteoconductive matrix seem to be the most promising emerging surgical options for bone repair. The incorporation of MSCs and/or BMPs into these biomaterials has been demonstrated to enhance their osteogenic capacity by accelerating bone formation and osteointegration when used for *in vivo* bone repair. [1, 89, 91].

2.5.2. Articular Cartilage

The healing of a cartilage tissue is challenging. Cartilage is basically formed by cells and extracellular matrix (ECM), mainly formed by the Type II collagen and proteoclycans. The configuration of the cells and ECM divides the cartilage into four different zones (superficial, transitional, the radial zone and the tidemark). To date the artificial structure of the cartilage with four zones is not achieved. The cell therapy for cartilage repair in a clinical setting was described in 1994 by Brittberg using autologous chondrocytes transplantation [93]. Another type of cell that can regenerate cartilage are the MSCs. These cells have been stimulated by the application of transforming growth factor (TGF)-β in order to obtain a chondrogenic differentiation [79].

The development of scaffolds for cartilage repair has been largely studied. The saturated aliphatic polyesters, PLA and PLGA have the ability to maintain chondrocytes phenotype and produce cartilage-specific ECM [94]. Nanotechnology may be used to mimic the cartilage structure. PLA or poly (ε–caprolactone) (PCL) nanofibrous scaffold has also been shown as a potential scaffold in cartilage research [95]. Hydrogels are also interesting polymers to be used for cartilage tissue engineering. They can absorb a large volume of aqueous solution and encapsulate cells. Hydrogels may be formed *in situ* within a defect site [96].

The use of signaling molecules, such as growth factors, is common to promote tissue growth in cartilage tissue engineering. Growth factors like the TGF-β superfamily, IGFs, FGFs, PDGFs and the EGF family have regulatory effects on chondrocytes or MSCs for cartilage tissue engineering. Growth factors such as IGF, FGF and PDGF mediate chondrocytic physiology, rather than promote chondrogenesis of MSCs. To enhance cartilage growth these factors commonly work in tandem with TGF-βs. A recent trend in cartilage tissue engineering is to administer a combination of growth factors to maximize their impact, as well as to simulate the *in vivo* growth factor environment [95]. It is important to note that the inflammatory environment of osteoarthritis has also been addressed. Gene therapy using IL-1 Ra and IL-10 to block inflammation and inhibit cartilage deterioration has been described [97]. Bioreactors to enhance the growth of cartilaginous constructs also have been described for cartilage tissue engineering [98].

2.5.3. Meniscus

The use of scaffold for meniscus tissue engineering has been described [99-102]. Polyurethane scaffolds with optimal mechanical properties and with optimal interconnective macro-porosity have been shown to facilitate ingrowth and differentiation of tissue into fibrocartilage. However, even these materials cannot prevent cartilage degeneration in animal models. Surface modification and/or seeding of cells into the scaffolds before implantation may offer a solution for this problem in the future [99]. A new biomaterial consisting of hyaluronic acid and polycaprolactone was used as a meniscus substitute in sheep to evaluate the properties of the implant material. The implants remained in position without tearing, and showed excellent tissue ingrowth to the capsule. Tissue integration was also observed between the original meniscus and the implant. However, graft compression and extrusion occurred. The histological investigation revealed tissue formation, cellular infiltration and vascularization [100]. Biodegradable PGA scaffolds in a meniscal shape were fabricated and implanted with expanded meniscal cells and, after total meniscectomy in rabbits, the implants formed neomenisci with the original scaffold shape maintained [101]. Few studies describe the effects of growth factors in the menisci repair, but TGF-β1 appears to be the most effective growth factor for use in scaffold-based approaches to tissue engineer the meniscus [102].

2.5.4. Tendons and Ligaments

Little is known about the use of scaffolds in regenerating tendons and ligaments. The direct administration of PDGF and IGF to injured ligaments has been shown to promote healing [103, 104]. Gene therapy to deliver PDGF to injured patellar ligaments also has been reported, resulting in increased collagen synthesis and angiogenesis [105].

2.5.5. Intervertebral Disc

Tissue engineering progress has demonstrated the feasibility of creating a composite intervertebral disc with both anulus fibrosus (AF) and nucleus pulposus

(NP) [106]. A tissue engineered AF was made from a PLA and PGA polymer with AF cells. NP cells were suspended in a solution of 2 percent alginate and injected into the empty center of the scaffold [106]. Others polymers have also been used for intervertebral disc research as Chitosan cross-linked with genipin, and gelatin/chondroitin-6-sulfate/hyaluronan tri-copolymer scaffold, and others [107, 108]. Several growth factors, including BMP-2; BMP-7, also known as osteogenic protein-1 (OP-1); growth and differentiation factor-5; TGF-β and IGF-1 were found to stimulate matrix production [109]. While anabolic proteins have been studied for intervertebral disc tissue engineering, the blocking of catabolic cytokines with IL-1 Ra has also been studied [109, 110].

2.6. Conclusion

The basics of musculoskeletal tissues and their natural regenerative processes have been known for many decades. However,fast growing basic science research and new concepts like stem cells has modified our understanding of their healing processes. The development of biological approaches has offered us new ways to intervene with the healing process and improve the outcomes. Thus, the concepts of stem cells, gene therapy and tissue engineering are introduced, and their applications in orthopaedics are discussed in this chapter. Although *in vitro* experiments and animal studies have been successfully conducted for most orthopaedic tissues and have shown a promising future, relatively few attempts and successes have been achieved in converting these results to human applications. More studies need to be done to investigate the potential problems and finally convert it from bench side to bedside.

References

1. Govender, S., C. Csimma, H.K. Genant, et al., *Recombinant human bone morphogenetic protein-2 for treatment of open tibial fractures: a prospective, controlled, randomized study of four hundred and fifty patients.* J Bone Joint Surg Am, 2002. **84-A**(12): 2123-34.
2. Ilizarov, G.A., *The tension-stress effect on the genesis and growth of tissues. Part I. The influence of stability of fixation and soft-tissue preservation.* Clin Orthop Relat Res, 1989(238): 249-81.
3. Iwasaki, M., H. Nakahara, K. Nakata, et al., *Regulation of proliferation and osteochondrogenic differentiation of periosteum-derived cells by transforming growth factor-beta and basic fibroblast growth factor.* J Bone Joint Surg Am, 1995. **77**(4): 543-54.
4. Schmidmaier, G., B. Wildemann, T. Gabelein, et al., *Synergistic effect of IGF-I and TGF-beta1 on fracture healing in rats: single versus combined application of IGF-I and TGF-beta1.* Acta Orthop Scand, 2003. **74**(5): 604-10.
5. Chadjichristos, C., C. Ghayor, M. Kypriotou, et al., *Sp1 and Sp3 transcription factors mediate interleukin-1 beta down-regulation of human type II collagen gene expression in articular chondrocytes.* J Biol Chem, 2003. **278**(41): 39762-72.
6. Pasternak, C., S. Wong, and E.L. Elson, *Mechanical function of dystrophin in muscle cells.* J Cell Biol, 1995. **128**(3): 355-61.
7. Garrett, W.E., Jr., A.V. Seaber, J. Boswick, et al., *Recovery of skeletal muscle after laceration and repair.* J Hand Surg [Am], 1984. **9**(5): 683-92.
8. Jackson, D.W. and J.A. Feagin, *Quadriceps contusions in young athletes. Relation of severity of injury to treatment and prognosis.* J Bone Joint Surg Am, 1973. **55**(1): 95-105.

9. Ryan, J.B., J.H. Wheeler, W.J. Hopkinson, et al., *Quadriceps contusions. West Point update*. Am J Sports Med, 1991. **19**(3): 299-304.
10. Lipscomb, A.B., E.D. Thomas, and R.K. Johnston, *Treatment of myositis ossificans traumatica in athletes*. Am J Sports Med, 1976. **4**(3): 111-20.
11. Beiner, J.M. and P. Jokl, *Muscle contusion injury and myositis ossificans traumatica*. Clin Orthop Relat Res, 2002(403 Suppl): S110-9.
12. Benjamin, M., E.J. Evans, and L. Copp, *The histology of tendon attachments to bone in man*. J Anat, 1986. **149**: 89-100.
13. Gelberman, R.H., D. Amiel, and F. Harwood, *Genetic expression for type I procollagen in the early stages of flexor tendon healing*. J Hand Surg [Am], 1992. **17**(3): 551-8.
14. Boyer, M.I., C.A. Goldfarb, and R.H. Gelberman, *Recent progress in flexor tendon healing. The modulation of tendon healing with rehabilitation variables*. J Hand Ther, 2005. **18**(2): 80-5; quiz 86.
15. Hannafin, J.A., S.P. Arnoczky, A. Hoonjan, et al., *Effect of stress deprivation and cyclic tensile loading on the material and morphologic properties of canine flexor digitorum profundus tendon: an in vitro study*. J Orthop Res, 1995. **13**(6): 907-14.
16. Frank, C., S.L. Woo, D. Amiel, et al., *Medial collateral ligament healing. A multidisciplinary assessment in rabbits*. Am J Sports Med, 1983. **11**(6): 379-89.
17. Baratz, M.E., F.H. Fu, and R. Mengato, *Meniscal tears: the effect of meniscectomy and of repair on intraarticular contact areas and stress in the human knee. A preliminary report*. Am J Sports Med, 1986. **14**(4): 270-5.
18. Levy, I.M., P.A. Torzilli, and R.F. Warren, *The effect of medial meniscectomy on anterior-posterior motion of the knee*. J Bone Joint Surg Am, 1982. **64**(6): 883-8.
19. Radin, E.L., F. de Lamotte, and P. Maquet, *Role of the menisci in the distribution of stress in the knee*. Clin Orthop Relat Res, 1984(185): 290-4.
20. Petersen, W. and B. Tillmann, *Collagenous fibril texture of the human knee joint menisci*. Anat Embryol (Berl), 1998. **197**(4): 317-24.
21. McDevitt, C.A. and R.J. Webber, *The ultrastructure and biochemistry of meniscal cartilage*. Clin Orthop Relat Res, 1990(252): 8-18.
22. Arnoczky, S.P. and R.F. Warren, *Microvasculature of the human meniscus*. Am J Sports Med, 1982. **10**(2): 90-5.
23. Berthiaume, M.J., J.P. Raynauld, J. Martel-Pelletier, et al., *Meniscal tear and extrusion are strongly associated with progression of symptomatic knee osteoarthritis as assessed by quantitative magnetic resonance imaging*. Ann Rheum Dis, 2005. **64**(4): 556-63.
24. Marchand, F. and A.M. Ahmed, *Investigation of the laminate structure of lumbar disc anulus fibrosus*. Spine, 1990. **15**(5): 402-10.
25. Chelberg, M.K., G.M. Banks, D.F. Geiger, et al., *Identification of heterogeneous cell populations in normal human intervertebral disc*. J Anat, 1995. **186 (Pt 1)**: 43-53.
26. Edelson, J.G. and H. Nathan, *Stages in the natural history of the vertebral endplates*. Spine, 1988. **13**(1): 21-6.
27. Boos, N., S. Weissbach, H. Rohrbach, et al., *Classification of age-related changes in lumbar intervertebral discs: 2002 Volvo Award in basic science*. Spine, 2002. **27**(23): 2631-44.
28. Twomey, L. and J. Taylor, *Age changes in lumbar intervertebral discs*. Acta Orthop Scand, 1985. **56**(6): 496-9.
29. Slack, J.M., *Stem cells in epithelial tissues*. Science, 2000. **287**(5457): 1431-3.
30. Anderson, D.J., F.H. Gage, and I.L. Weissman, *Can stem cells cross lineage boundaries?* Nat Med, 2001. **7**(4): 393-5.
31. Goel, A., S.S. Sangwan, R.C. Siwach, et al., *Percutaneous bone marrow grafting for the treatment of tibial non-union*. Injury, 2005. **36**(1): 203-6.
32. Siwach, R.C., S.S. Sangwan, R. Singh, et al., *Role of percutaneous bone marrow grafting in delayed unions, non-unions and poor regenerates*. Indian J Med Sci, 2001. **55**(6): 326-36.

33. Borden, M., M. Attawia, Y. Khan, et al., *Tissue-engineered bone formation in vivo using a novel sintered polymeric microsphere matrix*. J Bone Joint Surg Br, 2004. **86**(8): 1200-8.
34. Wright, V., H. Peng, A. Usas, et al., *BMP4-expressing muscle-derived stem cells differentiate into osteogenic lineage and improve bone healing in immunocompetent mice*. Mol Ther, 2002. **6**(2): 169-78.
35. Peng, H., V. Wright, A. Usas, et al., *Synergistic enhancement of bone formation and healing by stem cell-expressed VEGF and bone morphogenetic protein-4*. J Clin Invest, 2002. **110**(6): 751-9.
36. Shapiro, F., S. Koide, and M.J. Glimcher, *Cell origin and differentiation in the repair of full-thickness defects of articular cartilage*. J Bone Joint Surg Am, 1993. **75**(4): 532-53.
37. Majumdar, M.K., E. Wang, and E.A. Morris, *BMP-2 and BMP-9 promotes chondrogenic differentiation of human multipotential mesenchymal cells and overcomes the inhibitory effect of IL-1*. J Cell Physiol, 2001. **189**(3): 275-84.
38. Tamai, N., A. Myoui, M. Hirao, et al., *A new biotechnology for articular cartilage repair: subchondral implantation of a composite of interconnected porous hydroxyapatite, synthetic polymer (PLA-PEG), and bone morphogenetic protein-2 (rhBMP-2)*. Osteoarthritis Cartilage, 2005. **13**(5): 405-17.
39. Qu-Petersen, Z., B. Deasy, R. Jankowski, et al., *Identification of a novel population of muscle stem cells in mice: potential for muscle regeneration*. J Cell Biol, 2002. **157**(5): 851-64.
40. Jankowski, R.J., B.M. Deasy, B. Cao, et al., *The role of CD34 expression and cellular fusion in the regeneration capacity of myogenic progenitor cells*. J Cell Sci, 2002. **115**(Pt 22): 4361-74.
41. Yamasaki, T., M. Deie, R. Shinomiya, et al., *Meniscal regeneration using tissue engineering with a scaffold derived from a rat meniscus and mesenchymal stromal cells derived from rat bone marrow*. J Biomed Mater Res A, 2005. **75**(1): 23-30.
42. Juncosa-Melvin, N., G.P. Boivin, C. Gooch, et al., *The effect of autologous mesenchymal stem cells on the biomechanics and histology of gel-collagen sponge constructs used for rabbit patellar tendon repair*. Tissue Eng, 2006. **12**(2): 369-79.
43. Ge, Z., J.C. Goh, and E.H. Lee, *The effects of bone marrow-derived mesenchymal stem cells and fascia wrap application to anterior cruciate ligament tissue engineering*. Cell Transplant, 2005. **14**(10): 763-73.
44. Sakai, D., J. Mochida, T. Iwashina, et al., *Differentiation of mesenchymal stem cells transplanted to a rabbit degenerative disc model: potential and limitations for stem cell therapy in disc regeneration*. Spine, 2005. **30**(21): 2379-87.
45. Hannallah, D., B. Peterson, J.R. Lieberman, et al., *Gene therapy in orthopaedic surgery*. Instr Course Lect, 2003. **52**: 753-68.
46. Robbins, P.D. and S.C. Ghivizzani, *Viral vectors for gene therapy*. Pharmacol Ther, 1998. **80**(1): 35-47.
47. Bonadio, J., E. Smiley, P. Patil, et al., *Localized, direct plasmid gene delivery in vivo: prolonged therapy results in reproducible tissue regeneration*. Nat Med, 1999. **5**(7): 753-9.
48. Baltzer, A.W., C. Lattermann, J.D. Whalen, et al., *Potential role of direct adenoviral gene transfer in enhancing fracture repair*. Clin Orthop Relat Res, 2000(379 Suppl): S120-5.
49. Baltzer, A.W., C. Lattermann, J.D. Whalen, et al., *Genetic enhancement of fracture repair: healing of an experimental segmental defect by adenoviral transfer of the BMP-2 gene*. Gene Ther, 2000. **7**(9): 734-9.
50. Baltzer, A.W., C. Lattermann, J.D. Whalen, et al., *A gene therapy approach to accelerating bone healing. Evaluation of gene expression in a New Zealand white rabbit model*. Knee Surg Sports Traumatol Arthrosc, 1999. **7**(3): 197-202.

51. Musgrave, D.S., P. Bosch, S. Ghivizzani, et al., *Adenovirus-mediated direct gene therapy with bone morphogenetic protein-2 produces bone*. Bone, 1999. **24**(6): 541-7.
52. Christ, M., M. Lusky, F. Stoeckel, et al., *Gene therapy with recombinant adenovirus vectors: evaluation of the host immune response*. Immunol Lett, 1997. **57**(1-3): 19-25.
53. Yang, Y., F.A. Nunes, K. Berencsi, et al., *Cellular immunity to viral antigens limits E1-deleted adenoviruses for gene therapy*. Proc Natl Acad Sci U S A, 1994. **91**(10): 4407-11.
54. Lieberman, J.R., A. Daluiski, S. Stevenson, et al., *The effect of regional gene therapy with bone morphogenetic protein-2-producing bone-marrow cells on the repair of segmental femoral defects in rats*. J Bone Joint Surg Am, 1999. **81**(7): 905-17.
55. Trippel, S.B., S.C. Ghivizzani, and A.J. Nixon, *Gene-based approaches for the repair of articular cartilage*. Gene Ther, 2004. **11**(4): 351-9.
56. Mi, Z., S.C. Ghivizzani, E.R. Lechman, et al., *Adenovirus-mediated gene transfer of insulin-like growth factor 1 stimulates proteoglycan synthesis in rabbit joints*. Arthritis Rheum, 2000. **43**(11): 2563-70.
57. Saxer, R.A., S.J. Bent, B.D. Brower-Toland, et al., *Gene mediated insulin-like growth factor-I delivery to the synovium*. J Orthop Res, 2001. **19**(5): 759-67.
58. Kang, R., T. Marui, S.C. Ghivizzani, et al., *Ex vivo gene transfer to chondrocytes in full-thickness articular cartilage defects: a feasibility study*. Osteoarthritis Cartilage, 1997. **5**(2): 139-43.
59. Ahrens, M., T. Ankenbauer, D. Schroder, et al., *Expression of human bone morphogenetic proteins-2 or -4 in murine mesenchymal progenitor C3H10T1/2 cells induces differentiation into distinct mesenchymal cell lineages*. DNA Cell Biol, 1993. **12**(10): 871-80.
60. Hildebrand, K.A., C.B. Frank, and D.A. Hart, *Gene intervention in ligament and tendon: current status, challenges, future directions*. Gene Ther, 2004. **11**(4): 368-78.
61. Lou, J., Y. Tu, M. Burns, et al., *BMP-12 gene transfer augmentation of lacerated tendon repair*. J Orthop Res, 2001. **19**(6): 1199-202.
62. Nakamura, N., S.A. Timmermann, D.A. Hart, et al., *A comparison of in vivo gene delivery methods for antisense therapy in ligament healing*. Gene Ther, 1998. **5**(11): 1455-61.
63. Nakamura, N., D.A. Hart, R.S. Boorman, et al., *Decorin antisense gene therapy improves functional healing of early rabbit ligament scar with enhanced collagen fibrillogenesis in vivo*. J Orthop Res, 2000. **18**(4): 517-23.
64. Hart, D.A., N. Nakamura, L. Marchuk, et al., *Complexity of determining cause and effect in vivo after antisense gene therapy*. Clin Orthop, 2000(379 Suppl): S242-51.
65. Yurchenco, P.D., *Assembly of basement membranes*. Ann N Y Acad Sci, 1990. **580**: 195-213.
66. Barton-Davis, E.R., D.I. Shoturma, A. Musaro, et al., *Viral mediated expression of insulin-like growth factor I blocks the aging-related loss of skeletal muscle function*. Proc Natl Acad Sci U S A, 1998. **95**(26): 15603-7.
67. Kochanek, S., P.R. Clemens, K. Mitani, et al., *A new adenoviral vector: Replacement of all viral coding sequences with 28 kb of DNA independently expressing both full-length dystrophin and beta-galactosidase*. Proc Natl Acad Sci U S A, 1996. **93**(12): 5731-6.
68. Chen, H.H., L.M. Mack, R. Kelly, et al., *Persistence in muscle of an adenoviral vector that lacks all viral genes*. Proc Natl Acad Sci U S A, 1997. **94**(5): 1645-50.
69. Harper, S.Q., M.A. Hauser, C. DelloRusso, et al., *Modular flexibility of dystrophin: implications for gene therapy of Duchenne muscular dystrophy*. Nat Med, 2002. **8**(3): 253-61.

70. Watchko, J., T. O'Day, B. Wang, et al., *Adeno-associated virus vector-mediated minidystrophin gene therapy improves dystrophic muscle contractile function in mdx mice*. Hum Gene Ther, 2002. **13**(12): 1451-60.
71. Crawford, G.E., J.A. Faulkner, R.H. Crosbie, et al., *Assembly of the dystrophin-associated protein complex does not require the dystrophin COOH-terminal domain*. J Cell Biol, 2000. **150**(6): 1399-410.
72. Tinsley, J., N. Deconinck, R. Fisher, et al., *Expression of full-length utrophin prevents muscular dystrophy in mdx mice*. Nat Med, 1998. **4**(12): 1441-4.
73. Martinek, V., A. Usas, D. Pelinkovic, et al., *Genetic engineering of meniscal allografts*. Tissue Eng, 2002. **8**(1): 107-17.
74. Nishida, K., J.D. Kang, L.G. Gilbertson, et al., *Modulation of the biologic activity of the rabbit intervertebral disc by gene therapy: an in vivo study of adenovirus-mediated transfer of the human transforming growth factor beta 1 encoding gene*. Spine, 1999. **24**(23): 2419-25.
75. Wallach, C.J., S. Sobajima, Y. Watanabe, et al., *Gene transfer of the catabolic inhibitor TIMP-1 increases measured proteoglycans in cells from degenerated human intervertebral discs*. Spine, 2003. **28**(20): 2331-7.
76. Uematsu, K., K. Hattori, Y. Ishimoto, et al., *Cartilage regeneration using mesenchymal stem cells and a three-dimensional poly-lactic-glycolic acid (PLGA) scaffold*. Biomaterials, 2005. **26**(20): 4273-9.
77. Hutmacher, D.W. and A.J. Garcia, *Scaffold-based bone engineering by using genetically modified cells*. Gene, 2005. **347**(1): 1-10.
78. Pountos, I., E. Jones, C. Tzioupis, et al., *Growing bone and cartilage. The role of mesenchymal stem cells*. J Bone Joint Surg Br, 2006. **88**(4): 421-6.
79. Johnstone, B., T.M. Hering, A.I. Caplan, et al., *In vitro chondrogenesis of bone marrow-derived mesenchymal progenitor cells*. Exp Cell Res, 1998. **238**(1): 265-72.
80. Kawamura, K., C.R. Chu, S. Sobajima, et al., *Adenoviral-mediated transfer of TGF-beta1 but not IGF-1 induces chondrogenic differentiation of human mesenchymal stem cells in pellet cultures*. Exp Hematol, 2005. **33**(8): 865-72.
81. Sgaglione, N.A., *Biologic approaches to articular cartilage surgery: future trends*. Orthop Clin North Am, 2005. **36**(4): 485-95.
82. Quarto, R., M. Mastrogiacomo, R. Cancedda, et al., *Repair of large bone defects with the use of autologous bone marrow stromal cells*. N Engl J Med, 2001. **344**(5): 385-6.
83. Behrens, P., T. Bitter, B. Kurz, et al., *Matrix-associated autologous chondrocyte transplantation/implantation (MACT/MACI)–5-year follow-up*. Knee, 2006. **13**(3): 194-202.
84. Giannoudis, P.V., H. Dinopoulos, and E. Tsiridis, *Bone substitutes: an update*. Injury, 2005. **36 Suppl 3**: S20-7.
85. Kawaguchi, H., T. Kurokawa, K. Hanada, et al., *Stimulation of fracture repair by recombinant human basic fibroblast growth factor in normal and streptozotocin-diabetic rats*. Endocrinology, 1994. **135**(2): 774-81.
86. Schmidmaier, G., B. Wildemann, D. Ostapowicz, et al., *Long-term effects of local growth factor (IGF-I and TGF-beta 1) treatment on fracture healing. A safety study for using growth factors*. J Orthop Res, 2004. **22**(3): 514-9.
87. Andreassen, T.T. and H. Oxlund, *Local anabolic effects of growth hormone on intact bone and healing fractures in rats*. Calcif Tissue Int, 2003. **73**(3): 258-64.
88. Urist, M.R., *Bone: formation by autoinduction*. Science, 1965. **150**(698): 893-9.
89. Yamamoto, M., Y. Takahashi, and Y. Tabata, *Enhanced bone regeneration at a segmental bone defect by controlled release of bone morphogenetic protein-2 from a biodegradable hydrogel*. Tissue Eng, 2006. **12**(5): 1305-11.
90. Egermann, M., A.W. Baltzer, S. Adamaszek, et al., *Direct adenoviral transfer of bone morphogenetic protein-2 cDNA enhances fracture healing in osteoporotic sheep*. Hum Gene Ther, 2006. **17**(5): 507-17.

91. Rundle, C.H., N. Miyakoshi, Y. Kasukawa, et al., *In vivo bone formation in fracture repair induced by direct retroviral-based gene therapy with bone morphogenetic protein-4*. Bone, 2003. **32**(6): 591-601.
92. Bergsma, E.J., F.R. Rozema, R.R. Bos, et al., *Foreign body reactions to resorbable poly(L-lactide) bone plates and screws used for the fixation of unstable zygomatic fractures*. J Oral Maxillofac Surg, 1993. **51**(6): 666-70.
93. Brittberg, M., A. Lindahl, A. Nilsson, et al., *Treatment of deep cartilage defects in the knee with autologous chondrocyte transplantation*. N Engl J Med, 1994. **331**(14): 889-95.
94. Hunter, C.J. and M.E. Levenston, *Maturation and integration of tissue-engineered cartilages within an in vitro defect repair model*. Tissue Eng, 2004. **10**(5-6): 736-46.
95. Kuo, C.K., W.J. Li, R.L. Mauck, et al., *Cartilage tissue engineering: its potential and uses*. Curr Opin Rheumatol, 2006. **18**(1): 64-73.
96. Elisseeff, J., C. Puleo, F. Yang, et al., *Advances in skeletal tissue engineering with hydrogels*. Orthod Craniofac Res, 2005. **8**(3): 150-61.
97. Zhang, X., Z. Mao, and C. Yu, *Suppression of early experimental osteoarthritis by gene transfer of interleukin-1 receptor antagonist and interleukin-10*. J Orthop Res, 2004. **22**(4): 742-50.
98. Darling, E.M. and K.A. Athanasiou, *Articular cartilage bioreactors and bioprocesses*. Tissue Eng, 2003. **9**(1): 9-26.
99. Buma, P., N.N. Ramrattan, T.G. van Tienen, et al., *Tissue engineering of the meniscus*. Biomaterials, 2004. **25**(9): 1523-32.
100. Chiari, C., U. Koller, R. Dorotka, et al., *A tissue engineering approach to meniscus regeneration in a sheep model*. Osteoarthritis Cartilage, 2006.
101. Kang, S.W., S.M. Son, J.S. Lee, et al., *Regeneration of whole meniscus using meniscal cells and polymer scaffolds in a rabbit total meniscectomy model*. J Biomed Mater Res A, 2006. **77**(4): 659-71.
102. Pangborn, C.A. and K.A. Athanasiou, *Effects of growth factors on meniscal fibrochondrocytes*. Tissue Eng, 2005. **11**(7-8): 1141-8.
103. Hildebrand, K.A., S.L. Woo, D.W. Smith, et al., *The effects of platelet-derived growth factor-BB on healing of the rabbit medial collateral ligament. An in vivo study*. Am J Sports Med, 1998. **26**(4): 549-54.
104. Lynch, S.E., G.R. de Castilla, R.C. Williams, et al., *The effects of short-term application of a combination of platelet-derived and insulin-like growth factors on periodontal wound healing*. J Periodontol, 1991. **62**(7): 458-67.
105. Nakamura, N., K. Shino, T. Natsuume, et al., *Early biological effect of in vivo gene transfer of platelet-derived growth factor (PDGF)-B into healing patellar ligament*. Gene Ther, 1998. **5**(9): 1165-70.
106. Mizuno, H., A.K. Roy, C.A. Vacanti, et al., *Tissue-engineered composites of anulus fibrosus and nucleus pulposus for intervertebral disc replacement*. Spine, 2004. **29**(12): 1290-7; discussion 1297-8.
107. Mwale, F., M. Iordanova, C.N. Demers, et al., *Biological evaluation of chitosan salts cross-linked to genipin as a cell scaffold for disk tissue engineering*. Tissue Eng, 2005. **11**(1-2): 130-40.
108. Yang, S.H., P.Q. Chen, Y.F. Chen, et al., *An in-vitro study on regeneration of human nucleus pulposus by using gelatin/chondroitin-6-sulfate/hyaluronan tri-copolymer scaffold*. Artif Organs, 2005. **29**(10): 806-14.
109. Evans, C., *Potential biologic therapies for the intervertebral disc*. J Bone Joint Surg Am, 2006. **88 Suppl 2**: 95-8.
110. Le Maitre, C.L., A.J. Freemont, and J.A. Hoyland, *A preliminary in vitro study into the use of IL-1Ra gene therapy for the inhibition of intervertebral disc degeneration*. Int J Exp Pathol, 2006. **87**(1): 17-28.

3

Overview of Fracture Repair

Bruce Doll[1], Matthew Aleef[2], and Jeffrey O. Hollinger[3]

Abstract: Migration, adhesion, proliferation and differentiation of mesenchymal stem cells into osteoblasts, osteoclasts, chondroblasts, fibroblasts and endothelial cells characterize the cellular activities suspended within a collagenous matrix during fracture repair. Throughout life fracture repair is a dynamic process – orchestrated events directing the inflammatory response, chondrogenesis, osteogenesis and remodeling. These steps may involve many differently expressed genes. Fracture healing is also closely aligned with neo-angiogenesis. Matrix degradation and angiogenesis are concurrent processes supportive of endochondral bone formation. This chapter will focus on the biological hierarchy of bone and its capacity for repair. The cell and molecular biology of fracture repair will be considered as a context for proposed therapies for bone regeneration.

Keywords: fracture, bone, repair, skeletal injury, osteoblast, osteogenesis, healing

3.1. Fracture Wound Healing

Considerable information is available in the literature on bone morphogenesis, growth, remodeling and repair [1-3]. A review of all aspects of bone dynamics exceeds the intent of this chapter. However, understanding fracture healing is presented in the context of the events culminating in the creation, maintenance and responsiveness of osseous tissue to fracture. Successful fracture repair requires a coordinated and complex transcriptional program that integrates mechanical stimulus, signaling, angiogenesis and osteogenesis. However, the interdependence of these processes is not fully understood. Fracture healing entails an environment characterized by a supportive scaffold within and upon which pluripotent stem cells undergo proliferation and differentiation. Repair

[1]University of Pittsburgh, Pittsburgh, PA
[2]University of Pittsburgh Medical Center, Pittsburgh, PA
[3]Bone Tissue Engineering Center, Carnegie Mellon University, Pittsburgh, PA

From: *Orthopedic Biology and Medicine: Musculoskeletal Tissue Regeneration, Biological Materials and Methods*
Edited by W. S. Pietrzak © Humana Press, Totowa, NJ

activities depend upon the temporal and spatial distribution of appropriate osteogenic molecules, including extracellular matrix proteins. Given the enormous biomedical burden of skeletal injury, and the need to treat congenital, posttraumatic and postsurgical conditions in which bone regeneration is unsuccessful, understanding osteogenesis for skeletal repair has important clinical implications.

When bone is fractured cells and the cell mediators, in the form of extracellular signals (mechanical and chemical), collectively ensure the restoration of form and function. Fracture healing is a complex physiological process which involves the coordination of several different cell types. Cell activities bear partial resemblance to the molecular cascade characterizing natal bone formation. Elucidating the orchestrated events and the concurrent activation of osteogenesis and chondrogenesis that recapitulates mammalian embryological skeletal development is both complex and challenging. To this end, the chapter will focus upon the cell and molecular components of fracture healing.

3.1.1. Cellular Community

Within the osseous microstructure hierarchy of fracture repair, predominant members of the community include osteoblasts, osteoclasts and osteocytes. Chondroblasts and endothelial cells contribute a supporting roll to the mineralization process. The osteogenic cell community is supported by bone lining cells and an endothelial component. Each community has specific, interactive functions in bone physiological processes. Viability of these soteogenic cells depends upon a directed angiogenic response concurrent with the reparative mineralization activities of cells suspended in a collagenous matrix.

3.1.1.1. Osteoblasts

Osteoblasts arise from pluripotent mesenchymal progenitor cells that can also develop into adipocytes, myocytes and chondrocytes [4, 5]. Once the pluripotent progenitor cells have committed to the osteoblastic lineage they progress through several developmental stages of differentiation, proliferation, matrix maturation and mineralization. Proliferation of the pro-osteoblasts is primarily regulated by cell cycle-related genes, such as *c-fos, c-myc*, and *Ets-1*. Differentiation to the osteoblastic lineage appears more complex, involving at least three separate sets of genes concurrently expressed during this process: (a) the matrix-associated genes like Coll type I, fibronectin and osteonectin; (b) the osteoblast-specific genes, alkaline phosphatase (ALP) and osteopontin, and (c) transcription factors such as *Ets-2, Cbfα1/Runx2* (also implicated in tissue specific regulation of VEGF expression during the bone remodelling phase), *Dlx5*, and *osterix* [6, 7]. During the final stage osteoblast differentiation is characterized by expression of genes involved in matrix maturation and mineralization like collagen Type I, fibronectin, osteonectin, ALP, osteocalcin (OC), bone sialoproteins (BSP) and osteopontin (OPN) [8, 9].

Osteoblasts form bone. Mature osteoblastic cells are highly secretory. Type I collagen is the main secretory product, however; osteoblasts secrete other non-collagenous proteins including OP, OPN and BSP. Osteoblasts form bone by facilitating mineralization via probable concurrent pathways that are matrix dependent and matrix independent [10]. In any case osteoblasts are critically important in mineralization because they both secrete collagen and produce matrix vesicles.

3.1.1.2. Osteoclasts

The mature osteoclast is multinucleate, containing six to eight nuclei typically, but it can have many more. The cross sectional diameter varies from around 20 to several hundred microns. When actively resorbing bone an osteoclast appears flattened against the bone surface, or it may be highly contorted as it seals itself over the end of a spicule. Either scenario involves the establishment of tight contact along the peripheral cell margin with the bone to enable the highly acidic process of demineralization during repair and remodeling. The ruffled border is the most obvious organelle belying the cell's function. Adherence of osteoclasts to bone surfaces involves the interaction of membrane-associated $\alpha_v\beta_3$ integrin in clear zone membrane with OPN in exposed bone matrix surfaces. The ruffled border provides an extensive surface area of specialized plasma membrane through which acid is secreted and hydrolytic enzymes are released [11, 12]. Osteoclasts are phagocytic and bits of resorbed bone appear to be internalized.

Multinucleate osteoclasts are derived from fusion of migrating hemopoietic cells of the monocyte-macrophage lineage. The process requires orientation and contact with osteoblasts or stromal cells in the marrow (pre-osteoblasts) [13]. Osteoclasts are derived from myeloid lineage cells, and their differentiation is supported by various osteotropic factors, including the tumor necrosis factor (TNF) family member TNF-related activation-induced cytokine (TRANCE). Osteotropic factors, including PTH, PGE_2, 1,25$(OH)_2$ vitamin D_3 and IL-11, harmonize osteoclast formation through specific receptors on osteoblasts and stromal cells [14, 15].

Osteoclastogenesis requires cell-cell contact and signaling by osteotrophic factor(s) through specific receptors on osteoblasts and/or stromal cells, namely, the RANK-RANKL interaction. Current evidence indicates that RANK (on pre-osteoclasts) acts as the sole signaling receptor for RANKL (on osteoblasts), thereby inducing differentiation of pre-osteoclasts to fuse and develop into osteoclasts. The binding of cross-linking antibodies to the extracellular domain of RANK caused cell surface clustering of RANK, bypassing the need to interact with RANKL; a spleen culture model osteoclast formation was stimulated [16]. On the other hand, when Fab fragments of anti-RANK antibody were introduced, clustering was prevented. RANK-RANKL interaction was blocked. Osteoclasts did not develop. Subsequently it was found that soluble RANK, the extracellular domain of RANK, now called osteoprotegerin (OPG), also blocked osteoclast formation. RANKL/RANK/TRAF6 also signals through c-Src [17]. Targeted disruption of the c-Src gene causes osteopetrosis. Osteoclasts were shown to be present in c-Src -/- mice, but ruffled borders were absent [18-20]. However, hemotpoietic precursors from TRANCE-, RANK- or TRAF6-null mice can differentiate into osteoclasts, suggesting an alternative pathway for osteoclastogenesis, independent of TRANCE-,RANK- and TRAF6 –null mice (Fig. 3.3) [21].

3.1.1.3. Osteocytes

Within mature bone osteocytes are the most numerous cells and can display longevity matching the host. Due to the remote location of the cell in the mineralized matrix, isolation of the cells and preservation of their phenotype is difficult. Osteocytes are derived from osteoprogenitors, a fraction of which differentiate into active osteoblasts and subsequently are encased in osteoid. Osteoblasts synthesize osteoid, unmineralized bone matrix composed of collagen and other organic components. A fraction of the active osteoblasts become incorporated within the newly laid down matrix [22-25]. New osteocytes maintain direct contact with the overlying bone lining cells and osteoblasts, as well as with previous generations of osteocytes through cell processes that are created before and during matrix synthesis. The extended osteocytic network, comprised of cells interconnected by multiple cell processes and joined at gap junctions, forms a functional syncytium [26]. Transmission of mechanical signals to the osteocyte cytoskeleton via cell surface receptors can occur directly through the solid matrix structure of the tissue, as well as indirectly via fluid pressure and shear stresses imparted by fluid moving through the lacunocanalicular system due to load-induced fluid flow.

Bone is subjected to a dynamic environment in which functional adaptation is necessary for survival of the tissue and, ultimately, of the organism. Bone tissue health depends on the ability of bone cells to recognize and respond to mechanical and chemical stimuli, a process referred to as mechano-chemical transduction [27]. Remodeling activity, coordinated between osteocytes, osteoclasts and osteoblasts, provides a basis for adaptation. Osteocytes, the most abundant cells in bone, are actively involved in maintaining the bony matrix, and osteocyte death is eventually followed by matrix resorption. In addition, osteocytes are thought to be mechanosensors. Translation of mechanical signals at the cellular level may further involve triggering of integrin force receptors and/or changes in the conformation of membrane bound proteins that affect membrane fluidity and trafficking. Furthermore, chemical signals, modulated through diffusive, convective and active transport mechanisms, are transported intracellularly as well as through the extracellular fluid in which the cells are immersed. The lacunocanalicular system provides a facilitatory environment for transfer of exogenous and endogenous signals via mechanical, electrical and chemical mechanisms [26]. The cell signaling pathways leading to release of secondary messengers, transcription factors and finally gene expression are not yet fully elucidated.

3.2. Angiogenesis

The process of new blood vessel formation at the fracture is known as angiogenesis. It is a critical component of bone development and postnatal fracture repair, yet the progression of signals that couple osteogenic and angiogenic processes after bone injury remain to be elucidated. Bone fracture disrupts circulation, leading to acute necrosis and hypoxia of adjacent bone and marrow. However, these cell communities usually exhibit a favorable, orderly response to injury and ensure complete restoration of mechanical properties.

Early work by Rhinelander on fracture healing demonstrated an enhanced endosteal circulation subsequent to bone fracture [28]. Fracture repair involves a cascade of events. Following hemorrhage and release of thrombotic factors, tissue breakdown contributes mediators that modulate the migration of blood cells and mesenchymal cells. Blood supply and stability are two key elements that ensure the timely and accurate reconstitution of bone tissue. A cell mediated process of bone remodeling underlies the regenerative capacity of bone.

The study of bone induction in distraction osteogenesis has prompted the investigation of angiogenesis' role in bone regeneration. Using a distraction osteogenesis model, Fang administered TNP-470, a synthetic analog of fumagillin to rats. TNP 470 has been shown to block new capillary formation *in vivo* and inhibit endothelial cell proliferation *in vitro* [29-32]. They established that that both angiogenesis and a controlled mechanical environment were necessary for bone induction to occur during distraction. Furthermore, proper mechanical signaling may be a prerequisite for angiogenic and osteogenic programs to allow successful osteogenesis to occur [33].

3.2.1. Matrix Compositions

Bone is able to sense and respond to mechanical signals. Bone and cartilage cells exist in a complex biomechanical environment influenced by considerations of mechanical strain relative to the nature of the extracellular matrix. However, the mechanisms by which strain induces cellular behavior are only partly understood. Matrix deformation and interstitial fluid flow are the two most likely mechanisms by which mechanical loads are transduced to bone cells *in vivo*. Deformation of the matrix has the potential to induce cellular deformation leading to piezoelectric effects [34].

The rate and quality of the formation of extracellular matrix can be regulated by the application of mechanical strains of varying amplitudes and frequencies, and strain magnitude, frequency and size of fracture gap are determinants of fracture healing. Applied strains <5 percent and small hydrostatic pressures <0.5 MPa have been shown to stimulate intramembranous bone formation. Strains of 5 percent to 15 percent, and hydrostatic pressures >0.15 MPa stimulated endochondral bone formation, whereas strain magnitudes >15 percent resulted in the synthesis of fibrous tissue [35]. Two putative stretch activated channels have been identified in bone cells. Additionally, *in vitro* studies suggest that matrix deformation activates these channels.

Matrix deformation also induces endogenous electric fields. When bone is functionally loaded, electric currents are generated as a result of the piezoelectric properties of collagen [36]. Furthermore, relatively large electrokinetic currents, known as streaming potentials, are produced by the boundary interaction effects of charged constituents of fluids passing the mineral phase of the extracellular matrix in response to strain in the bone tissue [37]. Both *in vivo* and *in vitro* studies suggest that electric fields increase bone cell activity. Skeletal tissues respond to the physical demands of their environment by altering the synthesis and organization of the extracellular matrix. Physical environmental stimuli and manipulation result in physical environment stimulation contributing to fracture repair.

3.2.2. Phases of Wound Healing

Bone fracture healing occurs in a sequential progression of overlapping processes and requires the coordinated contributions of a variety of cellular activities. Tissue injury initiates the progression of bleeding, coagulation, inflammation, angiogenesis, repair and finally, remodeling of the damaged bone.

The manner of wound repair depends upon the mechanical stability of the fracture. Stabilizing a fracture with rigid internal fixation leads to primary bone healing. This process proceeds at a rigidly stable fracture site with the fracture surfaces held in contact. In contrast, unstable fractures undergo secondary fracture healing due to the presence of motion.

Primary bone healing involves a direct attempt by the cortex to reestablish itself. In these circumstances, when the fracture surfaces are rigidly held in contact, fracture healing can occur without a grossly visible callus. Primary bone healing is driven by remodeling osteoclasts and osteoblasts bridging the fracture gap and rejoining the fracture fragments [38]. This process seems to occur exclusively when there is anatomic restoration of the fracture fragments, by rigid internal fixation, and when the stability of fracture reduction is ensured by a substantial decrease in interfragmentary strain [39]. Fracture border apposition varies between direct contact and gaps along the fracture line. Where there is contact between bone ends, lamellar bone can form directly across the fracture line by extension of osteons. A cluster of osteoclasts cuts across the fracture line, osteoblasts following the osteoclasts then deposit new bone, and blood vessels follow the osteoblasts, configured as a cutting cone. New haversian systems are formed by the new bone matrix, enclosed osteocytes and blood vessels. Where gaps that prevent direct extension of osteons across the fracture site exist, osteoblasts fill the defects with woven bone. After the gap fills with woven bone, haversian remodeling begins reestablishing normal cortical bone structure. Discrete remodeling units called cutting cones, consisting of osteoclasts followed by osteoblasts and blood vessels, traverse the woven bone in the fracture gap. They deposit lamellar bone and reestablish the cortical bone blood supply across the fracture site without grossly visible fracture callus [39].

Most fractures worldwide are either not treated or are treated with a form of management that results in some degree of motion, such as cast immobilization, sling immobilization, external fixation or intramedullary fixation. Thus, primary fracture healing is rare and the majority of fractures heal via secondary fracture healing that involves the combination of intramembranous and endochondral ossification. When tissue damage takes place there is inevitably disruption of blood vessels in the bone, marrow, periosteum and surrounding tissue. This microvascular injury results in the extravasation of blood at the fracture site and formation of a hematoma. Vasoconstriction follows and the coagulation cascade is triggered to prevent further blood loss. Fibrin, the end product of both the intrinsic and extrinsic coagulation pathways, is the major component of the hematoma. The hematoma, mainly consisting of fibrin and fibronectin, is essential to wound healing as it provides a matrix into which cells then migrate. Evidence suggests that when the hematoma traps platelets, blood-borne cells and plasma proteins it provides a source of signaling molecules that have the capacity to initiate the pattern of cellular events that are critical to fracture healing [40]. Experimental work indicates that loss of the hematoma impairs or slows fracture healing [41]. This data suggests that the hematoma and an intact surrounding periosteal soft tissue envelope that contains the hematoma may facilitate the initial stages of wound healing. Platelets and inflammatory cells within the hematoma may release growth factors and cytokines such as Interleukin-1 and Interleukin-6. These growth factors and cytokines may be important in regulating early events in the fracture healing process, such as cell migration, proliferation and synthesis of the repair tissue matrix [42-45]. Platelets both contribute to coagulation and hemostasis, as well as to the inflammatory response. Degranulating platelets in the clot may release alpha granules that contain transforming growth factor beta (TGF-β) and platelet-derived growth factor (PDGF) that are important in regulating angiogenesis, chemotaxis, proliferation and differentiation of committed mesenchymal stem cells. Platelets also contain dense bodies that contain vasoactive amines with the capacity to enhance microvascular permeability [40].

Following coagulation and hematoma formation an inflammatory phase commences with the activation of complement and the initiation of the classical molecular cascade. This cascade leads to the infiltration of the wound with granulocytes approximately 24 to 48 hours after injury. Granulocytes are attracted by several chemotactic agents including complement component C5a, clotting factors, immunoglobulin G fragments and several cytokines that include TGF-β, PDGF and leukotriene B4. The granulocytes adhere to endothelial cells in the adjacent blood vessels via margination and actively move through the vessel wall via diapedesis. These inflammatory cells remove bacteria and foreign debris from the wound. Eventually macrophages become the primary producer of growth factors which govern the proliferation of extracellular matrix by fibroblasts, and proliferation of endothelial cells resulting in angiogenesis.

Eventually vascular proliferation occurs in the region of the fracture. Fibroblastic growth factors may be important mediators of angiogenesis in fracture healing [46]. Due to the initial destruction of the bone blood vessels, the bone ends are deprived of their blood supply and they become necrotic and reabsorbed as far as the junction of collaterals. The cells responsible for this function, the osteoclasts, come from a different cell line than the cells responsible for bone formation [47, 48]. Osteoclasts are derived from circulating monocytes in the blood and monocytic precursor cells from the bone marrow, whereas the osteoblasts develop from the undifferentiated mesenchymal cells that migrate into the fracture site.

Pluripotential mesenchymal cells, probably of common origin, form the fibrous tissue, cartilage and, eventually, bone at the fracture site. Some of these cells originate in the injured tissues, while others migrate to the injury site with the blood vessels. Cells from the cambium layer of the periosteum form the earliest bone. Due to the thicker and greater cellularity in children, periosteal cells have an especially prominent role in healing their fractures. With increasing age, the periosteum becomes thinner and contributes less to fracture healing. Osteoblasts from the endosteal surface also participate in bone formation, but surviving osteocytes do not appear to form repair tissue. The majority of cells responsible for osteogenesis during fracture healing appear in the fracture site with the granulation tissue that replaces the hematoma [47].

The mesenchymal cells at the fracture site proliferate, differentiate and produce the fracture callus consisting of bone, cartilage and fibrous tissue. Fibroblasts migrate into the wound after being stimulated by growth factors and then begin synthesizing collagen. Collagen synthesis begins with creation of procollagen alpha chains on membrane-bound ribosomes. Type I collagen, the major structural component of bones, consists of two alpha-1 chains and one alpha-2 chain, which then combine to form a triple helical molecule. Hydroxylation of proline and lysine amino acids contributes to the formation of this triple helix and only this triple helix may be exported from the cell. Disulfide bond cross-linking also occurs intracellularly. The entire procollagen is then packaged within secretory vesicles and transported to the cell surface where the procollagen is then cleaved into collagen at the cell membrane. This cleaving, which is performed by procollagen -C and -N peptidases, allows the release of collagen into the wound [49].

The fracture callus fills and surrounds the fracture site and, in the early stages of healing, can be divided into the hard callus and the soft callus. The bone formed initially at the periphery of the callus by intramembranous bone formation is the hard callus. The soft callus forms in the central regions with low oxygen tension and consists primarily of cartilage and fibrous tissue. Bone gradually replaces the cartilage through the process of endochondral ossification, enlarging the hard callus and increasing the stability of the fracture fragments. Calcification of fracture callus cartilage occurs via a mechanism almost identical to that in the growth plate. By nine days after the fracture there are many elongated, proliferating chondrocytes. Two weeks post-fracture, cell division declines and hypertrophic chondrocytes predominate. When observing these hypertrophic chondrocytes under electron microscopy, vesicularized bodies bud from the cell membranes. These bodies, known as matrix vesicles, travel to the extracellular matrix where they contribute in regulation of calcification. Investigations have shown that mitochondria within these cells store and release calcium for transport by matrix vesicles [50]. In addition, it has been demonstrated that matrix vesicles have the enzyme complement needed for proteolytic degradation of the matrix, which is a vital step in preparing the callus for calcification [51]. Matrix vesicles also possess phosphatases that are required to break down matrix phosphodiesters in order to release phosphate ions for precipitation with calcium. This process of calcification continues until new bone bridges the fracture site, re-establishing continuity between the cortical bone ends.

Analysis of fracture repair demonstrates a close correlation between the activation of genes for blood vessel, cartilage and bone-specific proteins in the cells, and the development of granulation tissue, cartilage and bone [52]. Thus, fracture repair is correlated with gene expression in the repair cells.

3.2.2.1. Gene Expression During Fracture Repair

The concurrent occurrence of chondrogenesis, endochondral ossification and intramembranous bone formation in different regions of the fracture callus indicates that local mediators and variations in the microenvironment determine what genes will be expressed and the type of tissue the repair cells form. Such local mediators include growth factors released from cells and platelets, acidic fibroblast growth factor, basic fibroblast growth factor and TGF-β may stimulate chondrocyte proliferation, cartilage formation, osteoblast proliferation and bone synthesis. In addition, TGF-β released from platelets immediately after injury may initiate the formation of the fracture callus and contribute to cartilage hypertrophy and calcification at the endochondral ossification front [52].

A number of hormones influence fracture healing. People with fractures have been shown to have lower serum levels of parathyroid hormone and calcitonin [53]. Parathyroid hormone may be systemically administered to enhance fracture healing by increasing bone mineral content, density and strength. In addition, it creates a lasting anabolic effect throughout the duration of fracture healing [54]. Calcitonin administration to fracture patients may provide benefit as well. It has been demonstrated that patients who receive calcitonin during fracture healing experience a benefit through the prevention of bone resorption [55]. The impact of growth hormone in fracture healing remains in doubt. Studies have suggested that deficiency in growth hormone adversely impacts fracture repair and that replacement of growth hormone may enhance healing [56, 57]. However, other research has shown that excess growth hormone may have little to no effect on fracture healing. In addition, the regular variation in the level of circulating growth hormone has little effect on fracture healing [58, 59]. Corticosteroids have been shown to impact fracture healing. Investigations have shown that corticosteroids may compromise fracture healing by possibly inhibiting differentiation of osteoblasts from mesenchymal cells [60]. Corticosteroids may also diminish the synthesis of bone organic matrix components [61]. Finally, extended corticosteroid exposure may decrease bone density and increase the likelihood of hip, distal radius, rib and vertebral fractures [62]. Insulin, anabolic steroids and thyroid hormone have also been described to improve the rate of fracture healing [63, 64].

As mineralization of fracture callus proceeds, the bone ends gradually become enveloped in a fusiform mass of callus containing increasing amounts of woven bone. The increasing mineral content is closely associated with increasing stiffness of the fracture callus [65]. Stability of the fracture fragments increase because of the internal and external callus formation, and eventually clinical union (where the fracture site is stable and pain free) occurs. Radiographic union occurs when plain radiographs show bone trabeculae or cortical bone crossing the fracture site, and often occurs later than clinical union. However, even at this stage healing is not complete. The immature fracture callus is weaker than normal bone, and it only gains full strength during remodeling.

3.2.3. Modeling and Remodeling

Modeling and remodeling processes have similarities and differences. Before we describe these processes and their individual elements, some fundamental definitions must be addressed.

Modeling is the process that shapes growing bones: " … modeling … alter(s) both the size and architecture [66, 67]." Remodeling maintains shape and patches blemishes in the adult skeleton, while responding to homeostatic demands to ensure calcium and phosphate balance. " … (R)emodeling … (is) replacement of older by newer tissue in a way that need not alter its gross architecture or size ….[66, 67]." Frost stated [66, 67]: "Growth determines size. Modeling molds the growing shape. Remodeling then maintains functional competence."

Appendicular bones grow in length and width. Physeal growth centers permit elongation, whereas the periosteal surface moves centrifugally, powered by osteoblastic deposition. Concurrently, endosteal growth proceeds centripetally, and osteoclastic activity slowly enlarges the zone of bone marrow. Appendicular bone growth maintains gross morphology.

The axial and craniofacial skeletons do not possess physeal growth centers. Therefore, bone growth for the vertebral bodies in the axial skeleton proceeds periosteally and includes an endosteal deposition-resorption component. The term "drifts" [66-69] emphasizes the waves of osteoblastic formation and osteoclastic resorption that move and mold bone.

Maintenance of bone shape and size in the adult skeleton is accomplished by the process of remodeling. Damaged bone (e.g., through micro-fracture or as a consequence of gross fracture) is removed, sculpted and replaced by osteoclasts and osteoblasts. [66, 67, 70].

Frost [66, 67] and Kimmel [71] describe macromodeling and mini modeling in the adult skeleton. Macromodeling increases the ability of bone to resist bending (by expanding periosteal and endosteal cortices), and mini modeling rearranges trabeculae to best adapt to functional demands.

When existing bone that becomes damaged and incurs micro-fractures is replaced with an equivalent amount of bone, the outcome is an identical-appearing bone that has been neither altered in size nor shape [72]. Frost defines this process (with some modification by the authors) as: "Remodeling maintains functional (competence of bone) [67] ... and ... serves the needs of replacement, maintenance and homeostasis [66]."

3.2.3.1. Micro-fracture Remodeling

Micro-fracture remodeling of damaged bone differs from fracture remodeling. Micro-fracture remodeling proceeds by a discrete and leisurely tempo of formation-resorption waves. Fracture remodeling is initiated as a consequence of an overwhelming biomechanical challenge that fractures bone. Fracture remodeling is an acute response crescendoing to restore form and function. The intensity of fracture healing is typified by inrushing peletons of cells and molecular signals squeezed in packets of time and called Regional area phenomenon (RAP). RAP has been eloquently described and reviewed by Frost [67]. We will come back to RAP and fracture remodeling later in the chapter.

The outcome from remodeling is the sculpting of existing and healing bone shape, either increasing or decreasing bulk, redirecting trabecular struts, patching blemishes, and either resorbing bone as a consequence of homeostatic demands or the need to restore form and function to bone that has fractured. Homeostatic demands are physiological and the activating signal can be humoral (e.g., parathyroid hormone: PTH). As a consequence of fracture, local biomechanical and molecular signals initiate and sustain the remodeling process.

Signals are received by osteoblasts. If there is a physiological requirement for increased levels of calcium, the humoral signal, parathyroid hormone (PTH) causes the osteoblast to leave the bone surface and, in the process, secrete an osteoclast cue [73].

The osteoclast binds to the bone by integrin-like binding, resorbs a volume of bone (~ 5 μm/day [74]), ceases activity and detaches. Osteoblasts may reattach to the bone at an osteopontin-rich cement line and deposit an osteoid matrix that calcifies. Osteoid is produced at a rate of ~1-2 μm per day and after about 20 μm are deposited (around 10 days), the osteoid mineralizes at ~1-2 μm per day [75].

3.2.3.2. Activation-Resorption-Formation

Remodeling (emphasis non-fracture remodeling) is divided into Activation-Resorption-Formation (ARF) [76]. Osteoblasts are activated; they move from the bone surface. Osteoclasts attach to the bone surface and resorb that surface. Following resorption the osteoclasts move away and are replaced by osteoblasts that deposit bone. While some of the cues that turn on and off functional activity of the cells have been elucidated, many more must be discovered.

Cell phenotypes, also referred to as cell packet [77], that are responsible for remodeling are known as the basic multicellular unit (BMU) and the temporal duration (i.e., life span) of a BMU is called sigma (Fig. 3.1) [74].

Remodeling results in ~25 percent of trabecular bone and about 3 percent of cortical bone to be removed and replaced each year (reviewed [78]). As a consequence of osteoporosis, the balance between osteoblastic formation and osteoclastic resorption becomes asynchronous: bone loss occurs and results in the clinical disease osteoporosis [79].

The duration of an active BMU (i.e., sigma) in cancellous and cortical bone is around two to eight months [78]. Sigma can be prolonged from two to 10 years in diseases such as osteoporosis and osteomalacia (reviewed [67]).

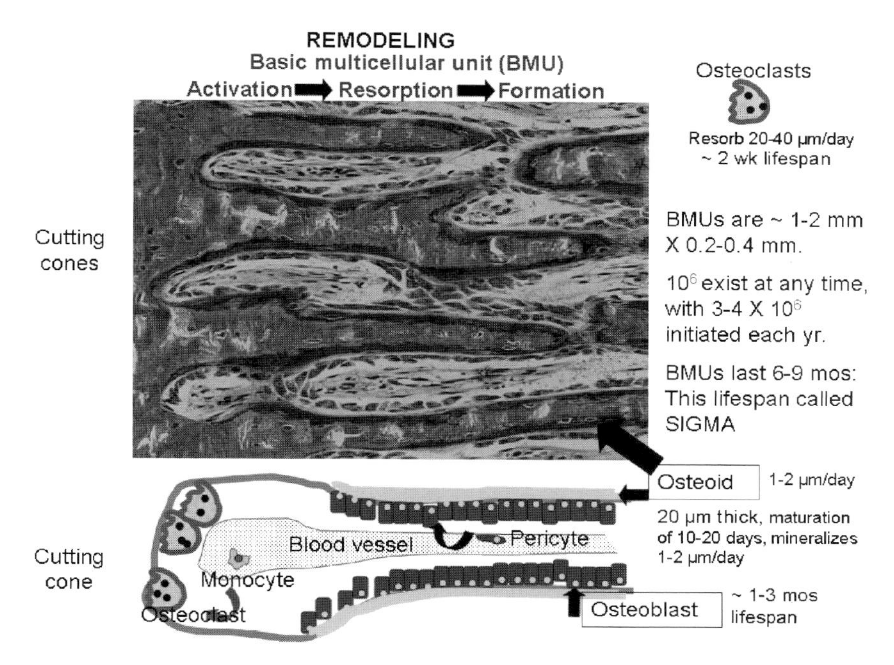

Fig. 3.1 *Remodeling: The Basic Multicellular unit (BMU) and Cutting Cones*: The cell phenotypes responsible for the BMU are responsible for remodeling and are known as the basic multicellular unit (BMU), and the temporal duration (i.e., life span) of a BMU is called sigma

The duration of an active BMU (i.e., sigma) in cancellous and cortical bone is around two to eight months. Sigma can be prolonged from two to 10 years in diseases such as osteoporosis and osteomalacia

The cutting cone is the hallmark of BMU cortical remodeling. It is approximately 2 mm in length, 0.2 mm wide, moves at a rate of about 20-40 μm/day, for a distance of 2-6 mm, and for a duration of two to eight months (sigma). Osteoclasts are in the front of the cutting cone, followed by osteoblasts **(With permission from S. Lynch, D.M.D., D.Sc.)**

The process of remodeling for trabecular (cancellous) and cortical bone is slightly different. Trabecular bone is trenched out by a BMU and cortical bone is burrowed out and the remnant is the cutting cone, which is eventually repaired with new bone.

The cutting cone is the hallmark of BMU cortical remodeling: approximately 2 mm in length, 0.2 mm wide, moving at a rate of about 20-40 μm/day, for a distance of 2-6 mm, and for a duration of two to eight months (sigma) [66-67, 78, 80-81]. Osteoclasts are in the front of the cutting cone, followed by osteoblasts. Osteoblasts have a life span of weeks to about three months. The center of each cutting cone includes a blood vessel, providing transit for monocytic precursors and pluripotential cells (e.g., pericytes) that can differentiate to osteoclast and osteoblast phenotypes, respectively (Fig. 3.2).

Bone remodeling may occur in an accelerated manner termed Regional Accelerated Phenomenon (RAP) [66]. A fracture healing site, a bone graft bed, may be considered a place where a RAP will occur. Remodeling in such a zone, according to Frost, may be 50 times the pace associated with homeostatic

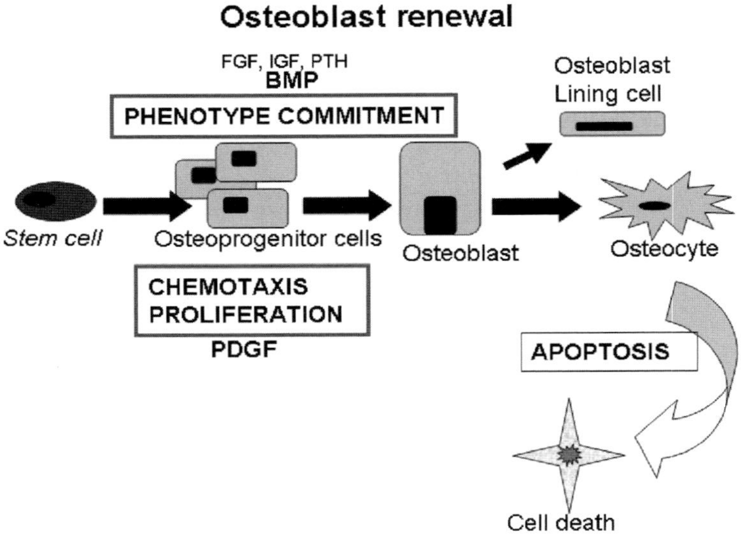

Osteoblast renewal

FGF, IGF, PTH
BMP
PHENOTYPE COMMITMENT
Osteoblast
Lining cell
Stem cell
Osteoprogenitor cells
Osteoblast
Osteocyte
CHEMOTAXIS
PROLIFERATION
PDGF
APOPTOSIS
Cell death

Fig. 3.2 *Osteoblast Renewal*: Osteoblasts have a life expectancy of about one to three months. Their renewal is crucial to maintain bone mass and replace bone resorbed by osteoclasts during remodeling and skeletal homeostasis. A cooperative interaction among growth factors such as the platelet-derived growth factor (PDGF) and bone morphogenetic proteins (BMP) ensures the continuous replenishment of osteoblasts. The process involves chemotaxis and mitogenesis of osteoblast progenitor cells by PDGF, followed by differentiation to osteoblasts by BMP **(With permission from S. Lynch, D.M.D., D.Sc.)**

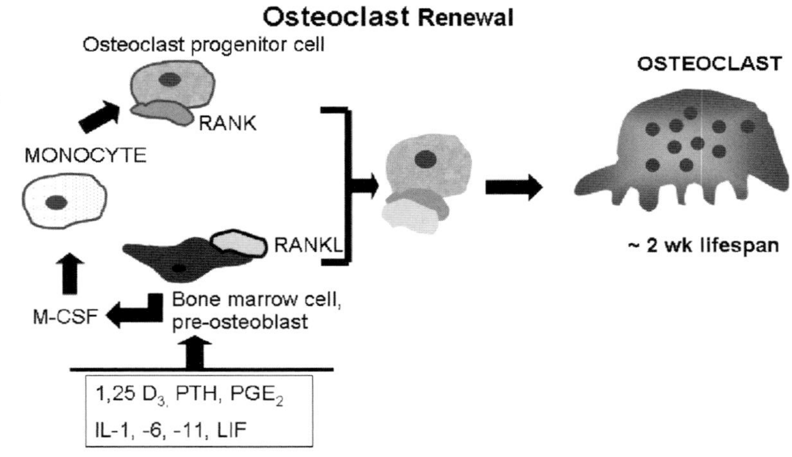

Fig. 3.3 *Osteoclast Renewal*: The osteoclast has about a two-week life expectancy, The renewal of osteoclasts requires the interaction between bone marrow pre-osteoblasts, and one of several secreted factors such as vitamin D 3 [1, 25], parathyroid hormone (PTH), prostaglandin E_2 (PGE_2), interleukin (IL) or lymphocyte initiating factor (LIF).

The stimulated progenitor may then express the soluble ligand known as RANK (RANKL) as well as monocyte colony stimulating factor (M-CSF), which promotes the expression of the RANK receptor by a blood-borne monocyte (i.e., osteoclast progenitor). Following binding between RANKL and RANK, the osteoclast progenitor matures into an osteoclast **(With permission from R Gruber, Ph.D.)**

remodeling. RAP at the fracture site continues until form and function are restored [66]. Locally administered therapies to enhance fracture healing and regeneration of osseous deficits may boost the tempo of RAP and restore healing deficits arising from aging, osteoporosis and diabetes, for example.

3.2.4. Approaches for Bone Grafting: Bone Grafts, Substitutes, Growth Factors

3.2.4.1. Bone Grafts

3.2.4.1.1. Autogenous bone: (i.e., autografts) is the most frequently used graft material for osseous clinical indications where bone deficits exist. Moreover, autografts are the benchmark against which alternatives may be compared. Autografts are free from disease transmission from donor to recipient. They lack immunological disparities and consequences. Further, autografts appear to have sufficient cells and biological factors to promote a predictably successful clinical outcome. However, in large gaps, unless transferred on its vascular pedicle with immediate reanastomosis, autogenous bone grafts must be revascularized and re-populated with osteogenic cells.

There is some speculation and argument whether autogenous grafts actually contain a satisfactory threshold quantity of viable cells that can be maintained following grafting. It is likely that most cells crucial to graft incorporation and remodeling are provided by the host bed, lured to the autograft by transferred biological signals in the autograft. These biological signals can include, for example, interleukins, cytokines and growth factors. The growth factors bone morphogenetic protein (BMP) and platelet-derived growth factor (PDGF) will be emphasized later in the chapter, being singled out for their especial therapeutic significance and the fact that only recombinant human (rh) BMP-2 and -7 and rhPDGF (BB homodimer) have approval for human use by the Food and Drug Agency (FDA).

The biological response at the autograft recipient site begins with hematoma formation. This is the accumulation of the localized vascular and cellular debris and vulnerary products. Inflammation follows and subsequently granulation tissue (also referred to as fibrovascular tissue) forms. Granulation tissue is a molecular-cell-matrix-rich nutrient pablum supporting healing.

Cortical grafts first undergo significant osteoclastic resorption of pre-existing matrix to accommodate the ingrowth of new blood vessels (i.e., neovascularization), while the more porous cancellous bone enables almost immediate graft incorporation. Depending on graft volume and location, resorption and replacement with host bone may take months to years [82].

The disadvantages of autografts include limited volume and shape of available donor bone. Also, the process of recovering autogenous bone is subject to donor site morbidity, including significant and prolonged pain (~30 percent of cases), donor bone weakness or fracture, additional operative time and blood loss and possible infection of an additional operative site [83].

Autogenous bone marrow also is used for grafting purposes to restore and regenerate skeletal defects. There is some controversy among surgeons regarding the success of freshly harvested bone marrow. A recent study of 60 patients with non-infected, non-unions undergoing bone marrow aspiration of their iliac crests resulted in union in 53 of 60 patients [84]. The study suggested that autogenous bone marrow can be effective, but efficacy will depend on the number and concentration of osteoprogenitor cells [84].

3.2.4.1.2. Allograft Preparations: Allograft materials are provided by a deceased donor to an immunologically matched recipient. A highly stringent process is used to screen donors to prevent disease transmission to the recipient. Reputable bone tissue banks belong to the American Association of Tissue Banks (AATB).

Cortical donor bone can be formulated into different shapes, such as rods, screws, spine cages and plates. Donor trabecular bone resembling bread croutons is a popular therapeutic modality.

Advantages offered by allogeneic bone preparations include versatility in shapes suitable for many bone applications (e.g., fixation, spine cages), as well as the elimination of a donor surgical site. Concern remains about disease transmission regardless of the stringency of the donor protocol. Moreover, there is a concern about lack of resorption in large allograft cortical segments.

Innovative preparations of allogeneic bone continue to expand the therapeutic envelope. This situation is especially underscored with allogeneic bone particulates that may or may not be demineralized and subsequently combined with carrier matrices such as hyaluronic acid, glycerin and calcium sulfate, for example.

3.2.4.1.3. Demineralized Bone Matrix: Demineralized bone matrix (DBM) is produced by the decalcification of cortical bone [85-86]. Demineralization removes the calcium and phosphate, leaving the extracellular matrix of primarily Type I collagen and nonstructural proteins.

DBM has little biomechanical strength. However, it can provide a permissive structure for host bone ingrowth (i.e., osteoconduction). Furthermore, DBM is noteworthy in its biological property of osteoinduction. Osteoinduction of DBM is due primarily to the content of BMPs and secondarily to other growth factors (e.g., vascular endothelial growth, PDGF, fibroblast growth factor, insulin-like growth factor and BMPs) that lead to angiogenesis and the chemotaxis, attachment, mitogenesis and differentiation of undifferentiated cells into osteoblasts [85, 87].

3.2.5.1. Osteoconductive Materials

Most osteoconductive materials used for bone healing consist of ceramics of calcium phosphate, calcium hydroxyapatite or calcium sulfate. These materials can serve as scaffolds that, in combination with a growth factor such as rhBMP, will stimulate osteoprogenitor cells to attach, proliferate and differentiate to osteoblasts.

3.2.5.1.1. Ceramics: Ceramic calcium phosphate is formed by heating and pressurizing stoichiometric ratios of calcium and phosphate. Hydroxyapatitic calcium phosphate (either laboratory synthesized, bovine derived, or as a coralline by-product) and tricalcium phosphate are the most widely used for bone repair. These materials are often included with autograft or allogeneic preparations as bone graft extenders or they can be used independently of bone grafts for cranioplasties, ridge augmentation and sinus lifts.

Ceramics are biocompatible, eliciting little to no inflammatory response, and there is no risk of disease transmission. Unlimited quantities are available. Further, the benefit to patients offered by ceramics is that a donor site is not required. Disadvantages of ceramics include low fracture resistance and poor tensile strength.

Ceramics have found a significant therapeutic niche in the craniofacial and axial skeletons. In the axial skeleton, there are data indicating comparable results between ceramic-autograft combinations versus only autografts for posterolateral fusions in idiopathic scoliosis [88]. Superior clinical outcome (~100 percent fusion rate) has been reported for anterior interbody fusion in the cervical spine using rigid internal fixation and ceramics [89].

A negative aspect of the hydroxyapatite-type ceramics is either a lack of or negligible resorption. Consequently, remaining material not resorbed prevents bone formation and may initiate a foreign body response.

3.2.5.1.2. Beta-tricalcium Phosphate: A biodegradable, porous beta-tricalcium phosphate (TCP) bone void filler has been developed to duplicate cancellous bone. In the craniofacial skeleton, especially for periodontal applications, beta-TCP is an osteoconductive matrix to deliver rhPDGF-BB for periodontal regeneration. This combination is the FDA-approved product GEM21S (BioMimetic Therapeutics, Inc. Franklin, TN).

3.2.5.2. *Growth Factors*

Growth factors either being developed or that have been developed for bone regenerative therapies include fibroblast growth factor (FGF), platelet-derived growth factor (PDGF), vascular endothelial growth factor (VEGF), bone morphogenetic protein (BMP) and insulin-like growth factor (IGF). We will emphasize recombinant human (rh) PDGF-BB and rhBMP-2 and -7 in this chapter since they are the only growth factors at the time of the writing of this chapter that have received FDA approval.

3.2.5.2.1. Platelet-Derived Growth Factor (PDGF): Recombinant human (rh) PDGF has been found to accelerate fracture repair and increase bone density. Howes, et al. studied subcutaneous implantation of demineralized bone matrix (DBM) augmented with PDGF in young and mature rats, and demonstrated reported induced bone formation and upregulated biochemical bone markers [123]. PDGF-DBM increased bone formation and associated bone markers in older animals by two-fold, compared to DBM alone. In the younger animals the impact of PDGF-amended DBM was not significant. Nash, et al. [90] delivered PDGF in a collagen gel to treat tibial osteotomies in rabbits. The authors reported a distinct increase in callus density and volume around the PDGF-treated osteotomies, compared to non-treated controls receiving only collagen. Indeed, PDGF-collagen-treated tibiae were not significantly different than unoperated, contralateral tibiae. Histologically, PDGF-collagen produced a more robust and advanced osteogenesis, both endosteally and periosteally, than collagen alone.

In another PDGF study Mitlak, et al. [91] reported on the substantial increase in bone density following treatment with rhPDGF or rhPDGF in combination with alendronate. Quantitative computerized tomography of axial and appendicular bones indicated significant enhancement in bone mass. Histologically, the PDGF recipients had a substantial increase in osteoblast number and lining osteoblasts, without a change in osteoclast number, when compared to the untreated group. Biomechanically, rats treated with PDGF had significantly enhanced vertebral body compressive strength and femoral shaft torsional stiffness. The combination of alendronate with PDGF further increased these indices.

Success with PDGF-BB in periodontics is underscored by the fundamental principles of bone wound biology. Specifically, PDGF is chemotactic and mitogenic for cells that will differentiate into osteoblasts, cementoblasts and periodontal-ligament cells. Moreover, the exogenous PDGF (in the GEM21S) and endogenous VEGF promote angiogenesis and vascularogenesis that will provide a normoxic and metabolically suitable environment for periodontal regeneration.

A prospective, masked and randomized controlled clinical trial tested the safety and effectiveness of rhPDGF-BB delivered with beta-TCP for advanced periodontal osseous defects [93]. Eleven clinical centers (total 180 subjects) treated patients requiring surgical treatment of 4 mm or greater intrabony periodontal defects. The rhPDGF-BB at 300 μg/ml caused a gain of clinical attachment level over beta-TCP alone after three months (3.8 mm versus 3.3 mm). By six months this finding was not statistically significant. The rhP-DGF-BB-treated sites had greater linear bone gain (2.6 mm versus 0.9 mm) and percent defect fill (57 percent versus 18 percent) than the sites receiving the beta-TCP with buffer at six months.

The favorable safety profile of PDGF-BB has been well established. This fact is based on the FDA clearance of Regranex, an rhPDGF-BB containing formulation for topical application in diabetic ulcers. Neither antibody formation nor immunologic responses was observed in patients receiving a daily dose of rhPDGF-BB over a time period of four months, based on six controlled clinical trials [92]. In addition, neither systemic reactivity nor gene toxicity was observed when tested using *in vivo* models.

3.2.5.3.2. Bone Morphogenetic Protein (BMP): Osteoinduction was coined by Urist [85, 87]. He defined osteoinduction (with slight modification by the authors) as: (t)he recruitment and differentiation of pluripotential mesenchymal-like cells at a non-bony site (e.g., heterotopic muscle site), and the subsequent differentiation into chondrocytes and osteoblasts and the formation of an ossicle. Urist recognized the capacity for bone to regenerate and hypothesized that a naturally occurring protein in bone was responsible for this effect and named the protein bone morphogenetic protein (BMP) [87].

During the next 25 years investigators identified a family of proteins with bone inducing properties. The BMPs are members of the larger TGF-beta super family. To date over 20 different BMPs have been isolated, but only some have the potential to induce formation of new bone. Currently, BMP-2 and -7 (also known as osteogenic protein-1: OP-1) have received FDA approval for clinical use.

BMP-7 (osteogenic protein-1; OP-1) has been used in a randomized controlled trial (122 patients with 124 tibial non-unions). The non-unions were at least nine months old and, clinically, there was no indication of progress in healing. Patients were treated with either an intramedullary nail and rhOP-1 in a Type I collagen carrier, or with autogenous bone graft alone. After nine months, 81 percent of the OP-1-treated patients and 85 percent of the autogenous bone graft-treated patients had healed (based on clinical criteria) [94].

In another study rhBMP-2 was used in a prospective randomized controlled trial (450 patients with open tibial fractures) [95]. Patients received either irrigation and debridement and treatment with a statically locked intramedullary (IM) nail, or supplementation with one of two doses of recombinant human BMP-2. After 12 months patients treated with the higher dose of BMP-2 had a 44 percent reduction in the risk of secondary interventions and had fewer IM nail fixation failures and fewer infections than patients who did not receive BMP [94].

3.2.5. Compromised Bone Healing: Osteoporosis, Geriatrics, Diabetes

The osteoporotic condition mutes the capacity to sustain the homeostatic remodeling cycle, where 25 percent of trabecular bone and 3 percent of cortical bone are resorbed and replaced each year [78]. Instead, osteoclastic resorption proceeds without compensatory osteoblastic-mediated bone formation and, consequently, in a lifetime, the aging process for women quietly steals up to 50 percent of their trabecular bone, while men lose about 25 percent of their bone [96]. From age 20 to 60 25 percent of the cortical bone in men is depleted, and 35 percent for women [96-97], with a concomitant loss of 80 to 90 percent in bone strength [98]. There is an overall risk of fracture of the hip, spine and distal forearm that will afflict 40 percent of women and 13 percent of men 50 years of age and older [99, http://www.osteo.org/2005]. Moreover, at least 25 million women in this country between 50- to 64–years-old [100], and 33 percent of women older than 65 will experience at least one vertebral fracture [101].

It is significant and noteworthy that the diabetic condition is often associated with compromised osseous healing and that bone in diabetic patients (even controlled diabetic patients) is osteopenic and osteoporotic (reviewed [102]). The vascular compromise in diabetics is well-known and recognized as a comorbidity factor, especially in cutaneous wound healing,that likely will severely strain the capacity for tissue to heal.

The reduction of healthy marrow elements that occurs as a consequence of aging or disease (e.g., osteoporosis, diabetes) is accompanied by a diminution of the cellular constituents, especially the osteogenic precursors. Moreover, in the osteoporotic condition there is a decreased quantity and activity of osteoblasts [103-104] and a decrease in signaling molecules, such as estrogen, IGH, TGF-beta and calcitropic hormones [105-110]. For postmenopausal women, osteoblast activity significantly decreases with estrogen depletion [106, 110, 111]. Moreover, osteoblasts from elderly donors are less responsive to soluble signals than osteoblasts from young donors [104, 112]. In addition, old osteoblast-like phenotypes in cell culture are three times less active than cells recovered from younger sources [113].

Furthermore, proliferation of human-derived cells of osteoblast phenotypes procured from donors of different ages revealed osteogenic capacity decreased commensurately with increasing donor age [114]. In addition, DBM from young donors is more osteoinductive than DBM derived from old donors, indicating a decrement of inductive factors in the DBM [115].

Significantly, there is data that bone healing is delayed in the aged individual [103-104, 112, 116-118]. In studies reported by Frost over 30 years ago, aging and osteoporosis were detailed clearly to retard remodeling dynamics [118], and using animal models, it was underscored that remodeling dynamics slow down with aging [120-122].

Howes, et al. determined an enhanced bone response in elderly rats when rhPDGF-BB was implanted subcutaneously with demineralized bone matrix (DBM) [123]. The DBM supplemented with rhPDGF-BB increased bone formation and upregulated biochemical bone markers. Moreover, the combination boosted bone formation and associated bone markers in older animals by two-fold, compared to DBM alone. In younger rats PDGF-amended DBM was not significant. The therapeutic opportunities are exciting for rhPDGH-BB to restore normal healing capacity for compromised bone healing in osteoporotic, geriatric and diabetic patients.

3.2.6. Conclusion

Fracture repair is a dynamic process. Regenerative capacities of prenatal bone development partially persist with the lifespan of the organism. However, inter- and intra-cellular signaling culminating in the postnatal fracture repair is confounded by the cumulative effects of internal and external factors. Comprehensive regenerative responses gradually yield to the cumulative influences of a compromised physiologic status. Thus, the discovery and exploitation of events in fracture repair is dependent upon our continued efforts to understand osteogenesis regarding the spatial, gradient and the temporal dependencies leading to bone repair.

Acknowledgements: Partial support for this work was provided by the NIDCR R01-DE15392 (JOH).

References

1. Aaron RK, Ciombor DM, Wang S, Simon B. Clinical biophysics: the promotion of skeletal repair by physical forces. Ann N Y Acad Sci 2006;1068:513-31.
2. Blair HC, Carrington JL. Bone cell precursors and the pathophysiology of bone loss. Ann N Y Acad Sci 2006;1068:244-9.
3. Khosla S, Eghbali-Fatourechi GZ. Circulating cells with osteogenic potential. Ann N Y Acad Sci 2006;1068:489-97.
4. Ellies DL, Krumlauf R. Bone formation: The nuclear matrix reloaded. Cell 2006;125(5):840-2.
5. Pountos I, Jones E, Tzioupis C, McGonagle D, Giannoudis PV. Growing bone and cartilage. The role of mesenchymal stem cells. J Bone Joint Surg Br 2006;88(4):421-6.
6. Deckers MM, van Bezooijen RL, van der Horst G, et al. Bone morphogenetic proteins stimulate angiogenesis through osteoblast-derived vascular endothelial growth factor A. Endocrinology 2002;143(4):1545-53.
7. Vortkamp A, Pathi S, Peretti GM, Caruso EM, Zaleske DJ, Tabin CJ. Recapitulation of signals regulating embryonic bone formation during postnatal growth and in fracture repair. Mech Dev 1998;71(1-2):65-76.
8. Gerstenfeld L, Cullilane D, Barnes G, Graves D, Einhorn T. Fracture healing as a post-natal developmental process: Molecular, spatial, and temporal aspects of its regulation. J Cell Biochem 2003;88:873-84.
9. Gerstenfeld LC, Einhorn TA. Developmental aspects of fracture healing and the use of pharmacological agents to alter healing. J Musculoskelet Neuronal Interact 2003;3(4):297-303; discussion 20-1.
10. Anderson HC. Matrix vesicles and calcification. Curr Rheumatol Rep 2003;5(3):222-6.
11. Miyauchi A, Alvarez J, Greenfield EM, et al. Binding of osteopontin to the osteoclast integrin alpha v beta 3. Osteoporos Int 1993;3 Suppl 1:132-5.
12. Ross FP, Chappel J, Alvarez JI, et al. Interactions between the bone matrix proteins osteopontin and bone sialoprotein and the osteoclast integrin alpha v beta 3 potentiate bone resorption. J Biol Chem 1993;268(13):9901-7.

13. Roodman GD. Cell biology of the osteoclast. Exp Hematol 1999;27(8):1229-41.
14. Reddy SV. Regulatory mechanisms operative in osteoclasts. Crit Rev Eukaryot Gene Expr 2004;14(4):255-70.
15. Arai S, Amizuka N, Azuma Y, Takeshita S, Kudo A. Osteoclastogenesis-related antigen, a novel molecule on mouse stromal cells, regulates osteoclastogenesis. J Bone Miner Res 2003;18(4):686-95.
16. Atkins GJ, Kostakis P, Pan B, et al. RANKL expression is related to the differentiation state of human osteoblasts. J Bone Miner Res 2003;18(6):1088-98.
17. Zhang YH, Heulsmann A, Tondravi MM, Mukherjee A, Abu-Amer Y. Tumor necrosis factor-alpha (TNF) stimulates RANKL-induced osteoclastogenesis via coupling of TNF type 1 receptor and RANK signaling pathways. J Biol Chem 2001;276(1):563-8.
18. Takahashi N. [Bone and bone related biochemical examinations. Bone and collagen related metabolites. Regulatory mechanisms of osteoclast differentiation and function]. Clin Calcium 2006;16(6):56-63.
19. Feng X. RANKing intracellular signaling in osteoclasts. IUBMB Life 2005;57(6):389-95.
20. Takayanagi H. Mechanistic insight into osteoclast differentiation in osteoimmunology. J Mol Med 2005;83(3):170-9.
21. Kim N, Kadono Y, Takami M, et al. Osteoclast differentiation independent of the TRANCE-RANK-TRAF6 axis. J Exp Med 2005;202(5):589-95.
22. Marotti G, Muglia MA, Palumbo C. Collagen texture and osteocyte distribution in lamellar bone. Ital J Anat Embryol 1995;100 Suppl 1:95-102.
23. Marotti G, Ferretti M, Remaggi F, Palumbo C. Quantitative evaluation on osteocyte canalicular density in human secondary osteons. Bone 1995;16(1):125-8.
24. Palumbo C. A three-dimensional ultrastructural study of osteoid-osteocytes in the tibia of chick embryos. Cell Tissue Res 1986;246(1):125-31.
25. Ferretti M, Muglia MA, Remaggi F, Cane V, Palumbo C. Histomorphometric study on the osteocyte lacuno-canalicular network in animals of different species. II. Parallel-fibered and lamellar bones. Ital J Anat Embryol 1999;104(3):121-31.
26. Aarden EM, Burger EH, Nijweide PJ. Function of osteocytes in bone. J Cell Biochem 1994;55(3):287-99.
27. Knothe Tate ML, Adamson JR, Tami AE, Bauer TW. The osteocyte. Int J Biochem Cell Biol 2004;36(1):1-8.
28. Rhinelander FW. Effects of medullary nailing on the normal blood supply of diaphyseal cortex. 1973. Clin Orthop Relat Res 1998(350):5-17.
29. Kusaka M, Sudo K, Matsutani E, et al. Cytostatic inhibition of endothelial cell growth by the angiogenesis inhibitor TNP-470 (AGM-1470). Br J Cancer 1994;69(2):212-6.
30. Folkman J, Ingber D. Inhibition of angiogenesis. Semin Cancer Biol 1992;3(2):89-96.
31. Kusaka M, Sudo K, Fujita T, et al. Potent anti-angiogenic action of AGM-1470: comparison to the fumagillin parent. Biochem Biophys Res Commun 1991;174(3):1070-6.
32. Ingber D, Fujita T, Kishimoto S, et al. Synthetic analogues of fumagillin that inhibit angiogenesis and suppress tumour growth. Nature 1990;348(6301):555-7.
33. Fang TD, Salim A, Xia W, et al. Angiogenesis is required for successful bone induction during distraction osteogenesis. J Bone Miner Res 2005;20(7):1114-24.
34. Mann FA, Payne JT. Bone healing. Semin Vet Med Surg (Small Anim) 1989;4(4):312-21.
35. Claes LE, Heigele CA, Neidlinger-Wilke C, et al. Effects of mechanical factors on the fracture healing process. Clin Orthop Relat Res 1998(355 Suppl):S132-47.
36. Chakkalakal DA, Lippiello L, Shindell RL, Connolly JF. Electrophysiology of direct current stimulation of fracture healing in canine radius. IEEE Trans Biomed Eng 1990;37(11):1048-58.
37. Walsh WR, Guzelsu N. Electrokinetic behavior of intact wet bone: compartmental model. J Orthop Res 1991;9(5):683-92.
38. Einhorn T. The cell and molecular biology of fracture healing. Clin Orthop Rel Res 1998;1(Suppl.):s7-s21.

39. McKibbin B. The biology of fracture healing in long bones. J Bone Joint Surg Br 1978;60-B(2):150-62.
40. Bolander ME. Regulation of fracture repair by growth factors. Proc Soc Exp Biol Med 1992;200(2):165-70.
41. Grundnes O, Reikeras O. The importance of the hematoma for fracture healing in rats. Acta Orthop Scand 1993;64(3):340-2.
42. Mark H, Penington A, Nannmark U, Morrison W, Messina A. Microvascular invasion during endochondral ossification in experimental fractures in rats. Bone 2004;35(2):535-42.
43. Wildemann B, Schmidmaier G, Brenner N, et al. Quantification, localization, and expression of IGF-I and TGF-beta1 during growth factor-stimulated fracture healing. Calcif Tissue Int 2004;74(4):388-97.
44. Einhorn T. Current concepts review. Enhancement of fracture healing. J Bone Joint Surg 1995;77-A(6):940-56.
45. Einhorn TA, Majeska RJ, Rush EB, Levine PM, Horowitz MC. The expression of cytokine activity by fracture callus. J Bone Miner Res 1995;10(8):1272-81.
46. Einhorn TA. The science of fracture healing. J Orthop Trauma 2005;19(10 Suppl):S4-6.
47. Buckwalter JA, Glimcher MJ, Cooper RR, Recker R. Bone biology. I: Structure, blood supply, cells, matrix, and mineralization. Instr Course Lect 1996;45:371-86.
48. Buckwalter JA, Glimcher MJ, Cooper RR, Recker R. Bone biology. II: Formation, form, modeling, remodeling, and regulation of cell function. Instr Course Lect 1996;45:387-99.
49. Muller PK, Kirsch E, Gauss-Muller V, Krieg T. Some aspects of the modulation and regulation of collagen synthesis in vitro. Mol Cell Biochem 1981;34(2):73-85.
50. Brighton CT, Hunt RM. Histochemical localization of calcium in the fracture callus with potassium pyroantimonate. Possible role of chondrocyte mitochondrial calcium in callus calcification. J Bone Joint Surg Am 1986;68(5):703-15.
51. Einhorn TA, Hirschman A, Kaplan C, Nashed R, Devlin VJ, Warman J. Neutral protein-degrading enzymes in experimental fracture callus: a preliminary report. J Orthop Res 1989;7(6):792-805.
52. Sandberg MM, Aro HT, Vuorio EI. Gene expression during bone repair. Clin Orthop Relat Res 1993(289):292-312.
53. Meller Y, Kestenbaum RS, Shany S, et al. Parathormone, calcitonin, and vitamin D metabolites during normal fracture healing in geriatric patients. Clin Orthop Relat Res 1985(199):272-9.
54. Alkhiary YM, Gerstenfeld LC, Krall E, et al. Enhancement of experimental fracture-healing by systemic administration of recombinant human parathyroid hormone (PTH 1-34). J Bone Joint Surg Am 2005;87(4):731-41.
55. Tsakalakos N, Magiasis B, Tsekoura M, Lyritis G. The effect of short-term calcitonin administration on biochemical bone markers in patients with acute immobilization following hip fracture. Osteoporos Int 1993;3(6):337-40.
56. Bak B, Jorgensen PH, Andreassen TT. The stimulating effect of growth hormone on fracture healing is dependent on onset and duration of administration. Clin Orthop Relat Res 1991(264):295-301.
57. Nielsen HM, Bak B, Jorgensen PH, Andreassen TT. Growth hormone promotes healing of tibial fractures in the rat. Acta Orthop Scand 1991;62(3):244-7.
58. Northmore-Ball MD, Wood MR, Meggitt BF. A biomechanical study of the effects of growth hormone in experimental fracture healing. J Bone Joint Surg Br 1980;62(3):391-6.
59. Carpenter JE, Hipp JA, Gerhart TN, Rudman CG, Hayes WC, Trippel SB. Failure of growth hormone to alter the biomechanics of fracture-healing in a rabbit model. J Bone Joint Surg Am 1992;74(3):359-67.
60. Simmons DJ, Kunin AS. Autoradiographic and biochemical investigations of the effect of cortisone on the bones of the rat. Clin Orthop Relat Res 1967;55:201-15.

61. Cruess RL, Sakai T. Effect of cortisone upon synthesis rates of some components of rat bone matrix. Clin Orthop Relat Res 1972;86:253-9.
62. Adinoff AD, Hollister JR. Steroid-induced fractures and bone loss in patients with asthma. N Engl J Med 1983;309(5):265-8.
63. Gandhi A, Beam HA, O'Connor JP, Parsons JR, Lin SS. The effects of local insulin delivery on diabetic fracture healing. Bone 2005;37(4):482-90.
64. Lyritis G, Papadopoulou Z, Nikiforidis P, Batrinos M, Varonos D. Effect of cortisone and an anabolic steroid upon plasma hydroxyproline during fracture healing in rabbits. Acta Orthop Scand 1975;46(1):25-30.
65. Aro HT, Wippermann BW, Hodgson SF, Wahner HW, Lewallen DG, Chao EY. Prediction of properties of fracture callus by measurement of mineral density using micro-bone densitometry. J Bone Joint Surg Am 1989;71(7):1020-30.
66. Frost HM. Intermediary Organization of the Skeleton. Vol. II. Boca Raton, FL: CRC Press; 1986.
67. Frost HM. Intermediary Organization of the Skeleton. Vol. I.; 1986.
68. Enlow DH. Principles of Bone Remodeling. Springfield: Thomas Publishing Co.; 1963.
69. Enlow D. Comparative study of facial growth in Homo and Macaca. Am J Phys Anthrop 1966;24:293-310.
70. Boyce B, Hughes D, Wright K, Xing L, Dai A. Recent advances in bone biology provide insight into the pathogenesis of bone diseases. Lab Invest 1999;79(2): 83-94.
71. Kimmel D. A paradigm for skeletal strength homeostasis. J Bone Joint Min Res 1993;8(2):515-22.
72. Geddes A. Animal models of bone disease. In: Bilezikian J, Raisz L, Rodan G, eds. Principles of Bone Biology. San Diego: Academic Press; 1996:1343-54.
73. Raisz L. Physiology and pathophysiology of bone remodeling. Clin Chem 1999;45(8B):1353-8.
74. Parfitt MA. The physiologic and clinical significance of bone histomorphometric data. In: Recker RR, ed. Bone Histomorphometry: Techniques and Interpretation. Boca Raton: CRC Press, Inc.; 1983:143-224.
75. Delmas PD, Malaval L. The proteins of bone. In: Mundy GR, ed. Physiology and Pharmacology of Bone. New York: Springer-Verlag; 1993:673-724.
76. Recker RR, ed. Bone Histomorphometry: Techniques and Interpretation. Boca Raton: CRC Press; 1983.
77. Frost H. Bone histomorphometry: Choice of marking agent and labeling schedule. In: Recker RR, ed. Bone Histomorphometry: Techniques and Interpretation. Boca Raton: CRC Press; 1983:37-52.
78. Parfitt AM. Osteonal and hemi-osteonal remodeling: The spatial and temporal framework for signal traffic in adult human bone. J Cell Biochem 1994;55: 273-86.
79. Parfitt AM, Villanueva AR, Foldes J, Rao DS. Relations between histologic indices of bone formation: implications for the pathogenesis of spinal osteoporosis. J Bone Min Res 1995;10(2):466-73.
80. Parfitt AM. Stereologic basis of bone histomorphometry; theory of quantitative microscopy and reconstruction of the third dimension. In: Recker RR, ed. Bone Histomorphometry: Techniques and Interpretation. Boca Raton: CRC Press, Inc.; 1983:54-87.
81. Parfitt M. Skeletal heterogeneity and the purposes of bone remodeling. In: Marcus R, Feldman D, Kelsey J, eds. Osteoporosis. San Diego: Academic Press; 1996:315-29.
82. Goldberg V, Akhavan S. Biology of bone grafts. In: Lieberman J, Friedleander G, eds. Bone Regeneration and Repair. Totawa: Humana Press; 2005:57-65.
83. Younger EM, Chapman MW. Morbidity of bone graft donor sites. J Orthop Trauma 1989;3:192-5.

84. Hernigou P, Poignard A, Beaujean F, Rouard H. Percutaneous autologous bone-marrow grafting for nonunions. Influence of the number and concentration of progenitor cells. J Bone Joint Surg 2005;87A(7):1430-7.
85. Urist MR. Bone: Formation by autoinduction. Science 1965;150:893-9.
86. Urist MR, Silverman MF, Buring K, Dubuc FL, Rosenburg JM. The bone induction principle. Clin Orthop Rel Res 1967; 53:243.
87. Urist MR, Strates BS. Bone morphogenetic protein. J Dent Res 1971;50:1392-406.
88. Delecrin J, Takahashi S, Gouin F, Passuti N. A synthetic porous ceramic as a bone graft substitute in the surgical management of scoliosis: a prospective, randomized study. Spine 2000;25(5):563-9.
89. McConnell JR, Freeman BJ, Debnath UK, et al. A randomized comparison of coralline hydroxyaptite with autograft in cervical interbody fusion. Spine 2003;28(4):317-23.
90. Nash TJ, Howlett CR, Martin C, Steele J, Johnson KA, Hicklin DJ. Effect of platelet-derived growth factor on tibial osteotomies in rabbits. Bone 1994;15(2):203-8.
91. Mitlak B, Finkelman R, Hill E, et al. The effect of systematically administered PDGF-BB on the rodent skeleton. J Bone Mineral Res 1996;11(2):238-47.
92. Smiell, J. M. Clinical safety of becaplermin (rhPDGF-BB) gel. Becaplermin Studies Group. Am J Surg 1998; 176 (2A): 68S-73S.
93. Nevins M, Giannobile WV, McGuire MH, et al. Platelet-derived growth factor stimulates bone fill and rate of attachment level gain: Results of a large multicenter randomized controlled trail. J Periodontol 2005;76:2205-15.
94. Friedlaender GE, Perry CR, Cole JD, et al. Osteogenic protein-1 (bone morphogenetic protein-7) in the treatment of tibial nonunions. J Bone Joint Surg Am 2001;83-A Suppl 1(Pt 2):S151-8.
95. Govender S, Csimma C, Genant H, et al. Recombinant human bone morphogenetic protein-2 for treatment of open tibial fractures: A prospective, controlled, randomized study of four hundred and fifty patients. J Bone Joint Surg 2002;84-A:2123-34.
96. Flemming LA. Osteoporosis: Clinical features, prevention, and treatment. J Gen Intern Med 1992;7:554-62.
97. Mazess RB. On aging bone loss. Clin Orthop Rel Res 1982;165:239-52.
98. Mosekilde L. Assessing bone quality - Animal models in preclinical osteoporosis research. Bone 1995;14(4(Suppl.)):3435-525.
99. Melton LJ. How many women have osteoporosis now? J Bone Min Res 1995;10:175-7.
100. Tosteson AN, Weinstein MC. Cost-effectiveness of hormone replacement therapy after menopause. Ballieres Clin Obstet Gynecol 1991;5:943-59.
101. Sagraves R. Estrogen therapy for postmenopausal symptoms and prevention of osteoporosis. J Clin Pharmacol 1995;35:2S-10S.
102. Thrailkill K, Lumpkin CK, Jr., Bunn R, Kemp S, Fowlkes J. Is insulin an anabolic agent in bone? Dissecting the diabetic bone for clues. AJP-Endo 2005;289:735-45.
103. Fleet JC, Cashman K, Cox K, Rosen V. The effects of aging on the bone inductive activity of recombinant human bone morphogenetic protein-2. Endocrinol 1996;137(11):4605-10.
104. Inoue K, Ohgushi H, Okumura M, Sempuku T, Tama S, Dohi Y. The effect of aging on bone formation in porous hydroxyapatite: Biochemical and histological analyses. J Bone Min Res 1997;12(6):989-94.
105. Gallagher JC. The pathogenesis of osteoporosis. Bone Mineral 1990;9:215-27.
106. Chestnut III CH. Osteoporosis and its treatment. N Engl J Med 1992;326:406-8.
107. Christiansen C. Prevention and treatment of osteoporosis: a review of current modalities. Bone 1992;13:S35-S9.
108. Papapoulos SE, Landman JO, Bijvoet OLM, et al. The use of bisphosphonates in treatment of osteoporosis. Bone 1992;13:S41-S9.

109. Nicolas V, Prewet A, Bettica P, et al. Age-related decreases in insulin-like growth factor-I and transforming growth factor-beta in femoral cortical bone from both men and women: Implications for bone loss with aging. J Clin Endocrinol Metab 1994;78(5):1011-6.
110. Masi L, Bilezikian JP. Osteoporosis: New hope for the future. Int J Fertil 1997;42(4):245-54.
111. Lindsay R. The burden of osteoporosis: cost. Bone 1995;98(2A):9-11.
112. Shirota T, Ohno K, Suzuki K, et al. The effect of aging on the healing of hydroxylapatite implants. J Oral Maxillofac Surg 1993;51(1):51-6.
113. Tsuji T, Hughes FJ, McCulloch CAG, Melcher AH. Effects of donor age on osteogenic cells of rat bone marrow *in vitro*. Mech Aging Develop 1990;51:121-32.
114. Evans C, Galasko SB, Ward C. Effect of donor age on the growth in vitro of cells obtained from human trabecular bone. J Orthop Res 1990;8(2):234-7.
115. Jergensen HE, Chua J, Kao RT, Kaban LB. Age effects on bone induction by demineralized bone powder. Clin Orthop 1991;268:253-9.
116. Caplan AI. The mesengenic process. Clin Plastic Surg 1994;21(3):429-35.
117. Quarto R, Thomas D, Liang T. Bone progenitor cell deficits and age-associated decline in bone repair capacity. Calcif Tissue Int 1995;56(2):123-9.
118. Caplan AI, Bruder SP. Cell and molecular engineering of bone regeneration. In: Lanza R, Langer R, Chick W, eds. Principles of Tissue Engineering. San Diego: Academic Press, Inc.; 1997:603-18.
119. Frost H. Mathematical Elements of Lamellar Bone Remodeling. Springfield, IL: Charles C. Thomas; 1969.
120. Detenbeck LC, Jowsey J. Normal aging in the bone of the adult dog. Clin Orthop Rel Res 1969;65:76-80.
121. Anderson C, Danylchuk KD. Appositional bone formation rates in the beagle. Am J Vet Res 1979;40:907-10.
122. Anderson C, Danylchuk DK. Age-related variations in cortical bone-remodeling measurements in male beagles 10 to 26 months of age. Am J Vet Res 1979;40:869-72.
123. Howes R, Bowness J, Grotendorst G, Martin G, Reddi A. Platelet-derived growth factor enhances demineralized bone matrix-induced cartilage and bone formation. Calcif Tissue Int 1988;42:34-8.

Section II

Hard Tissue Technologies

4

Autograft Bone

Takaaki Fujishiro[1], Hideo Kobayashi[2], and Thomas W. Bauer[2]

Abstract: Autograft is the gold standard for reconstructive orthopaedic surgery. Nonvascularized cortical autograft can provide structural support, and can become integrated around its periphery with bone in the insertion site, but is likely to remain largely necrotic and may eventually fracture. Vascularized cortical autografts integrate well with surrounding bone, but are associated with considerable morbidity at the harvest site. Iliac crest autograft has excellent osteogenic and osteoconductive properties, and has proven to be efficacious in many surgical procedures. Tissue harvested locally at the time of a spine operation avoids the morbidity associated with harvesting iliac crest, but "local autograft" preparations may contain substantial proportions of fibrous tissue and fibrocartilage, and may not be as osteogenic as iliac crest. Recent studies suggest that aspirated bone marrow with enrichment of osteoblast precursor populations may be a useful addition to other bone graft extender materials. The efficacy of autogenous growth factors isolated from platelet preparations for skeletal reconstruction has yet to be fully demonstrated.

Keywords: autograft; bone graft; history; cancellous bone; cortical bone; histology; bone marrow; platelet-rich plasma

4.1. Introduction

Autogenous (autologous) bone graft, or autograft bone, is defined as a tissue that has been harvested from one portion of the skeleton and transferred to another location in the same individual [1]. Autogenous bone grafts have been used frequently since the early 1900s, and are still considered to be the "gold standard" to which other graft materials are compared in reconstructive orthopaedic

[1]Department of Orthopaedic Surgery, Kobe University Graduate School of Medicine, Kobe, Japan
[2]Departments of Pathology and Orthopaedic Surgery, The Cleveland Clinic Foundation, Cleveland, OH

From: *Orthopedic Biology and Medicine: Musculoskeletal Tissue Regeneration, Biological Materials and Methods*
Edited by W. S. Pietrzak © Humana Press, Totowa, NJ

surgery. The advantages of autograft include optimum skeletal incorporation, no possibility of transmitting disease from one individual to another and histocompatibility. However, important disadvantages of autograft bone include morbidity associated with harvesting from the donor site, and limitations in the supply and quality of available tissue.

The purpose of this chapter is to summarize our current understanding of various autogenous bone graft preparations with particular focus on their properties, clinical applications and efficacy.

4.1.1. Brief History

According to de Boer [2] one of the first clinical autograft implantations was performed by Walther in 1820 [3], who replaced the surgically removed parts of the skull after trepanotomy. Autograft was used regularly during the first two decades of the 20th Century. For example, in 1923 Albee summarized his experience with 3,000 autogeneic bone graft operations [4]. Taylor, et al. reported one of the earliest vascularized fibular graft procedures in 1975 [5]. They used microvascular techniques to maintain vascularity of the contralateral fibula as it was transferred to a traumatic tibial defect. The authors demonstrated that revascularization was accomplished with preservation of blood flow to medullary and periosteal regions of the graft.

More recently aspirated bone marrow has been suggested to have value as a bone graft material. Connolly, et al. reported that percutaneous injections of 100 to 150 milliliters of non-heparinized bone marrow were successful in the treatment of 18 out of 20 tibial non-unions [6], and also suggested that intra-operative processing of bone marrow in order to concentrate the osteoblast progenitor cells may improve its efficacy as a bone graft [7].

4.1.2. Properties of Autograft Bone

Bone graft and bone graft substitute or extender materials have different biologic properties based, in part, on their composition. A bone graft material is considered to be osteogenic if it contains cells that contribute to subsequent bone formation. Properly harvested autograft contains mature osteoblasts and osteocytes, as well as osteoblast precursors that can potentially form new bone. A bone graft material is osteoconductive if it somehow promotes bone formation along its surface. The spicules of mineralized matrix in autograft can serve as a substrate on which direct bone formation can subsequently occur [8]. A bone graft material is osteoinductive if it induces stromal cells to differentiate into bone forming cells when it is placed into an extraskeletal site. Because mineralized autograft does not induce ectopic bone formation when it is placed into skeletal muscle, autograft is probably not osteoinductive in this classic sense, unless it is somehow demineralized. When autograft is placed into a skeletal site, it is gradually dissolved by osteoclasts. That process starts with demineralization by acid produced by osteoclasts, so autograft may have osteoinductive properties when used in the skeleton, although the release of osteoinductive proteins would be expected to be very slow.

The biologic properties of autograft depend, in part, on the site from which it has been harvested, the proportion of cortical to cancellous bone, the size and shape of the pieces of bone and the presence or absence of an intact vascular supply. Common preparations include cancellous, nonvascularized cortical, vascularized cortical and aspirated autologous bone marrow stromal cells. In addition, platelet-rich plasma or other preparations that are said to enrich autologous growth factors could also be considered autologous bone graft preparations, although the clinical efficacy of the latter two preparations is still unclear (see below).

4.2. Cortical Autograft

4.2.1. Nonvascularized Cortical Autograft

Nonvascularized cortical autograft is osteoconductive, but is thought to have few osteoinductive properties, and is not appreciably osteogenic [9-10]. However, autologous cortical grafts can provide structural support immediately after insertion. Like a bone infarct involving cortical bone, however, eventual osteoclastic resorption of the acellular bone matrix will weaken the construct, and eventual fracture is likely unless load-sharing new bone formation occurs.

Goldberg and Stevenson also studied biology of cortical bone grafts using other canine models [8]. The histological findings of cortical autografts showed that widespread necrosis and resorption of cortical bone was seen by the first two weeks after transplantation. The bone resorption increased until the sixth week and gradually declined to nearly normal levels by the end of one year. Appositional new bone formation was seen by three weeks and proceeded slowly; however, even at one year almost 40 percent of the original necrotic bone remained in these canine cortical autografts [8]. The marrow of the autogeneic graft was rapidly replaced by connective tissue and developed into normal marrow by nine months after transplantation. Enneking, et al. investigated the physical and biological aspects of repair in canine nonvascularized cortical autograft using a segmental fibular transplant model [11]. The experimental study showed that nonvascularized cortical autografts became osteoporotic and were mechanically deficient during the initial six weeks, and remained weakened until six to 12 months after transplantation.

4.2.1.1. Clinical Applications

Structural bone grafting is commonly used in orthopaedic reconstructive surgeries such as spinal fusion [12], bone grafting for osteonecrosis of the femoral head, revision arthroplasty when faced with extensive bone loss or repair of skeletal defects following the removal of tumor. The major source of nonvascularized cortical autograft is the fibula, although the use of rib or the anterior medial aspect of the tibia also has been described [12]. The iliac crest provides corticocancellous bone, but the mass and strength of the cortex is less than that of the fibula.

Autologous cortical bone grafts are often good choices for segmental defects of bone of >5 to 6 cm which require immediate structural support [13]. However, some surgeons suggest that autograft cortical bone may offer little advantage over allograft cortical bone when one considers donor site morbidity [1]. For example, Tang, et al. reported that, of 39 patients who had a free fibular graft harvested for treatment of avascular necrosis of the femoral head, 42 percent had a subjective sense of instability and 37 percent had a subjective sense of weakness in the lower extremity [14]. On the other hand, Yu, et al. evaluated the results of autogenous tibial strut grafts for anterior fusions in children with severe kyphosis and kyphoscoliosis regarding maintenance of correction, clinical outcome, graft fractures and donor site morbidity [12]. They concluded that their technique offered a reliable means of providing anterior support in the management of severe kyphosis with minimal donor site morbidity. Nelson, et al. reviewed 52 hips with Phemister bone grafting procedures for osteonecrosis of the femoral head [15] and concluded that the technique was not effective once collapse had occurred [16].

In general, the structural properties of autologous cortical bone graft, low risk of transmitting disease and histocompatibility are important potential advantages if the nonvascularized cortical autograft is used for an appropriate indication with good surgical techniques.

4.2.2. Vascularized Cortical Autograft

A vascularized cortical autograft is sometimes used in the management of skeletal defects larger than 5 to 6 cm, or those associated with poorly vascularized soft tissue related to traumatic bone loss [17], congenital pseudarthrosis of the tibia or forearm [18], necrosis of the femoral head [19-21] and long bone tumors [22].

The three sources for free vascularized bone autografts are the fibula, iliac crest [23] and rib [24], although limitations in mechanical properties, size, shape and vascular supply limit the efficacy of vascularized graft obtained from the iliac crest and rib.

Donor site complications of vascularized fibular grafts are usually minor, although donor site vascularity can be compromised when anatomic variation is not detected preoperatively [25]. On the other hand, recipient site complications include compromised vascularity, infection, nonunion of the graft-host junction sites and fatigue fracture of the graft [26]. The need of a well-trained surgical team to help with the microvascular surgery may also be a limitation of free vascularized bone grafts.

Vascularized cortical grafts heal rapidly at the host-graft interface, and their remodeling may be similar to that of normal bone. Doi, et al. investigated the healing mechanism of a free vascular-pedicle bone graft using canine vascularized rib grafts [10]. The experimental study suggested that more than 90 percent of the osteocytes may survive the transplantation when adequate vascular anastomosis and graft stability are achieved.

Dell, et al. compared the biological features of repair in nonvascularized and vascularized cortical autograft using a cortical bone graft canine model [27]. The histology of this controlled study showed that nonvascularized cortical grafts demonstrated empty lacunae and necrotic marrow elements at two weeks, but by six and 12 weeks the osteonal repair was quite apparent, with an admixture of necrotic osteons undergoing resorption or being replaced by newly formed bone. At 24 weeks the interstitial lamellae of the grafted bones remained necrotic. On the other hand, the vascularized cortical autografts showed viable osteocytes and normal marrow elements at all intervals, and demonstrated a mixture of regions with focal necrosis and viable bone at two weeks; however, by six and 12 weeks most of the interstitial lamellae in the vascularized grafts were visible with only a few necrotic osteons [27]. At 24 weeks the difference between the vascularized and nonvascularized grafts became less distinct, except the interstitial lamellae of the nonvascularized grafts remained necrotic.

4.2.2.1. Clinical Results

Vascularized cortical autografts have been used in numerous locations for a variety of difficult problems. In 2004 Yajima, et al. reported 20 patients with methicillin-resistant Staphylococcus aureus osteomyelitis and infected nonunion who had been treated with vascularized fibular grafts [17]. The authors described achieving primary union in 85 percent (17 of the 20 patients). The mean time required to obtain radiographic bone union was seven months in the femoral reconstruction group, and six months in the tibial reconstruction group. Marciniak, et al. followed,101 hips (86 patients) with osteonecrosis of the femoral head who had been treated with vascularized fibular grafting for a minimum of five years [21]. The authors showed radiographic evidence of an intact fibular graft at a median of eight-years follow-up in 42 hips (42 percent), while 57 hips (56 percent) had undergone total hip arthroplasty at a mean of three years after grafting. They believed that vascularized fibular grafting might potentially postpone the need for arthroplasty in young patients and offer the possibility of long-term benefits in selected patients. Kim, et al. compared the effectiveness of vascularized fibular grafting with that of nonvascularized fibular grafting for the prevention of progression and collapse of osteonecrotic lesions of the femoral head [20]. The authors showed that vascularized fibular grafting was associated with better clinical results and was more effective than nonvascularized fibular grafting for the prevention of collapse of the femoral head.

The study of clinically failed human cases cannot determine clinical efficacy of a technique in general, but in our evaluation of femoral heads removed at total joint replacement for failed treatment of osteonecrosis, we have had the opportunity to compare several different grafting procedures. In general, our retrieved specimens that received vascularized fibular autograft show histologic features of better incorporation than those that were treated with cortical allograft or with ProOsteon™ (Interpore, Corp) (Fig. 4.1) [1].

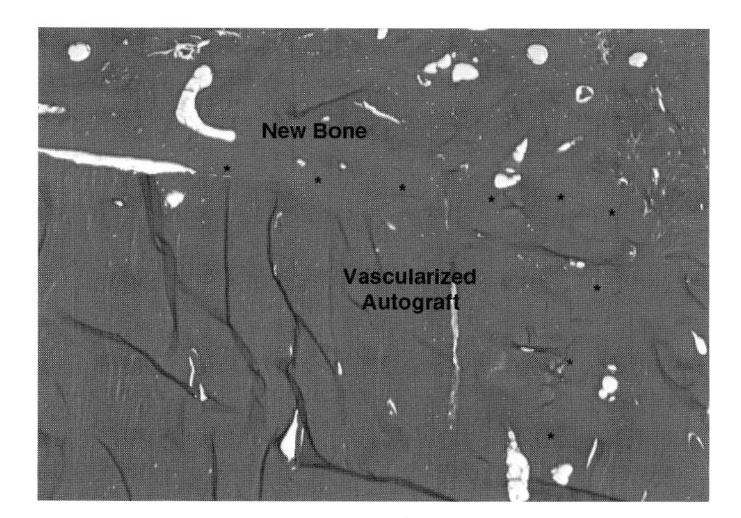

Fig. 4.1 A vascularized fibular autograft used to treat osteonecrosis of the femoral head is shown. Most of the graft is viable one year after implantation, and it has provided an osteoconductive surface for a few areas of new bone formation. The (*) symbols mark the interface between cortical autograft and new bone that has formed in the femoral head (*See Color Plates*)

Rose, et al. reported a retrospective case series of vascularized free fibula transfers for humeral reconstructions after oncologic resection [22]. The authors followed up with their patients for 68 months and showed 13 of the 15 patients went on to bony union, except two patients with asymptomatic fibrous unions. They concluded that vascularized free fibula transfer provided an effective and successful means of limb-preserving reconstruction after oncologic resection of the humerus, although healing time might be prolonged and refracture and other complications commonly were encountered.

Some studies have documented morbidity after harvesting free vascular grafts [25, 28]. For example, Vail and Urbaniak evaluated 247 donor limbs after free vascular fibular grafts to determine the prevalence of morbidity at the donor site and used Kaplan-Meier analysis to estimate the prevalence of each finding for the entire cohort over time [25]. The authors showed at least one of the indicators of morbidity in 47 of the 247 lower limbs (19 percent) at three months postoperatively, and 18 of the 74 limbs (24.3 percent) at five years. Thus, although vascularized cortical autografts work well for selected indications, they can be associated with longer time in the operating room (and, therefore, higher hospital cost) and graft site morbidity.

4.3. Cancellous Autograft

Cancellous autograft is useful in situations where the bone void does not require significant structural support. It can be added to acute fractures and to delayed or nonunion sites to promote healing of defects > 6 cm [13, 29, 30]. Cancellous bone can also be packed into metaphyseal defects, such as in fractures of the tibial plateau, plafond and distal radius [31-32]. Cancellous autograft is also commonly used to promote spinal fusion [33-34], in filling contained defects at revision arthroplasty [35] and in cranio-facial applications [36].

The major source of autogenous cancellous bone is the iliac crest. As noted above, autogenous cancellous bone, properly handled, is considered to be osteogenic [9, 37] and osteoconductive. It is easily revascularized and quickly integrated into the recipient site. It does not provide immediate structural support, but the rapidity with which autogenous cancellous bone stimulates new bone formation often contributes to the early stabilization of a fracture site. Although the graft material is extremely useful, significant morbidity accompanies the harvest procedure [13, 38]. Autograft harvested from other locations is also commonly used, especially in spine surgery (see discussion below).

4.3.1. Clinical Results

Iliac crest autograft can be considered the gold standard source of graft material for many orthopaedic surgeries. Hierholzer, et al. have treated patients with a delayed union or nonunion of a humeral shaft fracture with open reduction and internal fixation with a plate and autologous iliac crest bone graft or demineralized bone matrix allograft [39]. The authors showed osseous union in 100 percent of the 45 patients treated with autologous bone graft, and in 97 percent of the 33 patients treated with demineralized bone matrix, but 20 (44 percent) of the autologous bone graft recipients had donor site morbidity, including prolonged pain in the majority of patients and a superficial infection in one patient. The authors concluded that rigid plate fixation with either autologous cancellous bone graft or demineralized bone matrix could achieve healing of a humeral shaft nonunion, although harvest of the autologous bone graft was frequently associated with complications. Welton, et al. reviewed 47 acetabular reconstructions in 43 patients performed with the use of autologous morselized bone grafts because of acetabular bone stock loss [35]. The authors showed that the overall survival rate of these acetabular reconstructions, with revision as endpoint, was 94 percent at an average follow-up of 12.3 years, and concluded that reconstruction of acetabular bone loss with autologous morselized bone graft could be an attractive technique with a good potential for long-term success.

Iliac crest autograft is also commonly used for spinal surgery [34]. Schiffman, et al. evaluated 63 of 71 patients who underwent anterior lumbar interbody fusion with low profile interbody fusion cages filled with iliac autograft [30]. Their criteria for a successful fusion were lack of motion, anterior bridging bone and lack of lucencies on flexion/extension X-rays and/or contiguous bone through the cage using a thin-cut sagittal computed tomography scan. The authors showed 86 percent fusion rates of the 63 patients by at least 12-month follow-up examination, and 93 percent fusion rates in one-level procedures. The authors suggested that this procedure might be most beneficial for one-level patients.

Many previous studies have demonstrated relatively high complication rates after harvest of iliac crest bone grafts [13, 38], and the morbidity and limitations have motivated the search for bone graft alternatives [1, 13, 40]. Arrington, et al. reviewed 414 consecutive cases of iliac crest bone graft procedures retrospectively [38]. The authors identified 41 (10 percent) minor complications including superficial infections, superficial seromas and minor hematomas, and 24 (5.8 percent) major complications including herniation of abdominal contents through massive bone graft donor sites, vascular injuries, deep infections at the donor site, neurologic injuries, deep hematoma formation requiring surgical intervention,and iliac wing fractures. In a retrospective study of medical records of 88 consecutive patients who had undergone a total of 108 iliac crest bone grafting procedures for the treatment of chronic osteomyelitis, Ahlmann, et al. noted that harvest of a posterior iliac crest bone graft was associated with a significantly lower risk of postoperative complications than harvest of the anterior iliac crest [41].

The histologic features of incorporating cancellous autograft have been well described. For example, in several different types of canine autograft models, Goldberg and Stevenson noted that cancellous autografts were revascularized early, and that ingrowth of host blood vessels marked the beginning of graft resorption [8]. Resorption and new bone formation were seen throughout the interior of a cancellous graft by four weeks after the implantation, and new bone had replaced the majority of the original spongiosa by three months. The majority of cancellous autograft incorporation was completed, and the graft was completely resorbed and replaced by viable new bone by six months after implantation. More recently Togawa, et al. demonstrated histologic evidence of ongoing bone graft incorporation in all of nine patients who underwent core biopsies of tissue within radiographically successful intervertebral body fusion cages that had been packed with autograft obtained from iliac crest [42]. Their biopsies showed new bone formation and osteoid as well as cement (reversal) lines, illustrating the process of bone remodeling within these cages. Blood vessels were also present in all of the biopsies. Another case report showed histologic remodeling of autograft harvested from iliac crest and placed inside a human titanium mesh cage [33]. Many viable cells and normal lamella of trabecular bone were evident inside the mesh cage.

4.3.2. "Locally Harvested" Autograft

Cancellous autograft is most commonly harvested from the iliac crest, but other potential sources of autologous cancellous bone graft include proximal or distal tibia, distal radius, greater trochanter and even the vertebral body [13, 43]. In addition, spine surgeons commonly harvest bits of cancellous and cortical bone from local sources at the time of spine fusion surgery.

Raskin, et al. investigated the option of harvesting bone graft from the ipsilateral distal tibia or calcaneus and concluded that use of autologous bone graft harvested from these sites was a safe and reliable alternative to iliac crest bone graft harvest for operative procedures of the foot and ankle [43]. Shad, et al. reported that the use of local autograft to fill a cage for anterior cervical discectomy and fusion had several theoretical advantages over harvesting autograft from other locations, such as the lack of donor site morbidity [44]. However, to the best of our knowledge, there is no prospective study that compares clinical results or histology of locally harvested autograft with iliac crest autograft for spine fusion. Togawa, et al. evaluated the histology of retrieved, clinically failed intervertebral body fusion cages and showed that the 27 cages that had been packed with local autograft had a mean viable bone area of 38 percent, whereas the 25 cages that had been packed with iliac crest autograft had a mean viable bone area of 51 percent (Fig. 4.2) [45]. Many of the failed intervertebral body fusion cages that had been packed with locally harvested bone in the Togawa study also contained considerable fibrous tissue, fibrocartilage and hyaline cartilage (Fig. 4.3).

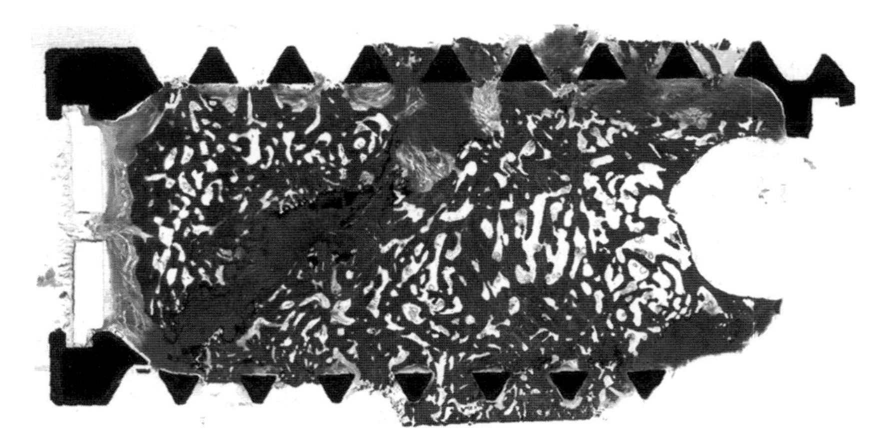

Fig. 4.2 The photomicrograph of histological sections through the center of a clinically failed intervertebral body fusion cage shows incorporated iliac crest autograft (*See Color Plates*)

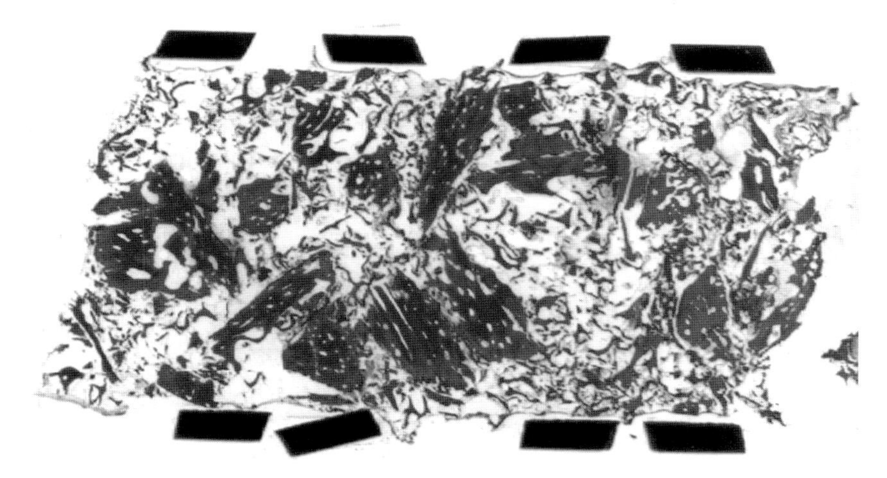

Fig. 4.3 The lower-magnification photomicrograph shows unincorporated iliac crest autograft in a Harms cage that had been used for cervical fusion, but failed shortly after insertion. Although this case was not clinically successful, it illustrates an appropriate combination of cortical and cancellous bone fragments prepared from iliac crest (*See Color Plates*)

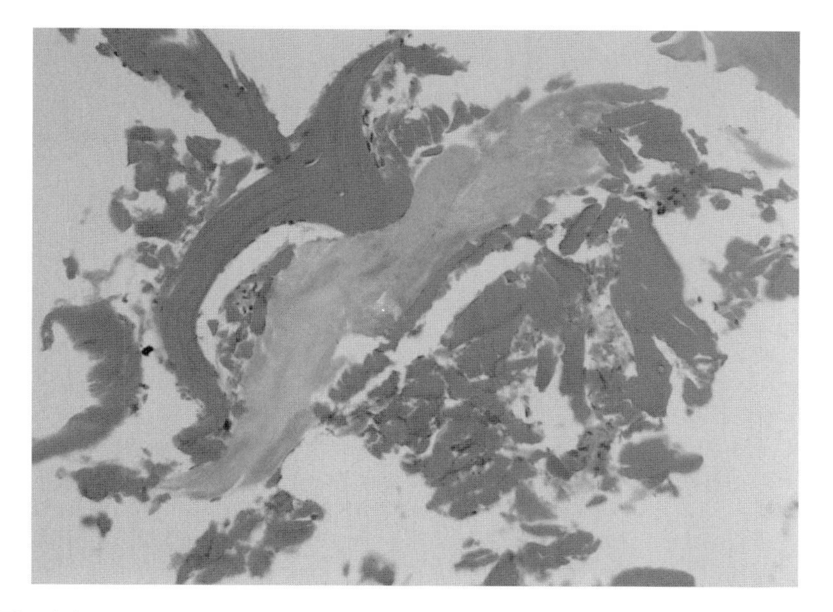

Fig. 4.4 The decalcified section of the shavings of one preparation of locally harvested autograft shows shavings of cancellous bone, almost completely devoid of cells. Fibrous tissue, hyaline cartilage and fibrocartilage were also present in this preparation (*See Color Plates*)

To better understand the variability of locally harvested autograft preparations, we histologically evaluated a sample of autograft that had been harvested, but not inserted into a cage at the time of human spine fusion. This preparation had been collected, milled and washed, as is common practice for some spine surgeons. Decalcified sections showed shavings of cancellous bone, almost completely devoid of cells (Fig. 4.4). Semiquantitative evaluation of multiple tissue blocks showed that only 40 percent of the autograft preparation contained spicules of bone with one dimension greater than 100 um (big enough to contain occasional osteocytes). Thirty percent of the preparation was composed of shavings of bone smaller than 100 um in maximum dimension (and, therefore, almost completely devoid of cells), 15 percent was composed of fibrous tissue, 10 percent was hyaline cartilage of either end plate or facet joint origin and 5 percent was fibrous tissue (Bauer TW and Togawa D, unpublished results). Almost all other cellular elements had been removed by the washing procedures. Many surgeons probably use different methods for harvesting local autograft than those described above, but these findings illustrate the variability likely to be found among locally harvested autograft preparations, and suggest that some preparations will be more biologically active than others. In general, it is desirable for cancellous autograft preparations to contain a few bits of cortical bone (as is the case in iliac crest preparations), and pieces of cancellous bone 1 to 2 mm in size. Although washing to remove fat and fibrous tissue is desirable, washing that removes bone marrow and stromal cells is undesirable.

4.4. Cells and other Autogenous Products

4.4.1. Aspirated Bone Marrow Stromal Cells

Aspirated bone marrow stromal cells are another source of autologous material. Injection of autologous bone marrow has been used to treat nonunion and delayed union of several bones [6, 46]. Connolly, et al. reported that 90 percent of delayed unions of the tibia united after utilization of this technique, and recommended waiting six to 12 weeks after the acute fracture to allow the initial inflammatory reaction and osteoclastic resorption to subside before injecting the autologous bone marrow [47]. Autologous bone marrow has also been proposed for the treatment of osteonecrosis of the femoral head [48-49].

Injection of autologous bone marrow offers several advantages including relatively simple technique and fewer complications at the donor and recipient sites than autograft harvested from the iliac crest [6, 47]. Studies by Muschler, et al. demonstrated that autologous osteogenic stem cell precursors could be harvested from iliac crest marrow and concentrated on autograft cancellous matrix to form a suitable graft substitute [50]. On the basis of these data they recommend that, when bone marrow is obtained with aspiration for use as a bone graft, the volume of aspiration from any one site should not be greater than two milliliters. A larger volume decreases the concentration of osteoblast progenitor cells because of dilution of the bone marrow sample with peripheral blood.

In vitro studies of bone marrow-derived osteoblastic progenitors have helped to define the potential role of these cells. For example, one study demonstrated that bone marrow aspirated from the vertebral body during pedicle screw preparation is comparable with that aspirated from the iliac crest with respect to providing osteogenic progenitor cells [51]. Niikura, et al. reported that cells derived from hemarthrosis caused by intra-articular osteochondral fractures could differentiate into osteoblast lineage *in vitro* [52].

4.4.2. Platelet-Rich Plasma (PRP), Autologous Growth Factor (AGF)

Platelet-rich plasma (PRP) or autologous growth factor (AGF) are autologous sources of platelets and growth factors that have been suggested as possible sources of factors that could be active in bone formation [53-54].

PRP is derived from autologous blood and is defined as a volume of plasma that has a platelet concentration that is typically a five-fold increase (~1,000,000/μl) above physiologic levels [54]. AGF is prepared by a concentration of platelets and has been shown to contain multiple growth factors, including Platelet Derived Growth Factor (PDGF) and TGF-β [55-57]. As far as we know only a few, uncontrolled studies have evaluated the use of AGF to enhance fusion rates in humans undergoing spine fusion. Lowery, et al. presented a retrospective review of 19 cases of anterior and posterolateral spinal fusions using AGF, in combination with autograft and coralline hydroxyapatite [58]. They reported a 100 percent fusion rate based on exploration of five cases, and on plain radiographs of 14 cases. Bose, et al. described a retrospective study of 60 cases of spinal fusion using AGF with autograft and reported a 96 percent fusion rate based on plain radiographs [59]. However, Carreon, et al. noted that AGF failed to increase the fusion rate, compared to autogenous bone graft alone [60]. Weiner, et al. reported that single-level intertransverse fusions showed a 62 percent single-level intertransverse fusion rate in 32 patients using autogenous iliac crest graft augmented with AGF, compared to a 91 percent fusion rate in a group with bone graft alone [61]. To the best of our knowledge, no prospective trials have demonstrated efficacy of PRP, PDGF or AGF, and several animal studies have shown that one preparation of PRP, as well as PDGF, actually inhibit (not stimulate) the new bone that is induced by demineralized bone allograft [62]. Thus, the clinical efficacy of these preparations has yet to be determined.

4.5. Future Trends and Needs

Current trends are to, whenever possible, avoid the morbidity of iliac crest harvesting by using bone graft substitutes, graft extenders or recombinant osteoinductive proteins. Harvested bone marrow stromal cells, sometimes enriched by differential filtration or adhesive properties, are also being used to supplement other graft materials. Future developments will likely include improved methods of inducing cells into osteogenic or chondrogenic differentiation, and using those cells in matrices that have been synthesized for specific clinical applications. We anticipate that in the future, low cost autograft substitutes will be available for selected, "low demand" clinical applications, but that more complex (and probably expensive), composite materials will be needed for more challenging applications. We hope that harvesting large segments of iliac crest, fibula and rib will be unnecessary in the future, but it is likely that components of autograft tissue (e.g., cells and/or growth factors) will be included in bone graft preparations for the foreseeable future.

4.6. Conclusion

Autogenous bone graft remains the gold standard for reconstructive orthopaedic surgery, although the morbidity involved with harvesting adequate iliac crest, rib or fibula is an important potential complication. Various types of other materials are becoming available as substitutes or extenders of bone graft, and will be described in other chapters. Carefully controlled clinical trials will be needed to help determine the most appropriate bone graft/substitute material for each specific clinical application.

References

1. Bauer TW, Muschler GF. Bone graft materials. An overview of the basic science. Clin Orthop Relat Res 2000(371):10-27.
2. de Boer HH. The history of bone grafts. Clin Orthop Relat Res 1988(226):292-8.
3. von Walther P. Wiedereinheilung der bei der Trapanation ausgebohrten Knochenscheibe. Journal der Chirurgie und Augen-Heilkunde 1821;2:571.
4. Albee FH. Fundamentals in bone transplantation. Experiences in three thousand bone graft operations. J Am Med Assn 1923;81:1429-32.
5. Taylor GI, Miller GD, Ham FJ. The free vascularized bone graft. A clinical extension of microvascular techniques. Plast Reconstr Surg 1975;55(5):533-44.
6. Connolly JF, Guse R, Tiedeman J, Dehne R. Autologous marrow injection as a substitute for operative grafting of tibial nonunions. Clin Orthop Relat Res 1991(266):259-70.
7. Connolly J, Guse R, Lippiello L, Dehne R. Development of an osteogenic bone-marrow preparation. J Bone Joint Surg Am 1989;71(5):684-91.
8. Goldberg VM, Stevenson S. Natural history of autografts and allografts. Clin Orthop Relat Res 1987(225):7-16.
9. Burwell RG. Studies In The Transplantation Of Bone. Vii. The Fresh Composite Homograft-Autograft Of Cancellous Bone; An Analysis Of Factors Leading To Osteogenesis In Marrow Transplants And In Marrow-Containing Bone Grafts. J Bone Joint Surg Br 1964;46:110-40.
10. Doi K, Tominaga S, Shibata T. Bone grafts with microvascular anastomoses of vascular pedicles: an experimental study in dogs. J Bone Joint Surg Am 1977;59(6):809-15.
11. Enneking WF, Burchardt H, Puhl JJ, Piotrowski G. Physical and biological aspects of repair in dog cortical-bone transplants. J Bone Joint Surg Am 1975;57(2):237-52.
12. Yu WD, Bernstein RM, Watts HG. Autogenous tibial strut grafts used in anterior spinal fusion for severe kyphosis and kyphoscoliosis. Spine 2003;28(7):699-705.
13. Finkemeier CG. Bone-grafting and bone-graft substitutes. J Bone Joint Surg Am 2002;84-A(3):454-64.
14. Tang CL, Mahoney JL, McKee MD, Richards RR, Waddell JP, Louie B. Donor site morbidity following vascularized fibular grafting. Microsurgery 1998;18(6):383-6.
15. Phemister DB. Treatment of the necrotic head of the femur in adults. J Bone Joint Surg Am 1949;31:55-66.
16. Nelson LM, Clark CR. Efficacy of phemister bone grafting in nontraumatic aseptic necrosis of the femoral head. J Arthroplasty 1993;8(3):253-8.
17. Yajima H, Kobata Y, Shigematsu K, Kawamura K, Kawate K, Tamai S, Takakura Y. Vascularized fibular grafting in the treatment of methicillin-resistant Staphylococcus aureus osteomyelitis and infected nonunion. J Reconstr Microsurg 2004;20(1):13-20.
18. Bae DS, Waters PM, Sampson CE. Use of free vascularized fibular graft for congenital ulnar pseudarthrosis: surgical decision making in the growing child. J Pediatr Orthop 2005;25(6):755-62.
19. Berend KR, Gunneson EE, Urbaniak JR. Free vascularized fibular grafting for the treatment of postcollapse osteonecrosis of the femoral head. J Bone Joint Surg Am 2003;85-A(6):987-93.
20. Kim SY, Kim YG, Kim PT, Ihn JC, Cho BC, Koo KH. Vascularized compared with nonvascularized fibular grafts for large osteonecrotic lesions of the femoral head. J Bone Joint Surg Am 2005;87(9):2012-8.

21. Marciniak D, Furey C, Shaffer JW. Osteonecrosis of the femoral head. A study of 101 hips treated with vascularized fibular grafting. J Bone Joint Surg Am 2005;87(4):742-7.
22. Rose PS, Shin AY, Bishop AT, Moran SL, Sim FH. Vascularized free fibula transfer for oncologic reconstruction of the humerus. Clin Orthop Relat Res 2005;438:80-4.
23. Gabl M, Reinhart C, Lutz M, Bodner G, Rudisch A, Hussl H, Pechlaner S. Vascularized bone graft from the iliac crest for the treatment of nonunion of the proximal part of the scaphoid with an avascular fragment. J Bone Joint Surg Am 1999;81(10):1414-28.
24. Wilden JA, Moran SL, Dekutoski MB, Bishop AT, Shin AY. Results of vascularized rib grafts in complex spinal reconstruction. J Bone Joint Surg Am 2006;88(4):832-9.
25. Vail TP, Urbaniak JR. Donor-site morbidity with use of vascularized autogenous fibular grafts. J Bone Joint Surg Am 1996;78(2):204-11.
26. Arai K, Toh S, Tsubo K, Nishikawa S, Narita S, Miura H. Complications of vascularized fibula graft for reconstruction of long bones. Plast Reconstr Surg 2002;109(7):2301-6.
27. Dell PC, Burchardt H, Glowczewskie FP, Jr. A roentgenographic, biomechanical, and histological evaluation of vascularized and nonvascularized segmental fibular canine autografts. J Bone Joint Surg Am 1985;67(1):105-12.
28. Lee EH, Goh JC, Helm R, Pho RW. Donor site morbidity following resection of the fibula. J Bone Joint Surg Br 1990;72(1):129-31.
29. Ring D, Allende C, Jafarnia K, Allende BT, Jupiter JB. Ununited diaphyseal forearm fractures with segmental defects: plate fixation and autogenous cancellous bone-grafting. J Bone Joint Surg Am 2004;86-A(11):2440-5.
30. Schiffman M, Brau SA, Henderson R, Gimmestad G. Bilateral implantation of low-profile interbody fusion cages: subsidence, lordosis, and fusion analysis. Spine J 2003;3(5):377-87.
31. Berkson EM, Virkus WW. High-energy tibial plateau fractures. J Am Acad Orthop Surg 2006;14(1):20-31.
32. Dickson KF, Montgomery S, Field J. High energy plafond fractures treated by a spanning external fixator initially and followed by a second stage open reduction internal fixation of the articular surface–preliminary report. Injury 2001;32 Suppl 4:SD92-8.
33. Akamaru T, Kawahara N, Tsuchiya H, Kobayashi T, Murakami H, Tomita K. Healing of autologous bone in a titanium mesh cage used in anterior column reconstruction after total spondylectomy. Spine 2002;27(13):E329-33.
34. Chen JF, Wu CT, Lee SC, Lee ST. Use of a polymethylmethacrylate cervical cage in the treatment of single-level cervical disc disease. J Neurosurg Spine 2005;3(1):24-8.
35. Welten ML, Schreurs BW, Buma P, Verdonschot N, Slooff TJ. Acetabular reconstruction with impacted morcellized cancellous bone autograft and cemented primary total hip arthroplasty: a 10- to 17-year follow-up study. J Arthroplasty 2000;15(7):819-24.
36. Tessier P, Kawamoto H, Matthews D, Posnick J, Raulo Y, Tulasne JF, Wolfe SA. Taking bone grafts from the anterior and posterior ilium–tools and techniques: II. A 6800-case experience in maxillofacial and craniofacial surgery. Plast Reconstr Surg 2005;116(5 Suppl):25S-37S; discussion 92S-94S.
37. Heslop BF, Zeiss IM, Nisbet NW. Studies on transference of bone. I. A comparison of autologous and homologous bone implants with reference to osteocyte survival, osteogenesis and host reaction. Br J Exp Pathol 1960;41:269-87.
38. Arrington ED, Smith WJ, Chambers HG, Bucknell AL, Davino NA. Complications of iliac crest bone graft harvesting. Clin Orthop Relat Res 1996(329):300-9.
39. Hierholzer C, Sama D, Toro JB, Peterson M, Helfet DL. Plate fixation of ununited humeral shaft fractures: effect of type of bone graft on healing. J Bone Joint Surg Am 2006;88(7):1442-7.

40. Fujishiro T, Bauer TW, Kobayashi N, Kobayashi H, Sunwoo M, Seim HBr, Turner AS. Histological evaluation of an impacted bone graft substitute composed of a combination of mineralized and demineralized allograft in a sheep vertebral bone defect. JBiomed Mater Res 2007;82A:538–544.
41. Ahlmann E, Patzakis M, Roidis N, Shepherd L, Holtom P. Comparison of anterior and posterior iliac crest bone grafts in terms of harvest-site morbidity and functional outcomes. J Bone Joint Surg Am 2002;84-A(5):716-20.
42. Togawa D, Bauer TW, Brantigan JW, Lowery GL. Bone graft incorporation in radiographically successful human intervertebral body fusion cages. Spine 2001;26(24):2744-50.
43. Raikin SM, Brislin K. Local bone graft harvested from the distal tibia or calcaneus for surgery of the foot and ankle. Foot Ankle Int 2005;26(6):449-53.
44. Shad A, Leach JC, Teddy PJ, Cadoux-Hudson TA. Use of the Solis cage and local autologous bone graft for anterior cervical discectomy and fusion: early technical experience. J Neurosurg Spine 2005;2(2):116-22.
45. Togawa D, Bauer TW, Lieberman IH, Sakai H. Lumbar intervertebral body fusion cages: histological evaluation of clinically failed cages retrieved from humans. J Bone Joint Surg Am 2004;86-A(1):70-9.
46. Hernigou P, Poignard A, Beaujean F, Rouard H. Percutaneous autologous bone-marrow grafting for nonunions. Influence of the number and concentration of progenitor cells. J Bone Joint Surg Am 2005;87(7):1430-7.
47. Connolly JF. Injectable bone marrow preparations to stimulate osteogenic repair. Clin Orthop Relat Res 1995(313):8-18.
48. Gangji V, Hauzeur JP, Matos C, De Maertelaer V, Toungouz M, Lambermont M. Treatment of osteonecrosis of the femoral head with implantation of autologous bone-marrow cells. A pilot study. J Bone Joint Surg Am 2004;86-A(6):1153-60.
49. Hernigou P, Beaujean F. Treatment of osteonecrosis with autologous bone marrow grafting. Clin Orthop Relat Res 2002(405):14-23.
50. Muschler GF, Boehm C, Easley K. Aspiration to obtain osteoblast progenitor cells from human bone marrow: the influence of aspiration volume. J Bone Joint Surg Am 1997;79(11):1699-709.
51. McLain RF, Fleming JE, Boehm CA, Muschler GF. Aspiration of osteoprogenitor cells for augmenting spinal fusion: comparison of progenitor cell concentrations from the vertebral body and iliac crest. J Bone Joint Surg Am 2005;87(12): 2655-61.
52. Niikura T, Miwa M, Sakai Y, Lee SY, Kuroda R, Fujishiro T, Kubo S, Doita M, Kurosaka M. Human hemarthrosis-derived progenitor cells can differentiate into osteoblast-like cells in vitro. Biochem Biophys Res Commun 2005;336(4): 1234-40.
53. Kim ES, Park EJ, Choung PH. Platelet concentration and its effect on bone formation in calvarial defects: an experimental study in rabbits. J Prosthet Dent 2001;86(4):428-33.
54. Marx RE, Carlson ER, Eichstaedt RM, Schimmele SR, Strauss JE, Georgeff KR. Platelet-rich plasma: Growth factor enhancement for bone grafts. Oral Surg Oral Med Oral Pathol Oral Radiol Endod 1998;85(6):638-46.
55. Canalis E, McCarthy TL, Centrella M. Effects of platelet-derived growth factor on bone formation in vitro. J Cell Physiol 1989;140(3):530-7.
56. Howes R, Bowness JM, Grotendorst GR, Martin GR, Reddi AH. Platelet-derived growth factor enhances demineralized bone matrix-induced cartilage and bone formation. Calcif Tissue Int 1988;42(1):34-8.
57. Noda M, Camilliere JJ. In vivo stimulation of bone formation by transforming growth factor-beta. Endocrinology 1989;124(6):2991-4.
58. Lowery GL, Kulkarni S, Pennisi AE. Use of autologous growth factors in lumbar spinal fusion. Bone 1999;25(2 Suppl):47S-50S.

59. Bose B, Balzarini MA. Bone graft gel: autologous growth factors used with autograft bone for lumbar spine fusions. Adv Ther 2002;19(4):170-5.
60. Carreon LY, Glassman SD, Anekstein Y, Puno RM. Platelet gel (AGF) fails to increase fusion rates in instrumented posterolateral fusions. Spine 2005;30(9): E243-6; discussion E247.
61. Weiner BK, Walker M. Efficacy of autologous growth factors in lumbar intertransverse fusions. Spine 2003;28(17):1968-70; discussion 1971.
62. Ranly DM, McMillan J, Keller T, Lohmann CH, Meunch T, Cochran DL, Schwartz Z, Boyan BD. Platelet-derived growth factor inhibits demineralized bone matrix-induced intramuscular cartilage and bone formation. A study of immunocompromised mice. J Bone Joint Surg Am 2005;87(9):2052-64.

5

Biology of Bone Allograft and Clinical Application

Victor M. Goldberg

Abstract: Bone allografts have become an accepted technology to replace bone loss as a result of tumor resection, trauma and failed total joint arthroplasty. Since fresh allograft invokes an immune rejection response, bone is usually processed by freezing or freeze-drying to reduce the immune response. The significance of biological events of incorporation include hemorrhage and inflammation, osteogenesis, osteoinduction, osteoconduction and effective remodeling to become a load bearing structure. The clinical parameters that enhance the chance of successful bone allograft incorporation are adherence to the American Association of Tissue Bank standards, appropriate graft selection for the clinical application, stable graft-host interface and preservation of the surrounding soft tissue and host blood supply. Cancellous allografts are usually completely incorporated, while cortical grafts remain an admixture of viable new bone and necrotic old bone for a prolonged period of time. Massive bone allografts used for reconstruction of the tumor resection have a long term successful outcome in about 80 percent of the procedures. Similar success is reported for its use in total joint revision surgery and other clinical applications.

The major complications reported for grafting procedures are infection, bone graft fracture, nonunion at the graft-host juncture and, rarely, massive allograft resorption. Although bone allografting is a successful procedure, future improved technology to regenerate bone includes the use of adjunctive growth factors, cell based and regional gene therapies. Ultimately tissue engineering techniques may be the most useful approach to regenerate bone.

Keywords: *allografts*, immune, osteoinduction, osteoconduction

---

Department of Orthopaedics, Case Medical Center, Cleveland, OH

From: *Orthopedic Biology and Medicine: Musculoskeletal Tissue Regeneration, Biological Materials and Methods*
Edited by W. S. Pietrzak © Humana Press, Totowa, NJ

5.1. Introduction

Bone allografts were initially used to replace bone and joint loss in tumors, however, during the last decade there has been a dramatic increase in the demand for bone allografts for reconstructing bone deficiencies caused by trauma, congenital abnormalities and, more frequently, as an adjunct to reconstruction in failed joint arthroplasties [1-4]. Bone allografts enjoy significant advantages when compared to autografts [5-6]. These include an unlimited amount of allograft material, no donor site morbidity and mechanical capabilities treating major defects such as pelvic column or proximal femoral loss. Massive osteochondral grafts are not available from autologous sources and host ligaments, muscles and other soft tissues can be re-attached to the allograft for biologic healing to restore stability and function. When allografts are interfaced with prosthetic devices, load sharing with normal translation of forces between the prosthetic implant and the host bone occurs. There are, however, a number of disadvantages to using bone allografts, including potential disease transmission and an unpredictable incidence of complications at the host-donor junction [7]. Allografts are replaced slowly and, therefore, unpredictably by the host bone and this may result in fractures and ultimate failures. Further, because of immunological rejection of fresh bone allografts, the grafts are processed and, therefore, are nonviable in regard to active bone-forming cells [6]. The treatment of massive bone loss with organic material has a definite advantage over synthetic implants. However, bone allografting must be a safe, predictable procedure.

Bone grafts activate a series of partially known biological phenomenon leading to progressive incorporation and through biomechanical loading to adaptive remodeling [8-9]. Bone allografts, whether fresh or processed, do trigger an immune response which has been shown to have an impact on the final clinical outcome [10-12]. It is important to understand the biologic sequence of bone allografting when selecting the appropriate bone graft, so that the surgeon can understand the potential clinical use and outcome of these procedures.

5.2. Basic Science

Bone graft incorporation is a complex physiological process that involves the host and the graft and, ultimately, results in the remodeling of the transplanted tissue in response to biomechanical loading [6, 13]. The success and rapidity of the incorporation depends upon the type of graft, its size, structure and fixation, vascularity of the host bed and its genetic compatibility with the receptor. The sequence of biological events are discrete, prolonged, but do occur in parallel. The biologic events include initial hemorrhage and inflammation, osteogenesis, osteoinduction, osteoconduction and, finally, remodeling. Hemorrhage and inflammation is the initial event in fresh and processed allografts and is similar to autograft; however an immune response may be seen early and, in wide genetic discrepancy, usually results in rapid resorption of the graft [9, 14].

Osteogenesis provided by viable osteocytes is only provided in fresh or vascularized autografts. In fresh allografts within the first 10 to 14 days, the donor cells are killed by the immune response of the host. By contrast, processed allografts, where the osteocytes are not viable, form new bone by providing a passive scaffolding (osteoconduction), or through bone morphogenic proteins (osteoinduction) [15].

Osteoconduction is a physiologic process whereby the bone graft supports the growth of host capillaries, vascular tissue and osteoprogenitor cells. Osteoconduction does not require live cells, but it does provide the appropriate surface to support vascularization and cellular ingrowth [6, 13]. Osteoinduction is the ability of extracellular bone matrix to induce donor osteoprogenitor cells to transform into osteoblasts and form new bone [16]. The differentiation of these cells is controlled by low molecular weight peptides known as bone morphogenic proteins. Demineralized bone provides effective osteoinduction, but does not require viable cells [5, 17].

Remodeling is a complex process influenced by the biology of the allograft and mechanical environment. Allografts incorporate more slowly and incompletely than autografts [18-19]. Morselized processed allografts are usually completely resorbed and replaced by new host bone, but large cortical cancellous allografts may never be completely remodeled, and remain an admixture of necrotic bone with viable host new bone for many years.

The immunogenicity of allografts has been shown to play an important role in successful graft incorporation [8-10, 14, 20]. Although a complete description of the immune responses to bone allografts is beyond this chapter, a summary of the important aspects is critical for the reader to understand the role immunogenicity plays in graft incorporation [12, 14, 21]. The antigens of the major histocompatibility complex (MHC) in humans appear to be principally responsible for recognition of the graft by the host. Class I and II antigens which are encoded by the genes from the MHC are both capable of activating T-cells. Extensive experimental and clinical data suggest that the HLA chromosomal complex is the major determinant of histocompatibility in humans [22]. Animals grafted with allogeneic bone (totally mismatched) show a stronger response than those receiving semi-allogeneic partially mismatched bone allografts, suggesting that the response to fresh bone allografts is directly related to the MHC [8-9]. The cells of all musculoskeletal tissues display Class I MHC antigens and some cells may display Class II antigens. Immune rejection of bone grafts has been shown to be similar to that of rejection for systemic organs [10]. The mechanisms in play include cell-mediated toxicity, antibody-mediated toxicity and antibody-dependent cell-mediated toxicity. Experimental and clinical studies have demonstrated that bone allografts may invoke all of these responses *in vivo*. Studies indicate that matching tissue of the host and modified allografts does reduce immunogenicity and improves allograft incorporation [8-9, 23]. The immune response appears to be directed toward the osteoinduction phase of bone graft incorporation [14].

Preservation of cancellous allografts using freezing or freeze-dried methods has been reported to improve their incorporation [24]. These grafts may be incorporated completely. They are primarily used as filler material for cavitary skeletal defects. Other preservation techniques such as decalcification and demineralization do provide some osteoinduction and osteoconduction, but are not as effective as frozen or freeze-dried methods for bone graft preservation [25].

Since fresh cortical allografts invoke a vigorous immune response, experimental and clinical use of this material has been confined to frozen or freeze-dried cortical allografts. The processing of these allografts by bone banks has insured safety of bone, as well as reducing the transmission of communicable diseases [26]. Central to the incorporation of cortical allografts is the stability of the graft-host junction. Excellent graft-host contact with a stable construct enhances union and incorporation of the bone [27]. Although the sterilization process is important in insuring safety of the bone, studies have demonstrated that radiation of more then 30kGy may destroy any osteoinductive function [28-29].

New preservation methodologies have recently been developed to enhance bone allograft incorporation. These include perforation of the graft which increases the available surface area for ingrowth and ongrowth of new bone, and provides easier access to the intramedullary canal [30-31]. Although the overall strength of these constructs decreases over the first four weeks, during the next four weeks the strength of the grafts returns to that of a non-perforated graft. Other approaches such as chemosterilized, autolyzed and antigenic extracted allogeneic bone provide inductive capabilities, but have little strength [13].

Basic science and preclinical studies have demonstrated that allograft incorporation is a complex process with significant variables that influence the ultimate incorporation and function of the graft. Both biological and mechanical issues are important in determining the clinical outcome for a bone grafting procedure. The well vascularized host bed is critical in providing a satisfactory host environment. Stable fixation and intimate host-bone graft contact is central to the successful incorporation of the bone graft. Bone grafts must be protected from full weight bearing until remodeling allows it to function fully in a loaded environment.

5.3. Clinical Applications

The demand for allograft bone has expanded recently because of the clinical needs to reconstruct bone deficiencies after excision of tumor, severe trauma, congenital abnormalities and reconstruction after failed joint arthroplasties. Although allograft surgery is successful, there are a number of significant complications that can lead to failure of the procedure. The immune response of the host, as previously discussed, may be the primary cause responsible for these complications. The reported complications that cause failure include infections, delayed healing, fractures and significant allograft resorption [2, 7]. Infection rates after major allograft reconstructive procedures have been reported as high as 14 percent [28, 32-33]. The problem does not appear to be the result of transfer of infection with the graft, as long as appropriate guidelines of bone banking are in place. Large structural allografts are more prone to infection because of the presence of large dead spaces and necrotic tissue that remain for a prolonged period of time.

Graft resorption is a major cause of clinical failures and, in hip revision procedures, has been reported as high as 36 percent [34]. Graft resorption may be the underlying cause of nonunion and fractures. It appears that bone resorption is mediated by cytokine production by activated immune cells. Clinical data suggest that antigen mismatching between donor and recipient may cause massive resorption and collapse of large osseous allografts [2, 7, 10]. Nonunions and fractures have been reported to vary from 9 percent to 23 percent [19, 35-36]. The intrinsic stability of the allograft-host bone junction is critical in enhancing bone healing. Intramedullary fixation appears to provide enhanced allograft protection, avoids cortical defects and reduces the opportunity for fractures to occur [37]. Most fractures occur approximately 24 months after implantation of the graft and most have occurred by four years [35]. In order to understand the causes of bone allograft failures, more retrieval analysis must be done with histological markers of immune responses to clarify many of these issues.

There are a number of long-term clinical studies reporting the outcomes of bone allografts used for reconstruction after tumor excision, or as an adjunct in revision total hip or total knee arthroplasty [18, 38-42]. One recent study of 1,082 patients treated for bone tumors with massive bone allografts reported an overall excellent or good result of 77 percent [2]. The initial success rate of the grafting procedure decreased significantly during the first four years, but thereafter graft survival was stable. Intercalary grafts had the best outcome, while alloarthrodesis had the worse. Complications had a significant influence on the ultimate outcome. Patients who ultimately developed an infection at the site of reconstruction only had a success rate of 12 percent.

The outcome of this and other studies using bone allografts in tumor reconstruction have developed guidelines which enhance the chances of a successful outcome [2, 7, 38]. The tissue bank chosen to provide the grafts should be in strict compliance with the standards for bone banking of the American Association of Tissue Banks. Sterility is critical in recovering the tissues and there must be an attempt to preserve the soft tissue attachment sites on the allograft bone. The bone should be catalogued with exact labeling of the type of allograft. There are a number of other critical elements that relate to the success or failure of the graft itself. These include proper sizing and shape of the graft to approximate the skeletal part that requires replacement, careful management and preservation of the soft tissue. The graft must be closely apposed to the host bone and the interface stable with internal fixation when necessary. Unabsorbable sutures should be used to reattach soft tissue to the host tissue. Prophylactic antibiotics during the hospital stay should be utilized as well as oral suppression for several months after the surgery. Careful clinical and radiographic follow-up is critical. If there is slow healing at the host-donor junction by one year, bone grafting utilizing autografts or bone inductive proteins should be considered. Recognition of allograft fractures is absolutely critical to the success of the procedure and can occur up to four years postoperatively. It should be aggressively treated with internal fixation and autogenous bone grafting when necessary. If these principles are followed, the long-term outcome of the bone allograft is successful in 80 percent of patients. However, with the development of improved metallic replacements, more modular type prosthetic devices are being used to reconstruct bone loss after tumor resection. The interaction of bone grafts with these implants has also gained wider use and may be the future, especially in older patients that require bone resection [43].

Much knowledge can be gained in regard to the natural history of bone allografts by studying autopsy retrieval specimens. One study by Enneking and Mindel extensively assessed 16 long-term retrieved specimens [18, 44]. Excellent healing was seen between soft tissues and the allograft surface. If a fracture occurred in the graft it did heal, and there was excellent union of the donor-recipient site when intrinsic stability was provided. The graft itself demonstrated significant areas of remodeling with necrotic bone, but also new viable bone which appeared to be advancing from the host. Other studies have demonstrated similar findings with successful grafts that were retrieved at autopsy [11, 19, 45]. However, when allografts were retrieved because of massive resorption, a significant number of chronic inflammatory cells were present which appeared to be participating in immune reaction to antigens present in the graft. Additional studies of retrieved allografts are important to clarify the role of all variables that affect the clinical outcome of large bone allografts used in tumor reconstruction.

Increasing failures as a result of bone loss from osteolysis particles has made use of allografts more common in revision total hip arthroplasty [4, 34, 42]. Many studies have reported the use of particulate and structural allografts to salvage severe bone loss associated with failed total hip arthroplasties [40, 46-54].

Morselized bone allografts are often used to repair contained acetabular or femoral bone defects at revision surgery [42, 47]. The grafts usually heal and incorporate into the host bone. Recent studies have reported the histological outcome of morselized bone allografts of the proximal femur during revision total hip arthroplasty. There were areas of dead bone surrounded by zones of partially revascularized viable cancellous bone seen throughout the bone allograft (Fig. 5.1).

Structural acetabular allografts are often used when multiple revisions of the acetabulum have led to severe loss of bone stock [50, 55]. Original studies on the use of structural acetabular allografts had not been encouraging [34]. However, recent studies have reported lower failure rates [48]. It has been suggested that the use of a rigidly fixed allograft to the host ilium markedly improves results. In addition, structural allografts used to provide support for acetabular components seem very effective if the graft involves less than 50 percent of the acetabulum, or with allografts supporting some load [4]. Information regarding biologic incorporation of these reconstructions is scarce;

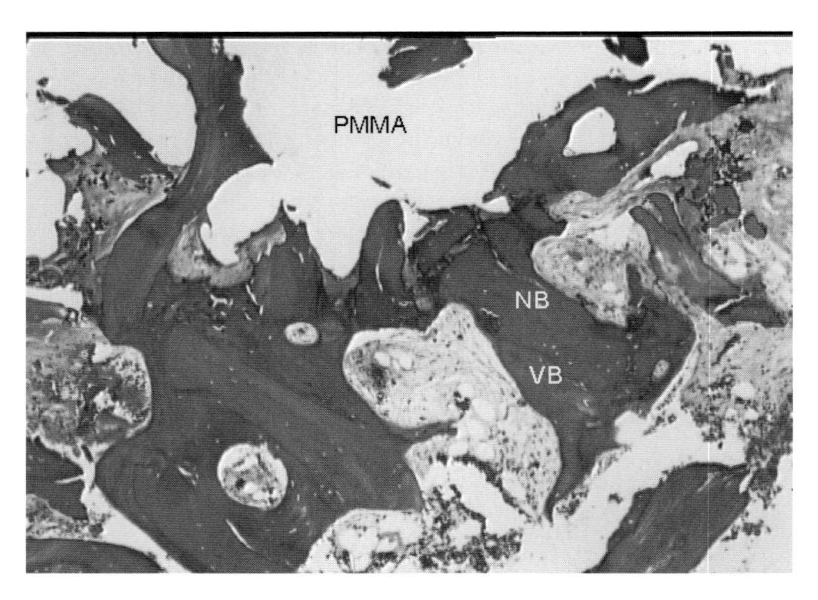

Fig. 5.1 Histological outcome of morselized bone allograft of the proximal femur obtained during revision total hip arthroplasty. Note areas of dead bone surrounded by zones of partially revascularized viable cancellous bone

however, studies have shown evidence of revascularization of allografts six months after surgery [52]. There is some data to indicate that at the time of re-revision the acetabular bone stock was sufficient to support an uncemented socket, suggesting that some bone restoration was achieved.

Cortical strut allografts have been used to restore continuity in a cortex with defects in revision total hip arthroplasty. The histological and mechanical response to these grafts in animals has been well documented [56]. Cortical strut grafts predictably unite to the host femur, remodel, mature and enhance the host bone. Clinical success with this type of allograft has been reported to be as high as 96 percent [53-54]. The main complications of allografts in revision total hip arthroplasty are infection, fracture, resorption and nonunion. Understanding the biology of incorporation of these bioimplants is important to predict, prevent and treat these complications.

The use of bone allografts for reconstructing total knee arthroplasty failures has some different issues when compared to the hip [4, 57]. Tissue and skin coverage, as well as ligament stability, are central when developing an approach to the use of allografts in revision total knee arthroplasty. Composite grafts, including the extensor mechanisms and bone, may be necessary under extreme circumstances [58]. Bone loss about the knee has also been classified [59]. This classification considers the location and extent of the bone defect. Small defects may be filled with morselized allograft and can expect a favorable result. Larger contained defects can also be managed by morselized allograft techniques [60]. Segmental defects usually require a large bone allograft combined with metal augments. Composite bone allograft prosthetic devices are also used with satisfactory outcomes. A number of studies have suggested a survival rate of approximately 70 to 75 percent at 10 years for uncontained defects for many of these challenging revisions [34, 61]. The ultimate success of bone allografts used around the knee is dependent upon the same principles that have been discussed previously for total hip revision. However, it is even more important for the surgeon to pay attention to the soft tissue bed to insure a successful outcome.

Other important areas for the use of bone allografts include spinal fusion and delayed and nonunion of fractures [62-64]. The principles of the application of allografting techniques in these areas is similar to the guidelines as discussed previously. The host bed provides important parameters for the healing of the graft. The local blood supply must be preserved to provide osteoprogenitor cells. Systemic variables also have an effect on the ultimate outcome of the bone allografting technique in these areas. Higher rates of failure have been demonstrated with patients who smoke or have diabetes [3]. Excessive use of nonsteroidal, anti-inflammatory drugs is also reported to have a negative impact on new bone formation [3]. Overall, the success or failure of any bone grafting technique is still influenced by the basic principles: preparation of the fusion bed, mechanical stability of the graft and choice of the appropriate bone grafting material.

5.4. Future Trends and Needs

Autologous bone graft is still the gold standard that provides the essential elements necessary to promote bone repair, namely, osteogenesis, osteoconduction and osteoinduction. However, the supply of autogenous bone is limited and significant morbidity can occur during the harvest. Bone allografts have advantages and disadvantages as previously noted, however, the main limitations include variable osteoinductive potential and the potential for immune response to foreign proteins and transmission of viral diseases. Because of these issues, other approaches to bone reconstitution have been explored [63, 65-67]. The future of bone repair in this century is in the development of effective growth factors such as bone morphogenic proteins, cell-based therapies, gene therapies and finally, as discussed in other areas of this book, tissue engineering and regional gene therapy. Recombinant BMP-2 has been approved by the Food and Drug Administration for anterior fusion of the spine [62, 64, 66]. BMP-7 in a collagen carrier has demonstrated significant efficacy in treating tibial nonunions [66, 68]. This is also approved by the FDA. Unfortunately, these BMPs are expensive and the exact dose required has not yet been defined. Future research in this area requires the identification of additional growth factors and cost-effective carriers.

The use of bone marrow aspirates and the recent identification of osseous osteoprogenitor cells (mesenchymal stem cells) that can differentiate into osteoblasts has been applied in clinical problems [69-71]. The cells are usually aspirated and recovered, purified from the iliac crest and delivered to the site of bone loss. Early data, both preclinical and clinical, suggest efficacy in tibial nonunions and other bone loss problems [6]. There are still a number of questions that require answers including the best delivery vehicle for these cells, the number and purity of the cells, as well as the delivery mechanisms. However, this is an important area of investigation and, combined with tissue engineering strategy, may be a useful approach to treat significant bone loss problems.

Gene therapy strategies are also attractive; however, a great deal of work is required to define the clinical application of this technology [65, 67]. Gene therapy requires a number of components for a successful outcome, including a cDNA that encodes for the specific protein, a vector that mediates entry of the genetic material into the cells, and target cells or tissues capable of transcribing and translating genetic information into protein. Preclinical studies to date have utilized cDNAs in coding osteoinductive growth factors. Some early success has been demonstrated with BMP-2, -7 and -9 in different models to evaluate this approach [72-74]. Gene therapy may be performed either in an *in vivo* or *ex vivo* approach. In the *in vivo* approach the vector with the cDNA is directly implanted into the anatomic site. In the *ex vivo* strategy cells are recovered from the patient, genetically manipulated and then re-implanted into a specific anatomic site. The *in vivo* approach is cost-effective and one step, however, the efficiency of the transfection is quite variable. An advantage of the *ex vivo* approach is that a specific cellular delivery vehicle is identified and the cells are easier to transfect and tissue culture. It is, however, time consuming and may not be cost-effective. Basic science and preclinical studies have demonstrated both approaches can be successful in reconstituting bone defects.

Finally, the interaction of tissue engineering, regional gene therapy and the *in vitro* development of viable large bone constructs is an area of future research [65]. Tissue engineering strategies that have been discussed in this book in other chapters require the development of appropriate cells, matrices and inductive growth factors. The interface of recombinant BMPs, with appropriate cells manipulated by *ex vivo* gene therapy strategies, may be an approach that could be successful. Future research efforts are required to identify the most efficient osteogenic growth factors and carrier combination for the different clinical applications. Gene therapy and its role in enhancing bone repair also requires additional studies. There are a number of other questions that are still outstanding. These include the osteoinductive potential of the BMPs, use of either *ex vivo* or *in vivo* gene therapy strategies, the different cellular delivery vehicle that must be used and, finally, how the carriers affect bone repair in both *ex vivo* and *in vivo* gene approaches. The methods of inducing new bone formation using these advanced technologies are available, but there is much work to be done to identify the systems that will provide the most cost-effective approaches to reconstituting large bone defects as a result of tumor resection, failure of joint replacement and trauma.

5.5. Conclusion

The surgeon, when considering graft options for skeletal reconstruction should evaluate the amount of bone loss, the load requirements and the biologic and biomechanical properties of available grafts. At the time of implantation processed bone allografts are nonviable structures. Biologic events induce a progressive incorporation of the graft, but also a possible immune response against foreign antigens. Because of their lack of viable cells, allografts prompt either an indolent chronic type of rejection or an immunologic state of tolerance in the host. When particulate morselized bone allografts are used to repair contained defects, mechanical strength is irrelevant. On the other hand, when segmental or structural grafts are indicated, the effects of different preservation methods on bone allograft strength should be considered. Risk of infection is decreased with different sterilization techniques, but may have potential biomechanical effects.

Future advances will include methods to preserve allograft viability and cellular and molecular biologic techniques for enhanced graft incorporation. Procedures to modulate the immune response or tissue-specific matching of donor and recipient also must be developed.

References

1. Ottolenghi CE: Massive osteoarticular bone grafts. *J Bone Joint Surg* 1966;48B:646-659.
2. Mankin HJ, Friedlaender GE, Tomford WW: Massive allograft transplantation following tumor resection. In *Bone Grafts and Bone Graft Substitutes*. American Academy of Orthopaedic Surgeons. 2006:39-48.
3. Erulkar JS, Grauer JN, Vaccaro AR et al: Spinal fusion and the role of bone grafts and substitutes. In *Bone Grafts and Bone Graft Substitutes*. American Academy of Orthopaedic Surgeons. 2006:49-56.
4. Long WJ, Trousdale RT: The use of allograft in adult hip and knee reconstruction. In *Bone Grafts and Bone Graft Substitutes*. American Academy of Orthopaedic Surgeons. 2006:57-68.
5. Bauer, TW, Muschler GF. Bone Graft Materials *Clin Orthop* 2000, 371:10-27.
6. Goldberg VM, Akhavan S: Biology of Bone Grafts in *Bone Grafts and Bone Graft Substitutes*. American Academy of Orthopaedic Surgeons. 2006:1-8.
7. Mankin HJ, Horniecek FJ, Gebhardt MC et al: Bone allograft transplantation from *Bone Regeneration and Repair: Biology and Clinical Applications*. Edited by J.R. Lieberman and G. E. Friedlaender, Humana Press Inc., Totowa NJ, 2005, 241-261.

8. Goldberg VM, Gos GD, Heiple KG et al: Improved acceptance of frozen bone allografts in genetically mismatched dogs by immunosuppression. *J Bone Joint Surg* 1984;66A:937-950.
9. Goldberg VM, Bos GD, Powell A et al: The effect of histocompatibility matching on canine frozen bone allograft. *J Bone Joint Surg*, 1983;65A:89-96.
10. Friedlaender GE: Bone allograft: The biological consequences of immunological events. *J Bone Joint Surg* 1991;73A:1119-1122.
11. Muscolo DL, Ayerza MA, Calabrese ME et al: HLA matching, radiographic score, and histologic findings in massive bone allografts. *Clin Orthop* 1996;326:115-126.
12. Muscolo DL, Ayerza MA, Goldberg VM: Allografts in *The Adult Hip* edited by J.J. Callaghan, A.G.Rosenberg and H.E.Rubash. Lippincott-Raven Pub. Philadelphia, Chapter 21, 2006. (in publication)
13. Goldberg VM, Akhavan S: Biology of bone grafts from *Bone Regeneration and Repair: Biology and Clinical Applications*. Edited by J.R. Lieberman and G.E. Friedlaender, Humana Press Inc., Totowa NJ, 2005,57-66.
14. Stevenson S, Horowitz M. Current concepts review. The response to bone allograft. *J Bone Joint Surg* 1992;74A:939-947.
15. Stevenson S, Li XQ, Davy DT et al: Critical biological determinants of incorporation of non-vascularized cortical bone grafts: Quantification of a complex process and structure. *J Bone Joint Surg* 1997;79A:1-16.
16. Reddi AH, Wientroub S, Muthukumaran N: Biological principles of bone induction. *Orthop Clin North Am* 1987;18:207-212.
17. Chakkalakal DA, Strates BS, Garvin KL et al: Demineralized bone matrix as a biological scaffold for bone repair. *Tissue Eng* 2001;7:161-177.
18. Enneking WF, Mindell ER: Observations on massive retrieved human allograft. *J Bone Joint Surg* 1991;73A:1123-1142.
19. Muscolo DL, Ayerza MA, Calabrese ME et al: Long term performance of massive allografts. In: Galante JO, Rosenberg AG, Callaghan JJ, eds. *Total hip revision surgery*. New York: Raven Press,1995;445-460.
20. Friedlaender GE, Strong DM, Tomford WW et al: Long term follow-up of patients with osteochondral allografts: A correlation between immunologic responses and clinical outcome *Orthop Clin North Am* 1999;30:583-590.
21. Albrechtsen D, Moen T, Thorsby E: HLA matching in clinical transplantation. *Transplant Proc* 1983;15:1120-1123.
22. Muscolo DL, Caletti E, Schajowicz F et al: Tissue-typing in human massive allograft of frozen bone. *J Bone Joint Surg* 1987;69A:583-595.
23. Goldberg VM, Powell A, Shaffer JS et al: Bone grafting: Role of histocompatibility in transplantation. *J Orthop Res* 1986;3:389-404.
24. Tomford WW, Thongphasuk J, Mankin HJ et al: Frozen musculoskeletal allografts. *J Bone Joint Surg* 1990;72A:657-663.
25. Gazdag AR, Lane JM, Glaser D et al: Alternatives to autogenous bone grafts: Efficacy and indications. *J Am Acad Orthop Surg* 1995;3:1-8.
26. American Association of Tissue Banks. Standards for Bone Banking. McLean VA. American Association of Tissue Banks, 2001.
27. Vandergriend RA: The effect of internal fixation on healing of large allgrafts. *J Bone Joint Surg* 1990;72A:657-663.
28. Tomford WW: Transmission of disease through transplantation of musculoskeletal allografts. *J Bone Joint Surg* 1995;77A:1742-1754.
29. Loty B, Courpied JP, Tomeno B et al: Bone allografts sterilized by irradiation: Biological properties, procurement and results of 150 massive allografts. *Int. Orthop* 1990;14:237-242.
30. Lewandronski K et al: Improved osteoinduction of cartical bone allografts: A study of the effects of laser perforation and partial demineralization *J Orthop Res* 1997;15(5):748-756.

31. Delloye C et al: Perforations of cortical bone allografts improved their incorporation. *Clin Orthop* 2002;396:240-247.
32. Dick HM, Stauch RJ: Infection of massive bone allografts. *Clin Orthop* 1994;306:46-53.
33. Lord F, Gebhardt MC, Tomford WW et al: Infection in bone allografts. *J Bone Joint Surg* 1988;70A:369-375.
34. Hamadouche M, Oakes DA, Berry DJ: Bone grafting for total joint arthroplasty from *Bone Regeneration and Repair* eds. J. Lieberman and G. Friedlaender, humana Press 2005:263-289.
35. Berry BH, Lord CF, Gebhardt MC et al: Fractures of allografts. *J Bone Joint Surg* 1990;72A:825-833.
36. Thompson RC, Pickvance EA, Garry D. Fractures in large-segment allograft. *J Bone Joint Surg* 1993;75A:1663-1673.
37. Muir P, Johnson KA: Tibial intercalary allograft incorporation: comparison of fixation with locked intramedullary nail and dynamic compression plate *J Orthop Res* 1995;13:132-137.
38. Mankin HJ, Beghardt MC, Jennings LC et al: Long-term results of allograft replacement in the management of bone tumors. *Clin Orthop* 1996;324:86-87.
39. Aho AJ, Ekfors T. Dean PB et al: Incorporation and clinical results of large allografts of the extremities and pelvis. *Clin Orthop* 1994;307:200-213.
40. Blackley HR, Davis AM, Hutchinson CR et al: Proximal femoral allografts for reconstruction of bone stock in revision arthroplasaty of the hip: A nine to fifteen year follow-up. *J Bone Joint Surg* 2001;83A:346-354.
41. Gitelis S. Heligman D, Quill G et al: The use of large allografts for tumor reconstruction and salvage of the failed total hip arthroplasty. *Clin Orthop* 1988;231:62-70.
42. Gross AE, Allen G, Lavoie G: Revision arthroplasty using allograft bone. Instruct Course Lect 1996;45:363-380.
43. Hejna MJ, Gitelis S: Allograft prosthetic composite replacements for bone tumors. *Sem Surg Oncol* 1997;13:18-24.
44. Enneking W, Campanacci D: Retrieved human allografts: A clinicopathological study. *J Bone Joint Surg* 2001;83A:971-986.
45. Gouin F, Passuit N, Verriele V et al: Histological features of large bone allografts. *J Bone Joint Surg* 1996;78B:38-41.
46. Allan DG, Lavoie GJ, McDonald S et al: Proximal femoral allografts in revision hip arthroplasty. *J Bone Joint Surg* 1991;73B:235-240.
47. Elting JJ, Zicat BA, Mikhail WEM et al: Impaction grafting: preliminary report of a new method for exchange femoral arthroplasty. *Orthopedics* 1995;18:107-112.
48. Gill TJ, Sledge JB, Muller ME: The management of severe acetabular bone loss using structural allograft and acetabular reinforcement devices. *J Arthroplasty* 2000;15:1-7.
49. Martin WR, Sutherland CJ: Complications of proximal femoral allografts n revision total hip arthroplasty. *Clin Orthop* 1995;295:161-167.
50. Paprosky WG, Bradford MS, Jablonsky WS: Acetabular reconstruction with massive acetabular allografts. Instruc Course Lect 1996;45:149-159.
51. Somers JFA, Timperley AJ, Norton M et al: Block allografts in revision total hip arthroplasty. *J Arthroplasty* 2002;17:562-568.
52. MacDonald SJ, Mehin R: Acetabular revision: Structural Grafts. In *Advanced Reconstruction Hip*. Eds. J. Lieberman, D. Berry, AAOS 2005, 335-342.
53. Emerson RH Jr, Malinin TI, Cuellar AD et al: Cortical strut allografts in the reconstruction of the femur in revision total hip arthroplasty: A basic science and clinical study. *Clin Orthop Relat Res* 1992;285:35-44.
54. Gross AE, Hutchison CR, Alexeeff M et al: Proximal femoral allografts for reconstruction of bone stock in revision arthroplasty of the hip. *Clin Orthop Relat Res* 1995;319:151-158.

55. Garbuz D, Morsi E, Gross AE: Revision of the acetabular component of a total hip arthroplasty with massive structural allograft. Study with a minimum five-year follow-up. *J Bone Joint Surg* 1996;78A:693-697.
56. Burchardt H, Busbee G, Enneking W: Repair of experimental autologous grafts of cortical bone. *J Bone Joint Surg* 1975;57A:814.
57. Bradley GW: Revision total knee arthroplasty by impaction bone grafting. *Clin Orthop Relat Res* 2000;371:113-118.
58. Burnett RSF, Berger RA, Della Valle CJ et al: Extensor mechanism allograft reconstruction after total knee arthroplasty. *J Bone Joint Surg* 2005;87A:175-194.
59. Engh GA, Rorabeck CH: Revision total knee arthroplasty. Baltimore MA. Williams and Wilkins, 1997.
60. Heyligers IC, van Haaren EH, Wuisman PI: Revision knee arthroplasty using impaction grafting and primary implants. *J Arthroplasty* 2001;16:533-537.
61. Clatworth MG, Balance J, Brick GW et al: The use of structural allograft for uncontained defects in revision total knee arthroplasty. A minimum five-year review. *J Bone Joint Surg* 2001;83A:404-411.
62. Boden SD, Kang J, Sandhu H et al: Use of recombinant human bone morphogenetic protein-2 to achieve posterolateral lumbar spine fusion in humans. A prospective, randomized clinical pilot trial. *Spine* 2002;27:2662-2673.
63. Lieberman JR, Daluiski A, Einhorn TA: The role of growth factors in the repair of bone: Biology and clinical applications. *J Bone Joint Surg* 2002;84A:10312-10344.
64. White AP, Weinstein MA, Patel TCh et al: Lumbar arthrodesis gene expression: A comparison of autograft with osteogenic protein-1. *Clin Orthop* 2004;429: 330-337.
65. Lieberman JR, Gamradt S: Novel bone repair options in the 21st century. In *Bone Grafts and Bone Graft Substitutes*. American Academy of Orthopaedic Surgeons 2006;69-80.
66. Einhorn TA: Clinical applications of recombinant human BMPs: Early experience and future development *J Bone Joint Surg* 2003;85A(supp 3):83-88.
67. Scadoto AA, Lieberman JR: Gene therapy for osteoinduction. *Orthop Clin North Am* 1999;30:625-633.
68. Friedlaender GEW, Perry CR, Cole JD et al: Osteogenic protein-1 (bone morphogenetic protein-7) in the treatment of tibial non-unions. *J Bone Joint Surg* 2001;83A(suppl 1):151-158.
69. Solchaga LA, Goldberg VM: Bone marrow and bone marrow products as osteogenic aids for bone repair. In *Bone Grafts and Bone Graft Substitutes*. American Academy of Orthopaedic Surgeons 2006:33-38.
70. Bruder SP, Fink DJ, Caplan AI: Mesenchymal stem cells in bone development, bone repair and skeletal regeneration therapy. *J Cell Biochem* 1994;56:283-294.
71. Bruder SP, Kraus KH, Goldberg VM et al: The effect of implants loaded with autologous mesenchymal stem cells on the healing of canine segmental bone defects. *J Bone Joint Surg* 1998;80A:985-996.
72. Dragoo JL, Choi JY, Lieberman JR et al: Bone induction by BMP-2 transduced stem cells derived from human fat. *J Orthop Res* 2003;21:622-629.
73. Hannallah D, Peterson B, Lieberman JR et al: Gene therapy in orthopaedic surgery. Instr Course Lect 2003;52:753-768.
74. Want JC, Kanim LE, Yoo S et al: Effect of regional gene therapy with bone morphogenetic protein-2 producing bone marrow cells on spinal fusion in rats. *J Bone Joint Surg* 2003;85A:905-911.

6

Demineralized Bone Matrix: Maximizing New Bone Formation for Successful Bone Implantation

Lloyd Wolfinbarger Jr.[1], Liisa M. Eisenlohr[1], and Katrina Ruth[2]

Abstract: The bone scaffold formed by ground cortical bone and cancellous chips creates the favorable environment required for bone-forming cells to be able to generate new bone; this property is called osteo*conductivity*. The demineralization of bone matrix exposes bone morphogenetic proteins (BMPs) and other bone growth promoting factors. Because of this, demineralized bone matrix (DBM) not only provides a scaffold for bone formation – meaning it is osteoconductive – but it also promotes differentiation of precursor cells into viable bone-forming cells, a process termed as osteo*inductivity*. It is important to emphasize that DBM can be osteoconductive without being osteoinductive and that more new bone formation does not necessarily equate to increased osteoinductivity. It is one thing to induce cells to differentiate along an osteoprogenitor pathway and quite another to cause the formation of new bone at an implant site. This chapter provides an overview of the various aspects that are important to the induction of new bone formation by DBM and examines the basic science behind the preparation of demineralized bone.

Various bioassays, both *in vivo* and *in vitro*, have been developed to measure the osteoinductive potential of ground demineralized bone products. The methodology and application of each assay are discussed, as are the effects of processing conditions, including sterilization, on the osteoinductivity of DBM.

Keywords: Demineralized bone matrix, DBM, demineralized freeze-dried bone allograft, DFDBA, bone morphogenetic protein, BMP, osteobiologic, osteoconductivity, osteoinductivity

---

[1]LifeNet Health, Virginia Beach, VA
[2]Smith and Nephew, Inc., Memphis, TN

From: *Orthopedic Biology and Medicine: Musculoskeletal Tissue Regeneration, Biological Materials and Methods*
Edited by W. S. Pietrzak © Humana Press, Totowa, NJ

6.1. Introduction

As early as 1889, the surgeon Nicholas Senn [1] reported using demineralized bone as a vehicle for the delivery of antiseptics in the treatment of bone cavities. In the 20th century, Leriche and Policard [2], Levander [3], LaCroix [4], and Huggins and Reddi [5, 6] established themselves as pioneers in the field of induced bone formation. The first unequivocal demonstration of matrix-induced bone formation was by Marshall Urist in 1965 for which he used preparations of allogeneic bone matrix implanted in muscle [7].

Due to its remarkable regenerative ability, bone is one of the most frequently implanted tissues in humans [8] and is routinely used for the repair of skeletal defects caused by trauma, neoplasia, and infection. Demineralized bone matrix (DBM), also commonly known as demineralized freeze-dried bone allograft (DFDBA), in particular is widely used in the repair of pathologies associated with trauma, skeletal defects, and periodontal diseases. Ground demineralized bone is, therefore, now widely available from commercial sources.

This chapter provides an overview of the various aspects important to the formation of new bone by DBM and examines the basic science behind the preparation of demineralized bone. The methodology and application of bioassays developed to measure the osteoinductive potential of ground demineralized bone products are discussed, as are the effects of processing conditions, including sterilization, on the osteoinductivity of DBM.

6.2. Remodeling in Demineralized Bone

Bone is a dynamic biological tissue composed of metabolically active cells that are integrated into a rigid framework [9]. Notably, the cellular and molecular events governing bone formation in the fetus, healing of a fractured bone, and induced bone remodeling after graft implantation all follow a virtually identical pattern. Bone fractured during life is repaired by a process involving osteoclasts attaching to the bone fragments, secreting acid to solubilize the mineral components of those bone fragments and proteolytic enzymes to digest the non-mineral components of those bone fragments. During the course of this cell-mediated demineralization, bone-forming cells (osteoblasts) or osteoprogenitor cells (cells capable of differentiating into osteoblast cells) are attracted to sites of demineralization whereupon these bone-forming cells begin to repair the damaged bone through new bone formation. It now seems obvious that if one wishes to promote the repair of bone in an individual, one only needs to demineralize bone and implant it at the site where new bone formation is desired. It is this simple observation that has led to what is now a considerable industry dedicated to the provision of demineralized bone-based materials for use in clinical pathologies to repair damaged bone. Under optimal circumstances, demineralized bone implantation replicates the stages of healing and remodeling outlined in Table 6.1 which recapitulates the process of natural bone formation [10].

Bone metabolism is regulated continually by a host of hormones and cellular factors. Among them are a series of proteins known as growth factors which are released from platelets, macrophages, and fibroblasts to act as signaling agents for other cells involved in bone formation and healing. These very specialized factors function as part of a vast cellular communications network to influence

Table 6.1 Stages of bone healing and remodeling [10]

Stage		Description	Development
Early Inflammatory Stage	I. Induction	Formation of hematoma at fracture site, triggering release of growth factors and cytokines	Immediate
	II. Inflammation	Recruitment of inflammatory cells, macrophages, and fibroblasts to the injury site under prostaglandin mediation	First two days
Repair Stage	III. Cartilage formation	Mitosis of mesenchymal cells and differentiation to chondrocytes; hypertrophy of chondrocytes and calcification; deposition of extracellular collagenous matrix; local angiogenesis	Day two to 18
	IV. Woven bone formation	Differentiation of osteoblasts; mineralization of extracellular matrix	Day 10 to week 16
Remodeling Stage	V. Lamellar bone formation	Bone resorption, remodeling, formation of lamellar bone, and hematopoietic marrow.	Months to years

Adapted from Kalfas, 2001 [9] and Rengachary, 2002 [10]

actual cell division, matrix synthesis, and tissue differentiation. They can induce mesenchymal-derived cells such as monocytes and fibroblasts to migrate, proliferate, and differentiate into bone cells. These growth factors include fibroblastic growth factors, insulin-like growth factors, platelet-derived growth factors, transforming growth factors, and bone morphogenetic proteins [9, 11].

Under optimal conditions for bone grafting, bone morphogenetic proteins (BMPs) are unlocked from bone matrix and exposed in order to engage in the process of osteoinductive new bone formation. This occurs, for example, during demineralization of ground bone particles to DBM. BMPs are members of the transforming growth factor-β (TGF-β) superfamily of glycoproteins, with more than a dozen individual BMP isoforms identified to date [12, 13]. By stimulating mesenchymal cells to differentiate into bone cells, BMP molecules – primarily isoforms 2, 4 and 7 – play a critical role in bone healing [14]. Marshall Urist first recognized the concept of induced new bone formation in 1965 [7] when he observed that a new ossicle had formed after implantation of demineralized bone matrix in a muscle pouch in the rat. Urist termed this phenomenon as the "bone-induction principle," later changing the name to bone morphogenetic protein when he identified the protein responsible for the effect. In 1988, Wozney and colleagues [15] determined the genetic sequence of BMP, which led to the discovery of its various isoforms. Based on this genetic information, it is now possible to produce various BMPs utilizing recombinant gene technology [14]. These proteins have already begun to form the basis for therapeutic applications that will advance the science of osteobiologics.

6.3. Methods for Measuring Osteoinductivity in Demineralized Bone

Numerous bioassays have been developed to assess the osteoinductive potential of ground demineralized bone products, and the ideal assay would allow the accurate prediction of the efficacy of the final product in clinical use for quality control purposes [16]. Bioassays that have been established for the evaluation of osteoinductive potential of ground demineralized bone include the following [8, 16, 17, 18, 19, 20, 21]:

- *In vitro* quantitative BMP ELISA assay
- *In vitro* alkaline phosphatase activity assay
- *In vivo* remineralization assay
- *In vivo* histology assay
- *In vivo* micro-CT analysis

Honsawek and colleagues [18] were able to demonstrate a correlation between the *in vitro* assay of extractable BMP-4 in demineralized bone matrix and more widely accepted assays for osteoinductivity and new bone formation. In this quantitative assay, the ground demineralized bone is solubilized using a proteolytic enzyme such as collagenase and the extractable BMP content determined using a standard, commercially available sandwich enzyme-linked immunosorbent assay (ELISA). In this particular study, extractable levels of BMP-4 were chosen for quantitation, although the levels of other BMPs such as BMP-2 and BMP-7 have been evaluated as well [21]. Although this assay method obviously does not ensure measurement of active protein only, the quantity of measured extractable BMP-4 paralleled the potential of DBM for new none formation as determined by the *in vivo* mouse bioassay. It is probable that the *in vitro* quantitative BMP ELISA assay method will be used in future studies in the determination of extractable quantities of a variety of BMP isoforms and detection of changes in the ratios of the different isoforms of BMP in bone between the various developmental stages of the individual.

A further *in vitro* assay, the alkaline phosphatase activity assay, makes use of the observation that increased levels of alkaline phosphatase (ALP) activity are found in areas of greater osteogenesis, a result of higher osteoblast activity [22]. Rehydrated demineralized ground bone is incubated with mammalian cells under cell culture conditions; non-demineralized ground bone is used as a control. ALP activity is then measured in the extracts of the cells using a standard protein assay to normalize the ALP activity to cell protein concentrations [19]. In cells induced to differentiate toward a chondroblastic or osteoblastic phenotype by the ground demineralized bone, levels of ALP activity will typically increase after three to five days, depending on whether the cells were of fibroblast or periosteal origin.

Attempts have been made to use increased cellular proliferation as a means to measure the presence or absence of growth and differentiation factors in demineralized bone in *in vitro* bioassays [23]. Although the presence of mitogenic factors (i.e., growth factors that stimulate cell proliferation) is likely to be of importance to the overall clinical utility of demineralized bone preparations, it is the differentiation factors (i.e., BMPs) that are presumed to be the most essential element of the bone-forming properties of DBM. In this regard, it should be noted that the doubling time of less differentiated cell populations such as fibroblasts is generally between 10 and 12 hours. The doubling time of osteoblastic cells, in contrast, typically lies at 35 to 40 hours. It might be expected, therefore, that proliferation of a population of less differentiated cells exposed to differentiation factors would decline over time as the cells are induced to differentiation along the osteogenic or chondrogenic lineage. Based on this premise, *in vitro* bioassays that intend to correlate increased cell proliferation with BMP activity will result in unexpected outcomes.

Zhang et al. [8, 17] have utilized the *in vitro* alkaline phosphatase activity assay as a means to study the proliferation and differentiation effects of commercially available DBM on cultured human periosteal (HPO) cells and fibroblasts derived from neonatal foreskin. HPO cells were chosen for study since osteoprogenitor cells found in areas of bone repair are often recruited from periosteal tissue; however, fibroblast cells work equally well and are more readily available in most laboratories. It is critical to limit the volume percent of fetal calf serum used in *in vitro* cell culture assays as growth and differentiation factors inherent to the serum can obscure the factors in demineralized bone preparations.

Alkaline phosphatase activity in confluent cell cultures of HPO cells exposed to DBM reached peak levels on day five of DBM treatment. In addition, a dose response study was conducted by incubating confluent cultures of HPO cells with a range of DBM amounts. Cultures receiving quantities of 5 to 10 mg of DBM exhibited the highest levels of ALP activity in cell extracts [8]. Results indicate that the addition of excessive quantities of DBM to the *in vitro* bioassay may have a detrimental effect on the culture cells; therefore, an optimal range should be established when utilizing this bioassay.

In vivo bioassays currently constitute the most commonly used assays for assessing the osteoinductive and bone-forming properties of demineralized bone. Two approaches are well published, the *in vivo* remineralization assay and the *in vivo* histology assay [8, 17]. In both bioassays, rehydrated demineralized ground bone is implanted into subdermal or muscle pouches of athymic (nude) mice or rats with the objective of stimulating new bone formation in the implant. The use of athymic mice or rats as xenogeneic models with human DBM overcomes problems of species limitations [24].

The sample is explanted and trimmed of excess soft tissue 28 to 35 days after implantation. In the case of the *in vivo* remineralization assay, the dried sample is ashed or solubilized in acid and the calcium content measured spectrophotometrically. The calcium content is expressed as the weight percent calcium of the explanted sample compared to the weight percent calcium of the original implanted material. The weight percent calcium of the original and explant samples are calculated using the following formula: calcium content / dry weight of the sample × 100 = weight percent calcium. The benefit of this analysis is that the entire explanted sample is measured. The limitation is that chondrocytes, precursors to the osteoblast lineage, do not contribute to the calcium content and the mineral content may be due to dystrophic calcification rather than mineralization of newly formed bone.

For the *in vivo* histology assay, samples are fixed for the preparation of histology slides. Histological evaluation requires the expertise of a skilled histologist or pathologist who, using histomorphometric methods, assigns the sample with a numeric value indicative of the amount of new bone formation in the sample. These values, usually expressed as percent new bone formation, can be conveyed relative to the cross-sectional area of the implanted demineralized bone or to the total cross-sectional area of the histological preparation assessed. The benefits of this method include the ability to visualize the cellular interactions with the implant material and make other observations of note (e.g., extent of angiogenesis and proximity of new bone growth to implanted material). The limitation is that several sections throughout the explanted material must be evaluated to ensure that an accurate representation is achieved.

Increasingly, researchers are utilizing micro-computed tomography (micro-CT) analysis to reap the benefits of both assessment methods, quantification of mineral content and three-dimensional (3-D) imaging of the entire sample [20]. This analytical tool remains cost prohibitive for commercial DBM providers to utilize as a screening tool for osteoinductivity, however.

In studies performed by Zhang and colleagues [8, 17] the primary *in vivo* assay methods were evaluated using commercially available human DBM. The site chosen for sample implantation showed a marked effect on the osteoinductivity of DBM. Calcium content of the explants as measured using the *in vivo* remineralization assay was used as the indicator of osteoinductivity/new bone formation in these studies. The increase in calcium content was higher in samples implanted in muscle pouches than subcutaneous pouches of the athymic mouse (increases of 10.0 ± 0.4 and 1.62 ± 0.27 weight percent of explant, respectively). The remineralization assay measures mineral deposition in the implanted materials over time, however, and is for that reason less reliable as a marker of induced new bone formation than the histological assessment method.

Calcium accumulation in the implanted sample increased in an approximately linear fashion over the course of the 35-day study. Day 28 was chosen as the time point of highest calcium accumulation attributable to remineralization without a considerable increase in dry weight due to mineral disposition as part of new bone formation [8]. This finding was corroborated by the results of the histological evaluation of the corresponding sample of the bilateral implants. Initial new bone formation was clearly visible and most of the cartilage was replaced by new bone with a significant rate of calcium deposition by day 28.

In a dose response study using a range of implanted DBM amounts in the athymic mouse model, the highest level of osteoinductivity (i.e., the greatest increase in calcium content) was obtained with 20 mg of DBM, correlating the results achieved with the *in vitro* alkaline phosphatase activity assay described previously [8]. Although the *in vivo* and *in vitro* assays measure different processes, they both have common features associated with the response of cells to demineralized ground bone. As shown in Fig. 6.1, a relationship between

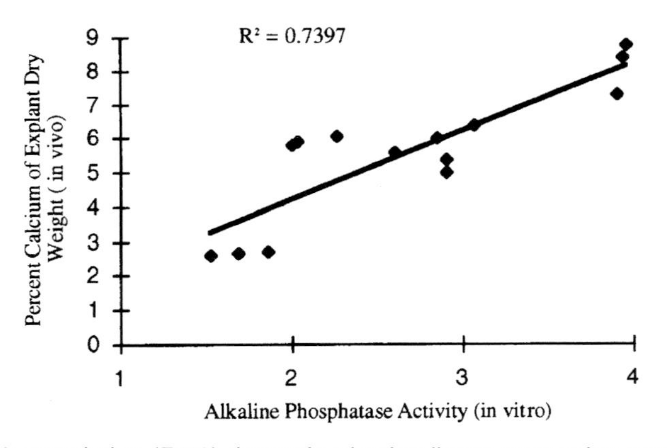

N = 14; correlation (74%) determined using linear regression analysis

Fig. 6.1 Correlation of ALP activity in HPO cells in *in vitro* alkaline phosphatase activity assay and calcium content of explanted DBM in *in vivo* remineralization assay [8]. ALP activity is expressed as units of enzyme (μmole p-nitrophenyl/min/mg protein)

ALP activity in the *in vitro* assay and the change in remineralization in the *in vivo* assay is evident. Although the *in vitro* and *in vivo* assays measure inherently different events, they possess common features associated with apparent response of cells to demineralized bone.

The widely used method of histological evaluation of bone formation in the *in vivo* histology assay is based on subjective estimation of the cross-sectional area of a sample in which bone formation has occurred. Attempts have been made to introduce some level of quantification through histomorphometric procedures; however, considerable differences remain in the way induced new bone formation is reported in published articles and technical reports. Individuals evaluating claims for the osteoinductivity of DBM preparations should be aware of these differences.

Utilizing the intramuscular DBM implantation protocol in the athymic mouse model, various groups report the amount of induced new bone formation as being as much as 100% to as little as 5% for equivalent ground demineralized bone material. Some groups compare induced new bone growth in a demineralized ground bone explant to a sample that has previously been shown to be osteoinductive. Explants that contain as much bone material as the control sample are said to be 100% osteoinductive. Other groups, in contrast, report the amount of new bone formation as a percentage of the cross-sectional area of the observed histological section of the explant. As the original implanted DBM particles usually occupy approximately 60% to 80% of the area of the histological section, quantitative histomorphometry rarely yields new bone values approximating 100%. For example, if one-half of the area that does not constitute the original implanted DBM (i.e., the remaining 40% or 20% of area, respectively) presents as new bone growth, this can be reported as 50% or as 10% (i.e., one-half of 40% or one-half of 20%), depending primarily on the packing density of the DBM particles or how the baseline of new bone formation is calculated. Clearly, the manner in which new bone formation is characterized has a significant impact on how the osteoinductive potential of a DBM preparation is perceived.

In light of the above observation, the quantifiable, more precise, and less time-consuming *in vitro* alkaline phosphatase activity assay is a good option for assessing osteoinductive potential of DBM, particularly when production and distribution of DBM for clinical use dictates rapid analysis. It is important to note, however, that although the *in vivo* rodent bioassay is perceived as the more comprehensive assessment, the ability of DBM to stimulate new bone formation in a muscle site has not been correlated with clinical outcomes.

6.4. Extent of Demineralization and Particle Size Affect Osteoinductivity Assessments

An unaddressed point in the assessment of the osteoinductive and/or osteoconductive potential of commercially available DBM is the likelihood of variability in bone obtained from different donors and generated using different processing methods. In both animal models and clinical studies, it has been suggested that the osteoinductivity of demineralized bone is primarily due to bone morphogenetic proteins and other noncollagenous proteins contained in the matrix [10, 13, 14, 25]. The role of the bone matrix itself should, however, not be disregarded. The hydroxyapatite component of bone may hinder the bioavailability of growth and differentiation factors such as BMP [17, 26]. Similarly, physical characteristics of DBM such as particle size, demineralization process, and other factors such as the age of the tissue donor and the recipient have also been suggested to affect the osteoinductivity and bone formation ability of demineralized ground bone [17, 27, 28].

6.5. Methods for Demineralizing Bone

Demineralized bone is defined by the American Association of Tissue Banks (AATB) as bone containing no more than 8% residual calcium as determined by a standard method [29]. Ground bone is demineralized by either stirring in acid with frequent changes of the acidic solution or stirring in large volumes of acid with no changes of the solution. In a third alternative the acid flows in a continuous stream through a device designed to retain the ground bone particles. With this latter technology ground bone is placed in a demineralization chamber and dilute hydrochloric acid is pumped through the chamber at a controlled flow rate that maintains continuous solubilization of the mineral phase of the bone. This process can be automated and the system closed to minimize the risk of contamination [16]. The continuous flow demineralization process has been further enhanced by "pulsing" the ground bone rapidly with acid, which improves the speed of the demineralization process and results in controlled residual calcium levels, but requires the validation of individual nomagrams for the pulsing processes.

The demineralization process utilizes one or more acid solutions at concentrations sufficient to extract bone mineral. Relatively strong acids such as hydrochloric acid may be used at a concentration of between approximately 0.1 and 3.0 N, while relatively weak acids including citric acid may be used at a concentration of between approximately 0.5 and 5.0 M. Typically, ground bone is demineralized using 0.5 to 0.6 N hydrochloric acid. Weak acids may be used in combination with strong acids to provide a demineralization solution with a specific pH, and the acid may be dissolved in solutions containing surfactants including anionic, cationic, and nonionic detergents as well as alcohol, defoamers, and buffers.

Hydroxyapatite, which constitutes the primary mineral component of bone tissue, is soluble only at pH values below approximately four. As it is exposed to dilute acid, hydroxyapatite dissolves and the resulting calcium phosphate eventually buffers the acid. Once the pH value rises above four, the demineralization process virtually ceases. Early demineralization efforts required frequent acid changes, leading to a greatly increased chance of contamination. Furthermore, poor control of the process had a detrimental effect on the activity of growth and differentiation factors in the bone matrix and did not always result in uniform demineralization or residual calcium contents.

6.5.1. Grinding

Prior to demineralization, the bone designated to be processed into DBM is typically ground using impact fragmentation or bone milling technology. The method by which bone is ground influences particle size range and geometry (Fig. 6.2) and affects the particle size and shape in the final product. Particle

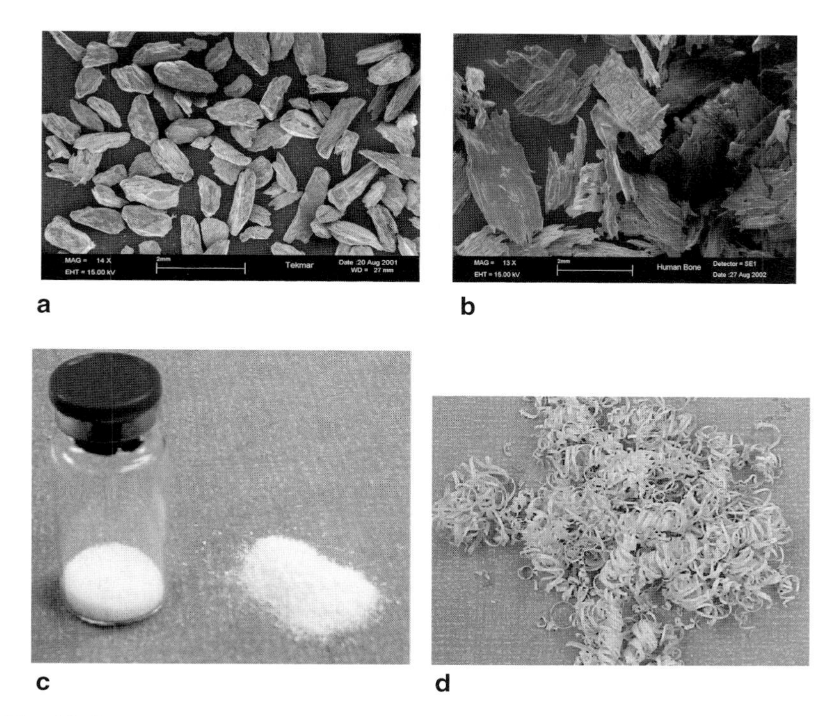

Fig. 6.2 Scanning electron photomicrograph of ground demineralized bone, 250 to 710 micrometer particle size range **(a)** and fiber bone **(b)**, and photographs of samples of demineralized ground bone particles **(c)** and cortical bone fibers **(d)**

size and shape have a significant impact on packing geometry, which is one of the central elements that contribute to the osteoconductive potential of ground demineralized bone. Alternatively, cortical bone may be shaved (skived) to produce bone fibers whose dimensions are determined by the length of bone shaft used, width of cutter, and angle of cutter teeth. These bone shavings may also be demineralized and provide a favorable geometry for osteoconduction and/or osteoinduction.

6.5.2. Demineralization

The rate of demineralization, that is, the grams of mineral solubilized per minute per unit mass of bone, can be increased or decreased as desired by varying numerous factors which include:

- Reaction temperature
- Concentration or normality of the acid solution
- Neutralization potential of the acid used (strong or weak)
- Volume of acid solution to the weight of bone
- Dissociation rate of the acid
- Delivery rate of the acid
- Acid solution exchange frequency
- Mass, volume, and density of the bone tissue to be demineralized
- Concentration of the hydroxyapatite in the bone
- Degree to which the bone has been cleaned of lipids and protein
- Surface area of the bone particles

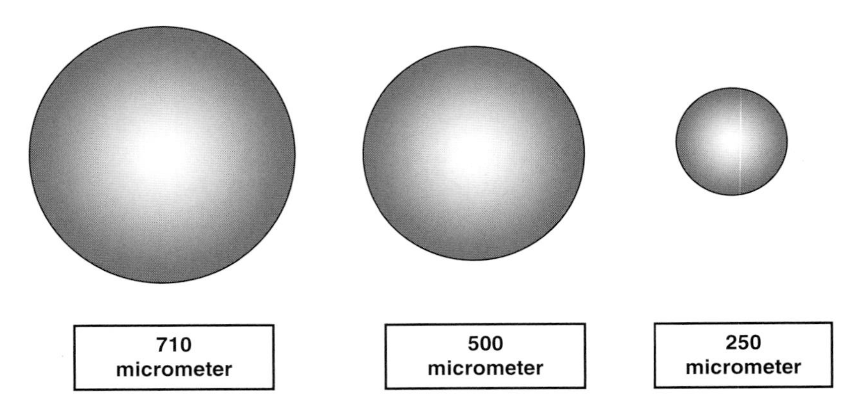

Fig. 6.3 Cartoon illustrating the relative particle size of ground bone and associated surface areas from which mineral will be solubilized during the demineralization process

- Particle size distribution of the bone
- Compaction of the bone
- Method of agitation of the demineralization process
- Degree to which a boundary layer resistance forms on the microporous surface of the bone particles

Accordingly, the demineralization rate may be accelerated by modifying one or more of the above factors, including increasing the reaction temperature, acid concentration, surface area of the bone, and/or the rate of agitation. Likewise, the demineralization rate can be decelerated by changing one or more of the above factors, for example, by decreasing the acid concentration, slowing the delivery of acid, and/or decreasing bone particle size. The collective, or bulk, demineralization rate of all bone particles in a given mixture of bone particle sizes is, evidently, the average of the individual rates of mineral solubilization from each discrete bone particle.

As depicted in Fig. 6.3, one would expect that a small bone particle will present less surface area from which minerals can be solubilized than a large bone particle; however, given a larger percentage of small bone particles in a given mixture (mass) of ground bone particles, the overall rate of demineralization may actually be accelerated due to the combined greater available surface area of all bone particles. Consequently, variable mixtures of small and large bone particles can be expected to yield variable rates of mineral solubilization given an equivalent flow or exposure time of demineralization solution. Figs. 6.4 and 6.5 are provided to illustrate the volumes, available surface areas, percentages of total mineral content and, hence, theoretical rates of demineralization that might occur as the demineralization process proceeds from the surface towards the interior of a bone particle.

Demineralization of bone tissue is essentially a surface-mediated solubilization reaction that proceeds from the outermost mineralized surface of the bone particle towards its center [30]. As this mineralized surface area decreases over time (Fig. 6.5a), the absolute amount of mineral available to be solubilized decreases in parallel as the demineralization process proceeds (Fig. 6.5b).

The actual amount of mineral that is solubilized during bulk demineralization over the course of a defined period of time or in a specific volume of acid is

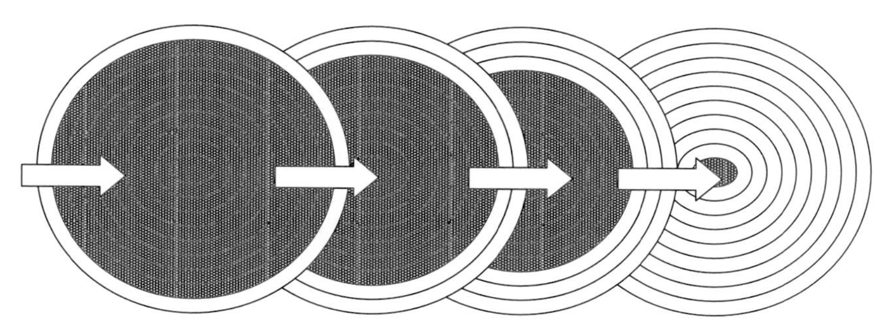

Fig. 6.4 Cartoon illustrating the demineralization of a theoretical 100 micrometer diameter bone particle in 10 micrometer increments. The figure is to be used in conjunction with the numerical values in Fig. 6.5

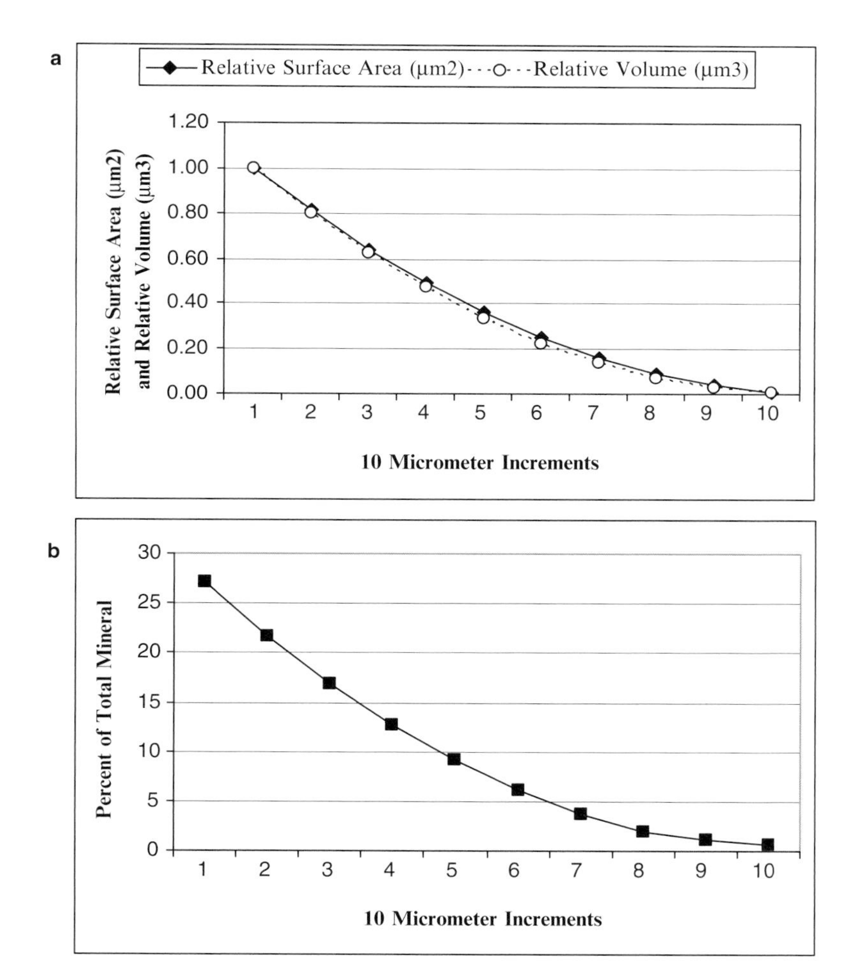

Fig. 6.5 **(a)** Relative surface area (in μm^2) and volume in (μm^3) of each successive 10 micrometer "shell" of the theoretical 100 micrometer diameter bone particle illustrated in Fig. 6.4. **(b)** Percentage of total solubilized mineral in each successive 10 micrometer "shell" of the theoretical 100 micrometer diameter bone particle illustrated in Fig. 6.4

difficult to calculate due to the irregular features of ground bone. The sequential steps during the demineralization of a particle are illustrated in Fig. 6.4. The figure depicts a theoretical sphere of bone that is 100 micrometers in diameter in which a series of concentric rings are used to indicate each 10 micrometer increment. Estimated values of the relative volume of bone tissue, the relative surface area, and the percent residual calcium in a given bone particle as each successive 10 micrometer increment is demineralized are shown in Fig. 6.5.

This theoretical example illustrates that approximately half the mineral content of a 100 micrometer bone particle lies in the outer 20 micrometers of bone particle. Accordingly, Fig. 6.5a illustrates the decrease in available surface area as demineralization progresses.

In view of the above postulation, if the rate of demineralization is truly a surface-related event, one can approximate the changing rate of demineralization based on the available surface area of the total population of bone particles. For example, based on the theoretical surface area depicted in Fig. 6.5a, the rate of demineralization would decline by approximately 5% for each 10 micrometer decrement in the diameter of the undemineralized portion of the bone particle. Consequently, approximately 87.5% of the available mineral in a bone particle will be removed within the first 50 micrometers of a bone particle of 100 micrometer diameter (Fig. 6.5b). Removing mineral to the depth of 70 micrometers will result in bone particles retaining only about 3% of their original mineral content. Although the spherical model does not account for cortical bone "porosity" due to the presence of the Haversian canal system, it provides an estimate of the extent of demineralization required to achieve a given desired weight percent residual calcium level such as 0.5 to 4.0%. This percent range in weight percent residual calcium in bone particles in the 250 to 710 micrometer particle size range has been described as producing maximally osteoinductive DBM [25]. However, it is important to emphasize that maximal osteoinductivity/new bone formation of DBM relies more on the bioavailability of the growth and differentiation factors and packing geometry of the DBM and, thus, the importance of demineralization lies in some crucial interaction between the DBM particles and the cells infiltrating them.

With knowledge of the physical and chemical characteristics of the bone particles, the demineralization process can be stopped when a desired residual calcium level has been reached. United States Patent numbers 6,189,537 and 6,305,379 exemplify methods for producing maximally osteoinductive bone based on average weight percent residual calcium [31, 32]. To establish an endpoint, the correlation between pH and desired residual calcium level was determined. Demineralization was standardized utilizing a representative bone sample of the same particle size range and total bone mass. The initial calcium concentration of the bone was determined; the bone was then demineralized at a constant rate while periodically sampling the eluent pH and the residual calcium in the bone particles at specific time intervals. As the eluent pH was found to correlate with a specific residual calcium level, a desired residual calcium level can be achieved by simply stopping the demineralization process once the pH of the eluent reaches the predetermined value.

The volume of acid that will be needed for the demineralization process can be approximated based on the initial weight of bone material. Approximately two-thirds of the dry weight of bone is inorganic mineral, the majority of which is hydroxyapatite (calcium phosphate) [33]. The projected weight of the soluble calcium phosphate allows the buffering capacity of the mineral component to be estimated which, in turn, allows an approximation of the acid equivalents required to reach a desired residual calcium level. Alternatively, by establishing the estimated acid equivalents required, it is possible to determine the amount of acid needed to reach a residual calcium level in a given mass of bone. By monitoring the calcium ion concentration or eluent pH during the demineralization process, the progress in the rate of demineralization can be monitored and calculated, thereby avoiding over-demineralization of the bone material.

6.5.3. Extent of Demineralization

In studies examining the relationship between residual calcium and osteoinductivity of DBM, Zhang and colleagues [17] determined that samples that contained approximately 2% residual calcium had the highest osteoinductivity of DBM. Samples with varying residual weight percent calcium content were implanted in the muscle pouch of athymic mice. The changes in calcium content of the explants over the original calcium content of the samples are shown in Fig. 6.6. Interestingly, non-demineralized bone matrix exhibited a decrease in calcium content of approximately 2.6% rather than additional mineralization.

These findings were substantiated in an *in vitro* alkaline phosphatase activity assay. DBM demineralized to 2% residual calcium content produced the highest level of ALP activity among the range of samples tested [17]. The reported results suggest that the residual calcium content is indicative of a complex mechanism by which DBM stimulates new bone growth. This target residual calcium level may represent an optimal level of BMP exposure without denaturing or inactivating the growth factors.

Studies comparing the extractable BMPs in ground bone demineralized to various percent residual calcium levels demonstrated an approximately linear relationship to extractability of BMPs versus extent or degree of demineralization (Fig. 6.7) [18]. BMPs were not extractable from non-demineralized ground bone, but were extracted in progressively larger amounts from bone particles that were increasingly demineralized. If BMP availability were the sole determinant of the ability of demineralized bone to induce cells to differentiate with subsequent new bone formation, one would not expect the data in Fig. 6.6. However, if BMPs were acid labile, one might expect the BMPs to be inactivated once sufficient bone mineral was dissolved and the buffering effect

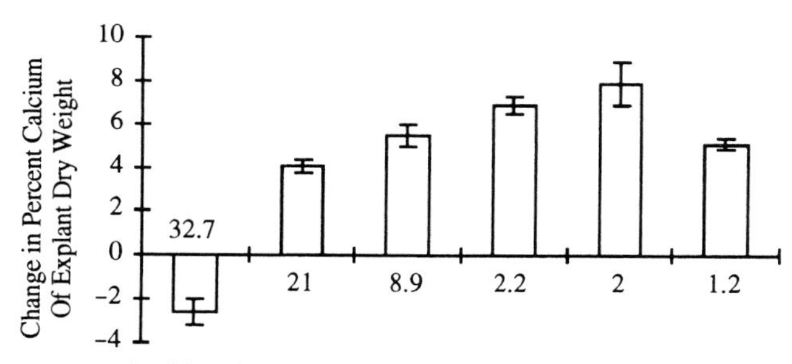

Fig. 6.6 Changes in percent residual calcium of explanted DBM (particle size 250 to 710 micrometers) containing variable levels of calcium at the time of implantation in an athymic mouse model. Calcium content of explants is expressed as change in weight percent residual calcium [17].

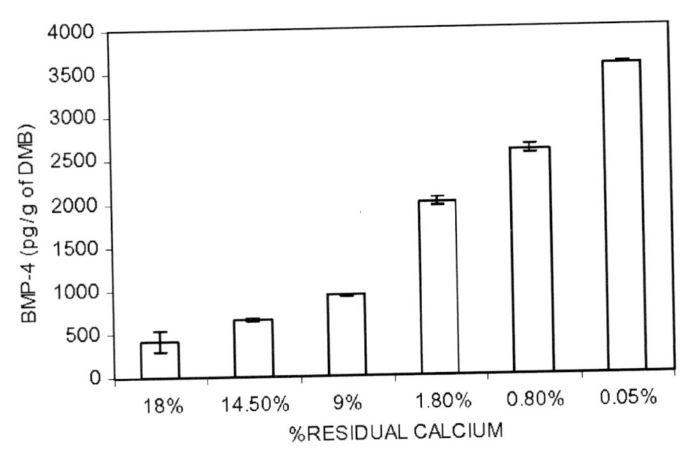

Fig. 6.7 Extractable BMP-4 as a function of extent or degree of demineralization of ground bone particles [18]. Residual calcium is expressed in weight percent

removed, so that the BMPs within the bone particles are exposed to the low pH of the bulk acid solution, i.e., a pH of ≤ 1.0.

6.5.4. Particle Size

Commercially available DBM is offered in a variety of size ranges, typically 125 to 250 micrometers (microns), 250 to 350 micrometers, 350 to 500 micrometers, and 500 to 710 micrometers. Size ranges are separated using mesh sieves and this procedure is usually performed prior to demineralization of the particles. The demineralization process may have an effect on particle size depending on the process employed, and processors generally do not verify particle size after demineralization and/or freeze-drying; therefore, actual particle sizes may not coincide completely with the description on the product label and package insert. Likewise, the calcium content stated is likely an average percent of residual calcium present within the range of bone particle sizes and not the weight percentage of calcium present within each particle of DBM.

Particle size plays an important role in the utility of DBM in various clinical applications. As an example, the more frequently processed bone particle size range for periodontal use is 250 to 710 micrometers. Bone particles that are smaller in size are assumed to be phagocytosed by macrophages, induce a local inflammatory response or disperse too rapidly from the implantation site [27]. Conversely, particles of a larger size do not allow for optimal packing geometry – and thus porosity – at the surgical site [16].

For the purpose of this discussion, porosity is defined as the ratio of the void space to the total volume of the implanted bone material. As illustrated in Fig. 6.8, the porosity of packed ground demineralized bone varies with the range of bone particle sizes in a mixture. A mixture with large bone particles will have larger spaces or pores between the individual particles than will a mixture of small bone particles; however, the total volume fraction of the pore space is greater in a mixture of small bone particles than a mixture of large bone particles. Combinations of large and small bone particles provide an effective means of controlling total volume fraction of the pore space volume

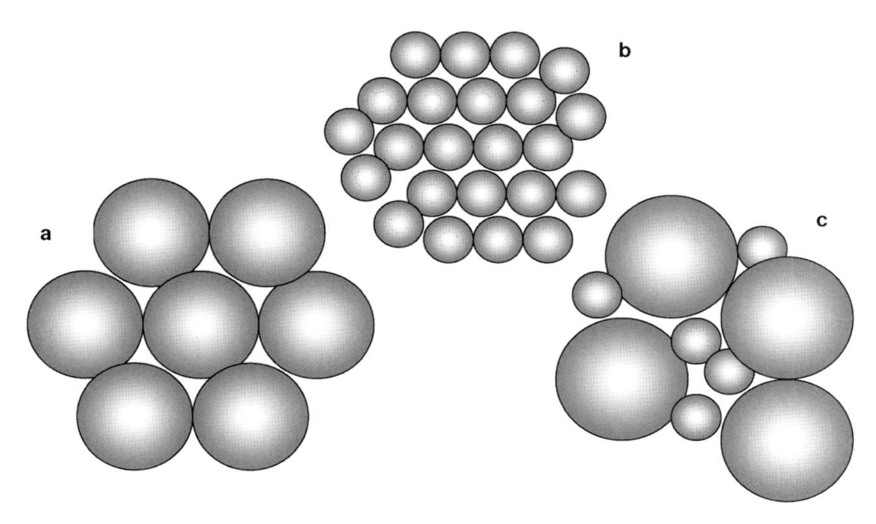

Fig. 6.8 Cartoon to illustrate the relative porosity and average pore size of spaces between bone particles (represented here as perfect spheres) as a function of bone particle size (a) and (b). The value of mixing bone particle sizes to control this porosity and average (with range) of pore sizes is illustrated in c

in mixtures of DBM. Porosity affects the permeability of a DBM mixture for cells migrating into the pore space. Consequently, it is possible to manage the osteoconductive properties of DBM by managing the porosity, both in regard to the volume of individual pores between the bone particles as well as the total available pore space volume in which new bone can be formed. This optimization of osteoconductivity of DBM is equally as important as bioavailability of BMPs (osteoinductivity) through control of the demineralization process.

Zhang et al. [17] examined the effects of particle size on the osteoinductivity of ground demineralized bone. Under both *in vivo* remineralization assay and *in vitro* alkaline phosphatase activity assay conditions, the research group found that ground demineralized bone retaining between 0.5 and 4.0 weight percent residual calcium and in the particle size range of 500 to 710 micrometers induced the highest level of new bone formation (see Fig. 6.9). The group noted that all samples had been demineralized for equal amounts of time, mimicking the actual demineralization process of commercially available DBM. As smaller particle sizes demineralize more quickly than larger bone particles, resulting in a lower residual calcium level in the small bone particles compared to large bone particles, additional experiments are warranted to compare particles of varying sizes, but equal residual calcium content. Additionally, a greater characterization of the bone fibers created by bone shaving (skiving) with respect to optimal packing density and demineralization are needed as well.

In the context of the discussion of porosity, it is important to consider how the induced new bone formation is currently assessed in the *in vivo* bioassay. Following implantation of DBM in the animal model, osteogenic precursor cells migrate into the available pore space volume between the packed demineralized bone particles. There, the precursor cells are induced to differentiate into osteoblast cells that excrete the molecules that will become osteoid, the organic matrix of the bone that subsequently undergoes mineralization. These

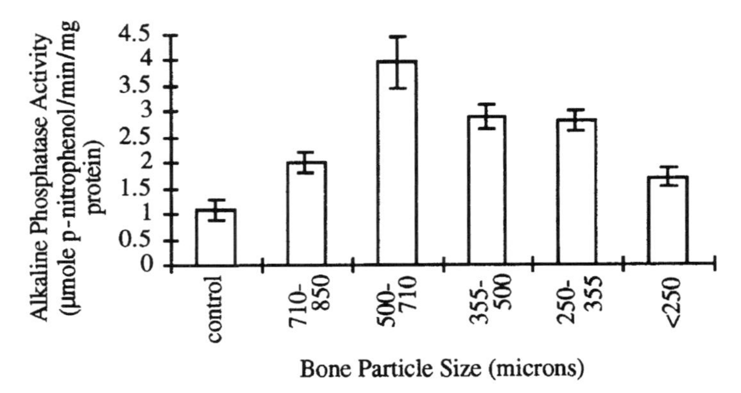

Fig. 6.9 Alkaline phosphatase levels in human periosteal cells incubated with ground demineralized bone particles (2% residual calcium). Control sample did not receive DBM. ALP assay performed on day 5 of incubation with DBM [17]

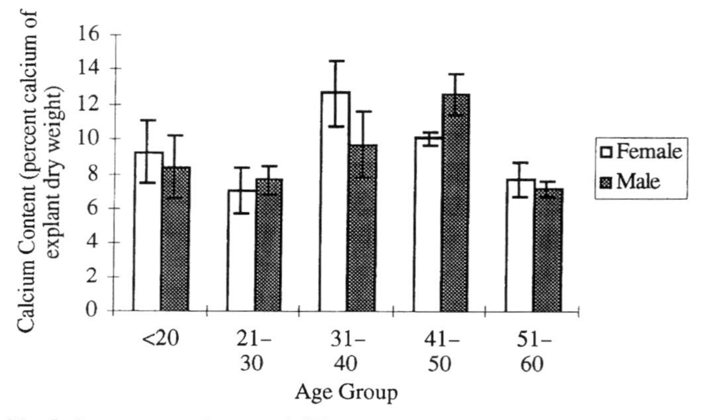

Fig. 6.10 Effect of donor age and gender on the osteoinductivity of DBM (2% residual calcium; particle size 250 to 710 µm) in an athymic mouse model. Calcium content of explants is expressed as weight percent calcium of explant dry weight [17]. Age group is expressed in years

molecules must become cross-linked to create osteoid before the molecules can diffuse from the osteoconductive environment. If the porosity of the DBM is too great, synthesized molecules can diffuse from the implant site prior to being incorporated. If the porosity is too small, cells will have difficulty in migrating into the individual spaces, and nutrient availability and waste removal will be limited.

6.5.5. Donor-Related Effects

DBM derived from all age groups of both male and female tissue donors were remineralized when implanted in the athymic mouse model system as shown by Zhang and colleagues [17, 34]. Donor gender and age-related effects on the osteoinductive potential were observed, but were not as conventionally expected. Female donors between the age of 31 to 40 years and male donors in

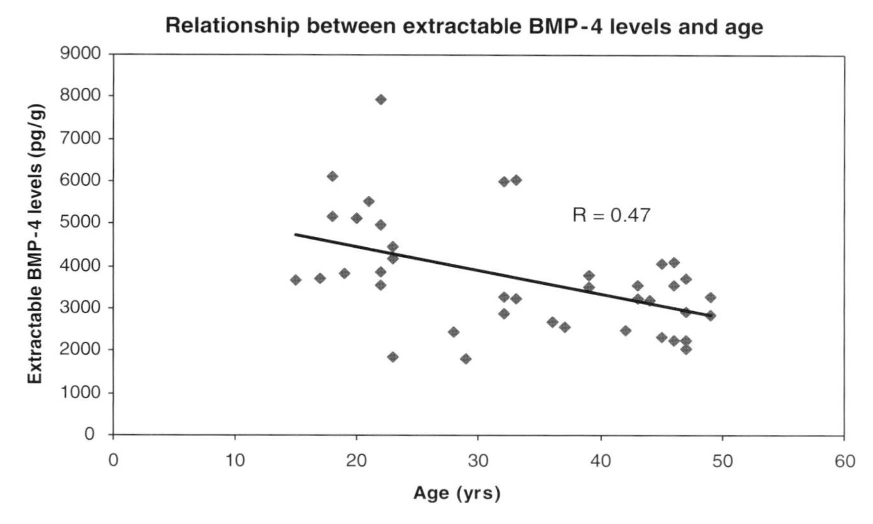

Fig. 6.11 Correlation of extractable BMP-4 from demineralized bone produced from donors of increasing age [18]

the age group of 41 to 50 years appeared more osteoinductive/osteoconductive than other groups tested, and there were no significant declines in osteoinductivity with donor age in either male or female donors. Nonetheless, observed differences may again be associated with differences in the processing of the demineralized bone rather than the actual characteristics of a tissue donor. Bone procured from male and female donors of all ages may, therefore, be expected to stimulate new bone formation when implanted in clinical applications [17, 34].

Other groups have reported an age-associated decrease in the osteoinductivity of DBM derived from young versus older donors [35]. However, one should consider the potential impact of the donor age ranges selected for presentation of the data, as this may affect the reported significance of donor age on osteoinductivity. Inherent donor variability would require very large samples across a wide age range to determine real age effects. When comparing BMP-4 extracted from bone tissue to the age of the bone tissue donors, Honsawek et al. [18] reported a gradual decline in extractable levels of BMP-4 from DBM as a function of donor age (Fig. 6.11). While the regression line does not exhibit a linear relationship ($R^2 = 0.47$), the slope is observably negative with increasing donor age.

6.5.6 Other Potential Factors

Multiple additional aspects may play a role in the complex mechanism by which DBM stimulates new bone growth [17]:

- *Residual calcium levels*. Residual mineral levels of DBM can be seen as a measure of the reproducibility of the demineralization process as well as a marker for the increased availability of active growth and differentiation factors. In addition, residual calcium may act as a nucleation site for the redeposition of calcium phosphates and, therefore, speed the rate of remineralization after implantation.

- *Degradation of the organic matrix.* During the demineralization process, the acidic environment most likely results in limited degradation of the organic collagen/proteoglycan matrix. The resulting degradation products may be responsible for stimulating cellular chemotaxis to the implant site and may act as sites to which cells attach.
- *Release of growth factors.* Whether growth and differentiation factors such as BMPs diffuse from the bone matrix or remain within the implant material to stimulate the differentiation of infiltrating cells into matrix- and bone-forming cells has not been completely determined to date. The application of recombinant BMPs to implant materials from which the BMPs are free to diffuse from the implant material may be one of the central elements distinguishing the mode of action of DBM from that of collagenous carriers of recombinant BMPs in the formation of bone at an implant site.
- *Preparation of the matrix.* Demineralized bone biomaterials used for different clinical applications may require different preparation methods. Particle size, extent of demineralization, bioavailability of growth and differentiation factors, packing geometry, and the presence or absence of a carrier may all play a role in the suitability of DBM products at various implantation sites. It should not be presumed that a given preparation of DBM or carrier-based DBM product or recombinant BMP/carrier product will serve equally well in all sites of clinical application.

6.6. Demineralized Bone Matrix Carrier Products

Although demineralized bone has been used in clinical applications for decades and has been shown in both *in vitro* and *in vivo* assays to be osteoinductive and to cause the formation of bone, it does have limitations. DBM, and most specifically particulate DBM, can be difficult to handle in the operating room. The small particles are flaky, do not adhere to each other, and can migrate from the implant site. Furthermore, DBM is typically provided in small quantities, that is, in volumes of 0.5 cc to 5 cc that correlate with the presumptive volume of the defect site into which the DBM is to be inserted. The use of these small graft volumes is less efficient for large bony defects of which the volume may be unknown prior to surgery. An additional problem with distribution of DBM in volume quantities lies in differences in the volume that a specific unit of weight of DBM will occupy depending on how the bone particles settle in the package over time. This variability in the volume of a DBM product due to settling frequently leads to complaints about insufficient product fill levels.

To overcome handling limitations, the variability in fill volume of DBM materials, and the need to extend the graft to fill larger voids, many companies offer DBM in combination with a carrier. Often, non-demineralized cancellous bone chips are used to extend the volume of the implant material and are added to DBM either by the manufacturer or by the physician at the time of surgery.

Carriers and extenders for DBM can be synthetic or biologic in origin [36]. Glycerol, hyaluronic acid, collagen, synthetic polymers, and autologous blood or blood components are examples of carriers used in commercially available osteobiologic products [36, 37, 38]. Handling characteristics such as malleability, resistance to graft migration, and viscosity are often manipulated by varying the ratio of carrier to DBM. Caution should be taken, however, when comparing the osteoinductive potential of carrier/DBM products with

DBM. For example, in the athymic mouse bioassay, 20 mg of DBM and 20 mg of carrier product should not necessarily be expected to perform equivalently. In most products, demineralized bone is the bioactive component of the product, which means that the DBM is the osteoinductive agent and variability in the content of DBM may also vary the bioactive component. Therefore, when comparing equal amounts of DMB and carrier product in either a biological or a clinical evaluation, there may be significantly less osteoinductive material in the carrier product. This should not be interpreted to denote that carrier products are less capable of stimulating new bone formation; nonetheless, researchers and clinicians should be aware of the differences between the carrier products and the appropriate control for them in *in vitro* and *in vivo* assessments. Some carrier products may use carriers that act synergistically with the DBM in improving osteoconductivity by helping to maintain porosity within the packed DBM matrix, enhancing cellular infiltration or promoting cellular activity in the synthesis of new matrix. Other carriers may serve only to lend better handling characteristics to DBM and will dissipate from the implant site rather quickly, leaving only the DBM to meet the osteoinductive and/or osteoconductive requirements of the procedure. In this regard, DBM and carrier products to which growth and differentiation factors have been added may have the advantage of greater levels of total or individual factors than DBM alone. These added growth and differentiation factors may also quickly dissipate from the implant site, however, reducing the overall and time-dependent bioavailability of these supplementary ingredients. Without the presence of DBM with its natural complement of growth and differentiation factors, carrier products with added growth and differentiation factors may quickly become only a scaffold in which infiltrating cells proliferate and grow without the capacity to stimulate these cells to differentiate and form bone.

Many surgeons have historically relied on autograft, taking bone and bone marrow from the iliac crest, as the gold standard for bone grafting. However, donor site morbidity presents the main disadvantage of this technique. In response, some products are leveraging the advantages of autograft in combination with demineralized bone. At the time of surgery a sample of the patient's own blood is prepared to concentrate the platelet-rich plasma component and is added to the DBM. Once the mixture clots, a semi-solid graft is formed that contains the patient's autologous growth factors together with the osteoinductive DBM. Similarly, bone marrow from the iliac crest can be aspirated and combined with DBM to make use of the bone marrow-derived stem cells with their growth and differentiation potential.

6.7. Optimizing Osteoinductivity and Safety of DBM

Maximally aseptic procurement techniques and efficient processing methods are essential for the production of safe and clinically effective osteoinductive bone material [16]. Relevant steps in the processing of demineralized bone matrix are described below.

6.7.1. Aseptic Recovery and Processing

Following consent of the donor family, donor tissue is procured using aseptic technique, then wrapped in sterile drapes and transported to the processing facility on ice. Although the specific method used in the procurement of bone tissue varies with the procurement agency, the objective is to retrieve and transport tissue in a manner that minimizes or prevents contamination or decomposition of the tissue. All recovered tissue is tested for microbiological contamination before the donor tissue is processed into grafts. Standard microbiological assays under aerobic and anaerobic conditions are utilized to culture and identify bacteria and fungi. Blood samples taken from each donor are tested for viral infectious agents and must meet or exceed Food and Drug Administration (FDA) regulations regarding donor tissue testing. It is also preferable that tissue banks comply with the standards established by the American Association of Tissue Banks (AATB).

6.7.2. Additional Cleaning Processes

To maximize allograft safety and osteoinductivity, bone tissue is first cleaned of cellular components. In addition to allograft cleaning, numerous tissue banks in the United States have developed processes to disinfect the tissue. These processes can use both mechanical and chemical methods to remove components such as lipids and cellular elements such as bone marrow, which are most likely to potentially harbor viral particles. In consequence, the potential of disease transmission is reduced. It is critical that the methods used to disinfect the bone tissue will not affect the osteoinductivity or osteoconductivity of the allograft and will not cause an inflammatory response at the implantation site. At the same time, removal of infective elements should be controlled and not result in stripping the bone of all of the proteinaceaous elements that protect the organic matrix of ground demineralized bone and contribute to the material's osteoinductive potential.

6.7.3. Sterilization of Bone Allograft

Human bone tissue for grafting is procured from deceased donors and, despite stringent procurement and processing methods, the risk remains that DBM might harbor microbial contaminants that are present in the tissue at the time of recovery. As there is no completely infallible way to exclude such donors, conscientious tissue banks are adopting sterilization procedures that do not adversely affect the performance of implanted allograft tissue.

The effects of a variety of sterilization methods on the osteoinductivity of demineralized bone matrix have been extensively studied in numerous animal models in which the DBM has been implanted at both heterotopic and orthotopic sites [39, 40, 41, 42, 43]. These methods included treatment with glutaraldehyde, formaldehyde, and ethylene oxide, as well as autoclaving and gamma irradiation. Of all sterilization methods examined, gamma irradiation demonstrated the most consistent results and appeared to be the most appropriate sterilizing method for demineralized bone in clinical use.

In further analyses the effect of gamma radiation at various temperatures on bone formation and remodeling were explored. In the experiments performed by Wientroub and Reddi [40] samples were maintained in ice water during irradiation. Preparations that had been irradiated with doses up to 25 kGy showed inductive properties that were similar to the non-irradiated control. Dziedzic-Goclawska and colleagues [41] irradiated DBM at room temperature or on dry ice (presumably −72 °C). While samples that were irradiated at room temperature had been completely resorbed five weeks after implantation into the muscle pouch of a rat, DBM irradiated on dry ice was osteoinductive and resorbed more slowly. DBM that had been treated with a dose of 35 kGy at −72 °C demonstrated new bone formation that was comparable to non-irradiated control samples [41]. These results led both groups to hypothesize that temperature may play a critical role in protecting osteoinductive properties of DBM against radiation damage.

In light of the finding that DBM irradiated at low temperatures was less susceptible to radiation damage, Crouch and colleagues undertook a study to examine the results of a range of absorbed gamma radiation doses on demineralized bone particles [44]. In this assay DBM particles were irradiated on dry ice at 7 kGy, 14 kGy, 21 kGy, and 30 kGy. Experimental samples were implanted in muscle pouches of athymic mice for 28 days and were then compared to the percentage of remineralization and new bone formation in non-irradiated control samples. The data demonstrated that gamma irradiation affected the implanted DBM in a way which allowed the interior of the particles to be resorbed and replaced with new bone (Fig. 6.12). This observation reinforces the need to separate the concepts of "osteoinductivity" and "new bone formation" stimulated by the implantation of a DBM material. Fig. 6.13 illustrates the resorption of implanted demineralized bone material at the site of implantation. This allows additional space for new bone formation to be made available without increasing the osteoinductivity *per se*. These data corroborate the results of experiments performed by Wientroub and Reddi, which suggested that irradiation of 30 to 50 kGy enhanced bone induction, leading to a higher level of mineralization than non-irradiated control samples in a heterotopic rat model [40]. The experimental samples irradiated at each dose did display significant osteoinductivity, however, regardless of the dose administered [44].

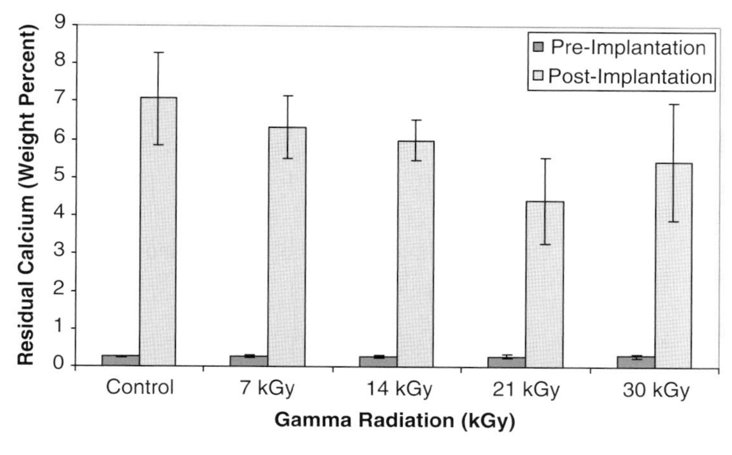

Fig. 6.12 Residual weight changes in percent residual calcium of DBM irradiated on dry ice [44]

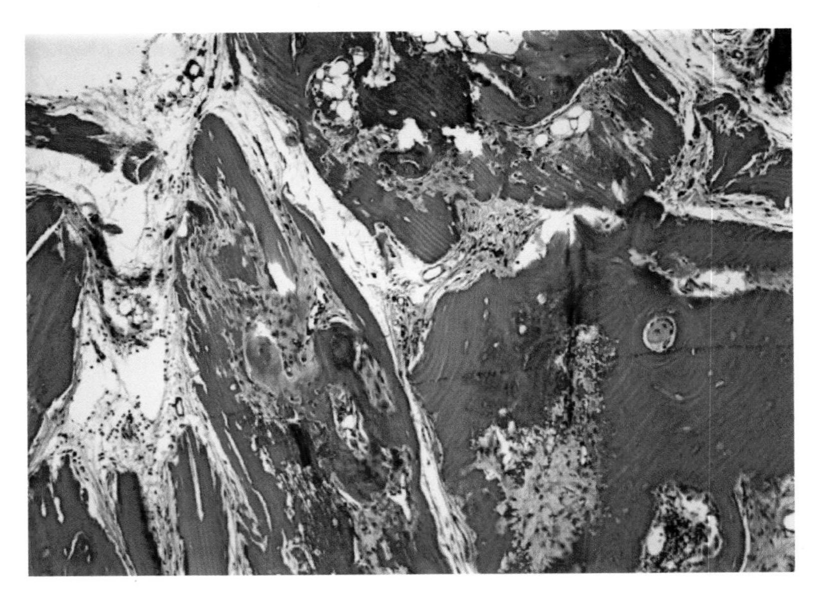

Fig. 6.13 Photograph of an H & E histologic preparation of gamma-irradiated DBM particle demonstrating the resorption of bone mineral to create additional space for new bone formation [44]. The implanted experimental sample was irradiated at 30 kGy; magnification is 100-fold

6.8. Future Trends and Needs

Osteoinductivity of demineralized ground bone is due in large part to BMPs and other noncollagenous proteins enclosed in the matrix. However, osteoinduction is not necessarily equivalent to new bone formation. The DBM must also be osteoconductive in order that induced or fully differentiated bone-forming cells may find an environment suitable for the formation of bone. To provide an osteoconductive environment DBM must also be comprised of particles of appropriate size and packing geometry, regardless of whether the DBM is implanted in a heterotopic or orthotopic site. Similar relationships have been reported for ceramic materials [45] in which comparisons of osteoconduction and osteoinduction have been correlated with the presence or absence of concavities or macropores in the induced formation of new bone. Development of methods for processing DBM from donor bone tissue that provide optimal levels of osteoinductivity and new bone formation, while minimizing the risk of infection or disease transmission, is, therefore, of importance.

When matching a graft to a clinical need, the surgeon must decide whether the issue is a loss of structure or a lack of osteoinduction or osteogenesis [46]. At this time there is no natural or synthetic substitute for an autologous graft that has osteogenic properties. Therefore, in poorly healing fractures that require new bone formation, such as a nonunion or delayed union with marginal vascularity of the grafting bed, autologous grafts or composites containing both autologous material and a graft substitute as carrier/extender are required. Recent clinical studies suggest that recombinant bone morphogenetic proteins can promote bone fusion even in the absence of autograft [47].

Even so, BMP preparations must be used judiciously as uncontrolled bone formation as well as the development of antibodies against a naturally present human protein may occur, raising concerns about the long-term effects of recombinant BMP use [47].

6.9. Conclusion

Demineralized bone matrix has been shown to possess both osteoconductive as well as osteoinductive properties. While the ground form in which it is typically available does not offer structural support, it is well suited for filling bone defects and cavities and can also be used with a carrier in combination with autologous bone marrow or platelet-rich plasma to enhance healing [46].

Based on studies performed by Zhang and colleagues [17] residual calcium levels of 2% are required for optimal osteoinductivity of demineralized ground bone in the 250 to 710 micrometer size range. Although it was to be expected that such donor-specific factors as age and gender would affect the osteoinductivity of DBM, these studies demonstrated that consistency in processing and controlled residual calcium levels leading to a consistent end product are more pertinent to the osteoinductive and bone-forming potential of demineralized ground bone than donor age or gender. Many tissue banks currently use controlled demineralization processes with the goal of achieving a consistently demineralized biomatrix that maximizes the osteoinductive potential of commercially available DBM.

Nonetheless, further developments, particularly in the area of assays for the objective and quantitative measurement of osteoinductivity in demineralized bone matrix, will be necessary. It is no longer adequate or acceptable to procure and process human tissue without stringent control of the resulting allografts' safety and efficacy for clinical use. Validation of processing procedures and standardization of testing for effectiveness in clinical applications are challenges that are currently being recognized and addressed by the tissue banking industry.

References

1. Senn N. On the healing of aseptic bone cavities by implantation of antiseptic decalcified bone. *Am J Med Sci.* 1889;98:219-240.
2. Leriche R, Policard A, eds. *The Normal and Pathological Physiology of Bone and its Problems*. London, England: Henry Kimpton; 1928.
3. Levander G. A study of bone regeneration. *Surg Gynecol Obstet.* 1938;67:705-714.
4. Lacroix P. Recent investigations on the growth of bone. *Nature.* 1945;156:576-577.
5. Reddi AH, Huggins CB. Biochemical sequences in the transformation of normal fibroblasts in adolescent rats. *Natl Acad Sci USA.* 1972;69:1601-1605.
6. Reddi AH. Cell biology and biochemistry of endochondral bone development. *Collagen Rel Res.* 1981;1:209-226.
7. Urist MR. Bone: formation by autoinduction. *Science.* 1965;150:893-899.
8. Zhang M, Powers RM Jr, Wolfinbarger L Jr. A quantitative assessment of osteoinductivity of human demineralized bone matrix. *J Periodontol.* 1997;68:1076-1084.
9. Kalfas IH. Principles of bone healing. *Neurosurg Focus.* 2001;10,Article 1.
10. Rengachary SS. Bone morphogenetic proteins: basic concepts. *Neurosurg Focus.* 2002;13:Article 2.
11. Pilitsis JG, Lucas DR, Rengachary SR. Bone healing and spinal fusion. *Neurosurg Focus.* 2002;13,Article 1.

12. Schmitt JM, Hwang K, Winn SR, Hollinger JO. Bone morphogenetic proteins: an update on basic biology and clinical relevance. *J Orthop Res.* 1999;17:269-278.
13. Walker DH, Wright NM. Bone morphogenetic proteins and spinal fusion. *Neurosurg Focus.* 2002;13:Article 3.
14. Lieberman JR, Daluiski A, Einhorn TA. The role of growth factors in the repair of bone. Biology and clinical applications. *J Bone Joint Surg Am.* 2002;84-A:1032-1044.
15. Wozney JM, Rosen V, Celeste AJ, et al. Novel regulators of bone formation: molecular clones and activities. *Science.* 242:1528-1534.
16. Wolfinbarger L Jr, Burkart M, Croft L, Linthurst A, Braendle L. Processing factors contributing to production of maximally osteoinductive demineralised ground bone for use in orthopaedic or periodontal applications. In: Phillips GO, Kearney JN, Strong DM, von Versen R, Nather A, eds. *Advances in Tissue Banking. Volume 3.* Singapore: World Scientific Publishing Co.; 1999;125-145.
17. Zhang M, Powers RM Jr, Wolfinbarger L Jr. Effect(s) of the demineralization process on the osteoinductivity of demineralized bone matrix. *J Periodontol.* 1997;68:1085-1092.
18. Honsawek S, Powers RM, Wolfinbarger L. Extractable bone morphogenetic protein and correlation with induced new bone formation in an *in vivo* assay in the athymic mouse model. *Cell Tissue Bank.* 2005;6:13-23.
19. Wolfinbarger L Jr, Zheng Y. An *in vitro* bioassay to assess biological activity in demineralized bone. *In Vitro Cell Dev Biol Anim.* 1993;29A:914-916.
20. Delling G, Hahn M, Bonse U, et al. New possibilities for structural analysis of bone biopsies using microcomputer tomography (muCT). *Pathologe.* 1995;16:342-347.
21. Murray SS, Brochmann EJ, Harker JO, King E, Lollis RJ, Khaliq SA. A statistical model to allow the phasing out of the animal testing of demineralised bone matrix products. *Altern Lab Anim.* 2007;35:405-409.
22. Pagini F, Francucci CM, Moro L. Markers of bone turnover: biochemical and clinical perspectives. *J Endocrinol Invest.* 2005;28:8-13.
23. Wergedal JE, Mohan S, Lundy M, Baylink DJ. Skeletal growth factor and other growth factors known to be present in bone matrix stimulate proliferation and protein synthesis in human bone. *J Bone Miner Res.* 1990;5:179-186.
24. Aspenberg P, Andolf E. Bone induction by fetal and adult human bone matrix in athymic rats. *Acta Orthop Scand.* 1989;60:195-199.
25. Urist MR, DeLange RJ, Finerman GA. Bone cell differentiation and growth factors. *Science.* 1983;220:680-686.
26. Urist MR, Strates BS. Bone formation in implants of partially and wholly demineralized bone matrix. Including observations on acetone-fixed intra and extracellular proteins. *Clin Orthop Relat Res.* 1970;71:271-278.
27. Syftestad G, Urist MR. Degradation of bone matrix morphogenetic activity by pulverization. *Clin Orthop Relat Res.* 1979;141:281-285.
28. Syftestad GT, Urist MR. Bone aging. *Clin Orthop Relat Res.* 1982;162:288-297.
29. American Association of Tissue Banks. *Standards for Tissue Banking.* 11th ed. Bethesda, MD: American Association of Tissue Banks; 2006.
30. Lewandrowski K, Tomford WW, Michaud NA, Schomaker KT, Deutsch TF. An electron microscopic study on the process of acid demineralization of cortical bone. *Calcif Tissue Int.* 1997;61:294-297.
31. Wolfinbarger L Jr, inventor; LifeNet, assignee. Process for producing osteoinductive bone, and osteoinductive bone produced thereby. US patent 6,189,537. February 20, 2001.
32. Wolfinbarger L Jr, inventor; LifeNet, assignee. Process for producing osteoinductive bone, and osteoinductive bone produced thereby. US patent 6,305,379. October 23, 2001.
33. Pietrzak WS, Woodell-May J. The composition of human cortical allograft bone derived from FDA/AATB-screened donors. *J Craniofac Surg.* 2005;16:579-585.

34. Traiandes K, Russell JL, Edwards JT, Stubbs HA, Shanahan IR, Knaack D. Donor age and gender effects on osteoinductivity of demineralized bone matrix. *J Biomed Mater Res B Appl Biomater*. 2004;70:21-29.
35. Schwartz Z, Somers A, Mellonig JT, et al. Ability of commercial demineralized freeze-dried bone allograft to induce new bone formation is dependent on donor age but not gender. *J Periodontol*. 1998;69:470-478.
36. Greenwald AS, Boden SD, Goldberg VM, et al, for the Committee on Biological Implants. Bone-graft substitutes: facts, fictions, and applications. *J Bone Joint Surg Am*. 2001;83-A:98-103.
37. Kassolis JD, Rosen PS, Reynolds MA. Alveolar ridge and sinus augmentation utilizing platelet-rich plasma in combination with freeze-dried bone allograft: case series. *J Periodontol*. 2000;71:1654-1661.
38. Cornell CN. Osteobiologics. *Bull Hosp Jt Dis*. 2004;62:13-17.
39. Munting E, Wilmart JF, Wijne A, Hennebert P, Delloye C. Effect of sterilization of osteoinduction. Comparison of five methods in demineralized rat bone. *Acta Orthop Scand*. 1988;59:34-38.
40. Wientroub S, Reddi AH. Influence of irradiation on the osteoinductive potential of demineralized bone matrix. *Calcif Tissue Int*. 1988;42:255-260.
41. Dziedzic-Goclawska A, Ostrowski K, Stachowicz W, Michalik J, Grzesik W. Effect of radiation sterilization on the osteoinductive properties and the rate of remodeling of bone implants preserved by lyophilization and deep-freezing. *Clin Orthop Relat Res*. 1991;Nov:30-37.
42. Ijiri S, Yamamuro T, Nakamura T, Kotani S, Notoya K. Effect of sterilization on bone morphogenetic protein. *J Orthop Res*. 1994;12:628-636.
43. Hallfeldt KKJ, Stützle H, Puhlmann M, Kessler S, Schweiberer L. Sterilization of partially demineralized bone matrix: the effects of different sterilization techniques on osteogenetic properties. *J Surg Res*. 1995;59:614-620.
44. Crouch K, Softic D, Wolfinbarger L. Effects of gamma irradiation on osteoinductivity of demineralized bone matrix. Presented at: 51st Orthopaedic Research Society Annual Meeting; Washington, DC; February 20-23, 2005.
45. Habibovic P, Yuan H, van den Doel M, Sees TM, van Blitterswijk CA, de Groot K. Relevance of osteoinductive biomaterials in critical-sized orthotopic defect. *J Orthop Res*. 2006;24:867-876.
46. Finkemeier CG. Bone-grafting and bone-graft substitutes. *J Bone Joint Surg Am*. 2002;84:454-464.
47. Walker DH, Wright NM. Bone morphogenetic proteins and spinal fusion. *Neurosurg Focus*. 2002;13:e3.

7

Deproteinized Bovine Bone Xenograft

Andreas Stavropoulos

Abstract: Deproteinized bovine bone (DBB) has a chemical composition and architectural geometry that is almost identical to that of human bone and can support new bone formation in direct contact to the graft. DBB grafts are widely used in dentistry in a variety of applications, and positive results have been generally observed after their application. However, an added clinical benefit from their use in association with dental implants and/or when used as adjuncts to guided tissue regeneration (GTR) in the treatment of periodontal intrabony defects cannot unequivocally be confirmed. It seems that DBB should be regarded as an osteocompatible filler material that may act as a space provision device rather than as a bone promoting substance, and the outcome of DBB grafting in terms of bone fill seems greatly dependent on the configuration and dimensions of the defect. Relevant *in vitro* and animal experiments, as well as human clinical studies in a variety of applications, are presented and discussed. The chapter also briefly describes the processing method of xenograft bone and its properties, and discusses the risk of disease transmission.

Keywords: Bone, bovine, devitalized, deproteinized, grafts, GTR, implants, osteoconduction, periodontology, regeneration, xenograft, xenotransplantation.

7.1. Introduction

Xenograft derives from the Greek word "xeno(s)" (= foreign) and graft, and means a graft of tissue taken from a donor of one species and transplanted into a recipient of another species. In the past the term *heterograft* was used to describe such a material [1]. Indeed, the first successful bone grafting operation ever, recorded in 1668 by the Dutch surgeon Job Janszoon van Meekeren, regarded a xenograft [2]. The account describes an incident where a section from the cranium of a dead dog was used to restore the defect in

Department of Periodontology and Oral Gerontology, School of Dentistry, University of Aarhus, Denmark

From: *Orthopedic Biology and Medicine: Musculoskeletal Tissue Regeneration, Biological Materials and Methods.*
Edited by W. S. Pietrzak © Humana Press, Totowa, NJ

the skull of a nobleman in Moscow who had received a heavy sword wound. The restoration was successful and the patient fully recovered; however, his troubles were not over because the Church found the method rather unchristian and pronounced an excommunication as long as "the forbidden section from the bones of a dog's head should remain united to the bones of a Christian man's head." Of course, the patient asked his surgeon to remove the graft, but the canine bone had firmly united with the human cranium, and the story concludes with the "unfortunate" (?) man having to flee Russia beyond the force of the excommunication!

During the last two centuries xenograft bone from a variety of species, including dog [3], monkeys [4], rabbit [5], calf [6-7], sheep [8], goose [9], eagle [9], as well as far more "exotic" materials, like ox and cow horns [10], ivory [11-13], sea algae [14] and corals from the Great Barrier Reef [15-16] have been transplanted into man. Although satisfactory treatment outcomes were occasionally reported, most of these materials produced rather poor results. For example, animal horns and ivory were found very resistant to incorporation into the host bone, and fresh xenograft bones – due to the antigenicity of the foreign tissue – consistently resulted in inflammation, fever, sequestration, resorption or other manifestations of rejection [17-18].

Amongst the above-mentioned xenograft materials, bovine bones have been the most preferred ones, basically because they are easily obtainable and there are no great ethical considerations regarding their use. Additionally they have the great advantage of practically unlimited availability of source/raw material. In the past fresh, fresh-frozen, freeze-dried (e.g. Boplant®, Squibb, New Brunswick, NJ, USA), and partially deproteinized and defatted (e.g. Kiel-bone; Surgibone®, Unilab Surgibone Inc., Canada; Navigraft™, Tutogen Medical GmbH, Neunkirchen am Brand, Germany) preparations have been used. Freeze-drying was thought to decrease the antigenicity of the material compared to that of fresh bone, thus rendering the graft more osteocompatible; however, implantation of freeze-dried bovine bone induced strong local inflammatory reactions postoperatively [19-20]. Partial removal of the organic component of bovine bone was also supposed to yield in an end-product with reduced antigenicity and a mild immune response [21], and successful treatment outcomes have been reported with such grafts in a variety of orthopedic [22-27] and dental [28-30] applications. In numerous other studies, however, disappointing results (e.g. high infection rates, nonunions, fibrous encapsulation, sequestration) have been observed after grafting with these materials [31-39], indicating inconsistencies in the production method. Today their use has been almost completely abandoned.

Recently, new processing and purification techniques have resulted in bovine bone products without the organic component (e.g. Bio-Oss®/Orthos®, Geistlich Söhne AG, Switzerland and Osteohealth, Shirley, New York, USA; Lubboc®/ Laddec®, Ost Development SA, France, Endobon®, Biomet Inc., Dordrecht, The Netherlands; OsteoGraf®/N, DENTSPLY Friadent Cera-Med, Lakewood, CO, USA, Cerabone®, aap Implantate AG, Berlin, Germany). In general, however, the use of such xenografts is limited in current orthopedic clinical practice [40-43]40-43) primarily because they have reduced mechanical strength/low fracture strength and cannot be used in load bearing applications [44-45]. On the other hand, there has recently been a great interest in these products in periodontology and dental implantology due to the increasing demand for alveolar and jaw bone regeneration. The current chapter will restrict itself in reviewing the use of deproteinized bovine bone grafts in association with various applications in dentistry.

7.2. Basic Science

Deproteinized bovine bone (DBB) belongs to the calcium phosphate (CaP) group of biomaterials. In general, the handling of the raw bovine bone material is aiming at the deactivation, destruction and removal of all unwanted organic substance (cells, proteins, fats, viruses and microbes) so that a pure inorganic matrix containing hydroxyapatite, and some of the minor and trace elements originally present in bone, such as Mg^{2+}, Na^{+}, CO_3^{2-}, is left behind [46-47]. This goal is achieved through several chemical purification processes, including strong alkaline baths, heat treatment and γ-irradiation. Nevertheless, differences in the purification steps and manipulation methods of the raw material do exist among the various proprietary technologies, leading to products with possibly variable biological behavior.

Depending on the temperature of the production process' heat treatment step, commercially available DBB products are basically of two types: unsintered (e.g. Bio-Oss®, Lubboc®/Laddec®) and sintered (e.g. OsteoGraf®/N, Endobon®, Cerabone®). Mass spectrometric analysis of the released gases has determined three ranges of mass loss of heat-treated bone [48]:

From room temperature to about 200° C, incorporated water is lost.
Above ca. 300° C, organic material like collagen, fat tissue, proteins start to burn, and at ca. 400° C, only the mineral phase is left.
Between 400° C and 900° C, carbonated apatite is lost.

Thus, heat treatment at 300° C does not affect crystallinity and yields an unsintered bovine bone mineral with a calcium and phosphorous content of 37 percent and 18 percent, respectively (Ca:P ratio = 2.1±0.1) [49] and consisting of small crystals of carbonate (CO_3^{2-}) hydroxyapatite (10-60 nm crystal size; 7 percent CO_3^{2-}-content) [50], similarly to normal (untreated) human bone tissue (Fig. 7.1). The resulting material also preserves the macroscopic structural characteristics of bovine bone (pore size 300 to 1,500 microns, total porosity 70 to 75 percent, specific surface area 97 m^2/gr) [51], and is comparable to human

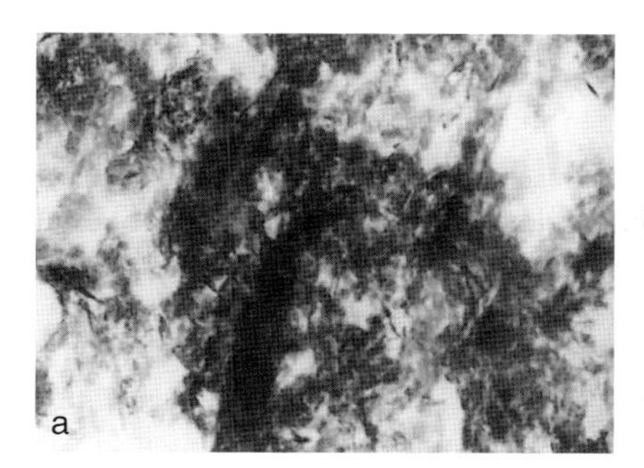

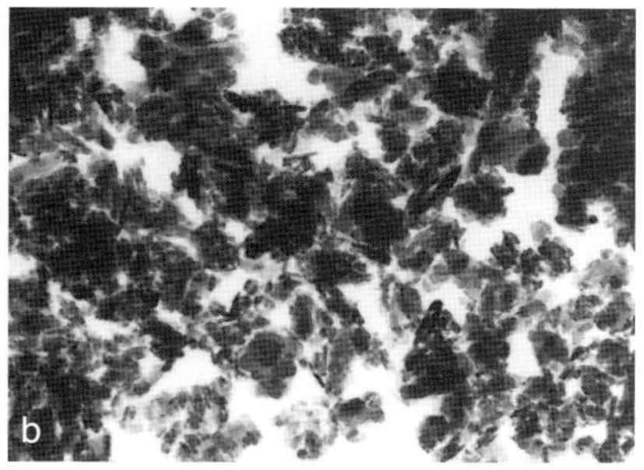

Fig. 7.1 The architecture of the unsintered DBB crystals (a) reflects the fine structure of human bone (b). TEM 100.000x (images provided by Geistlich Pharma AG, Wohlhusen, Switzerland)

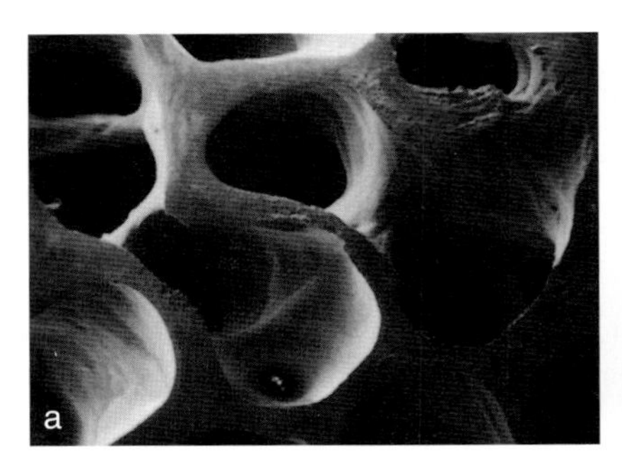

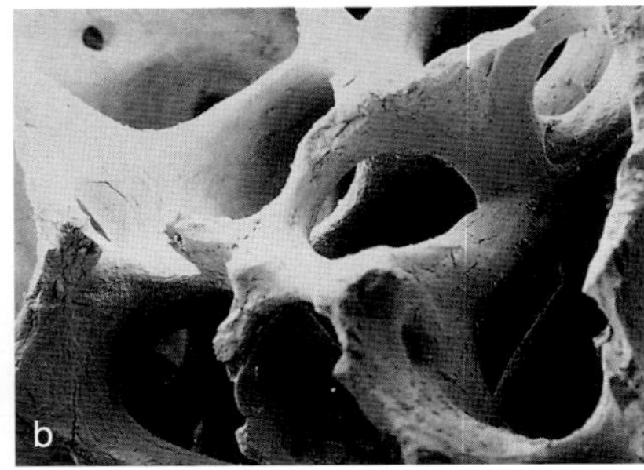

Fig. 7.2 The macro-porous mineral structure of unsintered DBB (a) is very similar to that of human bone (b). SEM 50x (images provided by Geistlich Pharma AG, Wohlhusen, Switzerland)

bone both morphologically (Fig. 7.2) and with regard to its mechanical properties [52]. When heating the material > 1,000 ° C, on the other hand, sintering occurs and the result is bone mineral consisting of large, CO_3^{2-}-deficient apatite crystals [45]. Additionally, in a recently published study evaluating a variety of CaP materials it was observed that sintering, apart from changes in crystallinity, also negatively affects the microporosity of the bovine bone since unsintered DBB was found to have statistically significant larger specific surface area than sintered DBB (79.7 m^2/g *versus* 0.7 m^2/g, respectively) [53].

Unsintered and sintered DBB, in theory, also differ with regard to their biodegradability. Cell-mediated biodegradation of a CaP biomaterial occurs under acidic conditions, and *in vitro* dissolution studies of CaP biomaterials are considered to be predictive of their *in vivo* dissolution or biodegradation. It has been found that the extent of dissolution of a CaP biomaterial depends on various structural characteristics such as particle size, porosity (microporosity and macroporosity), specific surface area and crystallinity (reflecting crystal size and perfection) [54-55]. Indeed, the extent of dissolution of unsintered DBB in acidic buffer was found to be greater than that of sintered bone [45].

Variables such as porosity, surface geometry and surface chemistry, and biodegradability are considered to play a decisive role in the capacity of a graft to support/promote bone formation [56]. Although there is no consensus and various pore size ranges have been suggested as being the most suitable, it is reasonable to expect that human bone possesses the ideal configuration. Thus, unsintered DBB seems to be an excellent substratum (perhaps better than sintered DBB), with appropriate chemical composition and architectural geometry, that may support tissue ingrowth, osteoprogenitor cell attachment, migration and proliferation, and phenotypic expression of bone cells (i.e., osteoconduction), leading to formation of new bone in direct apposition to the graft (i.e., bioactivity).

DBB is commercially available in particulate form of cancellous or cortical bone, with varying granule size (e.g. from 0.25-0.5 to 1.00-2.00 mm), or as cancellous bone blocks of various dimensions. Unsintered DBB also exists as a preformed block of graft particles supplemented with 10 percent of highly purified swine-skin collagen (Bio-Oss® Collagen, Geistlich Pharma AG, Wolhusen, Switzerland), which eases clinical handling (the block can be cut/shaped to the desired configuration and be transferred/applied to the desired place with forceps). Recently, a product containing sintered DBB (OsteoGraf®/N) coated with a 15-chain synthetic peptide (P-15), responsible for the cell binding domain of Type I collagen (PepGen P-15™, DENTSPLY Friadent Cera-Med, Lakewood, CO, USA), has become available. The vast majority of existing dental literature is on unsintered DBB (i.e., Bio-Oss®).

7.3. Pre-clinical Studies and Clinical Studies

7.3.1. In vitro Studies

In vitro studies have shown that unsintered DBB has the ability to support attachment, spreading, proliferation and matrix synthesis of isolated osteoblastic cells from rat calvariae [57-58], and that it also presents a favorable substrate for a three-dimensional cultivation of human osteoblast-like cells which were able to attach, divide and synthesize mature collagen [59]. Nevertheless, in the above-mentioned study by Stephan, et al. [58], maximum proliferation was found at 24 hours whereas, at the following time points, the proliferation of osteoblasts had decreased more than 50 percent of the 24-hour value. Osteoblast-like cells cultured with sintered DBB exhibited increased DNA and collagenous protein synthesis and increased alkaline phosphatase activity, suggesting that sintered DBB may also be an acceptable substrate for growth and differentiation of osteoblast-like cells [60]. Furthermore, sintered DBB coated with P-15 showed an increased attachment of human dermal fibroblasts [61] and periodontal ligament cells [62] which formed three-dimensional colonies with cellular bridges between adjacent particles having tissue-like structure, and had increased DNA production compared with cells on uncoated DBB. When osteoblasts derived from human iliac crest were seeded on the three DBB types and cell proliferation and viability were evaluated, sintered DBB coated with P-15 showed the highest proliferation and differentiation rate, while unsintered DBB showed the lowest [63]. Similarly, when osteoblasts from human alveolar bone were cultured on the surface of sintered DBB/P-15 or unsintered DBB and evaluated with respect to cell attachment, proliferation and osteogenic differentiation, those cultured on sintered DBB/P-15 showed a continuous increase in DNA content, protein synthesis and alkaline phosphatase activity, while cells cultured on unsintered DBB showed a decrease in DNA content from day six to day 21, and in protein synthesis on day 21; alkaline phosphatase levels of activity were at the lowest on day 21 [64].

In another recent *in vitro* study the ability of unsintered DBB (Bio-Oss®) and sintered DBB (OsteoGraf®/N) to undergo osteoclastic resorption was evaluated [65]. Although, both materials were found to support osteoclast attachment, some spreading and survival in culture, only unsintered DBB showed large scallop-edged resorption pits with trails and exposed collagen when examined by SEM – although not to the same extent as unprocessed natural bone material.

7.3.2. Risk of Disease Transmission

In the above-mentioned study by Taylor, et al. [65], X-ray photoelectron spectroscopic analysis revealed the presence of nitrogen in the surface layers of unsintered DBB and some areas of the material were positively stained for bovine Type I collagen after it had been exposed to osteoclastic activity, suggesting that there is residual protein in that product. A similar assumption was previously made by Schwartz, et al. [66] who, following solvent extraction, gel electrophoresis (SDS-PAGE) and silver staining and Western blotting, alleged the presence of the proteins transforming growth factor-beta (TGF-β) and bone morphogenetic protein-2 (BMP-2) in Bio-Oss®. When these extracts were implanted in combination with inactive demineralized freeze-dried bone allograft (DFDBA) in the calf muscle of nude mice, similar amounts of bone formation (i.e., osteoinduction) with those achieved by active DFDBA were observed. Also, in a short communication, Honig, et al. [67] claimed presence of protein remnants, based on the observation that Bio-Oss® was strongly reactive to Coomassie-blue staining, a dye which is normally used as a reagent for detecting protein. These observations have raised concerns regarding the safety of the product. Prions, which are mainly composed of an altered normal protein, cause Creutzfeldt-Jakob disease (CJD) in humans and bovine spongiform encephalopathy (BSE) in cattle, and the new variant CJD (vCJD) in humans appears to be caused through consumption of infectious bovine food products. Therefore, the use of unsintered DBB for grafting raises the question, to what degree can such material be considered completely free of proteins and what is the risk of transmission of the disease to humans? Sintered DBB is not under question because of its production process (heating >1,000° C). In this context, however, it has to be mentioned that none of the vCJD patients had a history of surgery [68] and that, to date, there are no reported cases of disease transfer through dental use of bovine bone xenografts.

Unfortunately, no marker currently exists to screen potential donors/animals for CJD/BSE. At present the only way to irrevocably establish diagnosis is postmortem brain biopsy, and the final test for the presence of CJD/BSE-contaminating agent is inoculation of animals with donor tissue which, unfortunately, includes a long latency and survival period [69-71].

In a recent paper [72] the safety of unsintered DBB (Bio-Oss®) was evaluated, experimentally as well as statistically, and compared to the risk calculated for sintered DBB (Osteograf®/N). To determine the prion inactivation capacity of the alkaline treatment used in the manufacturing process of Bio-Oss®, the authors treated BSE brain homogenates from confirmed Swiss cases of BSE and then checked for the presence of PrP^{Sc} (the disease-specific form of the prion protein) by Western blotting. The risk assessment was based on a system of safety requirements for products made from cattle, goats or sheep published by the German Federal Health Authority [73-74]. Risk evaluation includes all relevant aspects of production and application, such as origin and feeding of the animals, type of tissue used for production, processing steps for inactivation of prions, amount of raw material needed for the production of one daily dose, number of daily doses and method of application. The German risk assessment also induces the worst-case assumption that there are no species barriers between humans and animals, an issue that still remains open. The probability of humans contracting CJD spontaneously is less than one in 1 million, which corresponds to a value of 20 in the German system. During risk calculation, for example, use of animals from countries with no cases of BSE gives a factor of six, while use of animals of unknown origin gives a factor of one. Regarding the type of tissue, bone is amongst the tissues bearing the least risk of infection with a factor of eight, while spinal bone marrow gets a factor zero as this tissue contains high concentrations of prions in infected animals. The results of the experiment indicated complete inactivation of PrP^{Sc}, while risk assessment produced value ranges of 26 to 38.7 for unsintered DBB, and of 24.5 to 26.3 for sintered DBB. In a previously published risk assessment, a factor of 30 was calculated for sintered DBB, which is much less than that posed by the risk of death related to lightning, tornadoes or similar rare events [75]. The finding that Bio-Oss® is free from any protein content was confirmed in another recent study where the material was thoroughly examined with a variety of tests, including Bio-Rad protein micro-assay, SDS-PAGE and silver staining, and Western blotting [50]. According to these authors, the 60-65 kDa bands observed in the Western blotting analysis by Schwartz, et al. [66] and interpreted as evidence of the presence of a high molecular complex of TGF-β in Bio-Oss®, seem to be rather artifactual, while staining of Bio-Oss® with Coomassie-blue seems to be due the CO_3^{-2} content of the product. However, none of the above-mentioned studies [50, 72] commented on the results of the osseoinduction test performed in the study by Schwartz, et al. [66].

7.3.3. Experimental and Clinical Studies on Bone Regeneration (Defects, Sinus Augmentations and Implants)

There is a plethora of clinical studies reporting that DBB facilitated bone healing and implant osseointegration when grafted in extraction sockets, regardless of the implantation regimen (i.e., immediately after tooth extraction or after some period allowing for soft tissue healing) [76-79], in jaw bone defects [80] or when used as onlay grafts [81-82]. DBB grafting, alone or in combination with other materials (most often autogenous bone), for augmenting the maxillary sinus and simultaneous or delayed implant placement (i.e., 1- or 2-stage sinus lifts) [83-92] has also yielded excellent results, with implant survival rates of 92 percent to 97 percent [93-96] which are similar to those achieved with autogenous bone grafting or to those reported for implants placed in pristine bone [97-98]. Similarly, successful clinical results were observed/reported when DBB was applied in combination with non-resorbable or resorbable membrane barriers according to the principle of guided tissue regeneration (GTR) (often under the terms of guided bone regeneration (GBR) or guided bone augmentation (GBA)), in association with immediate or delayed-immediate implants placed in extraction sockets and presenting a dehiscence or intrabony defect, with implants placed in narrow ridges resulting in exposed implant threads [99-111], in association with vertical bone augmentation and 1- or 2-stage sinus lifts, [83, 90, 112-121] or treatment of peri-implantitis [122]. Acceptable clinical results were also achieved when unsintered DBB was used as interpositional graft during orthognathic surgery [123], and it is claimed that covering of onlay block grafts with unsintered DBB may reduce their resorption [124].

Although clinical success is the goal of all therapeutic procedures, interpreting biological events based solely on clinical evaluation and/or clinical success criteria may lead to erroneous conclusions and/or incorrect treatment approaches. For example, bone fill in periodontal intrabony defects, as demonstrated in radiographs, was formerly accepted to indicate periodontal regeneration, and regrowth of alveolar bone was believed to be necessary for the re-establishment of a connective tissue attachment on the previously diseased portion of the root. Consequently, treatment modalities aiming at stimulating bone growth were often utilized (for review see [125-126]). However, today it is well documented that the re-establishment of a connective tissue attachment on a root surface and the regeneration of alveolar bone are unrelated phenomena [127-130], and that radiographic changes (e.g., bone fill/regrowth) after treatment do not necessarily indicate changes in the fibrous attachment level, and a long junctional epithelium may be lining the root surface [131-133].

Thus, histological documentation on the sequence of events and/or the treatment outcome is essential. Obviously, human histological data obtained from controlled clinical trials would provide the most convincing evidence for the potential of a procedure to facilitate bone regeneration. However, such studies are rather difficult to conduct and may be ethically questionable for many; thus histological evidence from humans is usually limited to case reports. Indeed, there are several publications [80, 82-84, 87, 92-93, 95, 112-113, 118, 120, 134-138] with histological evaluation of "bone core" biopsies mainly from DBB grafted sinuses but also from other types of defects. In all of the biopsies, variable amounts of new bone – values from 15 percent up to 42 percent have been reported in sinus biopsies – in contact with the DBB particles were observed, while a variable amount of the graft was embedded in soft fibrovascular connective tissue; the graft particles always constituted a significant portion of the biopsy. In one report, larger amounts of bone could be observed in biopsies harvested from sinuses augmented with sintered DBB combined with autogenous bone than from those grafted with only sintered DBB [83], but in another report similar amounts of bone were observed after unsintered DBB+autogenous bone (80 percent DBB; 20 percent autog) or only unsintered DBB grafting [93]. Another report claimed that sinuses grafted with sintered DBB coated with P-15 showed enhanced bone formation within a shorter time interval, compared with those augmented with a composite graft material consisting of sintered DBB+demineralized freeze-dried bone allograft [84]. However, due to problems such as missing/incomplete description of the exact site of biopsy harvesting and/or biopsy dimensions, no correlation of biopsy length with the pre-existing alveolar bone height, variable graft combinations, different healing/evaluation periods, inconsistency in the method of histomorphometric assessment, and generally a limited number of units (i.e., patients/biopsies), a collective coherent interpretation of the results regarding the effect of DBB on bone formation is rather difficult. Actually, in a recently published systematic review of clinical studies reporting histomorphometric data from sinus augmentation procedures with a variety of grafting materials, it was concluded that DBB seemed to produce amongst the lowest amounts of bone, but it was also stated that firm conclusions could not be drawn because there were substantial differences between the studies [139]. On the other hand, it became obvious from those data that both sintered and unsintered DBB persist for a long period of time {up to six years [80]), and that DBB particles occupy a substantial portion of the grafted space. Apparently some resorption of the DBB might had occurred, since osteoclast-like cells were occasionally observed in the vicinity of the graft particles; obviously, no firm conclusion on the rate of resorption could be drawn, since there was no information on the amount of DBB at "baseline" (i.e., at the time of grafting).

To objectively evaluate the genuine nature of DBB's effect on bore healing, the results of animal experiments must be considered. Indeed, the results of various animal experimental models report that DBB promotes bone formation when implanted in surgically created calvarial [49, 140-141], jaw bone [142] and tibial [143-145] defects in rabbits, calvarial defects in pigs [146-148], jaw bone defects in dogs [149-151] or in elevated sinuses in chimpanzees [152-154], compared with non-grafted control defects. DBB has also been shown to facilitate the osseointegration of implants placed in tibial defects [155] and alveolar defects [156] in dogs and in combination with sinus lift procedures in experimental animals, both when implants were inserted simultaneously or consecutively [157-163].

In a recent study, for example, cylindrical defects (3.5 mm in diameter × 8 mm deep) in the edentulous mandibular alveolar ridge in dogs were grafted with unsintered DBB or left empty to serve as controls [151]. After three months almost complete regeneration could be observed in the non-augmented defects (mineralized bone 39 percent, marrow 61 percent), but a 0.8 mm invagination existed in the surface of the reformed crestal bone. Defects grafted with DBB also presented a bridge of new bone that sealed the marginal entrance of the defect (i.e., complete fill of the defect), however, exhibited less wound shrinkage with only a minimal invagination of 0.1 mm. The new bone consisted of thin trabeculae that had grown from the margins of the defect in direct contact with most of the DBB particles, which occasionally – mainly in the lateral/apical portions and in the coronal bridge – were completely incorporated into the new bone. However, a considerable portion of the graft – mainly in the central segment of the defect – was surrounded by fibrovascular connective tissue. Mineralized bone and bone marrow made up 47 percent and 26 percent, respectively, of the newly formed tissue, while DBB occupied 27 percent of the total tissue volume inside the defect. In another recent study Thorwarth, et al. [147] created 10 mm × 10 mm cylindrical defects in the frontal bone in pigs and grafted them with either unsintered DBB (Bio-Oss®) or sintered DBB (OsteoGraf®/N), or with autogenous bone, or left them empty to serve as controls. The authors reported that after 26 weeks of healing there was virtually complete bone fill in the Bio-Oss® grafted sites, with DBB particles enclosed in newly formed bone covering the whole cross section area of the defect, while new bone formation in the OsteoGraf®/N treated sites extended to the lower two-thirds of the originally created defect. The difference in new mineralized bone between Bio-Oss® treated sites and those filled with OsteoGraf®/N was found to be statistically significant (44 percent versus 32 percent of the defect space, respectively); however, this difference should be interpreted with care because of the limited number of animals/sites included in the study. Regarding the amount of residual graft material, both unsintered and sintered DBB did not reduce during the course of the study, and occupied a considerable portion of the defect (Bio-Oss®: 41 percent to 44 percent, OsteoGraf®/N: 19 percent to 21 percent). Bone fill in the sites grafted with autogenous bone was complete, while approximated 75 percent of the defect area in originally empty controls. Using the same experimental model, Thorwarth, et al. [146] observed that coating sintered DBB with P-15 significantly accelerates bone formation during early stages of healing (from one to three months) as compared with uncoated sintered DBB, but there was no difference between the two groups after six months (mineralized bone fill ~40 percent versus ~37 percent, respectively). On the other hand, P-15 did not influence the biodegradation rate of sintered DBB, which again occupied a considerable portion

(~41 percent to 43 percent) of the defect after six months. Similarly, accelerated bone formation was observed during early stages of healing (from one to two months) when autogenous bone was added in unsintered DBB (25 percent autog:75 percent DBB), while there was no difference between the groups (i.e., autog + DBB vs. DBB solo) after three and six months [148].

On the other hand some reports have yielded compromised results after using DBB. For instance, unsintered and sintered DBB failed to exhibit any osteoconductive or osteoinductive effect when placed as onlay grafts on the rat maxilla and, instead, led to a foreign body reaction [164]. In other reports from experiments in rabbits, sheep and goats, DBB grafted defects did not perform better than empty controls in terms of bone regeneration [165-169]. For example, in a series of experiments in goats, Merkx, et al. [167-168, 170] created full thickness, critical-size, cylindrical bone defects in the frontal bone of the animals and filled them with autogenous or unsintered DBB grafts in various combinations, or left them empty to serve as controls. After 24 weeks of healing, it was observed that DBB granules did not stimulate osteoconduction when compared with the empty controls, but resulted to an extensive osteoclastic activity, and that the new bone basically "pushed" the graft particles outwards. DBB blocks performed a bit better, but again larger amounts of bone formation were observed in control defects. Defects grafted with particulated or block cancelous autogenous bone performed equally well (i.e., healed completely), while cortical bone block seemed more reliable than cortical chips. When a composite graft consisting of particulate autogenous cancellous bone/unsintered DBB graft was used, all defects were completely bridged after six to 12 weeks of healing, while composite grafts consisting of particulate autogenous cortical bone/unsintered DBB did not bridge even after 24 weeks of healing.

The failure of DBB-filled defects to enhance bone healing when compared to non-grafted controls as observed in the above-mentioned studies is difficult to explain, but may be due to differences in the experimental models regarding defect site, dimensions and configuration, as well as differences in healing times. Indeed, when evaluating the results following application of candidate technologies for regeneration in animal models and in order to reasonably extract information transferable into clinical situations, defect dimensions and configuration should be critically considered. Of course, an essential parameter is that the model satisfies criteria for a critical size defect [171]. Such a defect will not resolve within the lifetime of the animal unless subject to a regenerative technology. Use of lesser defects may only detract from our understanding of wound healing/regeneration and it is imperative, in this context, to point out that "lifetime of the animal" implies/signifies the duration of the experiment! Nevertheless, defect size *per se* plays an important role; obviously, during a given period of time, small/smaller critical size defects subjected to regenerative treatment (e.g., GTR) will heal with larger amounts of bone in terms of percent of defect fill, than large/larger critical size defects subjected to the same regenerative treatment (Fig. 7.3a and 7.3b). Indeed, absolute values (e.g., height, volume) of bone formation are rarely reported, something that would somewhat ease comparisons between studies. Similarly, defect configuration is an important parameter and healing of a 3-wall self-contained defect appears greatly influenced by the vascular and cellular resources from the surrounding bony walls circumscribing the defect, and it is obvious that

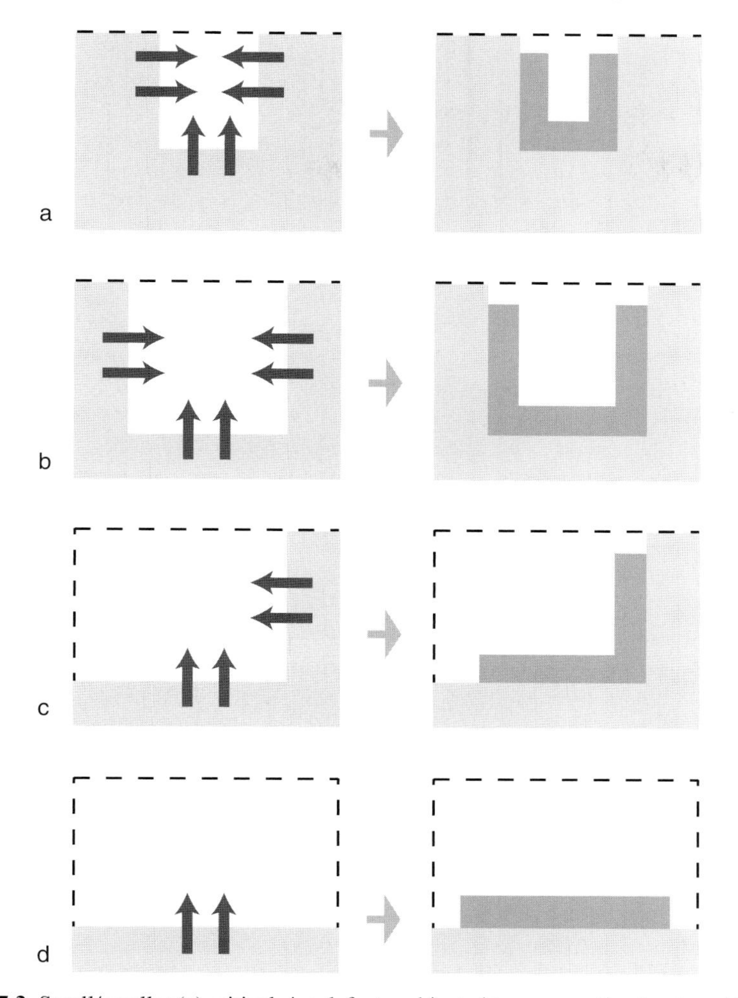

Fig. 7.3 Small/smaller (a) critical size defects subjected to regenerative treatment (e.g., covered with a membrane: dotted line) will heal with larger amounts of bone in terms of percent of defect fill than large/larger (b) critical size defects subjected to the same treatment during the same amount of time. Similarly, a 3-wall defect (b) subjected to regenerative treatment will present more bone fill than a 2- wall (c) or 1-wall (d) defect subjected to the same regenerative treatment during the same period of time (*See Color Plates*)

the distribution and contribution of tissue resources is dramatically altered and reduced in 2- and 1-wall defects. Obviously, during a given period of time, a 3-wall defect subjected to regenerative treatment will present more bone fill than a 2- or 1-wall defect of similar dimensions subjected to the same regenerative treatment (Figs. 7.3b, 7.3c and 7.3d).

In perspective, our laboratory has developed and characterized the "capsule model" in rats, which offers superior discriminating capabilities for testing the bone promoting potential of various biomaterials. The model comprises the placement of a rigid, hemispherical polytetrafluoroethylene (PTFE) capsule on the lateral surface of the mandibular ramus, on either side of the jaw in rats, with its open part facing the bone surface (Fig. 7.4). The capsule has

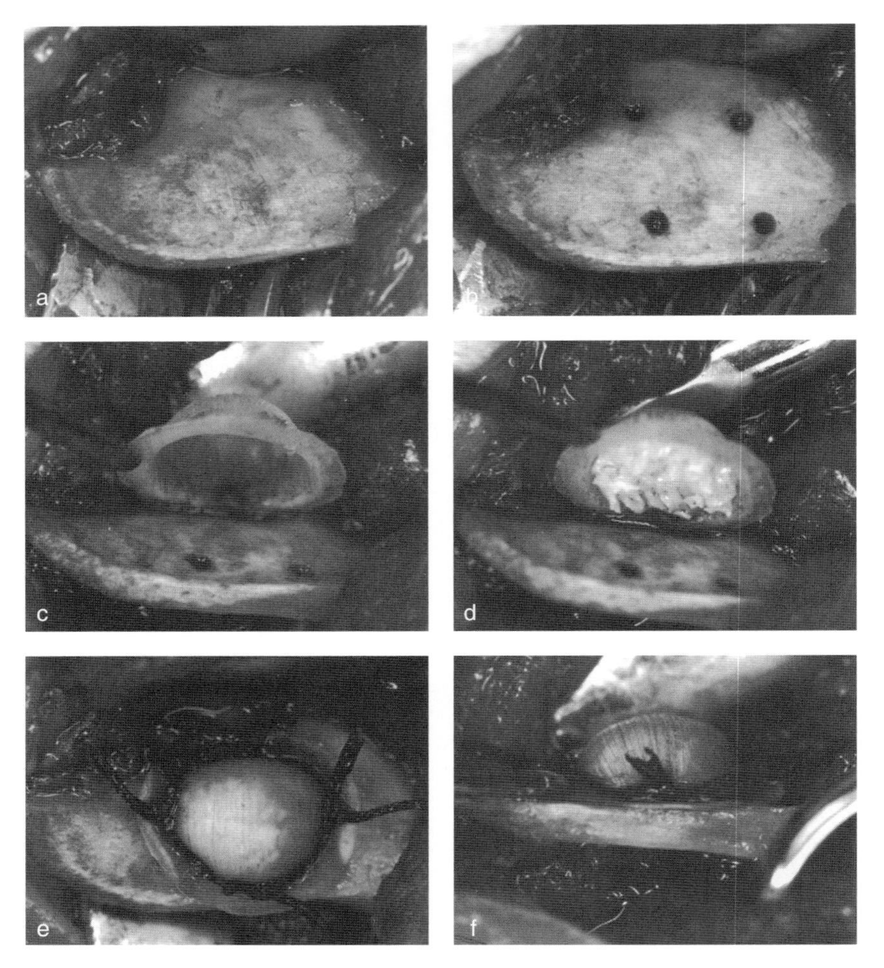

Fig. 7.4 The mandibular ramus is exposed (a) and four holes are drilled (b). A Teflon capsule is then placed and may be either left empty to serve as control (c) or be filled with biomaterial under testing (e.g., DBB) (d). The capsule is stabilized by means of sutures passing through the collar of the capsule and the holes in the ramus (e), and thus a tight adaptation of the capsule onto the bone surface can be achieved (f) (*See Color Plates*)

a peripheral collar that allows close adaptation and stabilization of the device on the bone surface by means of sutures passing through holes drilled in the ramous. In this way, a secluded space is created adjacent to an essentially uninjured bone surface and, at the same time, the surrounding soft connective tissues are excluded from participating in the healing process. The rigid non-collapsible capsule with a standardized volume creates an experimental region that is clearly defined and unchangeable throughout the course of the study period, and identical in the different experimental groups. The capsules may be filled with various grafts, biomaterials and/or bioactive substances, or may be left empty to serve as controls. It has been shown that when such empty capsules are placed, continuous bone formation occurs predictably for at least four to six months after capsule placement, until the capsules are eventually filled up with newly formed bone after a period of six to 12 months [172-174] (Fig. 7.5). When choosing a shorter observation period, a material's bioactivity on the formation of bone tissue can be readily discriminated. The amount of bone formed under "optimal" conditions (i.e., in empty capsules) for a given observation period reflects the intrinsic bone forming potential of the model for this specific time period, and may serve as the standard during evaluation of the results. Thus, capsules receiving materials that favor bone regeneration will either present larger amounts of newly formed bone at a given time-point (for example, after four months) or fill the capsule earlier (or both) compared to originally empty control capsules. The fact that the space inside the capsule is voluminous compared with the anatomy of the region (the height of the capsule is 3 mm and the thickness of the ramus of an adult rat at that particular region is less than 0.5 mm), offers superior possibilities to distinguish between osteo-promotive versus osteo-inhibitory substances, in a rather economical set-up. Materials that "fail" the "capsule model test" should be critically evaluated for their potential to promote bone formation, since rats generally are considered to have better regenerative potential than higher animals and humans. Conversely, materials that "pass" this challenging test may be worthwhile to test in more clinically relevant models.

The potential of unsintered DBB (Bio-Oss®) to promote bone formation has been evaluated with the "capsule model" [173-175]. DBB filled capsules presented limited amounts of new bone after four months of healing when compared with the originally empty control capsules (12 percent of the total

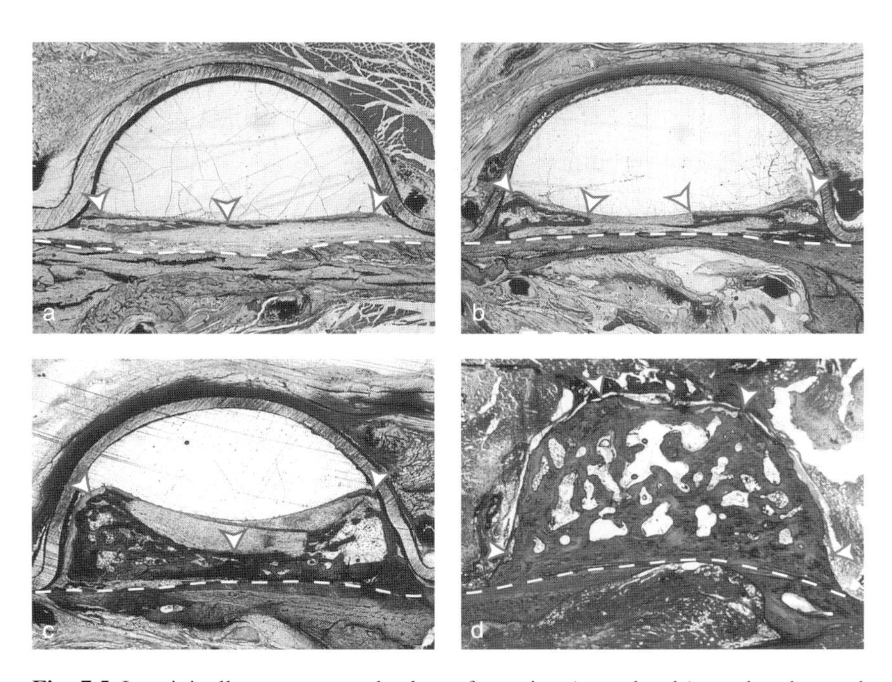

Fig. 7.5 In originally empty capsules bone formation (arrowheads) can be observed already after one month of healing (a), and increasing amounts of new bone are formed after two (b) and four months (c), until 12 months (d) where the capsules are almost entirely filled out with bone. The dotted line indicates the level of pristine bone (*See Color Plates*)

capsule space in the grafted specimens versus 39 percent in the controls) [173], while extending the healing period up to one year, did not have a dramatic change in terms of bone formation inside the DBB filled capsules (average bone fill: 23 percent; average height of new bone: 1.4 mm) [174] (Figs. 7.5 and 7.6). The newly formed bone inside the DBB grafted capsules was in continuity with the preexisting host bone, had a dense appearance with few marrow spaces and had grown in direct contact with DBB particles, which in many cases were totally incorporated into bone. However, bone formation was confined to the lower part of the capsule and extended only a limited distance from the preexisting bone surface. In the remaining major part of the space originally created by the capsule (i.e., at a larger distance from the host bone), the graft particles remained embedded in fibrovascular connective tissue. The osteocyte lacunae in the graft particles were empty and there were no signs of progressive resorption of the particles or extensive bone formation. On the other hand, this newly formed bone seemed to be stable on a long-term basis, since the amounts of bone observed six months after capsule removal (average bone fill: 21.5 percent; average bone height: 1.3 mm) were similar to those formed under the capsules after one year [175], which is in accordance with findings in other animal studies [162, 176].

In recently published animal and human studies a similar "pattern" of bone formation was observed after applying DBB in various types of bone defect, and the DBB+GTR combination resulted in less amounts of new bone/bone

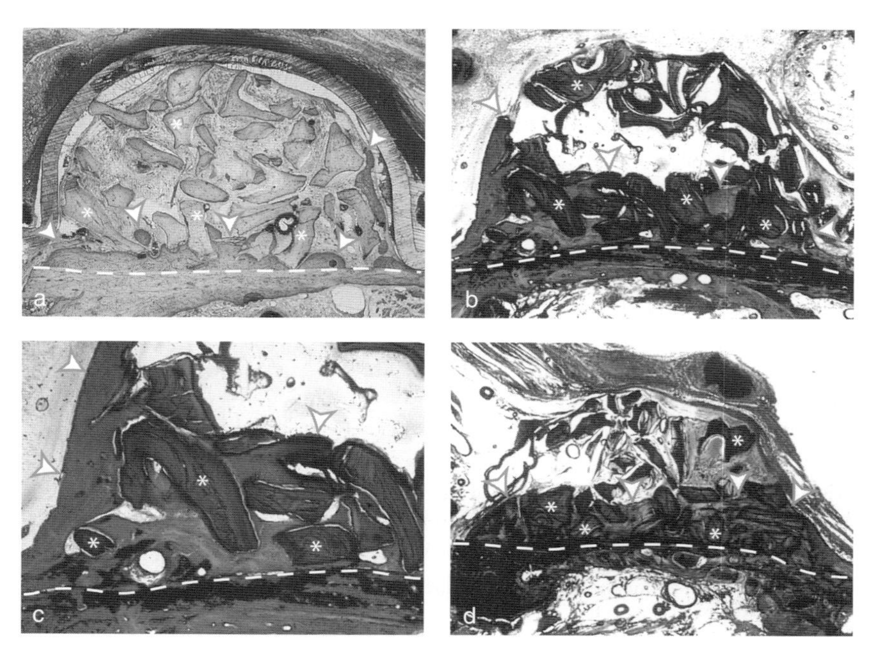

Fig. 7.6 Limited amounts of bone (arrowheads) confined in the vicinity of the pristine bone (dotted line) are observed inside capsules grafted with unsintered DBB after four (a) or 12months (b) of healing. The new bone grows in continuity with the host bone and in contact with the DBB particles (stars) (c), which occupy the major portion of the capsules. The amount of new bone remains basically stable for at least six months after capsule removal (d) (*See Color Plates*)

fill than what was observed in only GTR treated sites [125, 150, 177-181]. For instance. Carmagnola, et al. [178] prepared cylindrical defects in the edentulous mandible of Labrador dogs, which were either filled with unsintered DBB or left empty, and subsequently covered with a resorbable membrane. After three months of healing the major portion (56 percent) of the DBB treated defects was occupied by graft particles embedded in a cell-rich fibrous connective tissue, whereas the control defects were totally filled (99 percent) with new bone. When the same authors [179] examined cylindrical biopsies taken from extraction sockets of patients previously treated with a combination of DBB and a resorbable membrane, they observed that 77 percent of the area was occupied by residual graft particles and connective tissue, even after a mean period of seven months. Extraction sites treated only with a membrane, on the other hand, were totally filled with bone after only four months. In both these studies the new bone formation was in continuity with the preexisting bone and was confined to the periphery of the defects, whereas in the central portion of the lesions, the space was occupied by graft particles embedded in fibrovascular connective tissue.

Collectively, the findings of these studies [125, 150, 173-174, 177-181] suggest that, under optimal conditions for healing (i.e., well protected defects with secured space provision for GTR/GBR), DBB grafting does not enhance bone formation but, in fact, it may inhibit osseous healing. It appears that new bone formation tends to be confined to the vicinity of the host bone even with prolonged periods of healing. Therefore, it is reasonable to presume that a narrow defect filled with DBB may heal completely, while a wider one may not; similarly, a self-contained or 3-wall defect will heal more readily than a 2- or 1-wall defect. This assumption, in turn, may explain the positive results observed in the publications mentioned at the beginning of this section, where DBB grafted defects were found to be filled out with new bone. It is possible that the defects in those studies have had sufficiently small dimensions and/or favorable configuration to allow them to be filled out solely by the rather limited bone formation occurring adjacent to the host bone. Thus, a concept of DBB acting as a space provision device for tissue ingrowth rather than a bone promoting substance emerges from these observations. This view is also supported by observations in an animal experiment, where DBB in combination with GTR with collagen membranes was used to augment peri-implant defects in dogs [182]. In that study, vertical bone regeneration reached a higher level in DBB+GTR treated sites, compared with sites treated only with GTR. However, horizontal bone growth at a level located 1 mm from the base of the defect was similar in both situations. Obviously, the graft supported the soft collagen membrane that kept its position at a coronal level and, thereby, the space under the device was preserved, allowing for more tissue ingrowth in the GTR+DBB sites; in the GTR sites, the unsupported membrane partially collapsed into the defect (at the coronal level) and the space available for bone formation was decreased. In the apical portion of the defect, on the other hand, where the position of the membrane was ensured by the morphology of the defect and the anatomy of the region (i.e., space provision was achieved), the addition of DBB did not enhance bone formation. Indeed, the relative importance of space provision alongside that of tissue occlusion for GTR/GBR procedures has been recently elucidated [183-185].

The view that DBB acts as a bone filler material occupying a substantial portion of the grafted space, along with the fact that it persists in the area for a long period of time, raises concerns regarding to the true effect of DBB grafting on osseointegration of dental implants (i.e., the amount of bone-to-implant contact: BIC), as well as on the long-term outcome of treatment. Results of animal experiments, however, show that a similar amount of osseointegration of implants is achieved when the implants are inserted in DBB augmented sites or in native bone [155-156, 162]. Likewise, an implant removed from a patient six months after maxillary sinus augmentation with unsintered DBB demonstrated comparable BIC in the residual alveolar process (63 percent) as in the augmented part (73 percent) [92]. An interesting observation made in several studies [92, 155-156, 162, 182, 186-187] is that although the DBB particles occupy a substantial portion of the augmented defect/site, the xenograft was rarely found to be in direct contact with the implant surface. This indicates that during the early phase of healing, a tissue was formed on the titanium surface that prevented the graft particles from establishing a permanent presence in this location. With respect to the long-term outcome of implant treatment in association with DBB grafting, as already mentioned, survival rates similar to those reported for implants placed in pristine bone have been observed. This may be explained by the finding that bone formed in association with DBB remains stable on a long-term basis [162, 175-176]. However, the amount of bone-to-implant contact that is necessary to obtain and sustain osseointegration and trouble-free implant function is not yet determined. Indeed, in a review paper on augmentation procedures for the rehabilitation of deficient edentulous ridges with oral implants, published from the 1st European Association of Osseointegration Consensus Conference, it was concluded that "as the quantity of initial available bone before the augmentation procedure is very rarely specified in the various clinical studies, it is difficult to assert whether the success of implants relies on the augmented tissue or on the residual native bone" [188]. An important issue related to the long-term outcome of treatment is whether the DBB/regenerated bone tissue-blend may be more susceptible to destruction in the event of peri-implantitis. Currently, studies are being conducted in our laboratory to answer this question.

7.3.4. Experimental and Clinical Studies on Periodontal Regeneration

Bovine bone was introduced in periodontology during the first half of the 20th Century and many of its "versions" (e.g., boiled, Kielbone® etc.) were used in treating intrabony defects. Although some complications (e.g., sequestration) were reported [38, 189] improved clinical results (i.e., probing pocket depth (PPD) reduction, clinical attachment level (CAL) gain and radiographic bone fill) were observed [28-30, 190, 192]. More recently, it was claimed that implanting unsintered DBB into intrabony periodontal defects in dogs enhances bone regeneration, as compared with only surgically treated control defects [193], while implantation of unsintered DBB into periodontal defects in humans resulted in improved clinical parameters (decreased PPD, increased CAL and moderate defect fill [194-196]). As already mentioned, the rationale to stimulate bone regeneration was based on the assumption that clinical improvements and radiographic bone fill in periodontal intrabony defects indicates periodontal regeneration, and on the belief that regrowth of alveolar bone was necessary for the re-establishment of a connective tissue attachment on the previously diseased portion of the root. This assumption implied that the cells responsible for periodontal regeneration reside in bone. However, according to the current understanding of periodontal wound healing, the cells responsible for periodontal regeneration (i.e., *de novo* formation of a periodontal attachment including new cementum, a functionally oriented periodontal ligament, and alveolar bone) do not reside in bone tissue, but in the periodontal ligament itself (for review see [197]). Thus, the rationale for placing bone grafts in osseous periodontal defects to promote bone healing and, thereby, periodontal regeneration is indeed questionable.

On the other hand, considerable histologic and clinical evidence gathered over the last two decades has unequivocally proved that the regeneration of periodontal tissues lost as a result of periodontitis can be achieved in humans by means of guided tissue regeneration (GTR) (for review see [198]). Briefly, the GTR technique involves the surgical placement of a physical barrier (membrane) around the tooth, which covers the defect and thereby prevents epithelium and gingival connective tissue from coming in contact with the root surface and invading the defect space during healing. At the same time a secluded space is created and cells from the remaining periodontal ligament with the capacity to regenerate the lost tissues are allowed to re-populate the wound. A critical issue in GTR is that the space underneath the barrier is preserved for an adequate period of time during healing to allow complete periodontal regeneration to occur (i.e., formation of new cementum, periodontal ligament, *and* alveolar bone). In cases where the membrane collapses into the defects or towards the roots, reduced amounts of bone are formed, apparently due to a lack of space for tissue invasion/formation [199-201]. Thus, the placement of a bone graft under the barrier to compensate for the lack of space-keeping effect of the currently available membranes and prevent collapse and/or to promote bone formation, may be useful.

Indeed, there are several publications reporting on the outcome of treatment of periodontal intrabony defects with DBB (alone or in combination with autogenous bone or enamel matrix proteins (EMD)) used as adjunct to GTR. In previously published case series, CAL gains of 2.2–5.3 mm, PPD reductions of 2.9–6.7 mm, and residual PPDs of 3.5–5.2 mm were reported six to 12 months following treatment of intrabony defects with various types of resorbable membranes in combination with unsintered DBB (Bio-Oss®) [194-195, 202-209]. Also, findings from controlled clinical studies have indicated that treatment of intrabony defects with DBB+GTR may result in significantly higher CAL gains, PPD reductions and radiographic bone fill, compared with that obtained following access flap surgery [202, 210-213]. In the largest of these studies, including 124 patients in 10 centers in seven countries, the combined treatment had an added benefit of 0.8±0.3 mm of CAL gain over that obtained with flap surgery alone [212]. However, conflicting results have been reported when the DBB+GTR combination regimen was evaluated against only GTR in the treatment of intrabony defects. In a recent study a significantly larger CAL gain was observed after DBB+GTR, as compared with GTR, with a collagen membrane only (5.1 mm versus 4.0 mm, respectively) [214]. Yet, in another randomized controlled clinical trial, Stavropoulos, et al. did not find any difference in the clinical and radiographical improvements obtained with these two treatment modalities (CAL gain, DBB+GTR: 2.5 mm; GTR: 2.9 mm) [211].

The findings of the latter study are, in fact, in accordance with the results of a recently published systematic review evaluating a variety of bone grafts and/or substitutes as adjuncts to GTR that also failed to find any added clinical benefit of the combination treatment over that achieved by using only a membrane [215]. In this context, care should be taken when interpreting the results of periodontal regenerative therapy in combination with a bone graft/substitute. While improvement in clinical parameters can result in actual gain in attachment, placeing a bone graft into a defect may impede penetration of the periodontal probe without necessarily having induced any true gain in attachment. Similarly, radiographic data assessing bone fill after GTR, in combination with a mineralized bone graft as DBB should also be interpreted with caution since these grafts are barely distinguishable from the host bone in the radiographs, and grafts appearing on radiographs may not necessarily be incorporated in bone.

In a few of the above-mentioned clinical reports some of the roots (deemed as irrational to keep prior to treatment) were removed with surrounding tissues after six to nine months of healing and were processed for histological evaluation of the outcome of DBB+GTR treatment [194, 204-205, 207, 216]. In many instances it could be observed that epithelial downgrowth was prevented and variable amounts of new cementum, new attachment and new bone had been formed, but the connective tissue fibers of the "new" periodontal ligament were mostly oriented parallel to the root surface. Bone was never observed in contact with the root (i.e., no ankylosis) but had often formed in contact with DBB particles, while a substantial portion of the defect was occupied by graft particles embedded in a periodontal ligament-like connective tissue; this connective tissue was occasionally extending deep inside the DBB/regenerated bone network (Fig. 7.7) [205]. In a 4-cases report, where unsintered DBB was combined with intraoral autogenous bone and GTR in intrabony defects, the healing result after nine months was consistent with new attachment formation on the root and bone regeneration, but a major portion of the regenerated osseous tissue was occupied by deproteinized bone particles [203]. Some reports have also included evaluation of biopsies from sites treated with only DBB grafting [194, 207, 217], and more or less similar results with those obtained after the combined treatment – apparently related to a space provision function of the graft – were observed. However, as mentioned in the previous section of this chapter, the configuration of the defect must be considered when evaluating histological data, since the spatial distribution of tissue resources surrounding the defect plays an important role in the healing process; obviously, this also applies in the case of periodontal defects. Unfortunately, in the majority of the above-mentioned reports limited information is provided on the precise morphology of the defect and on the methodology of tissue/biopsy sampling, histological sectioning and evaluation; this renders an objective evaluation of the results difficult. In another report Paolantonio, et al. [216] took a core biopsy from the interdental area of a site treated eight months earlier with DBB and a collagen membrane, and found that some amount of periodontal regeneration had occurred only in the vicinity of the pre-existing lingual alveolar plate, while the majority of the defect space was occupied by DBB particles embedded in connective tissue. These authors concluded that "from a histologic point of view, the clinical appearance of bone regeneration is not always confirmed in the part of the defect far from the bony walls."

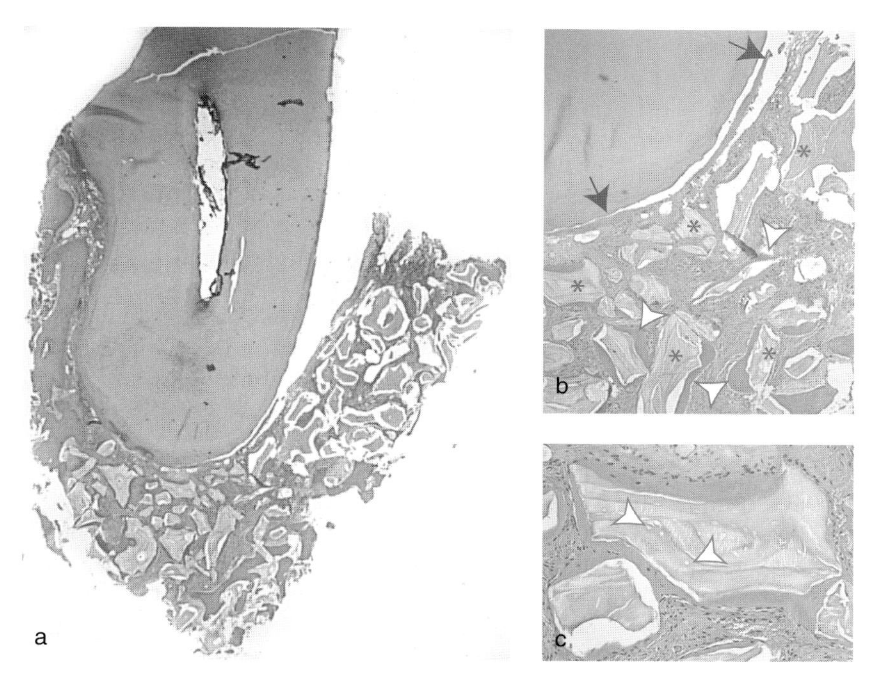

Fig. 7.7 Overview of a root with neighboring tissues, removed six months after treatment with unsintered DBB+GTR (a). New cementum (arrows) with inserting collagen fibers and a new bone-like tissue (arrowheads) in direct contact with DBB particles (star) can be observed (b). A substantial portion of the defect was occupied by graft particles with empty osteocytic lacunae (arrowheads) embedded in a periodontal ligament-like connective tissue (c) (*See Color Plates*)

In a recent experimental study in dogs [218], surgically created 1-wall, box-type defects (7 mm deep × 4 mm wide) were treated with unsintered DBB (Bio-Oss®) and a collagen membrane, and the result was evaluated histologically after six months of healing.

New cementum with inserting collagen fibers and new bone formation could be observed in all specimens. The regenerated bone was in continuity with the preexisting alveolar bone in the base and lateral walls of the defect, and in many instances was in contact with the DBB particles. The new bone was never found to be in contact with the root surface, i.e. no ankylosis was observed. However, bone formation was not constantly juxtaposed to the new cementum (or the denuded root surface), but its continuity was often "interrupted" by DBB particles embedded in a widened periodontal ligament-like connective tissue. This connective tissue was occasionally extending deep inside the DBB/regenerated bone network. By means of linear measurements, new cementum formation was estimated to be approximately 30 percent of the length of the previously denuded root surface, while bone formation reached up to 60 percent of the defect height. In another similar study in dogs [219] where the same DBB+GTR combination was compared to only GTR for the treatment of surgically induced 2-wall (5 mm deep × 5 mm wide) intrabony defects with the lingual bone wall preserved, the authors reported that periodontal regeneration occurred to a statistically significant greater extent (higher level) in sites receiving the combination regimen, compared with those treated only with a membrane. Yet, this study suffers from poor histological documentation. Collectively, the data from the currently existing animal and human histological studies show that some amounts of periodontal regeneration can be achieved when DBB is used as an adjunct to GTR. However, those histological results must be put in perspective with those of previous animal and human studies where complete periodontal regeneration has, indeed, been achieved by means of GTR without the use of a bone graft (for review see [197;198]).

The results of the clinical and histological studies presented above, where the combination treatment did not yield a clear added benefit, as well as the findings of the animal experiments presented in the previous section, where it was shown that DBB does not enhance bone formation but rather acts as a filler material, question whether DBB is beneficial as adjunct to GTR in the treatment of intrabony periodontal defects. However, an important aspect in such a discussion should also be the long-term effect of therapy. In a recent publication, the results after five years from DBB+GTR treatment of human intrabony defects were reported [220]. The significant clinical improvements obtained after treatment in a group of 11 patients remained basically stable and only a few patients had lost part of the CAL gain obtained one year after surgery – 36.6 percent experienced a CAL loss ≥1 mm and 9.1 percent showed a CAL loss ≥2 mm – whereas 63.7 percent of the sites presented with a CAL gain ≥4 mm, compared to baseline values. To date, there is no histological evidence on the long-term result of DBB in periodontal defects, but it is reasonable to expect that graft particles will also be present in treated periodontal sites for a long time, similarly to what has been observed for other type of bone defects treated with DBB [80, 82]. The results observed in the study of Stavropoulos and Karring [220] suggest that the mere presence of DBB particles in the reformed periodontal tissues may have no influence on the stability of the improved clinical conditions. This view is supported by the results of an animal experiment showing that the presence of graft particles did not hinder normal orthodontic tooth movement through extraction defects grafted with unsintered DBB [221].

7.4. Future Trends – DBB as a Carrier for Growth Factors

In reviewing the literature presented above it becomes apparent that DBB does not posses the ability to enhance bone formation and it acts rather as a space providing device. However, due to its favorable structural characteristics and excellent osteocompatibility, the combination of DBB with a substance capable of promoting bone formation may be useful. Indeed, DBB has been used as a carrier and/or controlled release device for biologically active substances such as growth factors for bone [160, 222-225] and/or periodontal regeneration [226-228], and promising results have been reported. However, an extensive review on this topic is beyond the scope of this chapter, and only a couple of examples will be given. For instance, Sigurdsson, et al. [228] utilized supra-alveolar critical size defects in dogs and found more periodontal regeneration when unsintered DBB was used as a carrier for rhBMP-2, than when canine demineralized bone matrix, poly(D,L-lactide-co-glycolide) microparticles (PLGA) or PLA were used. The combined use of unsintered DBB with enamel matrix proteins (EMD) versus only EMD [226], or versus unsintered DBB mixed with an autogenous fibrin/fibronectin system (AFFS) [227] for the treatment of intrabony defects, was compared in split-mouth clinical studies. At six-month reentry, statistically significant greater PPD reduction, CAL gain and defect fill were observed following the combined treatment, compared with only EMD, while there were no differences between the DBB+EMD and DBB+AFFS combinations. A histological report from three cases treated with DBB+EMD showed that this combination treatment is compatible with some amounts of periodontal regeneration; obviously, the relative contribution of the two components (DBB or EMD) in the observed result could not be evaluated [217].

7.5. Conclusions

DBB has a chemical composition and architectural geometry that is almost identical to that of human bone and can support tissue ingrowth, osteoprogenitor cell attachment, proliferation and new bone formation in direct contact to the graft. However, the material has reduced mechanical strength and low fracture strength, and cannot be used in load bearing applications. Although positive results have been observed after DBB grafting in association with dental implants, showing survival rates similar to those achieved with autogenous bone or to those reported for implants placed in pristine bone, an added clinical benefit from its use cannot unequivocally be confirmed. Similarly, an added benefit from the use of DBB as an adjunct to GTR in the treatment of periodontal defects cannot be established. Results from controlled experimental studies have shown that, under optimal conditions for healing (i.e., well protected defects with secured space provision for GTR/GBR), DBB grafting does not enhance bone formation, but it may inhibit osseous healing. New bone formation in DBB grafted defects tends to be confined to the vicinity of the host bone even with prolonged periods of healing, and the DBB particles occupy a substantial portion of the grafted space. Thus, DBB should be regarded as an osteocompatible filler material that may act as a space provision device rather than as a bone promoting substance, and the outcome of DBB grafting in terms of bone fill seems greatly dependent on the configuration and dimensions of the defect. In association with GTR, DBB grafting may exert a positive effect on the healing outcome by supporting the membrane and providing the space for tissue ingrowth in defects with small dimensions, but with an unfavorable morphology that involves a risk for membrane collapse. DBB should not be regarded as biodegradable material and will be present in the grafted space for a very long period of time; however, this fact does not seem to produce any undesirable events. Due to its production method, the risk of transmission of vCJD to humans is practically nonexistent and DBB grafting should be regarded as a safe procedure.

References

1. Gorer PA, Loutit JF, Micklem HS. Proposed revision of "transplantese". Nature. 1961;189:1024-25.
2. van Meekeren J. Heel en geneeskonstige aanmerkingen. Commelijn. 1668.

3. Ricard MA. Réparation d'une perte de substance de la voûte cranienne par la greffe osseuse immédiate. Gaz Hopitaux. 1891;64:785-86.
4. Küttner D. Die Transplantation aus dem Affen und ihre Dauererfolge. Wien Med Wochenschr. 1917;64:1449-52.
5. Reynier MP. Réparation des pertes osseuses craniennes dans les plaies de guerre, greffes hétéroplastiques. Bull Acad Med. 1915;73:753-67.
6. Senn N. On the healing of aseptic bone cavities by implantation of antiseptic decalcified bone. J Med Sci (Am). 1889;98:219-43.
7. Grekoff J. Über die Deckung von Schädeldefekten mit ausgeglühtem Knochen. Zentralbl Chir. 1898;39:969-73.
8. Babcock WW. "Soup Bone" implant for the correction of defects of the skull and face. JAMA 69, 352-355. 1917. Ref Type: Generic
9. Jaksch R. Zur Frage der Deckung von Knochendefekten des Schädels nach der Trepanation. Wien Med Wochenschr. 1889;38:1435-37.
10. Rehn E. Über halbe Gelenktransplantation mit Horn. Zentralbl Chir. 1913;40:1185-86.
11. Hughes CW. Rate of absorption and callus stimulating properties of cow horn, ivory, beef bone and autogenous bone. Surg Gynecol Obstet. 1943;76:665.
12. Magnusson PB. Holding fractures with absorbable materials-ivory plates and screws. JAMA. 1913;61:1514.
13. Mauclaire P. Prosthese d'ivoire pour réparer les pertes de substance du crâne. Soc Chir Bull Mem. 1916;42:1191.
14. Weibrich G, Gnoth SH, Kunkel M, Trettin R, Werner HD, Wagner W. Röntgenspektrometrischer Vergleich der aktuell verfügbaren Knochenersatzmateri alien. Mund Kiefer Gesichtschir. 1999;3:92-97.
15. Holmes RE. Bone regeneration within a coraline hydroxyapatite implant. Plast Reconstr Surg. 1979;63:626-33.
16. Holmes RE. A coralline hydroxyapatite bone graft substitute: preliminary report. Clin Orthop. 1984;188:252-62.
17. Burchardt H. The biology of bone graft repair. Clin Orthop. 1983;174:28-42.
18. Salama R. Xenogeneic bone grafting in humans. Clin Orthop. 1983;174:113-21.
19. Heiple KG, Kendrick RE, Herndon CH, Chase SW. A critical evaluation of processed calf bone. J Bone Joint Surg Am. 1967;49:1119-27.
20. Pieron AP, Bigelow D, Hamonic M. Bone grafting with Boplant. Results in thirty-three cases. J Bone Joint Surg Br. 1968;50:364-68.
21. Elves MW, Salama R. A study of the development of cytotoxic antibodies produced in recipients of xenografts (heterografts) of iliac bone. J Bone Joint Surg Br. 1974;56:331-39.
22. Cantore G, Fortuna A. Intersomatic fusion with calf bone "Kiel bone splint" in the anterior surgical approaach for the treatment of myelopathy in cervical spondylosis. Acta Neurochir (Wien). 1969;20:59-61.
23. Goran A, Murthy KK. Fracture dislocation of the cervical spine. Value of anterior approach with bovine bone interbody fusion. Spine. 1978;3:95-102.
24. Jackson JW. Surgical approaches to the anterior aspect of the spinal column. Ann R Coll Surg Engl. 1971;48:83-98.
25. Salama R, Weissman SL. The clinical use of combined xenografts of bone and autologous red marrow. A preliminary report. J Bone Joint Surg Br. 1978;60:111-15.
26. Siqueira EB, Kranzler LI. Cervical Interbody fusion using calf bone. Surg Neurol. 1982;18:37-39.
27. Taheri ZE, Gueramy M. Experience with calf bone in cervical interbody spinal fusion. J Neurosurg. 1972;36:67-71.
28. Nielsen IM, Ellegaard B, Karring T. Kielbone in new attachment attempts in Humans. J Periodontol. 1981;52:723-28.
29. Older LB. The use of heterogenous bovine bone implants in the treatment of periodontal pockets. An experimental study in humans. J Periodontol. 1967;38:539-49.
30. Sigurdson A. Orala benimplantat. Sven Tandlak Tidskr. 1972;65:33-40.

31. Christiansen JV, Hindmarsh T, Levander B, Lofgren H, Olsson T, ReinholtFP. Comparative vascular evaluation by MRI of autologous and bovine grafts. In: Schoutens A, Arlet J, Gardeniers JWM, Hughes SPF, eds. Bone Circulation in Normal and Pathological Condition. New York: Plenum Press; 1993: 137-40.
32. Espersen JO, Buhl M, Eriksen EF, Fode K, Klaerke A, Kroyer L et al. Treatment of cervical disc disease using Cloward's technique. I. General results, effect of different operative methods and complications in 1,106 patients. Acta Neurochir (Wien). 1984;70:97-114.
33. Lofgren H, Johannsson V, Olsson T, Ryd L, Levander B. Rigid fusion after cloward operation for cervical disc disease using autograft, allograft, or xenograft: a randomized study with radiostereometric and clinical follow-up assessment. Spine. 2000;25:1908-16.
34. McMurray GN. The evaluation of Kiel bone in spinal fusions. J Bone Joint Surg Br. 1982;64:101-4.
35. Ramani PS, Kalbag RM, Sengupta RP. Cervical spinal interbody fusion with Kiel bone. Br J Surg. 1975;62:147-50.
36. Rawlinson JN. Morbidity after anterior cervical decompression and fusion. The influence of the donor site on recovery, and the results of a trial of surgibone compared to autologous bone. Acta Neurochir (Wien). 1994;131:106-18.
37. Sutter B, Friehs G, Pendl G, Tolly E. Bovine dowels for anterior cervical fusion: experience in 66 patients with a note on postoperative CT and MRI appearance. Acta Neurochir (Wien). 1995;137:192-98.
38. Melcher AH. The use of heterogenous anorganic bone as an implant material in oral procedures. Oral Surg Oral Med Oral Pathol. 1962;15:996-1000.
39. Nielsen IM, Ellegaard B, Karring T. Kielbone in healing interradicular lesions in monkeys. J Periodontal Res. 1980;15:328-37.
40. Baer W, Schaller P, Carl HD. Spongy hydroxyapatite in hand surgery–a five year follow-up. J Hand Surg [Br]. 2002;27:101-3.
41. Briem D, Linhart W, Lehmann W, Meenen NM, Rueger JM. Langzeitergebnisse nach Anwendung einer porösen Hydroxylapatitkeramik (Endobon) zur operativen Versorgung von Tibiakopffrakturen. Unfallchirurg. 2002;105:128-33.
42. Helber MU, Ulrich C. Metaphysärer Defektersatz mit Hydroxylapatitkeramik - 3- bis 4-Jahresnachuntersuchungsergebnisse. Unfallchirurg. 2000;103:749-53.
43. Werber KD, Brauer RB, Weiss W, Becker K. Osseous integration of bovine hydroxyapatite ceramic in metaphyseal bone defects of the distal radius. J Hand Surg [Am]. 2000;25:833-41.
44. Jarcho M. Calcium phosphate ceramics as hard tissue prosthetics. Clin Orthop Relat Res. 1981;259-78.
45. LeGeros RZ. Properties of osteoconductive biomaterials: calcium phosphates. Clin Orthop Relat Res. 2002;81-98.
46. LeGeros RZ. Apatites in biological systems. ProgCrystal Growth Charact. 1981;4:1-45.
47. LeGeros RZ. CaP in Oral Biology and Medicine. In: Meyers H, ed. Monographs in Oral Sciences. Basel: Karger; 1991.
48. Peters F, Schwarz K, Epple M. The structure of bone studied with synchrotron X-ray diffraction, X-ray absorption spectroscopy and thermal analysis. Thermochim Acta. 2000;361:131-38.
49. Jensen SS, Aaboe M, Pinholt EM, Hjorting-Hansen E, Melsen F, Ruyter IE. Tissue reaction and material characteristics of four bone substitutes. Int J Oral Maxillofac Implants. 1996;11:55-66.
50. Benke D, Olah A, Mohler H. Protein-chemical analysis of Bio-Oss bone substitute and evidence on its carbonate content. Biomaterials. 2001;22:1005-12.
51. Peetz M. Characterization of xenogeneic bone mineral. In: Boyne PJ, ed. Osseous Reconstruction of the Maxilla and the Mandible: Surgical Techniques using Titanium Mesh and Bone Mineral. Carol Stream, IL: Quintessence Publishing; 1997: 87-93.

52. Spector M. Basic principles of tissue engineering. In: Lynch SEGRJMRE, ed. Tissue engineering: applications in maxillofacial surgery and periodontics. Carol Stream, IL, USA: Quintessence Publishing Co. Inc.; 1998: 3-16.
53. Weibrich G, Trettin R, Gnoth SH, Gotz H, Duschner H, Wagner W. Bestimmung der Größe der spezifischen Oberfläche von Knochenersatzmaterialien mittels Gasadsorption. Mund Kiefer Gesichtschir. 2000;4:148-52.
54. LeGeros RZ. Biodegradation and bioresorption of calcium phosphate ceramics. Clin Mater. 1993;14:65-88.
55. Koerten HK, van der MJ. Degradation of calcium phosphate ceramics. J Biomed Mater Res. 1999;44:78-86.
56. Bauer TW, Muschler GF. Bone graft materials. An overview of the basic science. Clin Orthop Relat Res. 2000;10-27.
57. Hofman S, Sidqui M, Abensur D, Valentini P, Missika P. Effects of Laddec on the formation of calcified bone matrix in rat calvariae cells culture. Biomaterials. 1999;20:1155-66.
58. Stephan EB, Jiang D, Lynch S, Bush P, Dziak R. Anorganic bovine bone supports osteoblastic cell attachment and proliferation. J Periodontol. 1999;70:364-69.
59. Acil Y, Terheyden H, Dunsche A, Fleiner B, Jepsen S. Three-dimensional cultivation of human osteoblast-like cells on highly porous natural bone mineral. J Biomed Mater Res. 2000;51:703-10.
60. Matsumoto T, Kawakami M, Kuribayashi K, Takenaka T, Minamide A, Tamaki T. Effects of sintered bovine bone on cell proliferation, collagen synthesis, and osteoblastic expression in MC3T3-E1 osteoblast-like cells. J Orthop Res. 1999;17:586-92.
61. Qian JJ, Bhatnagar RS. Enhanced cell attachment to anorganic bone mineral in the presence of a synthetic peptide related to collagen. J Biomed Mater Res. 1996;31:545-54.
62. Bhatnagar RS, Qian JJ, Wedrychowska A, Sadeghi M, Wu YM, Smith N. Design of biomimetic habitats for tissue engineering with P-15, a synthetic peptide analogue of collagen. Tissue Eng. 1999;5:53-65.
63. Kubler A, Neugebauer J, Oh JH, Scheer M, Zoller JE. Growth and proliferation of human osteoblasts on different bone graft substitutes: an in vitro study. Implant Dent. 2004;13:171-79.
64. Turhani D, Weissenbock M, Watzinger E, Yerit K, Cvikl B, Ewers R et al. Invitro study of adherent mandibular osteoblast-like cells on carrier materials. Int J Oral Maxillofac Surg. 2005;34:543-50.
65. Taylor JC, Cuff SE, Leger JP, Morra A, Anderson GI. In vitro osteoclast resorption of bone substitute biomaterials used for implant site augmentation: a pilot study. Int J Oral Maxillofac Implants. 2002;17:321-30.
66. Schwartz Z, Weesner T, van DS, Cochran DL, Mellonig JT, Lohmann CH et al. Ability of deproteinized cancellous bovine bone to induce new bone formation. J Periodontol. 2000;71:1258-69.
67. Honig JF, Merten HA, Heinemann DE. Risk of transmission of agents associated with Creutzfeldt-Jakob disease and bovine spongiform encephalopathy. Plast Reconstr Surg. 1999;103:1324-25.
68. Will RG, Ironside JW, Zeidler M, Cousens SN, Estibeiro K, Alperovitch A et al. A new variant of Creutzfeldt-Jakob disease in the UK. Lancet. 1996;347:921-25.
69. Asher DM, Gibbs CJ, Jr., Sulima MP, Bacote A, Amyx H, Gajdusek DC. Transmission of human spongiform encephalopathies to experimental animals: comparison of the chimpanzee and squirrel monkey. Dev Biol Stand. 1993;80:9-13.
70. Lantos PL. From slow virus to prion: a review of transmissible spongiform encephalopathies. Histopathology. 1992;20:1-11.
71. WHO. Public health issues related to animal and human spongiform encephalopathies: Memorandum from a WHO meeting. Bulletin of the World Health Organization. 1992;70:183-90.

72. Wenz B, Oesch B, Horst M. Analysis of the risk of transmitting bovine spongiform encephalopathy through bone grafts derived from bovine bone. Biomaterials. 2001;22:1599-606.
73. Bundesgesundheitsamt. Bekanntmachung der Sicherheitsanforderungen an Arzneimittel aus KoK rperbestandteilen von Rind, Schaf oder Ziege zur Vemeidung des Risikos einer UG bertragung von BSE bzw. Scrapie. Bundesanzeiger. 1994;40:1851-55.
74. Bundesgesundheitsamt. Bekanntmachung über die Zulassung und Registrierung von Arzneimitteln. Bundesanzeiger. 1996;67:4158-62.
75. Sogal A, Tofe AJ. Risk assessment of bovine spongiform encephalopathy transmission through bone graft material derived from bovine bone used for dental applications. J Periodontol. 1999;70:1053-63.
76. Artzi Z, Nemcovsky CE. The application of deproteinized bovine bone mineral for ridge preservation prior to implantation. Clinical and histological observations in a case report. J Periodontol. 1998;69:1062-67.
77. Artzi Z, Tal H, Dayan D. Porous bovine bone mineral in healing of human extraction sockets. Part 1: histomorphometric evaluations at 9 months. J Periodontol. 2000;71:1015-23.
78. Artzi Z, Tal H, Dayan D. Porous bovine bone mineral in healing of human extraction sockets: 2. Histochemical observations at 9 months. J Periodontol. 2001;72:152-59.
79. van Steenberghe D., Callens A, Geers L, Jacobs R. The clinical use of deproteinized bovine bone mineral on bone regeneration in conjunction with immediate implant installation. Clin Oral Implants Res. 2000;11:210-216.
80. Schlegel AK, Donath K. BIO-OSS–a resorbable bone substitute? J Long Term Eff Med Implants. 1998;8:201-9.
81. Maiorana C, Santoro F, Rabagliati M, Salina S. Evaluation of the use of iliac cancellous bone and anorganic bovine bone in the reconstruction of the atrophic maxilla with titanium mesh: a clinical and histologic investigation. Int J Oral Maxillofac Implants. 2001;16:427-32.
82. Skoglund A, Hising P, Young C. A clinical and histologic examination in humans of the osseous response to implanted natural bone mineral. Int J Oral Maxillofac Implants. 1997;12:194-99.
83. Froum SJ, Tarnow DP, Wallace SS, Rohrer MD, Cho SC. Sinus floor elevation using anorganic bovine bone matrix (OsteoGraf/N) with and without autogenous bone: a clinical, histologic, radiographic, and histomorphometric analysis–Part 2 of an ongoing prospective study. Int J Periodontics Restorative Dent. 1998;18:528-43.
84. Krauser JT, Rohrer MD, Wallace SS. Human histologic and histomorphometric analysis comparing OsteoGraf/N with PepGen P-15 in the maxillary sinus elevation procedure: a case report. Implant Dent. 2000;9:298-302.
85. Fugazzotto PA, Vlassis J. Long-term success of sinus augmentation using various surgical approaches and grafting materials. Int J Oral Maxillofac Implants. 1998;13:52-58.
86. Hallman M, Lundgren S, Sennerby L. Histologic analysis of clinical biopsies taken 6 months and 3 years after maxillary sinus floor augmentation with 80 percent bovine hydroxyapatite and 20 percent autogenous bone mixed with fibrin glue. Clin Implant Dent Relat Res. 2001;3:87-96.
87. Hallman M, Cederlund A, Lindskog S, Lundgren S, Sennerby L. A clinical histologic study of bovine hydroxyapatite in combination with autogenous bone and fibrin glue for maxillary sinus floor augmentation. Results after 6 to 8 months of healing. Clin Oral Implants Res. 2001;12:135-43.
88. Hurzeler MB, Kirsch A, Ackermann KL, Quinones CR. Reconstruction of the severely resorbed maxilla with dental implants in the augmented maxillary sinus: a 5-year clinical investigation. Int J Oral Maxillofac Implants. 1996;11:466-75.

89. Maiorana C, Redemagni M, Rabagliati M, Salina S. Treatment of maxillary ridge resorption by sinus augmentation with iliac cancellous bone, anorganic bovine bone, and endosseous implants: a clinical and histologic report. Int J Oral Maxillofac Implants. 2000;15:873-78.
90. Tawil G, Mawla M. Sinus floor elevation using a bovine bone mineral (Bio-Oss) with or without the concomitant use of a bilayered collagen barrier (Bio-Gide): a clinical report of immediate and delayed implant placement. Int J Oral Maxillofac Implants. 2001;16:713-21.
91. Valentini P, Abensur D. Maxillary sinus floor elevation for implant placement with demineralized freeze-dried bone and bovine bone (Bio-Oss): a clinical study of 20 patients. Int J Periodontics Restorative Dent. 1997;17:232-41.
92. Valentini P, Abensur D, Densari D, Graziani JN, Hammerle C. Histological evaluation of Bio-Oss in a 2-stage sinus floor elevation and implantation procedure. A human case report. Clin Oral Implants Res. 1998;9:59-64.
93. Hallman M, Sennerby L, Lundgren S. A clinical and histologic evaluation of implant integration in the posterior maxilla after sinus floor augmentation with autogenous bone, bovine hydroxyapatite, or a 20:80 mixture. Int J Oral Maxillofac Implants. 2002;17:635-43.
94. Hising P, Bolin A, Branting C. Reconstruction of severely resorbed alveolar ridge crests with dental implants using a bovine bone mineral for augmentation. Int J Oral Maxillofac Implants. 2001;16:90-97.
95. Valentini P, Abensur DJ. Maxillary sinus grafting with an organic bovine bone: a clinical report of long-term results. Int J Oral Maxillofac Implants. 2003;18:556-60.
96. Maiorana C, Sigurta D, Mirandola A, Garlini G, Santoro F. Sinus elevation with alloplasts or xenogenic materials and implants: an up-to-4-year clinical and radiologic follow-up. Int J Oral Maxillofac Implants. 2006;21:426-32.
97. Del Fabbro M, Testori T, Francetti L, Weinstein R. Systematic review of survival rates for implants placed in the grafted maxillary sinus. Int J Periodontics Restorative Dent. 2004;24:565-77.
98. Wallace SS, Froum SJ. Effect of maxillary sinus augmentation on the survival of endosseous dental implants. A systematic review. Ann Periodontol. 2003;8:328-43.
99. Mayfield LJ, Skoglund A, Hising P, Lang NP, Attstrom R. Evaluation following functional loading of titanium fixtures placed in ridges augmented by deproteinized bone mineral. A human case study. Clin Oral Implants Res. 2001;12:508-14.
100. Zitzmann NU, Scharer P, Marinello CP. Long-term results of implants treated with guided bone regeneration: a 5-year prospective study. Int J Oral Maxillofac Implants. 2001;16:355-66.
101. Dies F, Etienne D, Abboud NB, Ouhayoun JP. Bone regeneration in extraction sites after immediate placement of an e-PTFE membrane with or without a biomaterial. A report on 12 consecutive cases. Clin Oral Implants Res. 1996;7:277-85.
102. Lorenzoni M, Pertl C, Keil C, Wegscheider WA. Treatment of peri-implant defects with guided bone regeneration: a comparative clinical study with various membranes and bone grafts. Int J Oral Maxillofac Implants. 1998;13:639-46.
103. Zitzmann NU, Naef R, Scharer P. Resorbable versus nonresorbable membranes in combination with Bio-Oss for guided bone regeneration. Int J Oral Maxillofac Implants. 1997;12:844-52.
104. Carpio L, Loza J, Lynch S, Genco R. Guided bone regeneration around endosseous implants with anorganic bovine bone mineral. A randomized controlled trial comparing bioabsorbable versus non-resorbable barriers. J Periodontol. 2000;71:1743-49.
105. Hammerle CH, Lang NP. Single stage surgery combining transmucosal implant placement with guided bone regeneration and bioresorbable materials. Clin Oral Implants Res. 2001;12:9-18.
106. Zitzmann NU, Scharer P, Marinello CP, Schupbach P, Berglundh T. Alveolar ridge augmentation with Bio-Oss: a histologic study in humans. Int J Periodontics Restorative Dent. 2001;21:288-95.

107. Cornelini R, Cangini F, Martuscelli G, Wennstrom J. Deproteinized bovine bone and biodegradable barrier membranes to support healing following immediate placement of transmucosal implants: a short-term controlled clinical trial. Int J Periodontics Restorative Dent. 2004;24:555-63.
108. Moses O, Pitaru S, Artzi Z, Nemcovsky CE. Healing of dehiscence-type defects in implants placed together with different barrier membranes: a comparative clinical study. Clin Oral Implants Res. 2005;16:210-219.
109. Norton MR, Odell EW, Thompson ID, Cook RJ. Efficacy of bovine bone mineral for alveolar augmentation: a human histologic study. Clin Oral Implants Res. 2003;14:775-83.
110. Nemcovsky CE, Artzi Z, Moses O, Gelernter I. Healing of marginal defects at implants placed in fresh extraction sockets or after 4-6 weeks of healing. A comparative study. Clin Oral Implants Res. 2002;13:410-419.
111. De Boever AL, De Boever JA. Guided bone regeneration around non-submerged implants in narrow alveolar ridges: a prospective long-term clinical study. Clinical Oral Implants Research. 2005;16:549-56.
112. Yildirim M, Spiekermann H, Biesterfeld S, Edelhoff D. Maxillary sinus augmentation using xenogenic bone substitute material Bio-Oss in combination with venous blood. A histologic and histomorphometric study in humans. Clin Oral Implants Res. 2000;11:217-29.
113. Artzi Z, Nemcovsky CE, Tal H, Dayan D. Histopathological morphometric evaluation of 2 different hydroxyapatite-bone derivatives in sinus augmentation procedures: a comparative study in humans. J Periodontol. 2001;72:911-20.
114. Rodoni LR, Glauser R, Feloutzis A, Hammerle CH. Implants in the posterior maxilla: a comparative clinical and radiologic study. Int J Oral Maxillofac Implants. 2005;20:231-37.
115. Hallman M, Nordin T. Sinus floor augmentation with bovine hydroxyapatite mixed with fibrin glue and later placement of nonsubmerged implants: a retrospective study in 50 patients. Int J Oral Maxillofac Implants. 2004;19:222-27.
116. John HD, Wenz B. Histomorphometric analysis of natural bone mineral for maxillary sinus augmentation. Int J Oral Maxillofac Implants. 2004;19:199-207.
117. Scarano A, Pecora G, Piattelli M, Piattelli A. Osseointegration in a sinus augmented with bovine porous bone mineral: histological results in an implant retrieved 4 years after insertion. A case report. J Periodontol. 2004;75:1161-66.
118. Artzi Z, Dayan D, Alpern Y, Nemcovsky CE. Vertical ridge augmentation using xenogenic material supported by a configured titanium mesh: clinicohistopathologic and histochemical study. Int J Oral Maxillofac Implants. 2003;18:440-446.
119. Fugazzotto PA. GBR using bovine bone matrix and resorbable and nonresorbable membranes. Part 2: Clinical results. Int J Periodontics Restorative Dent. 2003;23:599-605.
120. Philippart P, Daubie V, Pochet R. Sinus grafting using recombinant human tissue factor, platelet-rich plasma gel, autologous bone, and anorganic bovine bone mineral xenograft: histologic analysis and case reports. Int J Oral Maxillofac Implants. 2005;20:274-81.
121. Toffler M. Osteotome-mediated sinus floor elevation: a clinical report. Int J Oral Maxillofac Implants. 2004;19:266-73.
122. Schwarz F, Bieling K, Latz T, Nuesry E, Becker J. Healing of intrabony periimplantitis defects following application of a nanocrystalline hydroxyapatite (Ostim) or a bovine-derived xenograft (Bio-Oss) in combination with a collagen membrane (Bio-Gide). A case series. J Clin Periodontol. 2006;33:491-99.
123. Hislop WS, Finlay PM, Moos KF. A preliminary study into the uses of anorganic bone in oral and maxillofacial surgery. Br J Oral Maxillofac Surg. 1993;31:149-53.
124. Maiorana C, Beretta M, Salina S, Santoro F. Reduction of autogenous bone graft resorption by means of bio-oss coverage: a prospective study. Int J Periodontics Restorative Dent. 2005;25:19-25.

125. Hammerle CH, Olah AJ, Schmid J, Fluckiger L, Gogolewski S, Winkler JR et al. The biological effect of natural bone mineral on bone neoformation on the rabbit skull. Clin Oral Implants Res. 1997;8:198-207.
126. Nasr HF, Aichelmann-Reidy ME, Yukna RA. Bone and bone substitutes. Periodontol 2000. 1999;19:74-86.
127. Karring T, Nyman S, Thilander B, Magnusson I. Bone regeneration in orthodontically produced alveolar bone dehiscences. J Periodontal Res. 1982;17:309-15.
128. Lindhe J, Nyman S, Karring T. Connective tissue reattachment as related to presence or absence of alveolar bone. J Clin Periodontol. 1984;11:33-40.
129. Nyman S, Karring T. Regeneration of surgically removed buccal alveolar bone in dogs. J Periodontal Res. 1979;14:86-92.
130. Thilander B, Nyman S, Karring T, Magnusson I. Bone regeneration in alveolar bone dehiscences related to orthodontic tooth movements. Eur J Orthod. 1983;5:105-14.
131. Caton J, Zander HA. Osseous repair of an infrabony pocket without new attachment of connective tissue. J Clin Periodontol. 1976;3:54-58.
132. Caton J, Nyman S, Zander H. Histometric evaluation of periodontal surgery. II. Connective tissue attachment levels after four regenerative procedures. J Clin Periodontol. 1980;7:224-31.
133. Listgarten MA, Rosenberg MM. Histological study of repair following new attachment procedures in human periodontal lesions. J Periodontol. 1979;50:333-44.
134. Ewers R, Goriwoda W, Schopper C, Moser D, Spassova E. Histologic findings at augmented bone areas supplied with two different bone substitute materials combined with sinus floor lifting. Report of one case. Clin Oral Implants Res. 2004;15:96-100.
135. Valentini P, Abensur D, Wenz B, Peetz M, Schenk R. Sinus grafting with porous bone mineral (Bio-Oss) for implant placement: a 5-year study on 15 patients. Int J Periodontics Restorative Dent. 2000;20:245-53.
136. Wallace SS, Froum SJ, Tarnow DP. Histologic evaluation of a sinus elevation procedure: a clinical report. Int J Periodontics Restorative Dent. 1996;16:46-51.
137. Wallace SS, Froum SJ, Cho SC, Elian N, Monteiro D, Kim BS et al. Sinus augmentation utilizing anorganic bovine bone (Bio-Oss) with absorbable and nonabsorbable membranes placed over the lateral window: histomorphometric and clinical analyses. Int J Periodontics Restorative Dent. 2005;25:551-59.
138. Yildirim M, Spiekermann H, Handt S, Edelhoff D. Maxillary sinus augmentation with the xenograft Bio-Oss and autogenous intraoral bone for qualitative improvement of the implant site: a histologic and histomorphometric clinical study in humans. Int J Oral Maxillofac Implants. 2001;16:23-33.
139. Merkx MA, Maltha JC, Stoelinga PJ. Assessment of the value of anorganic bone additives in sinus floor augmentation: a review of clinical reports. Int J Oral Maxillofac Surg. 2003;32:1-6.
140. Klinge B, Alberius P, Isaksson S, Jonsson J. Osseous response to implanted natural bone mineral and synthetic hydroxylapatite ceramic in the repair of experimental skull bone defects. J Oral Maxillofac Surg. 1992;50:241-49.
141. Thaller SR, Hoyt J, Borjeson K, Dart A, Tesluk H. Reconstruction of calvarial defects with anorganic bovine bone mineral (Bio-Oss) in a rabbit model. J Craniofac Surg. 1993;4:79-84.
142. Young C, Sandstedt P, Skoglund A. A comparative study of anorganic xenogenic bone and autogenous bone implants for bone regeneration in rabbits. Int J Oral Maxillofac Implants. 1999;14:72-76.
143. Schmitt JM, Buck DC, Joh SP, Lynch SE, Hollinger JO. Comparison of porous bone mineral and biologically active glass in critical-sized defects. J Periodontol. 1997;68:1043-53.
144. Al Ruhaimi KA. Bone graft substitutes: a comparative qualitative histologic review of current osteoconductive grafting materials. Int J Oral Maxillofac Implants. 2001;16:105-14.

145. Scarano A, Iezzi G, Petrone G, Orsini G, Degidi M, Strocchi R et al. Cortical bone regeneration with a synthetic cell-binding peptide: a histologic and histomorphometric pilot study. Implant Dent. 2003;12:318-24.
146. Thorwarth M, Schultze-Mosgau S, Wehrhan F, Kessler P, Srour S, Wiltfang J et al. Bioactivation of an anorganic bone matrix by P-15 peptide for the promotion of early bone formation. Biomaterials. 2005;26:5648-57.
147. Thorwarth M, Wehrhan F, Srour S, Schultze-Mosgau S, Felszeghy E, Bader RD et al. Evaluation of substitutes for bone: Comparison of microradiographic and histological assessments. Br J Oral Maxillofac Surg. 2006.
148. Thorwarth M, Schlegel KA, Wehrhan F, Srour S, Schultze-Mosgau S. Acceleration of de novo bone formation following application of autogenous bone to particulated anorganic bovine material in vivo. Oral Surg Oral Med Oral Pathol Oral Radiol Endod. 2006;101:309-16.
149. Barboza EP, de Souza RO, Caula AL, Neto LG, Caula FO, Duarte ME. Bone regeneration of localized chronic alveolar defects utilizing cell binding peptide associated with anorganic bovine-derived bone mineral: a clinical and histological study. J Periodontol. 2002;73:1153-59.
150. Artzi Z, Givol N, Rohrer MD, Nemcovsky CE, Prasad HS, Tal H. Qualitative and quantitative expression of bovine bone mineral in experimental bone defects. Part 2: Morphometric analysis. J Periodontol. 2003;74:1153-60.
151. Cardaropoli G, Araujo M, Hayacibara R, Sukekava F, Lindhe J. Healing of extraction sockets and surgically produced - augmented and non-augmented - defects in the alveolar ridge. An experimental study in the dog. J Clin Periodontol. 2005;32:435-40.
152. Margolin MD, Cogan AG, Taylor M, Buck D, McAllister TN, Toth C et al. Maxillary sinus augmentation in the non-human primate: a comparative radiographic and histologic study between recombinant human osteogenic protein-1 and natural bone mineral. J Periodontol. 1998;69:911-19.
153. McAllister BS, Margolin MD, Cogan AG, Taylor M, Wollins J. Residual lateral wall defects following sinus grafting with recombinant human osteogenic protein-1 or Bio-Oss in the chimpanzee. Int J Periodontics Restorative Dent. 1998;18:227-39.
154. McAllister BS, Margolin MD, Cogan AG, Buck D, Hollinger JO, Lynch SE. Eighteen-month radiographic and histologic evaluation of sinus grafting with anorganic bovine bone in the chimpanzee. Int J Oral Maxillofac Implants. 1999;14:361-68.
155. Berglundh T, Lindhe J. Healing around implants placed in bone defects treated with Bio-Oss. An experimental study in the dog. Clin Oral Implants Res. 1997;8:117-24.
156. Botticelli D, Berglundh T, Lindhe J. The influence of a biomaterial on the closure of a marginal hard tissue defect adjacent to implants. An experimental study in the dog. Clinical Oral Implants Research. 2004;15:285-92.
157. Haas R, Mailath G, Dortbudak O, Watzek G. Bovine hydroxyapatite for maxillary sinus augmentation: analysis of interfacial bond strength of dental implants using pull-out tests. Clin Oral Implants Res. 1998;9:117-22.
158. Haas R, Donath K, Fodinger M, Watzek G. Bovine hydroxyapatite for maxillary sinus grafting: comparative histomorphometric findings in sheep. Clin Oral Implants Res. 1998;9:107-16.
159. Hurzeler MB, Quinones CR, Kirsch A, Gloker C, Schupbach P, Strub JR et al. Maxillary sinus augmentation using different grafting materials and dental implants in monkeys. Part I. Evaluation of anorganic bovine-derived bone matrix. Clin Oral Implants Res. 1997;8:476-86.
160. Terheyden H, Jepsen S, Moller B, Tucker MM, Rueger DC. Sinus floor augmentation with simultaneous placement of dental implants using a combination of deproteinized bone xenografts and recombinant human osteogenic protein-1. A histometric study in miniature pigs. Clin Oral Implants Res. 1999;10:510-521.

161. Wetzel AC, Stich H, Caffesse RG. Bone apposition onto oral implants in the sinus area filled with different grafting materials. A histological study in beagle dogs. Clin Oral Implants Res. 1995;6:155-63.
162. Schlegel KA, Fichtner G, Schultze-Mosgau S, Wiltfang J. Histologic findings in sinus augmentation with autogenous bone chips versus a bovine bone substitute. Int J Oral Maxillofac Implants. 2003;18:53-58.
163. Rahmani M, Shimada E, Rokni S, Deporter DA, Adegbembo AO, Valiquette N et al. Osteotome sinus elevation and simultaneous placement of porous-surfaced dental implants: a morphometric study in rabbits. Clin Oral Implants Res. 2005;16:692-99.
164. Pinholt EM, Bang G, Haanaes HR. Alveolar ridge augmentation in rats by Bio-Oss. Scand J Dent Res. 1991;99:154-61.
165. Mandelkow HK, Hallfeldt KK, Kessler SB, Gayk M, Siebeck M, Schweiberer L. Knochenneubildung nach Implantation verschiedener Hydroxylapatitkeramiken. Tierexperimentelle Studie am Bohrlochmodell der Schaftstibia. Unfallchirurg. 1990;93:376-79.
166. Fukuta K, Har-Shai Y, Collares MV, Lichten JB, Jackson IT. Comparison of inorganic bovine bone mineral particles with porous hydroxyapatite granules and cranial bone dust in the reconstruction of full-thickness skull defect. J Craniofac Surg. 1992;3:25-29.
167. Merkx MA, Maltha JC, Freihofer HP, Kuijpers-Jagtman AM. Incorporation of particulated bone implants in the facial skeleton. Biomaterials. 1999;20:2029-35.
168. Merkx MA, Maltha JC, Freihofer HP, Kuijpers-Jagtman AM. Incorporation of three types of bone block implants in the facial skeleton. Biomaterials. 1999;20:639-45.
169. Aghaloo TL, Moy PK, Freymiller EG. Evaluation of platelet-rich plasma in combination with anorganic bovine bone in the rabbit cranium: a pilot study. Int J Oral Maxillofac Implants. 2004;19:59-65.
170. Merkx MA, Maltha JC, Freihofer HP. Incorporation of composite bone implants in the facial skeleton. Clin Oral Implants Res. 2000;11:422-29.
171. Schmitz JP, Hollinger JO. The critical size defect as an experimental model for craniomandibulofacial nonunions. Clin Orthop Relat Res. 1986;299-308.
172. Lioubavina N, Kostopoulos L, Wenzel A, Karring T. Long-term stability of jaw bone tuberosities formed by "guided tissue regeneration". Clin Oral Implants Res. 1999;10:477-86.
173. Stavropoulos A, Kostopoulos L, Mardas N, Nyengaard JR, Karring T. Deproteinized bovine bone used as an adjunct to guided bone augmentation: an experimental study in the rat. Clin Implant Dent Relat Res. 2001;3:156-65.
174. Stavropoulos A, Kostopoulos L, Nyengaard JR, Karring T. Deproteinized bovine bone (Bio-Oss) and bioactive glass (Biogran) arrest bone formation when used as an adjunct to guided tissue regeneration (GTR): an experimental study in the rat. J Clin Periodontol. 2003;30:636-43.
175. Stavropoulos A, Kostopoulos L, Nyengaard JR, Karring T. Fate of bone formed by guided tissue regeneration with or without grafting of Bio-Oss or Biogran. An experimental study in the rat. J Clin Periodontol. 2004;31:30-39.
176. Xu H, Shimizu Y, Asai S, Ooya K. Grafting of deproteinized bone particles inhibits bone resorption after maxillary sinus floor elevation. Clinical Oral Implants Research. 2004;15:126-33.
177. Araujo MG, Sonohara M, Hayacibara R, Cardaropoli G, Lindhe J. Lateral ridge augmentation by the use of grafts comprised of autologous bone or a biomaterial. An experiment in the dog. J Clin Periodontol. 2002;29:1122-31.
178. Carmagnola D, Berglundh T, Lindhe J. The effect of a fibrin glue on the integration of Bio-Oss with bone tissue. A experimental study in labrador dogs. J Clin Periodontol. 2002;29:377-83.

179. Carmagnola D, Adriaens P, Berglundh T. Healing of human extraction sockets filled with Bio-Oss. Clin Oral Implants Res. 2003;14:137-43.
180. Schmid J, Hammerle CH, Fluckiger L, Winkler JR, Olah AJ, Gogolewski S et al. Blood-filled spaces with and without filler materials in guided bone regeneration. A comparative experimental study in the rabbit using bioresorbable membranes. Clin Oral Implants Res. 1997;8:75-81.
181. Slotte C, Lundgren D. Augmentation of calvarial tissue using non-permeable silicone domes and bovine bone mineral. An experimental study in the rat. Clin Oral Implants Res. 1999;10:468-76.
182. Hockers T, Abensur D, Valentini P, Legrand R, Hammerle CH. The combined use of bioresorbable membranes and xenografts or autografts in the treatment of bone defects around implants. A study in beagle dogs. Clin Oral Implants Res. 1999;10:487-98.
183. Polimeni G, Koo KT, Qahash M, Xiropaidis AV, Albandar JM, Wikesjo UM. Prognostic factors for alveolar regeneration: effect of tissue occlusion on alveolar bone regeneration with guided tissue regeneration. J Clin Periodontol. 2004;31:730-735.
184. Polimeni G, Koo KT, Qahash M, Xiropaidis AV, Albandar JM, Wikesjo UM. Prognostic factors for alveolar regeneration: effect of a space-providing biomaterial on guided tissue regeneration. J Clin Periodontol. 2004;31:725-29.
185. Wikesjo UM, Lim WH, Thomson RC, Hardwick WR. Periodontal repair in dogs: gingival tissue occlusion, a critical requirement for GTR? J Clin Periodontol. 2003;30:655-64.
186. Hammerle CH, Chiantella GC, Karring T, Lang NP. The effect of a deproteinized bovine bone mineral on bone regeneration around titanium dental implants. Clin Oral Implants Res. 1998;9:151-62.
187. Schou S, Holmstrup P, Jorgensen T, Skovgaard LT, Stoltze K, Hjorting-Hansen E et al. Anorganic porous bovine-derived bone mineral (Bio-Oss((R))) and ePTFE membrane in the treatment of peri-implantitis in cynomolgus monkeys. Clinical Oral Implants Research. 2003;14:535-47.
188. Chiapasco M, Ferrini F, Casentini P, Accardi S, Zaniboni M. Dental implants placed in expanded narrow edentulous ridges with the Extension Crest device. A 1-3-year multicenter follow-up study. Clin Oral Implants Res. 2006;17:265-72.
189. Patur B, Glickman I. Clinical and roentgenographic evaluation of the post-treatment healing of infrabony pockets. J Periodontol. 1962;33:164-71.
190. Beube FE, Silvers HF. Influence of devitalized heterogenous bone-powder on regeneration of alveolar and maxillary bone of dogs. J Dent Res. 1934;14:15-19.
191. Beube FE. Observations on the formation of cementum, periodontal membrane and bone, 20 months postperatively, with the use of boiled cow bone powder. J Dent Res. 1942;21:2989-299.
192. Scopp IW, Morgan FH, Dooner JJ, Fredrics HJ, Heyman RA. Bovine bone (Boplant) implants for intrabony oral lesions. Periodontics. 1966;4:169-76.
193. Clergeau LP, Danan M, Clergeau-Guerithault S, Brion M. Healing response to anorganic bone implantation in periodontal intrabony defects in dogs. Part I. Bone regeneration. A microradiographic study. J Periodontol. 1996;67:140-149.
194. Camelo M, Nevins ML, Schenk RK, Simion M, Rasperini G, Lynch SE et al. Clinical, radiographic, and histologic evaluation of human periodontal defects treated with Bio-Oss and Bio-Gide. Int J Periodontics Restorative Dent. 1998;18:321-31.
195. Hutchens LH, Jr. The use of a bovine bone mineral in periodontal osseous defects: case reports. Compend Contin Educ Dent. 1999;20:365-4.
196. Richardson CR, Mellonig JT, Brunsvold MA, McDonnell HT, Cochran DL. Clinical evaluation of Bio-Oss: a bovine-derived xenograft for the treatment of periodontal osseous defects in humans. J Clin Periodontol. 1999;26:421-28.

197. Karring T, Nyman S, Gottlow J, Laurell L. Development of the biological concept of guided tissue regeneration–animal and human studies. Periodontol 2000. 1993;1:26-35.
198. Stavropoulos A. Guided tissue regeneration in combination with deproteinized bovine bone and gentamicin. PhD thesis ed. Aarhus, Denmark: 2002.
199. Caton J, Wagener C, Polson A, Nyman S, Frantz B, Bouwsma O et al. Guided tissue regeneration in interproximal defects in the monkey. Int J Periodontics Restorative Dent. 1992;12:266-77.
200. Gottlow J, Nyman S, Karring T, Lindhe J. New attachment formation as the result of controlled tissue regeneration. J Clin Periodontol. 1984;11:494-503.
201. Sallum EA, Sallum AW, Nociti FH, Jr., Marcantonio RA, de TS. New attachment achieved by guided tissue regeneration using a bioresorbable polylactic acid membrane in dogs. Int J Periodontics Restorative Dent. 1998;18:502-10.
202. Camelo M, Lekovic V, Weinlaender M, Nedic M, Vasilic N, Wolinsky E et al. A controlled re-entry study on the effectiveness of bovine porous bone mineral used in combination with a collagen membrane of porcine origin in the treatment of intrabony defects in humans. Journal of Clinical Periodontology. 2000;27:889-96.
203. Camelo M, Nevins ML, Lynch SE, Schenk RK, Simion M, Nevins M. Periodontal regeneration with an autogenous bone-Bio-Oss composite graft and a Bio-Gide membrane. Int J Periodontics Restorative Dent. 2001;21:109-19.
204. Mellonig JT. Human histologic evaluation of a bovine-derived bone xenograft in the treatment of periodontal osseous defects. Int J Periodontics Restorative Dent. 2000;20:19-29.
205. Sculean A, Stavropoulos A, Windisch P, Keglevich T, Karring T, Gera I. Healing of human intrabony defects following regenerative periodontal therapy with a bovine-derived xenograft and guided tissue regeneration. Clin Oral Investig. 2004;8:70-74.
206. Lundgren D, Slotte C. Reconstruction of anatomically complicated periodontal defects using a bioresorbable GTR barrier supported by bone mineral. A 6-month follow-up study of 6 cases. J Clin Periodontol. 1999;26:56-62.
207. Nevins ML, Camelo M, Lynch SE, Schenk RK, Nevins M. Evaluation of periodontal regeneration following grafting intrabony defects with bio-oss collagen: a human histologic report. Int J Periodontics Restorative Dent. 2003;23:9-17.
208. Zitzmann NU, Rateitschak-Pluss E, Marinello CP. Treatment of angular bone defects with a composite bone grafting material in combination with a collagen membrane. J Periodontol. 2003;74:687-94.
209. Pietruska MD. A comparative study on the use of Bio-Oss and enamel matrix derivative (Emdogain) in the treatment of periodontal bone defects. Eur J Oral Sci. 2001;109:178-81.
210. Sculean A, Berakdar M, Chiantella GC, Donos N, Arweiler NB, Brecx M. Healing of intrabony defects following treatment with a bovine-derived xenograft and collagen membrane. A controlled clinical study. J Clin Periodontol. 2003;30:73-80.
211. Stavropoulos A, Karring ES, Kostopoulos L, Karring T. Deproteinized bovine bone and gentamicin as an adjunct to GTR in the treatment of intrabony defects: a randomized controlled clinical study. J Clin Periodontol. 2003;30:486-95.
212. Tonetti M, Cortellini P, Lang NP, Suvan E, Adriaens P, Dubravec D et al. Clinical outcomes following treatment of human intrabony defects with GTR/bone replacement material or access flap alone. A multicenter randomized controlled clinical trial. Journal of Clinical Periodontology. 2004;31:770-776.
213. Sculean A, Chiantella GC, Windisch P, Arweiler NB, Brecx M, Gera I. Healing of intra-bony defects following treatment with a composite bovine-derived xenograft (Bio-Oss Collagen) in combination with a collagen membrane (Bio-Gide PERIO). J Clin Periodontol. 2005;32:720-724.
214. Paolantonio M. Combined periodontal regenerative technique in human intrabony defects by collagen membranes and anorganic bovine bone. A controlled clinical study. J Periodontol. 2002;73:158-66.

215. Murphy KG, Gunsolley JC. Guided tissue regeneration for the treatment of periodontal intrabony and furcation defects. A systematic review. Ann Periodontol. 2003;8:266-302.
216. Paolantonio M, Scarano A, di PG, Tumini V, d'Archivio D, Piattelli A. Periodontal healing in humans using anorganic bovine bone and bovine peritoneum-derived collagen membrane: a clinical and histologic case report. Int J Periodontics Restorative Dent. 2001;21:505-15.
217. Sculean A, Windisch P, Keglevich T, Chiantella GC, Gera I, Donos N. Clinical and histologic evaluation of human intrabony defects treated with an enamel matrix protein derivative combined with a bovine-derived xenograft. Int J Periodontics Restorative Dent. 2003;23:47-55.
218. Sakata J, Abe H, Ohazama A, Okubo K, Nagashima C, Suzuki M et al. Effects of combined treatment with porous bovine inorganic bone grafts and bilayer porcine collagen membrane on refractory one-wall intrabony defects. Int J Periodontics Restorative Dent. 2006;26:161-69.
219. Yamada S, Shima N, Kitamura H, Sugito H. Effect of porous xenographic bone graft with collagen barrier membrane on periodontal regeneration. Int J Periodontics Restorative Dent. 2002;22:389-97.
220. Stavropoulos A, Karring T. Five-year results of guided tissue regeneration in combination with deproteinized bovine bone (Bio-Oss) in the treatment of intrabony periodontal defects: a case series report. Clin Oral Investig. 2005;9:271-77.
221. Araujo MG, Carmagnola D, Berglundh T, Thilander B, Lindhe J. Orthodontic movement in bone defects augmented with Bio-Oss. An experimental study in dogs. J Clin Periodontol. 2001;28:73-80.
222. Boyne PJ, Shabahang S. An evaluation of bone induction delivery materials in conjunction with root-form implant placement. Int J Periodontics Restorative Dent. 2001;21:333-43.
223. Jiang D, Dziak R, Lynch SE, Stephan EB. Modification of an osteoconductive anorganic bovine bone mineral matrix with growth factors. J Periodontol. 1999;70:834-39.
224. Terheyden H, Jepsen S, Vogeler S, Tucker M, Rueger DC. Recombinant human osteogenic protein 1 in the rat mandibular augmentation model: differences in morphology of the newly formed bone are dependent on the type of carrier. Mund Kiefer Gesichtschir. 1997;1:272-75.
225. Terheyden H, Jepsen S, Rueger DR. Mandibular reconstruction in miniature pigs with prefabricated vascularized bone grafts using recombinant human osteogenic protein-1: a preliminary study. Int J Oral Maxillofac Surg. 1999;28:461-63.
226. Lekovic V, Camargo PM, Weinlaender M, Nedic M, Aleksic Z, Kenney EB. A comparison between enamel matrix proteins used alone or in combination with bovine porous bone mineral in the treatment of intrabony periodontal defects in humans. J Periodontol. 2000;71:1110-1116.
227. Lekovic V, Camargo PM, Weinlaender M, Vasilic N, Djordjevic M, Kenney EB. The use of bovine porous bone mineral in combination with enamel matrix proteins or with an autologous fibrinogen/fibronectin system in the treatment of intrabony periodontal defects in humans. J Periodontol. 2001;72:1157-63.
228. Sigurdsson TJ, Nygaard L, Tatakis DN, Fu E, Turek TJ, Jin L et al. Periodontal repair in dogs: evaluation of rhBMP-2 carriers. Int J Periodontics Restorative Dent. 1996;16:524-37.

8

Bioactive Bioceramics

Racquel Z. LeGeros[1], Guy Daculsi[2], and John P. LeGeros[1]

Abstract: Bioactive bioceramics as alternative to autografts and allografts include: bioactive glass, calcium carbonate (natural coral), calcium sulfate and calcium phosphates of biologic (derived from bovine bone, coral and marine algae) or synthetic origin. These bioceramics are available as granules or blocks (dense or porous), specially designed shapes (wedges, cylinders), cements or as coatings on orthopedic or dental implants. Properties of bone that are emulated by bioceramics include: interconnecting porosity, degradation and osteoconductivity. Osteoinductivity is introduced by mixing the bioceramics with osteogenic molecules (e.g., growth factors, demineralized bone matrix). Some calcium phosphate-based bioceramics were observed to have osteoinductive properties attributed to yet-to-be-defined critical geometry. Difference in composition and syntheses or processing methods affect the properties of the bioceramics. Applications of these bioceramics are described. The applications are limited to non-load bearing areas because of the poor mechanical strengths of these bioceramics. In addition to their application as bone graft substitutes or autograft extenders, some of these bioceramics are efficient carriers for growth factors or drugs, and as scaffolds for tissue engineering.

Keywords: bioactive glass, calcium carbonate, calcium sulfate, calcium phosphates, calcium phosphate cements, implant coatings

8.1. Introduction

Ceramics (from Greek, '*keramos*') refers to inorganic non-metallic materials. Their common uses dating back to prehistoric times are as ceramic potteries and dishes. Industrial ceramics include abrasives (silica, alumina), nuclear fuels

[1]Calcium Phosphate Research Laboratory, Department of Biomaterials & Biomimetics, New York University College of Dentistry, New York, NY
[2]INSERM, Faculte de Chirurgie Dentaire, Universite de Nantes, Nantes, France

From: *Orthopedic Biology and Medicine: Musculoskeletal Tissue Regeneration, Biological Materials and Methods.*
Edited by W. S. Pietrzak © Humana Press, Totowa, NJ

(uranium oxide), magnetic ceramics, semiconductors, coatings for rockets, etc. Ceramics used in restorative dentistry include porcelain crowns, glass-ionomer cements, etc.

Archeological findings show several types of materials used in prehistoric times to replace missing teeth including animal bones (ox), shells, corals, ivory, wood, metals (gold and silver), etc [1]. In modern times materials used to repair, replace or substitute for missing bones and teeth include: human bones, bovine bone-derived materials, coral and coral-transformed materials, metals (titanium, titanium alloy and stainless steel), ceramics and polymers. These materials are classified as: (a) autografts (bone from the same patient obtained from another site), (b) allografts (freeze-dried mineralized or demineralized bone matrix processed from cadavers) and (c) alloplasts (synthetic materials including those of biologic origin). While autografts remain the gold standard, allografts are most frequently used by medical and dental clinicians. However, the shortcomings [2,3] of autografts (limited supply, additional surgery and trauma, expensive, potential complications) and allografts (expensive, potential for disease transmission, unpredictability of results due to complicated processing methods) provided the strong impetus for the development of synthetic bone graft materials including those of biologic origin (e.g., coral-derived, bovine bone-derived).

Bioceramics describe a host of ceramics (including bioactive glasses) that are "specially designed and fabricated for the repair and reconstruction of diseased, damaged, missing or worn out parts of the body" [4,5].

Based on the nature of the attachment of the bioceramics to the tissue (bone), bioceramics are described as either: (1) bioinert or nearly inert (does not bond directly with the bone and exhibit a fibrous layer at the interface, forms a weak bioceramic/bone interface) or, (2) bioactive (directly attaches to the bone by chemical bonding with the bone, forms a strong interface) [4-7]. Commercial bioinert bioceramics include alumina (Al_2O_3) and zirconia (Zr_2O_3) that are used for both dental and orthopedic applications [8, 9].

Currently used bioactive bioceramics are either of biologic or synthetic origin. Bioceramics of biologic origin include: natural coral, coral converted to hydroxyapatite, apatite from bovine bone or apatite derived from marine algae (Table 8.1). Completely synthetic materials include specially formulated glasses (silica-based or phosphate based), calcium sulfate (plaster of Paris) and different types of calcium phosphates (Table 8.1).

Calcium phosphate (CaP) bioceramics include: calcium deficient apatite (CDA), hydroxyapatite (HA), beta-tricalcium phosphate (β-TCP) and biphasic calcium phosphate (BCP) – an intimate mixture of HA and β-TCP. Bioactive bioceramics are available as powders, granules, pellets and blocks (dense or porous), as cements (CPC), as composites (CaP/polymer) and as coatings on orthopedic and dental implants.

This chapter focuses on the bioactive bioceramics, their properties and applications, expanding on reviews published previously [4,10-24]. Properties of bone that are emulated in the development of bioactive bioceramics are also briefly described.

Table 8.1a Commercial bioactive bone grafts

Biologic origin
Natural coral, $CaCO_3$
Biocoral ®(Inoteb, France)
Coralline HA (complete conversion of $CaCO_3$ to HA)
Interpore 200, ProOsteon 200®, ProOsteon 500® (Interpore Int, CA)
Corraline HA /$CaCO_3$ (partial conversion of $CaCO_3$)
Prosteon™ 200R, ProOsteton™ 500R (Interpore Int, CA)
Bovine bone apatite, unsintered
BioOss® (EdGeitslich, Switzerland
Bovine bone apatite, sintered
Endobon® (Merck, Germany)
Osteograf®-N (Ceramed,CO)
Synthetic
Bioactive glass
Bioglass ®(US Biomaterials, FL)
Ceravital® (Germany)
Cerabone A-W® (Japan)
Calcium sulfate (CS), $CaSO_4$•$2H_2O$
OsteoSet® (Wright Medical, TN)
Jax™ (Smith & Nephew, TN)
$CaSO_4$•$1/2H_2O$ (CSH), mixed with diluent
BonePLAST™ (Interpore Cross, CA)
MIIG™ (Wright Medical, TN)
CSH + DBM
ALLOMATRIX^{TR} (Wright Medical, TN)
*CSH coated with PLA
*BoneGen-^{TR} (Orthogen BioLok, NJ)

DMB – demineralized bone matrix (human bone); PLA – polylactic acid

Table 8.1b Commercial bone grafts: Calcium phosphates (synthetic).

Calcium deficient apatite	
Osteogen® (Impladent,NY)	
Ceramic HA, $Ca_{10}(PO_4)_6(OH)_2$	
Calcitite®	
Osteograf® (Ceramed, CO)	
Bioroc® (Depuy-Bioland, France)	
HA (Japan)	
β-TCP, $Ca_3(PO_4)_2$	
Vitoss® (OrthoVita Inc PA)	
BCP (HA+β-TCP); HA/β-TCP rat io	
60/40; 20/80	MBCP® (Biomatlante, France)
20/80	Tribone 80® (Strycker Europe)
60/40	Osteosynt® (Einco Ltd, Brazil)
60/40	Triosite® (Zimmer, IND)
60/40	4Bone® (MIS Israel)
60/40	OptiMX® (Exactech USA)
55/45	Eurocer® 400 (Depuy-Bioland, France)
65/35	Eurocer® 200 (Depuy-Bioland, France)

(continued)

Table 8.1b (continued)

Composites
BCP/Collagen
Allograft® (Zimmer, IN)
BCP/HPMC
MBCP® Gel (Biomatlante France)
BCP/Fibrin
Tricos® (Baxter BioSciences BioSurgery)
BCP/Silicon
Flex™HA (Xomed, FL))
CHA/collagen
Healos™ (Orquest Inc, CA)
HA/$CaSO_4$
Hapset® (Lifecore, MINN)
HA/polyethylene
HAPEX® (Gyrus, TN)
$CaSO_4$/DMB
Allomatrix^{TR} Wright Medical, Memphis, TN

8.2. Basic Science

8.2.1. General Properties of Bone

Bone may be simply described as a biocomposite consisting of organic and mineral phases. The organic phase consists mostly of collagen (Type 1) and minor amounts of important non-collageneous proteins including proteoglycans, bone morphogenetic proteins (BMPs) and other growth factors responsible for inducing bone formation. The inorganic phase previously idealized as hydroxyapatite, $Ca_{10}(PO_4)_2(OH)_2$ [25,26] was later identified as an impure HA, essentially a carbonate substituted apatite (CHA) with other minor but important constituents (e.g., magnesium) [27-29], similar to some mineral carbonate apatites like dahllite [30]. Bone also contains bone-forming cells (osteoblasts) and bone-resorbing cells (osteoclasts) and various osteoinductive growth factors and molecules. Critical physico-biochemical properties of bone include (1) interconnecting porosity (macro- and micro-porosity), (2) biodegradability (remodeling), (3) bioactivity, (4) osteoconductivity and (5) osteoinductivity. Pore size in normal cortical bone ranges from 1 to 10 μm, and 200 to 400 μm in trabecular bone. To promote bone formation, repair or regeneration, the size and interconnection of the porosity is critical for the diffusion of nutrients, cell attachment, migration, proliferation and differentiation and tissue ingrowths to promote bone formation, repair and regeneration.

8.2.2. General Properties of Bioceramics Approximating Bone Properties

Development of bioactive ceramics in recent years has tried to mimic some of the properties of bone by adjusting the composition, introducing interconnecting porosity and incorporating osteoinductive factors or molecules.

8.2.2.1. Porosity

Interconnecting macro-porosity (100 to 500 μm) allows tissue ingrowths and microporosity (1 to 10 μ) allows ingrowths of blood vessels [31, 32]. For bioceramics from biologic origin, e.g., HA derived from coral, or derived from bovine bone, the original interconnecting porosity of coral or bone is preserved during the processing (Fig. 8.1). In the case of synthetic bioceramics, macro-porosity is introduced by the addition of porogens (e.g., naphthalene, H_2O_2, sugar, starch, polymers, etc), then evolution of the porogens at initial temperature of firing (100° C) before the final sintering temperature (1,000 to 1,200° C) [33, 34]. Other means of creating interconnecting macro-porosity is by foaming method [35]. For synthetic bioceramics and sintered bone bioceramics, microporosity (spaces between the crystals) and crystal size depends on the final sintering temperature and the process of sintering [36] as shown in Fig. 8.2.

8.2.2.2. Degradation and Dissolution

Degradation of biomaterials *in vivo* (biodegradation) is cell-mediated by macrophages and osteoclasts (bone-resorbing cells) that promote acidic conditions [37-39]. *In vitro*, dissolution in acidic buffer may be predictive of the in vivo degradation or dissolution of the biomaterials [40]. *In vitro* or *in vivo* dissolution of a bioceramic material depends on its composition, particle size, porosity (micro- and macro-porosity), specific surface area and crystallinity (reflecting crystal size and perfection) [40-44]. Figure 8.3 shows the difference in the *in vitro* dissolution characteristics for some commercial bioceramics of similar but not identical compositions:

Unsintered bovine bone apatite (Bio-Oss®) >> sintered bovine bone apatite (Osteograf® N)

coralline HA (Interpore 200) > ceramic HA (Calcitite®).

In both cases, the difference in dissolution properties is due to the difference in apatite crystal size and difference in minor composition (CO_3^{2-} content is

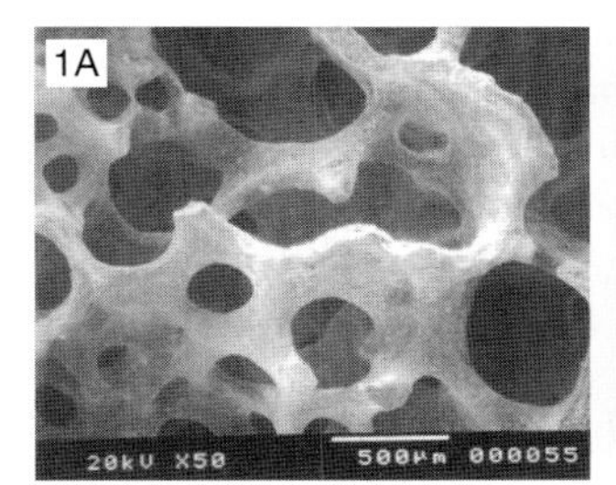

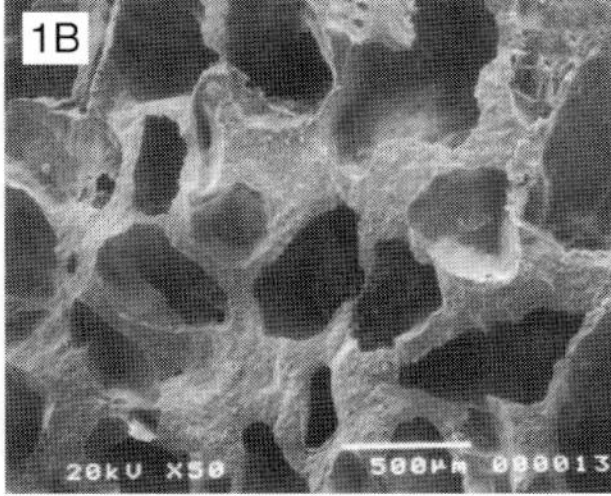

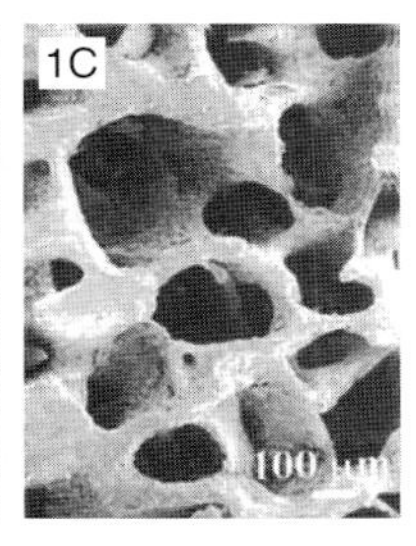

Fig. 8.1 SEM images showing comparative interconnecting macro-porosity in (A) bovine bone, sintered (Endobone, Merck), (B) biphasic calcium phosphate (MBCP®, Biomatlante, France) and (C) coralline HA (Interpore 200, Interpore, CA)

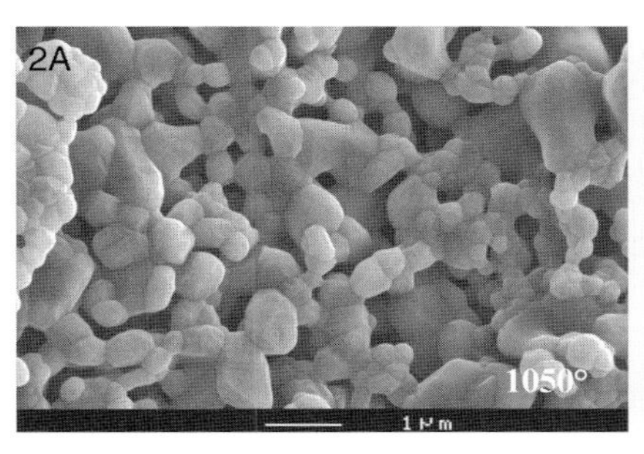

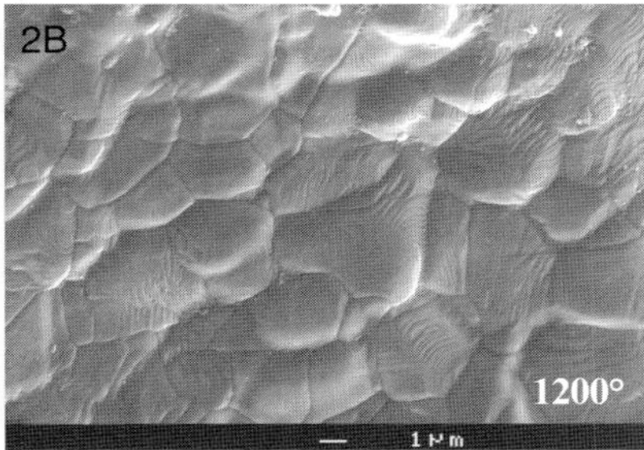

Fig. 8.2 SEM images showing the effect of sintering temperature on the microporosity of bioceramics: (A) sintered at 1,050° C and (b) sintered at 1,200° C [36]

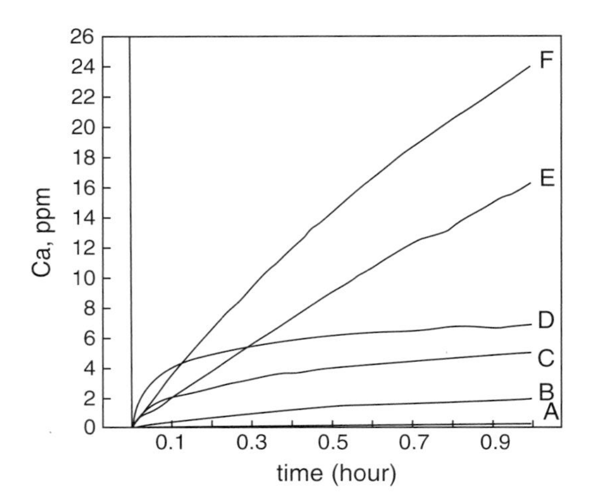

Fig. 8.3 Comparative dissolution properties of different bioceramics (powdered and sieved to obtain similar particle size) in Tris buffer (pH 7.3, 37° C) reflected by the release of calcium ions (Ca^{2+}, in ppm) with time. (A) bioactive glass (Perioglass^{R}); (B) coralline HA (Interpore 200), (C) sintered bovine bone apatite (Osteograf® N), (D) sintered bovine bone apatite (BonAp, experimental), (E) unsintered bovine bone apatite (BioOss®); and (F) coral, $CaCO_3$ (Biocorail®) [42]

less in sintered compared to unsintered bovine bone (Fig. 8.4); coralline HA contains Mg^{2+} and CO_3^{2-} while ceramic HA does not) [20, 44]. Mg^{2+} and CO_3^{2-} ions incorporated in apatite are known to cause a decrease in crystallinity and increase in solubility of synthetic and biologic apatites [27, 28].

The difference in preparation methods (described in Section C) also causes difference in crystal size (Figs. 8.4 and 8.5) and in composition (Figs. 8.5, 8.6, 8.7) that, in turn, affect their dissolution properties. For example, the bioceramics below are listed in the order of *decreasing* crystal size and *increasing* solubility.

CeramicHA >> corallineHA
sintered bone apatite >> unsintered bone apatite.
Bioglass >> A-W glass

Among bioceramics of diverse composition, but with very similar particle size (powdered and sieved samples), the extent of *in vitro* dissolution decreases in the following order [42]:

Calcium sulfate > coral (calcium carbonate) >> bioactive glass >> unsintered bovine bone apatite > sintered bone apatite >> coralline HA > ceramic HA.

Initial rate of dissolution, d[Ca]/dt in acetate buffer (0.1 M KAc, pH 6, 37 °C) was determined to be:

(A) HA (Calcitite®), 5.2; (B) β-TCP, 10.2; (C) bovine bone mineral (BioOss®); (D) calcium carbonate, 69.4; and (E) calcium sulfate hemihydrate, 113.9 ppm Ca/min.

In the case of synthetic calcium phosphate biomaterials, the extent of dissolution decreases in the order:

β-TCP > BCP > HA

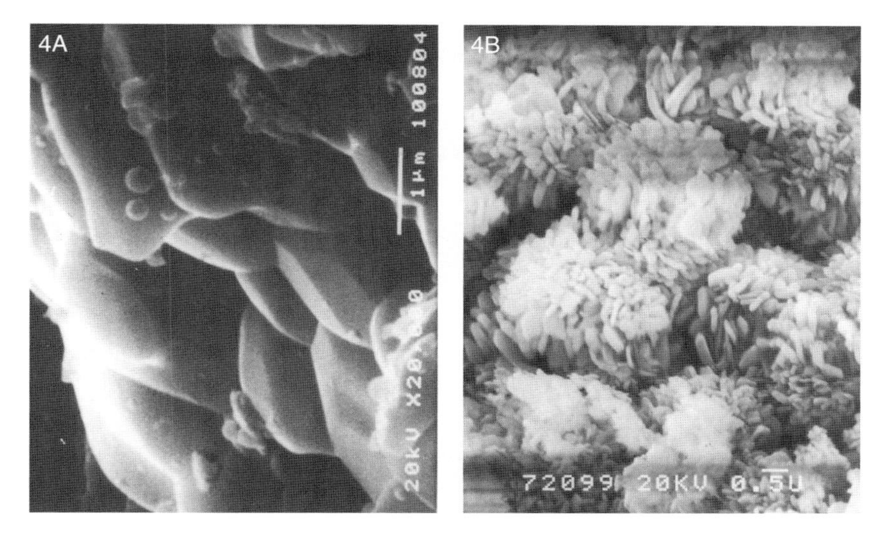

Fig. 8.4 SEM images showing comparative crystal size of apatite from (A) dense HA, sintered at 1,100° C (Calcitite) and (B) coralline HA (Interpore 200) [21]

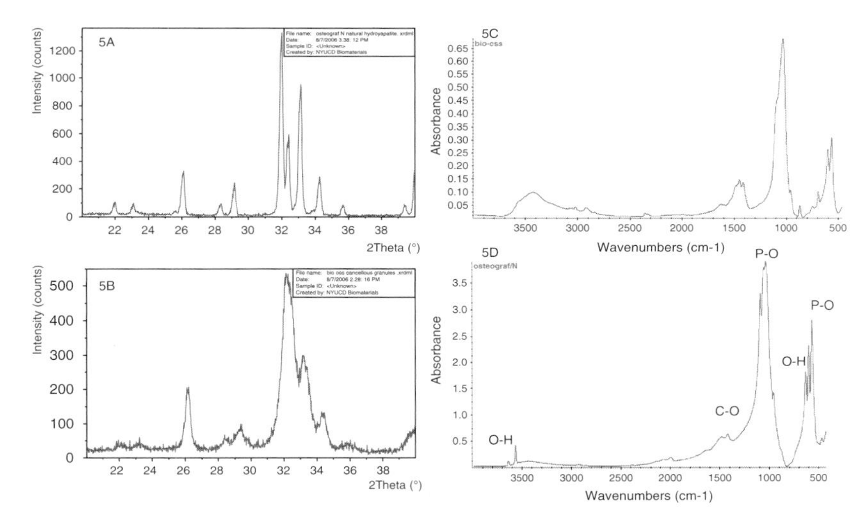

Fig. 8.5 X-ray diffraction (XRD) profiles of: (A) unsintered (BioOss®) and (B) sintered (Osteograf® N) bovine bone apatite showing difference in crystallite size (B>>A) as reflected by the broadening of the XRD peaks: the broader the peaks the smaller the crystal size

FT-IR spectra of: (C) unsintered and (D) sintered bovine bone apatite showing difference in carbonate content (C>>D) and crystallite size (D>>C) reflected by the higher resolution of absorption bands (D>>C). Sintering causes loss of carbonate (as CO_2) and crystal growth

With biphasic calcium phosphates (BCP), the extent of degradation *in vitro* and *in vivo* depends on the HA/β-TCP weight ratio of the BCP: the higher the ratio, the less the extent of dissolution/degradation since β-TCP is much more soluble than HA [36-40, 45. 46].

In vitro cell-mediated degradation of bioceramics parallels that of *in vitro* dissolution properties. For example, osteoclast activity was found to increase

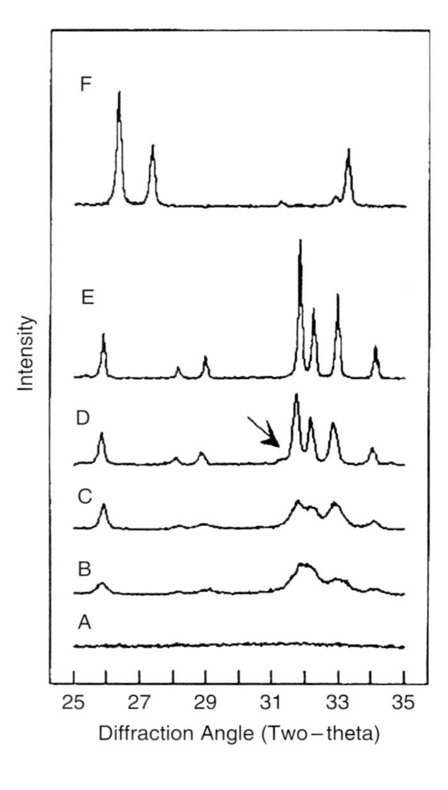

Fig. 8.6 XRD profiles of different bioceramics: (A) bioglass (Perioglas®); (B) unsintered bovine bone apatite (BioOss®); (C) calcium-deficient apatite (Osteogen®); (D) coralline HA (Interpore® 200); (E) HA (Calcitite®) and (F) calcium carbonate, aragonite form (Biocorail®) [42]

in the order [47]: HA < β-TCP < $CaCO_3$, which parallels the order of their solubility. The amount of bone formation appears to also be related to the extent of biodegradation [43]: bioglass > A-W glass > HA again paralleling the *in vitro* dissolution of these materials mentioned above.

Substitutions in the apatite structure (e.g., CO_3^{2-}-for-PO_4^{3-}, F^--for-$(OH)^-$, Mg^{2+}-for-Ca^{2+}, silicate for phosphate) or in the tricalcium phosphate structure (Mg^{2+}-for-Ca^{2+}) affect *in vitro* dissolution whether solution- or cell-mediated [28, 48-52].

In the case of plasma-sprayed 'HA' coating on orthopedic or dental implants, the biodegradation of the coating depends on the ratio of HA/ACP: the lower the ratio the greater the rate of degradation of the coating since amorphous calcium phosphate (ACP) is considerably more soluble than HA [28, 40, 53, 54].

The factors that influence dissolution properties *in vitro* (composition, micro- and macro-porosity, particle size, surface area, surface topography) are also operative *in vivo*.

8.2.2.3. Bioactivity

Bioactivity is defined as the property of the material to develop a direct, adherent and strong bonding with the bone tissue [4, 5, 7]. *In vitro*, formation of carbonate apatite (CHA) on material surfaces after suspension in simulated body fluid (SBF) has been used as a criterion for determining its bioactivity [55]. *In vivo*, nanocrystals of CHA intimately associated with an organic phase, have been observed on surfaces of calcium phosphate ceramics implanted in nonosseous [56] and osseous sites [45] as shown in Fig. 8.8. Besides calcium phosphates, other calcium releasing materials such as calcium carbonate

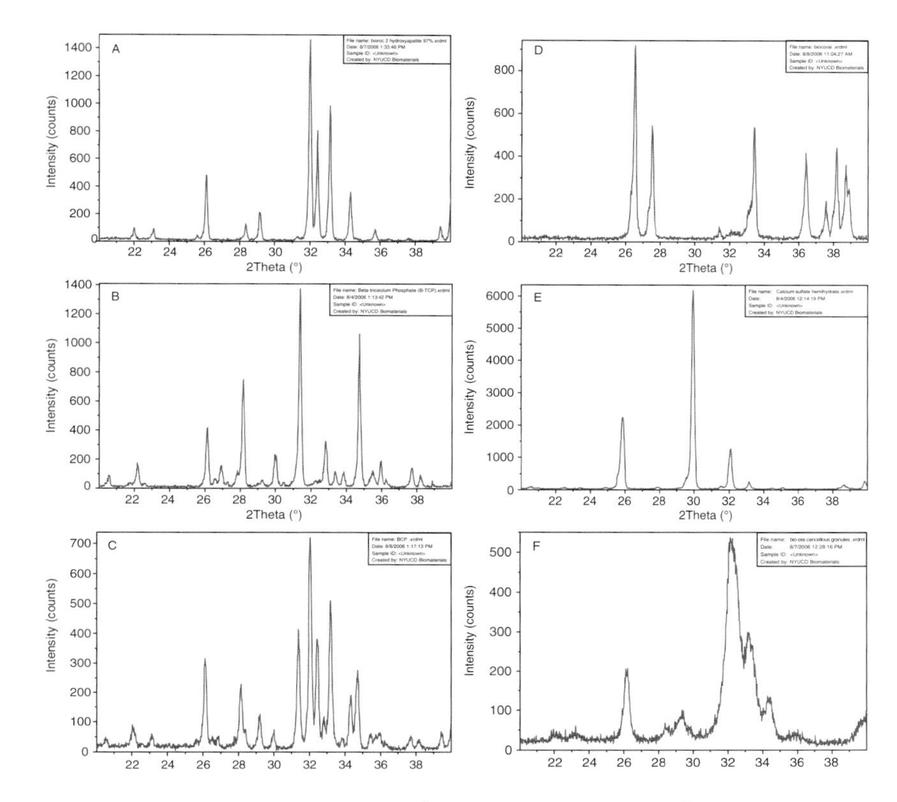

Fig. 8.7 XRD profiles of: (A) HA; (B) β-TCP; (C) BCP (60HA/40β-TCP); (D) calcium sulfate hemihydrate, $CaSO_4.1/2H_2O$; (E) calcium carbonate, $CaCO_3$, aragonite form. and (F) bovine bone mineral

(natural coral), calcium sulfate and bioactive glass-ceramics form a carbonate apatite layer to which the new bone firmly attaches itself (Fig. 8.9).

The formation of CHA on surfaces of Ca-releasing bioceramics is thought to be a cell-mediated dissolution and precipitation process [45, 57-59]. Cellular activity associated with acidic environment (e.g., macrophages, osteoclasts) [37, 39] induces partial dissolution of the bioceramic and liberation of Ca or Ca and P ions onto the microenvironment. The liberated ions increase the supersaturation of the biologic fluid causing precipitation incorporating other ions, e.g., CO_3^{2-}, Mg^{2+}, Na^+, etc. from the biologic fluid resulting in the formation of CHA nanocrystals on the surface of the dissolving bioceramic crystals (Fig. 8.8). This initial action may trigger a mineralization of the extracellular matrix leading to bone formation. The enrichment of the Ca or Ca and P ions in the microenvironment seems to promote bone mineralization and enhance bone formation [38, 57-59].

8.2.2.4. Osteoconductivity

Osteoconductivity is a property of a biomaterial to serve as a scaffold or template guiding the formation of new bone (Fig. 8.10). Osteoconductive bioceramics allow attachment, proliferation, migration and phenotypic expression of bone cells leading to formation of new bone in direct apposition to the bioactive biomaterials [22, 43].

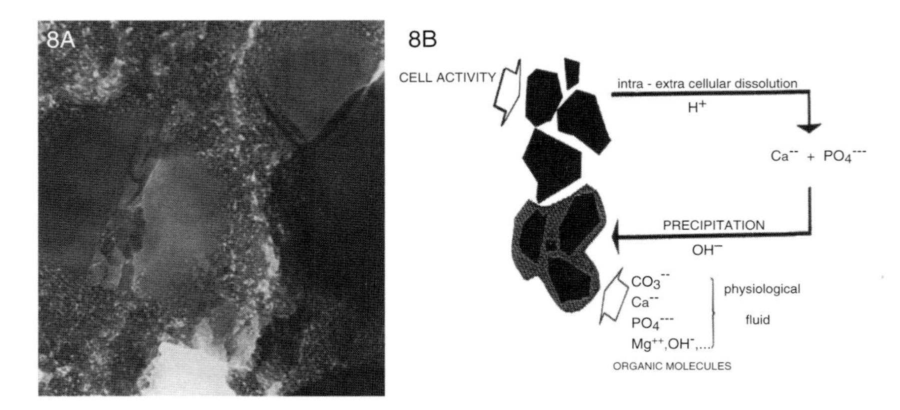

Fig. 8.8 (A) Nanocrystals of carbonate apatite (CHA) associated with larger bioceramic crystals after implantation of BCP. (B) Schematic representation of the dissolution/precipitation processes occurring after implantation of calcium phosphate bioceramic (BCP) in rabbit [45, 46, 57]. Cell (osteoclast) interaction with the BCP ceramics causes partial dissolution of the β-TCP- releasing Ca^{2+} and PO_4^{3-} onto the microenvironment increasing the supersaturation of the biologic fluid with respect to apatite leading to the precipitation of the nano-carbonate apatite crystals similar to bone apatite [57-59]

8.2.2.5. *Osteoinductivity*

The concept of osteoinductivity, first introduced by Urist [60], is the ability of the biomaterial implanted in non-bone forming sites (subcutaneously or in the muscle) in animals, to induce *de novo* bone formation. Osteoinductivity is introduced with the bioceramics by the incorporation of materials such as demineralized bone matrix (DBM) or growth factors (BMPs, platelet-rich factors, etc).

It has been generally accepted that bioactive ceramics (e.g., calcium phosphates) are osteoconductive but not osteoinductive by themselves [10, 22]. However, some animal studies observed possible osteoinductive properties of some calcium phosphate bioceramics (porous β-TCP, porous HA, coralline HA) [61-65]. Ripamonti, et al. [63, 64] and Kuboki, et al. [62] suggested that the geometry of the bioceramics is critical for osteoinductivity. Reddi [66] explained this phenomenon as the property of the bioceramic with particular geometry to trap the circulating growth factors (BMP), thus making the bioceramic osteoinductive. Recently, Le Nihouhannen, et al. [67] observed in back-scattered electron (BSE) images, ectopic bone formation with Haversian structures in close contact with the remaining macroporous biphasic calcium phosphate MBCP (MBCP™ Biomatlante, France) after six months implantation in dorsal muscles of sheep. The MBCP had a composition of 60HA/40TCP, granule size 1 to 2 mm, total porosity 70 percent, size of macropore 450±49 μm, size of micropore 0.43±0.2 μm, specific surface area, 1.8 ±0.1 m^3/g. Kuboki, et al. [60] also speculated that the geometry may be critical for the efficient transport and delivery of the BMP growth factor. To date, the 'appropriate geometry' that would allow the bioceramics to trap or concentrate the critical amount of growth factors to make them osteoinductive is not known and is an intriguing subject of several investigations. It is also not known whether there are other factors, in addition to appropriate geometry of the bioceramic scaffolds, that would make them efficient carriers for growth factors.

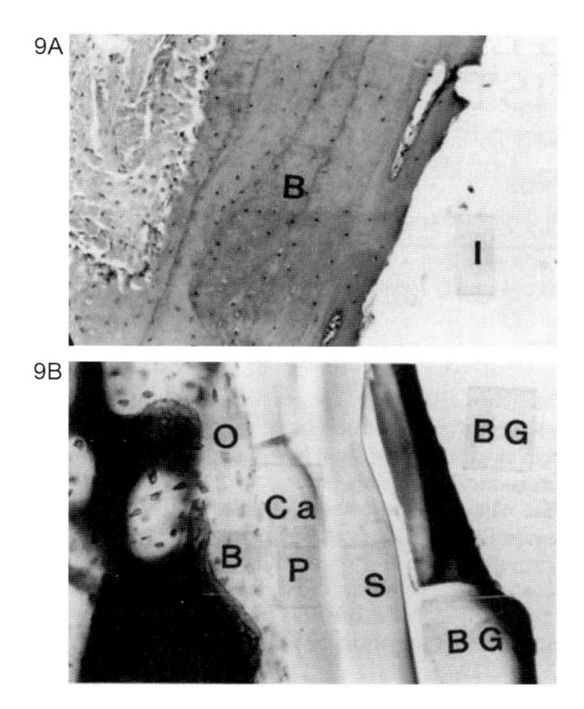

Fig. 8.9 SEM images showing interface between (A) bioglass (I) and host bone (B); and (B) silica-rich (S) and calcium phosphate (Ca,P) layers. The newly formed bone (B) is attached to the CaP layer [20]

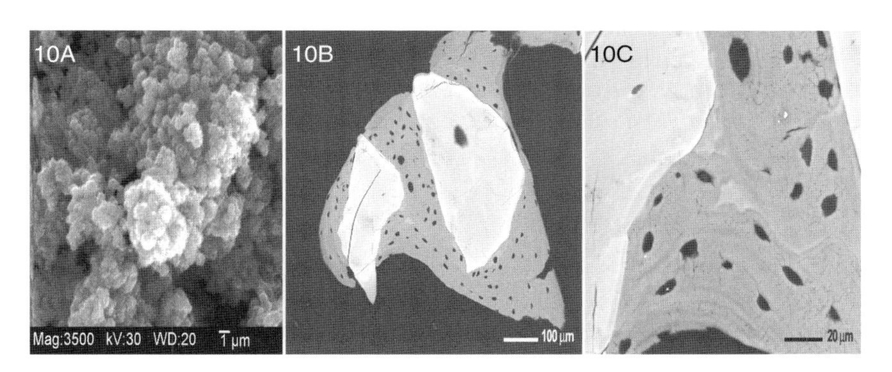

Fig. 8.10 SEM of Mg-substituted β-TCP (Mg- β-TCP) before (A) and after (B,C) implantation in surgically created defect in rabbit showing its osteoconductive property [22]

8.2.3. Bioactive Bioceramics

8.2.3.1. Bioactive Glass Ceramics

Hench pioneered the development of glass ceramics described as 'bioactive' because it allowed the formation of new bone on its surface and provided a uniquely strong interface with the host bone [36]. The bioactivity of the glass depends on its composition [4]. The bioactive glass ceramic developed by Hench is available commercially (Bioglass®, US Biomaterials, Fl) and is prepared by melting together SiO_2 (network former), Na_2O/K_2O and CaO (network modifiers) and P_2O_5 (internal nucleant for surface apatite formation) in specific proportions (45 percent SiO_2, 24.5 percent CaO, 24.5 percent Na_2O and 6 percent P_2O_5). Other bioactive glass ceramics of different formulations were subsequently developed: Cerabone^{R}A-W containing crystalline hydroxy or fluoride-containing apatite, $Ca_{10}(PO_4)_6(O,F)_2$, and wollastonite, CaO.SiO_2, developed by Kokubo in Japan [68], and Ceravital^R developed by Broemer and Deutcher in Germany and described by Gross, et al. [69].

Non-silicate glasses of the system CaO-P_2O_5 were originally developed for processing of dental crowns [70]. An experimental calcium phosphate glass (CPG) based on the system CaO-CaF_2–P_2O_5-MgO-ZnO with Ca/P molar ratio ranging from 0.2 to 1.2 was developed by LeGeros and Lee [71].The biodegradation of these CPGs can be controlled by changing the Ca/P ratio of the glass. Recent animal studies showed the potential of this material for bone repair [72].

8.2.3.2. Calcium Sulfate, Plaster of Paris.

The use of plaster of Paris (calcium sulfate hemihydrate, $CaSO_4{\bullet}1/2H_2O$) as filler for bone defects was first reported by Dreesmann in 1892 [73]. A surge of interest in calcium sulfate in recent years resulted in the development and commercialization of surgical grade calcium sulfate dihydrate pellets, $CaSO_4{\bullet}2H_2O$ (OSTEOSET®, Wright Medical, Arlington, TN). Commercial calcium sulfate products are available as calcium sulfate dihydrate ($CaSO_4{\bullet}2H_2O$) pellet or as calcium sulfate hemihydrate, ($CaSO_4{\bullet}1/2H_2O$) powder provided in a kit with a diluent (distilled H_2O) that hardens when mixed. Calcium sulfate mixed with demineralized bone matrix (86 percent by volume) is available as an osteoinductive putty (Allomatrix™, Wright Medical TN).

A new calcium sulfate product, Bone-Gen-TR^{TR} (Orthogen Corporation, BioLok International, NJ) was developed by Ricci, et al. [74]. This product, a composite of calcium sulfate hemihydrate (CSH) and poly lactic acid (PLLA) with a CSH/PLLA ratio of 96/4, is described as a time-release calcium sulfate. Compared to calcium sulfate alone, which completely biodegrades in four to five weeks, the composite product completely biodegrades in 16 weeks [74].

8.2.4. Bioceramics of Biologic Origin

8.2.4.1. Natural Coral (Calcium Carbonate)

The commercial product, Biocoral® (Bio-CC® 1-1, Inoteb, France) is obtained from natural coral (reef-building species, *Porites*) that has been processed to remove the organic phase. The mineral phase of the coral consists of calcium carbonate ($CaCO_3$) with the aragonite structure. It has interconnecting macroporosity similar to that of trabecular bone.

8.2.4.2. Coral-derived Hydroxyapatite, Coralline HA

Coralline HA is obtained by the hydrothermal conversion of natural coral (calcium carbonate, $CaCO_3$ in aragonite form) to apatite (coralline HA) in the presence of ammonium phosphate under pressure of about 200 psi and reaction temperature of about 365 ° C [75]. This process preserves the inherent interconnecting macro-porosity of the coral before the conversion (Fig. 8.1). The resulting coralline HA is mixed with a small amount of magnesium-substituted tricalcium phosphate, Mg-βTCP (Fig. 8.6) and contains a small amount of carbonate and strontium [20, 44]. Commercial coralline HA (Interpore 200, Pro Osteon™ 500, ProOsteon™® 200, Interpore, CA) is obtained from coral

Porites and *Goniopora* species differing in porosity and pore size: *Goniospora*, average pore size of 500 μm and average porosity of 65 percent; *Porites*, average pore size of 200 μm and average porosity of 50 percent. The original process (complete conversion of $CaCO_3$) was modified to allow only partial conversion of the $CaCO_3$ (about 15 percent) resulting in an apatite coating layer (2 to 10 μm in thickness) to provide more resorbable products (Pro Osteon™ 500R, ProOsteon™ 200R). The resorption rate was reported to be months to years for completely converted products and weeks to months for the partially converted products described as resorbable [76].

8.2.4.3. Bovine-derived Apatite

Bovine-derived materials are prepared by removing the organic phase and the bone mineral (carbonate apatite) is either unsintered (BioOss®,EdGeitslich, Switzerland) [77] or sintered (Ostegraft N®, Ceramed, CO; Endobon®, Merck, Darmstad, Germany) [78]. The unsintered and sintered bone mineral differ in crystallinity reflecting crystal size (sintered >> unsintered) and dissolution properties (unsintered>>sintered) as shown in Figs. 8-3 and 8-5. The sintering process causes the loss of carbonate (Fig. 8.5) and causes an increase in crystal size (Fig. 8.5) of the bone apatite. The loss in carbonate and increase in crystal size account for the lower solubility of the sintered bone mineral (e.g., Endobon®, Merck, Germany), compared to the unsintered one (e.g., BioOss®. EdGeitslich Switzerland).

8.2.5. Synthetic Calcium Phosphates

The first successful medical application of calcium phosphate (ambiguously described as 'triple calcium phosphate') was reported by Albee in 1920 [79]. Albee used 'triple calcium phosphate,' presumably a chemical reagent. Nery, et al. reported successful treatment of surgically created periodontal defects using a calcium phosphate he described as 'porous tricalcium phosphate, TCP' [80]. X-ray diffraction analysis of this material by LeGeros in 1986 [20] revealed that Nery's 'TCP' was actually a mixture of 80HA and 20 β-TCP, prompting Nery to rename his material and others like it (i.e., mixtures of HA and β-TCP) as biphasic calcium phosphate, BCP [46]. Initial basic studies on BCP [58, 81] and focused studies on its potential applications [39, 46, 82-88] led to the commercialization of BCP.

Commercial calcium phosphate products currently available are: calcium deficient apatite (CDA); hydroxyapatite (HA), $Ca_{10}(PO_4)_6(OH)_2$; beta-tricalcium phosphate (β-TCP), $Ca_3(PO_4)_2$, and biphasic calcium phosphate (BCP), an intimate mixture of HA and β-TCP, with various HA/β-TCP weight ratios (Table 8.1).

8.2.5.1. Calcium-deficient Apatite, CDA

Pure HA has a Ca/P molar ratio of 1.67. Calcium deficient apatite, CDA, has a Ca/P molar ratio lower than 1.67 and may be represented by the formula: $(Ca,Na)_{10}(HPO_4)(PO_4)_5(OH)_2$. CDA is prepared by precipitation at neutral pH or by hydrolysis of calcium phosphate dihydrate (DCPD), $CaHPO_4{\bullet}2H_2O$ or dicalciumphosphate anhydrous (DCPA), $CaHPO_4$ [28]. CDA is much more soluble than either coralline HA or ceramic HA (Fig. 8.3). Besides its limited use in dentistry, it is used as one of the components of calcium phosphate cements (Table 8.2) [23].

Table 8.2a Commercial cements

Self-setting
Bioactive glass-based
Cortoss® (Orthovita, PA)
Nova-Bone® (US Biomaterials Corp, FL)
Calcium phosphate based
SRS® (Norian Corp, CA)
Bone Source® (Stryker, Howmedica NJ)
α-BSM® (ETEX Corpation, Cambridge, MA)
Biopex® (Mitsubishi Mat, Japan)

Table 8.2b Commercial calcium phosphate (CPC): composition

Cements	Powder Component	Set Product
Self-setting		
α-BSM® (ETEX,Cambridge,MA)	ACP, DCPD	HAp
SRS® Skeletal Repair System, (Norian, Synthes)	α-TCP, $CaCO_3$, MCPM	CHA
BoneSource® (Stryker, Howmedica, NJ)	TTCP, DCPA	HAp
Cementek® (Teknimed, France)	α-TCP,TTCP,MCPM	HAp
BiocementD® (Merck GmBH, Germany)	α-TCP, DCPA,$CaCO_3$, HAp	CHA•
Biopex® (Mitsubishi Materials, Japan)	α-TCP, DCPA, $CaCO_3$, Hap	CHA

ACP: amorphous calcium phosphate; DCPD: dicalcium phosphate dihydrate, $CaHPO_4.2H_2O$; DCPA: dicalcium phosphate anhydrous, $CaHPO_4$; α-TCP: α-tricalcium phosphate; MCPM: monocalciumphosphate monohydrate, $CaH_4(PO_4)_2$•H_2O, HAP: apatitic calcium phosphate; CHA: carbonate-substituted hydroxyapatite; HAp – calcium-deficient apatite.
Biocement® D and Biopex® have similar composition of the powder components but differ in the composition of their liquid components

8.2.5.2. Calcium Hydroxyapatite (HA), Ceramic HA

Ceramic HA, $Ca_{10}(PO_4)_6(OH)_2$ is prepared by precipitating at high pH and sintering the precipitated product above 1,000° C [11,15,18,28,89]. HA was the first calcium phosphate product that became commercially available and was used in dentistry and medicine in dense and porous forms. Of all the calcium phosphate-based bioceramics, HA is the least soluble (Fig. 8.3).

A composite of HA and high molecular weight polyethylene was developed by Bonfield [90] and is now available (HAPEX®, Gyrus, TN) for use as ear implant and in orthopedic prosthesis. Experimental composite of HA with collagen is being developed as bone graft material [92].

Besides its application in dentistry and medicine, HA is now currently used as an alternative abrasive for orthopedic and dental implants. As an abrasive, HA leaves a clean surface, compared to the alumina abrasive [92], and appears to impart bioactive property to the implant surface [92-94] shown in Fig. 8.11.

8.2.5.3. Beta-Tricalcium phosphate (β-TCP)

β-TCP, $Ca_3(PO_4)_2$ is prepared by sintering precipitated calcium deficient apatite with a Ca/P molar ratio of about 1.5. It can also be prepared by solid state reaction between appropriate amounts of $CaHPO_4$ and $CaCO_3$ or CaO [28, 36, 89]. Commercial porous β-TCP (Vitoss®, Orthovita, PA) has undergone preclinical studies and limited clinical studies for orthopedic application.

8.2.5.4. Biphasic Calcium Phosphate, BCP

BCP is prepared by sintering precipitated calcium deficient apatite (Ca/P molar ratio between 1.55 and 1.65), resulting in an intimate mixture of HA and βTCP [28, 36]. The HA/βTCP weight ratio of the BCP depends on the calcium deficiency of the precipitated apatite before sintering. Successful application of BCP was attributed to controlled bioactivity manipulated by controlling the HA/βTCP ratio because of the preferential dissolution of the βTCP component of BCP [45, 46, 58, 81]. Biodegradation or dissolution of BCP depends on

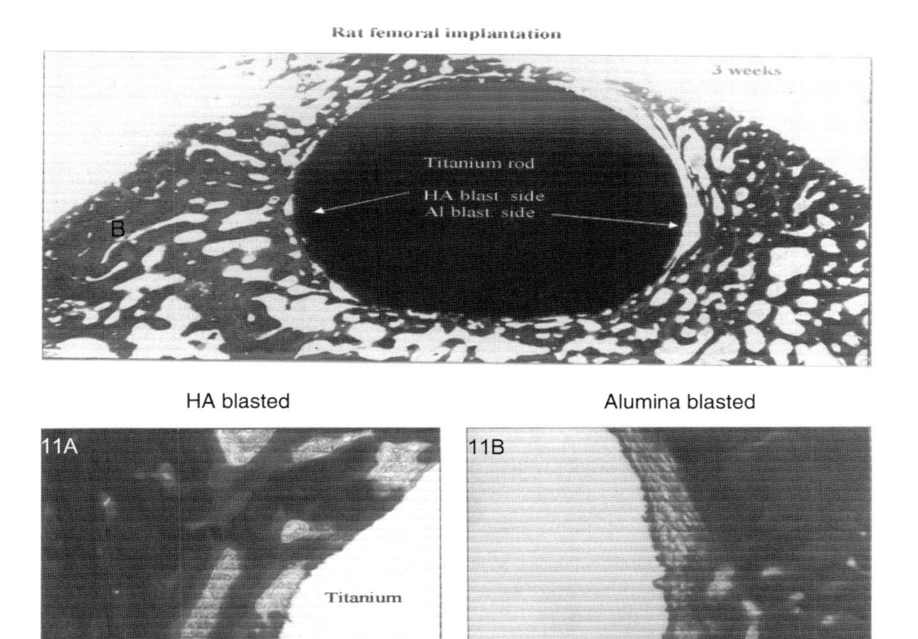

Fig. 8.11 Histologic images showing the difference in interface between the Ti alloy surface (A) grit-blasted with apatitic abrasive (MCD, HiMed, New York) and (B) grit-blasted with alumina abrasive. Newly formed bone is directly apposed to the implant side grit-blasted with apatitic abrasive while non-mineralized fibrous tissue is on the interface between the bone and the Ti alloy surface grit-blasted with alumina [93]

the processing and sintering methods that affect the crystallinity and porosity. Thus, BCPs of equivalent HA/βTCP ratio may exhibit different biodegradation properties [36].

A composite of BCP (80HA/20β-TCP) with silicone (Flex™ HA, Xomed,FL) is available as an ear implant, replacing damaged ear ossicles. A composite of BCP (65HA/35β-TCP) with bovine-derived collagen in a 1:1 ratio (Collagraft®, Zimmer Corporation, Warsaw, IN) is used with autogenous bone marrow aspirate [12, 13, 17, 95].

8.2.6. Calcium Phosphate Cements

The concept of calcium phosphate cements (CPC) was first introduced by LeGeros, et al. in 1982 [96] showing that apatitic calcium phosphate mixed with calcium hydroxide and dilute phosphoric acid can form a cement and may have potential for restorative dentistry or as bone cement. Brown and Chow obtained the first patent on CPC in 1986 based on tetracalcium phosphate (TTCP) and dicalcium phosphate anhydrous (DCPA) as the powder component and sodium phosphate solution as the liquid component [97]. Other CPC formulations were developed with varying components of the powder and liquid components [23, 98-102]. The setting time depends on the composition of the powder and liquid components and on the powder/liquid ratio. The composition of the product after setting depends on the composition of powder and liquid components (Table 8.2).

8.2.7. Calcium Phosphate Coatings on Orthopedic and Dental Implants

Although calcium phosphate bioceramics have many desirable properties, they do not have the mechanical strength to be used in load bearing areas. Orthopedic and dental implants with calcium phosphate coatings (principally, plasma sprayed 'HA' coating was developed commercially to combine the strength of the metal (titanium, titanium alloy, stainless steel) with the bioactivity of the calcium phosphate coating [15,18,103]. However, due to the high temperature (>10,000° C) involved in the plasma spray process, the resulting coating is quite different from the initial HA materials [53, 54,103]. The principal coating components are HA and amorphous calcium phosphate (ACP). The HA/ACP ratio varies from one manufacturer to the other and even from one lot to another from the same manufacturer [53, 54, 104] due to the difference in parameters used in the plasma spray process. In addition, the HA/ACP ratio is significantly lower in the coating layer closest to the metal substrate, compared to the HA/ACP ratio in the coating layer closest to the surface [28, 54].

8.2.8. Bioceramic Scaffolds for Tissue Engineering and Carriers for Growth Factors and Drugs

8.2.8.1 Bioceramic Scaffolds

Tissue engineering for bone regeneration requires appropriate scaffolds for seeding the cells before implantation in the defect sites [105-108]. Studies on different scaffolds used in tissue engineering demonstrated that composition and particle size influence the amount of new bone formation. Livingstone, et al. [105] used BCP (MBCP®, Biomatlante, France) of varying HA/βTCP ratios as scaffolds for adult mesenchymal stem cells. These authors demonstrated that BCP with 20HA/80βTCP was more efficient in growing new bone, compared to 100 percent βTCP or BCP with higher HA/βTCP ratios. Mankani, et al.

[106], also using BCP (Triosite®, Zimmer, IN) as scaffolds for human bone marrow stromal cells, demonstrated that BCP particles of 0.2 to 0.25 mm size had the greatest bone formation in four and 10 weeks implantation subcutaneously in Bg-NuXID mice while larger or smaller particles showed less extensive bone formation. Texeira, et al. [106] showed that chondrocytes seeded on BCP (MBCP®, Biomatlante) attached and proliferated.

8.2.8.2. Bioceramics as Carriers of Growth Factors

Kuboki, et al. [62] suggested that the geometry of the porous ceramic HA scaffold was important for the efficiency in transporting BMPs. BCP with fibrin (Tissucol®, Baxter) has been used in the reconstruction in chronic otitis media surgery [110] undergoing clinical testing [83]. Studies on A-W glass ceramic with fibrin has also been reported [111].

8.2.8.3. Bioceramics for Drug Delivery

HA has been used for the delivery of bisphosphonate drug [112,113] and antibiotics [114,115]. Calcium sulfate with antibiotic (tobramycin) was found effective in healing non-unions [116].

8.3. Review of Pre-clinical Studies

8.3.1. Calcium Sulfate

Earlier studies reviewed by Alexander, et al. in 1987 [10] concluded that calcium sulfate was biocompatible, does not cause inflammatory reaction, does not inhibit bone formation and is replaced by new bone, but that the rate of resorption was more rapid than the rate of new bone formation. Clinical studies using calcium sulfate alone or calcium sulfate mixed with demineralized bone matrix or mixed with autogenous bone or mixed with BMP reported that calcium sulfate alone was just as effective as when mixed with DBM or with autogenous bone [13, 17, 24, 117]. Walsh, et al. [118] compared bone healing and bone quality in defects filled with calcium sulfate pellets (OSTEOSET®, Wright Medical, TN) or calcium sulfate pellets combined with autograft using a sheep model. Their results showed incomplete healing in defects filled with calcium sulfate pellets alone. Furthermore, although calcium sulfate alone showed similar results compared with autograft and calcium sulfate pellets based on the total area of new bone in the defect, the quality of the bone in the calcium sulfate pellets alone group was thicker and less mature. *In vitro*, these authors observed a pH decrease (from pH of 7.4 to 5.1) when calcium phosphate pellets were stirred in phosphate buffered solution for 24 hours. These authors concluded that the calcium sulfate pellet "may not only act as a filler but also as an accelerator of the healing process through a pH-dependent pathway or other unknown mechanism."

A new calcium sulfate product, Bone-Gen-TR^{TR} (Orthogen Corporation, BioLok International, NJ) was developed by Ricci, et al. [74]. This product, a composite of calcium sulfate and polylactic acid (PLLA) with a calcium sulfate/PLLA ratio of 96.4, is described as a time-release calcium phosphate. Using a sheep model, Mamidwar and Ricci [74] determined the degradation of calcium sulphate alone and the calcium sulfate/PLLA composite. Calcium sulfate alone completely biodegraded in four to fiv weeks while the composite product completely biodegraded in 16 weeks. Animal and human studies are in progress for this material.

8.3.2. Coralline HA

The efficacy of coralline HA in several orthopedic applications had been shown in many animal studies reviewed by Shors [76]. Several animal studies showed that coralline HA mixed with autografts (in a 1:1 ratio) or with bone marrow was more successful in posterior lumbar fusion than coralline apatite alone.

8.3.3. Calcium Phosphate Bioceramics

Preclinical studies of porous βTCP (Vitoss®, Orthovita, PA) with and without bone marrow aspirate and as a graft extender showed its use in various indications: fractures of the calcaneus, tibial plateau, humerus, distal radius; wedge osteotomies of the tibia; knee prostheses and actabular revisions; backfilling of iliac crest donor sites, and anterior and posterolateral spinal fusion procedures [13]. Using a βTCP product manufactured in Japan (Olympus Optical Co. Ltd), implanted in animals showed the gradual degradation of the βTCP and its replacement by mature new bone [119].

BCP in a polymer (hydroxymethylcellulose) carrier (MBCP®-gel, Biomatlante, France) was recently developed. As the polymer dissolves, it leaves spaces between the BCP granules providing the macro-porosity and the scaffold for the newly forming bone [87]. The mechanical strength of the cement increased as the new bone formed, replacing MBCP. BCP mixed with bone marrow was successful in bone reconstruction in irradiated areas in a dog study [84].

8.3.4. Calcium Phosphate Cements

One significant advantage of injecTablecement is its ability to assume the shape and size of the defect and the ability to be replaced by the new forming bone in a shorter time than the granules. The efficiency of a certain CPC (Biopex®, Mitsubishi Materials, Japan) was investigated using 50 Chinese mountain sheep in which the femoral necks were osteotomized and divided into three groups of treatment: untreated, treated with CPC and treated with PMMA cement [120]. Maximum load to fixation failure was highest for the PMMA group after three weeks and highest for the CPC group after 12 weeks.

One disadvantage of current CPC cements, besides low mechanical strength, is the lack of porosity of the set cement. A recent formulation of a CPC that provides a macro-porous structure after it sets (Fig. 8.12) is being developed [121] and tested in animals [102]. The creation of macro-porosity is based on the mixture of different calcium phosphates that biodegrade at different rates.

8.4. Clinical Review: Applications of Bioactive Bioceramics

8.4.1. Natural Coral

Applications of natural coral (Biocoral®, Inoteb, France) have included bone filling for defects in orthopedics, craniofacial, periodontal defects and neurosurgery and are also recommended for repair of osteoporotic fracture [16,121-124]. A study by Vuola, et al. [124] in iliac crest defect in human patients monitored for an average of 2.1 years showed that healing of the bone defect was not complete and that at least 50 percent of the implanted coral still remained. Addition of bone morphogenetic protein was shown to induce bone ingrowths into the pores of the coral [125].

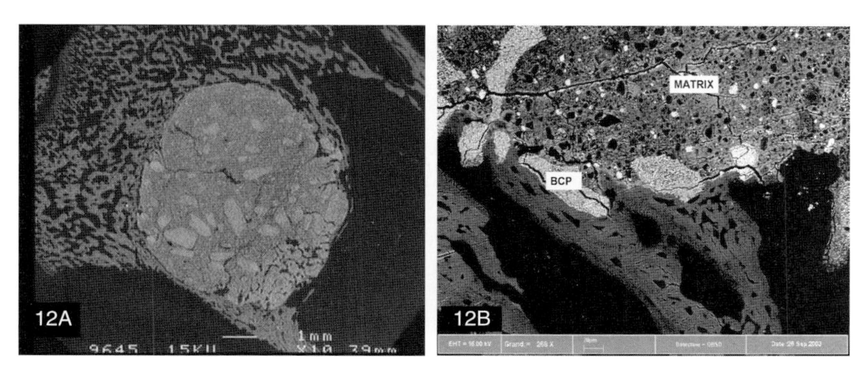

Fig. 8.12 SEM images comparing (A) macro-porous calcium phosphate cement, MCPC and (B) traditional calcium phosphate cement showing macro-porous structure of MCPC cement and ingrowths of new bone inside the MCPC (B) and the dense structure of traditional CPC (A) [102]

8.4.2. Bioactive Glass

Bioactive glass (silica-based) has been used as middle ear prosthesis to replace one or more ossicles of the middle ear that have been lost due to disease or trauma, as periodontal implants (Perioglas™, US Biomaterials, FL) and maxillofacial implants [126]. AW glass (Cerabone®A-W, Kyocera) is stronger and less soluble than bioactive glass because of a difference in composition (AW glass contains HA, or F-substituted HA and wollastonite) and crystallinity (bioactive glass gives an amorphous XRD profile). Cerabone®A-W has been successful clinically as artificial vertebrae, intervertebral spacers, iliac spacers, bone fillers, etc. [127].

8.4.3. Coralline HA

Coralline HA has been used clinically for the past 20 years. Shors [76] reviewed successful clinical applications of completely converted coral (Interpore HA 500 and HA 200, Pro Osteon™ 500, Interpore, CA) for periodontal, maxillofacial, plastic and orthopedic surgery (treatment of fractures, tumors, spinal fusion). Biopsies of implanted resorbable products (Pro Osteon™ 500R, Pro Osteon™ 200R) for posterolateral lumbar spinal fusion showed bone regeneration and significant implant resorption.

8.4.4. Calcium Sulfate

Plaster of Paris has been used in various orthopedic (craniofacial, long bone defects, spinal fusions, osteochondral defects, benign bone lesions) and dental (mandibular defects) applications in animals and humans [13,128,129].

8.4.5. Calcium Phosphates

The early medical and dental applications of β-TCP was reviewed by Metzger, et al. [130]. Reports on clinical studies of recent β-TCP commercial products were not available to date.

The use of BCP in orthopedics has gained wide acceptance in recent years [82-88, 107,121]. There are now several commercial BCP products with varying

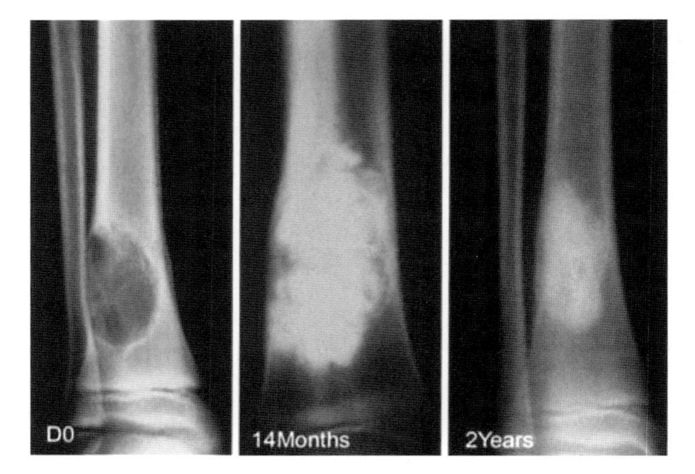

Fig. 8.13 Radiographic images of bone defect before and after 14 months and two years implantation of BCP (MBCP™, Biomatlante)

HA/βTCP ratio (Table 8.1b), the most popular product having the 60HA/40βTCP ratio. An example of a successful application of macroporous BCP (MBCP®, Biomatlante, France) in a large bone defect is shown in Fig. 8.13.

8.4.6. Calcium Phosphate Cements

Clinical studies of the different cements [19, 23, 97-102,131) have shown promising results in many dental and orthopedic applications including treatment of bone tumor, osteoporotic bone fracture and other fractures (compression fracture, femoral neck, distal end or radius fractures, spine fracture), stabilization of hip prostheses and bone graft substitute for filling bone defect after harvesting aulogous bone graft in the iliac crest. CPCs were shown to be vehicles for drug delivery of antibiotics, anticancer drugs and anti-inflammatory drugs, as well as delivery system for BMPs or biologically active peptides.

8.4.7. Calcium Phosphate Coatings (plasma sprayed 'HA')

Multicenter clinical studies demonstrated that orthopedic or dental implants with plasma sprayed HA coatings showed accelerated skeletal fixation [103,132]. However, because the solubility of ACP is considerably greater than that of HA, coatings with low HA/ACP ratio may result in premature degradation causing delamination of the coating, leading to implant loosening and even failure [53].

8.5. Future Trends

Animal studies on substituted apatites for bone repair [133,134] showed that fluoride-substituted carbonate apatite (CFA) promoted the formation of more mature bone, compared to carbonate-substituted apatite (CHA) or fluoride-substituted apatite (FA). Magnesium-substituted tricalcium phosphate, TCMP or Mg-βTCP, demonstrated favorable bone growth in surgically created defects in animals [50]. In addition, BCP consisting of apatite and Mg-TCP [28] can be prepared at low temperature (below 100° C) and may be an alternative to current BCP prepared at high temperature (1,000 to 1,200° C) for future investigations *In vitro* studies on silicon-substituted apatite showed higher dissolution compared to silicon-free apatite (HA) [51]. Webster, et al. [52] demonstrated that *in vitro* cell adhesion was greater with ytrrium-substituted apatite than the other substituted apatites tested. Other *in vitro* cell culture studies showed that cell response (proliferation, differentiation) was greater for F-substituted apatite, compared to F-free apatites [48].

Calcium phosphate cements that provide a macro-porous structure when it sets *in vivo* may be more efficient than the current or traditional CPCs.

Disadvantages of the plasma-sprayed HA coating method include inhomogeneity in composition of the coating (consisting of HA, ACP and minor amounts of α-TCP, β-TCP and sometimes even CaO) and nonuniformity of coating coverage for implants of complex geometry and porosity. In addition, since the plasma spray method involves very high temperature, it is not possible to incorporate bioactive molecules. An alternative coating method is the precipitation method already being used by some orthopedic company for their implants (e.g., Peri-apatite™, coating on orthopedic implants, Stryker Orthopedics). Another method of depositing thin coatings of nano-apatite crystals on dental implants used by 3i (communication with Implant Innovations Inc., Florida). Coating methods such as the electrochemical deposition method (pulse modulated) [135,136] or precipitation method [137] are low temperature methods (37 to 95° C) that provide a uniform coating even on implants with complex geometry and porosity and homogeneous coating composition. In addition, low temperature coating method can allow the incorporation of growth factors or antibiotics.

8.6. Conclusion

The bioactive ceramics described above differ in their biodegradation properties and their efficiencies to form new bone. These differences may be attributed to difference in origin (biologic or synthetic), composition (calcium carbonate vs. calcium sulfate vs. several types of calcium phosphates) and in preparation methods All the bioactive bioceramics described in this chapter cannot be used in load bearing areas because they lack sufficient mechanical strength. Some of the bioceramics are stronger than others (e.g., A-W glass ceramic > bioglass; coralline HA > macroporous HA, β-TCP, or BCP). *In vivo* performance of some of the bioceramics (e.g., calcium sulfate, some BCPs, some CPCs) is claimed to be equal to that of autografts. Some of the bioceramics (e.g., coralline HA, HA and BCP with appropriate geometry) demonstrated their ability to trap circulating growth factors and thus become osteoinductive. Some of the bioceramics tested were shown to be efficient as scaffolds for transport of cells and/or growth factors for bone regeneration in tissue engineering Table 8.3.

Improvement of current bioceramics or development of new ones should take into consideration some of the properties of the bioactive ceramics described here.

Table 8.3 Clinical applications of bioceramics

Applications	Bioceramics	Refs.
Bone graft substitute, osteotomy, periodontal defects, neurosurgery,osteoporotic fracture	natural coral	[16, 122-124]
Craniofacial, periodontal defects, osteochondral defects, bone lesions, spinal fusions	calcium sulfate (CS)	[13, 17,128,129]
Middle ear prosthesis, peridontal defects, sinus lifts	Bioglass	[5,126]
Vertebral prostheses, bone defect filler, fractures revision surgery (hip prosthesis), spine fusion	A-W glass ceramic	[68,127]
Bone graft substitute, sinus grafting, periodontal defects	Bovine bone	[77, 78]
bone augmentation (alveolar), dental, orthopedic	HA	
bone graft substitute, fractures, spinal fusion, dental	β-TCP	[12,15,18,20, 21,119,130]
Middle ear prosthesis	HA/PE; BCP/silicone	[90]
Oral, periodontal, plastic, orthopedic surgery, tumors, cysts,delayed unions, non-union	coralline HA	[14, 76,122,124,125]
Spine fusion, revision surgery (hip prosthesis), Fractures. correction of scoliosis, pseudoarthrosis, opthalmic implant, bone graft substitute, trauma surgery	BCP	[46,82-88]
Chronic otitis media surgery	BCP/fibrin	[110]
Bone filler (bone tumor, bone cyst, periodontal defects, replacement for autogenous graft from obtained from iliac crest), fractures (osteoporotic), spine fusion, bone graft substitute	CPC	[23,98-101]
Scaffold for tissue engineering, growth factor carrier	HA, coralline HA, BCP BCP,CPC	[62-65,105-109]
Drug delivery	HA, CS, CPC	[13,112-116]
Coatings on orthopedic and dental implants	HA	[54,103,104,132]
Barrier membrane for guided tissue regeneration	HA/CS	
Other applications		
Abrasives for orthopedic and dental implants	HA, BCP	[92-94]

Bioglass, silica based; A-W glass ceramic, contains crystalline OH- and F-apatite; HA – calcium hydroxyapatite, $Ca_{10}(PO_4)_6(OH)_2$; β-TCP, beta-tricalcium phosphate, β-$Ca_3(PO_4)_2$; CS, calcium sulfate dihydrate ($CaSO_4.2H_2O$) or hemihydrate ($CaSO_4.1/2H_2O$); PE, high molecular weight polyethylene; BCP, biphasic calcium phosphate (intimate mixture of HA and β-TCP); CPC, calcium phosphate cement

Acknowledgments: It is a pleasure to acknowledge the professional collaboration of the following colleagues for some of the work cited in this chapter: Drs. R. Rohanizadeh, D. Mijares, S. Lin, and Prof. C. Teixeira (New York University College of Dentistry); Prof. T Sakae (Nihon University School of Dentistry at Matsudo), Dr. T. Ookubo (Japan Institute for Advanced Dentistry, Nagasaki), Prof. A. Gatti (University of Modena, Italy), Prof. R. Kijkowka (Technological University of Krakow) and the technical assistance of Ms. F. Yao and Ms. Q. Xi in the preparation of some of the figures for this chapter. The support of research grants from NIDCR/NIH, Calcium Phosphate Research Funds and L. Linkow Professorship Research Funds for some of our work cited in this chapter is gratefully acknowledged.

References

1. Ring ME. Dentistry: An Illustrated History. New York, Abradale Press 1985;15-36.
2. Banwart JC, Asher MA, Hassanein RS. Iliac crest bone graft harvest donor site morbidity. A statistical evaluation. Spine 1995;20:1055-1060.
3. Younger EM, Chapman MW (1989). Morbidity at bone graft donor sites. J Orthop Trauma 1989;3:192-195.
4. Hench LL. Bioceramics: From concept to clinics. J Am Ceram Soc 1991;74:1487-1570.
5. Hench LL, Paschall HA. Direct bonding of bioactive glass ceramics to bone and muscle. J Biomed Mater Res 1973;4:25-42.
6. Hench LL, Wilson JW. Surface active biomaterials. Science 1984;226:251-254.
7. Osborn JF, Newesely H:The material science of calcium phosphate ceramic. Biomaterials 1980; 1:108-111.
8. Christel P (1992). Biocompatibility of surgical-grade dense polycrystalline alumina. Clin Orthop 1992;282:210-218.
9. Hulbert SF. History of Bioceramics. Ceramics Int 1982;8:131-140.
10. Alexander H, Parsons JR, Ricci JL, Bajpai PK, Weiss AB. Calcium based ceramics and composites in bone reconstruction. ICRC Critical Reviews in Biocompatibility 1987;4: 43-77.
11. Aoki H. Science and Medical Applications of Hydroxyapatite. Tokyo, Takayama Press, 1991.
12. Boyan B, McMillan J, Lohmann CH, Schwartz Z. Bone graft substitutes; Basic information for successful clinical use with special focus on synthetic graft substitutes. In: Laurencin CT (ed). Bone Graft Substitutes. 2003; 231-259.
13. Bucholz RW. Nonallograft osteoconductive bone graft substitutes. Clin Orthop Rel Res 2002;395: 44-52.
14. Damien E. Revell PA. Coralline hydroxyapatite bone graft substitute: A review of experimental studies and biomedical applications. J Appl Biomat Biomech 2004;2:65-75.
15. deGroot K. Ceramics of calcium phosphates: Preparation and properties. In: Bioceramics of Calcium Phosphates. Boca Raton, CRC Press, 1983; 100-114.
16. Demers C. Hamdy CR, Corsi K, Chellat F, Tabrizian M, Yahia L. Natural coral exoskeleton as a bone graft substitute: A review. Biomed Mater Eng 2002;12:15-35.
17. Haggard WO, Richelsoph KC, Parr JE. Calcium sulfate-based bone void substitutes. In: Laurencin CT (ed). Bone Graft Substitutes. ASTM Mono6, 2003; 260-270.
18. Jarcho M. Calcium phosphate ceramics as hard tissue prosthetics. Clin Orthop Rel Res 1981;157: 259-278.
19. Larsson S, Bauer TW. Use of injecTablecalcium phosphate cement for fracture fixation: A review. Clin Orhop Rel Res 2002;395: 23-32
20. LeGeros RZ. Calcium phosphate materials. In: NIH-NIDR State of the Science Conference on Dental Materials, September 1986. Adv Dent Res 1988;3:164-180.

21. LeGeros RZ. Materials for bone repair, augmentation and implant coatings. In: Niwa S, Perren SM, Hattori T (eds). Biomechanics in Orthopedics. Springer-Verlag, Tokyo, 1992;147-174.
22. LeGeros RZ. Properties of osteoconductive biomaterials: Calcium phosphates. Clin Orfhop Rel Res 2002;395: 81-98.
23. Niwa S, LeGeros RZ. InjecTablecalcium phosphate cements for repair of bone defects. In: Lewandrowski K-U, Wise DL, Trantolo DJ, Gresser, JD et al (eds). Tissue Engineering and Biodegradable Equivalents: Scientific and Clinical Applications. (Marcel Dekker Inc, New York) 2002;385-500.
24. Ricci JL, Alexander H, Nadami P. Biological mechanisms of calcium sulfate replacement by bone. In Davis J (ed) Toronto, emsquared inc. 2001; 332-345.
25. Beevers CA, McIntyre D. The atomic structure of fluorapatite and its relation to that of tooth and bone mineral. Mineral Mag 1946;27:254-259.
26. Kay MI, Young RA, Posner AS. Crystal structure of hydroxyapatite. Nature 1964;294:1050-1053.
27. LeGeros RZ. Apatites in biological systems. Prog. Crystal Growth Charact 1981;4:1-45.
28. LeGeros RZ. Calcium Phosphates in Oral Biology and Medicine. Monographs in Oral Biology. H. Myers (ed). Vol. 15. Karger, Basel,1991.
29. Rey C, Renugopalakrishnan V, Collins B. Fourier transform infrared spectroscopic study of the carbonate ions in bone mineral during aging. Calcif Tissue Int 1991;49:251-258.
30. McConnell D. The crystal chemistry of carbonate apatites and their relationship to the composition of calcified tissue. J Dent Res 1952;31:53-63.
31. Klawitter JJ. A Basic Investigation of Bone Growth in Porous Materials. PhD Thesis. Clemson, Clemson University 1979.
32. Tsuruga E, Takita H, Itoh H, Wakisaka Y, Kuboki Y. Pore size of porous hydroxyapatite as the cell-substratum controls BMP-induced osteogenesis. J Biochem 1997;121:317-324,
33. Hubbard W. Physiological Calcium Phosphates as Orthopedic Biomaterials. PhD thesis, Marquette University, 1974.
34. Li S, De Wijn JR, Li J, Layrolle P, deGroot K. Macroporous biphasic calcium phosphate scaffold with high permeabiity/porosity ratio. Tissue Eng 2003;9:535-548.
35. Munar M, Udoh K, Nakagawa M, Matsuya S, Ishikawa K. Three dimensional interconnected pore scaffold as bone defect filler: The effects of sintering temperatures on the physical properties of α-TCP. J Jpn Soc Dent Mat Dev 2003;22:147.
36. LeGeros RZ, Lin S, Rohanizadeh R, Mijares D, LeGeros JP. Biphasic calcium phosphates: Preparation and properties. J Mater Sci. Mat Med 2003;14: 201-209.
37. Baron R, Neff L, Louvard D. Cell mediated extracellular acidification and bone resorption: Evidence for a low pH in resorbing laculnae and localization of 100kD lysosomal membrane protein at the osteoclast ruffled border. J Cell Biol 1985;101:2210-2222.
38. Davies JE. In vitro modeling of the bone/implant interface. Anat Rec 1996;245: 426-445.
39. Heymann D, Guicheux J, Rousselle AV. Ultrastructural evidence in vitro of osteoclast-induced degradation of calcium phosphate ceramic by simultaneous resorption and phagocytosis mechanisms. Histol Histopathol 2001;16:37-44.
40. LeGeros RZ (1993). Biodegradation and bioresorption of calcium phosphate ceramics. Clin Mat 1993;14:65-88.
41. Koerten HK, van der Meulen J. Degradation of calcium phsophate ceramics. J Biomed Mater Res 1999;44:78-86.
42. LeGeros RZ, Bautista C, Styner D, LeGeros JP,Vijayraghavan TV, Retino M, Valdecanas A. Comparative properties of bioactive bone graft materials. Bioceramics 1995:8: 81-87.
43. Oonishi H, Hench LL, Wilson J, Sugihara F. Quantitative comparison of bone growth behavior in granules of Bioglass[R], A-W glass –ceramic, and hydroxyapatite. J Biomed Mater Res 2000;51:37-46.

44. LeGeros RZ, Orly I, Gregoire M, Kazimiroff J. Comparative in vitro properties of HA ceramic and coralline HA. Apatite Vol 1. Japanese Association of Apatite Science 1992;229-235.
45. LeGeros RZ, Daculsi G. In vivo transformation *of* biphasic calcium phosphate ceramics: Ultrastructural and physico-chemical characterizations. In: Yamamuro T, Hench L, Wilson -Hench J (eds). Handbook of Bioactive Ceramics Vol 11. CRC Press, Boca Raton, 1990;17-28.
46. Nery EB, LeGeros RZ, Lynch KL, Lee K. Tissue response to biphasic calcium phosphate ceramic with different ratios of HA/β?-TCP in periodontal osseous defects. J Periodontol 1992;63:729-735.
47. Ohgushi H, Okumura M, Tamai s, Shors EC and Caplan AI. Marrow cel induced osteogenesis in porous hydroxyapatite and tricalcium phosphate: a comparative histomorphometric study of ectopic bone formation. J Biomed Mater Res 1990;24:1563-1570.
48. Frondoza CG, LeGeros RZ, Hungerford DS. Effect of bovine bone-derived materials on human osteoblast-like cells in vitro. Bioceramics 1998;11:289-291.
49. Fujimori Y, Mishima H, Sugaya K, Sakae T, LeGeros RZ, Koawa Y, Nagura H. In vitro interactions of osteoclast-like cells and hydroxyapatite ceramics. Bioceramics 1998:11:335-338.
50. LeGeros RZ, Gatti AM, Kijkowska R, Mijares DQ, LeGeros JP. Mg-substituted tricalcium phosphates: formation and properties. Key Engineer Mater 2004; 254-256:127-130.
51. Porter AE, Buckland T, Hing K, Best SM, Bonfield W. Comparison of in vitro dissolution processes in hydroxyapatite and silicon-substituted hydroxyapatite bioceramics. Biomaterials 2003;24:4609-4620.
52. Webster TJ, Ergun C, Doremus RH, Bizios R. Hydroxylapatite with substituted magnesium, zinc, cadmium and yttrium II: Mechanisms of osteoblast adhesion. J Biomed Mater Res 2002;59:312-317.
53. LeGeros RZ, Kim YE, Kijkowska R, Zurita V, Bleiwas C, Huang PY, Edwards B, Dimaano F, LeGeros JP. HA/ACP ratios in calcium phosphate coatings on dental and orthopedic implants: Effect on properties. Bioceramics 1998; 11:181-184.
54. LeGeros RZ, LeGeros JP, Kim Y, Kijkowska R, Zheng R, Bautista C, Wong JL. Calcium phosphates in plasma-sprayed HA coatings. Ceramic Transactions 1995;48:173-189.
55. Kokubo T. Formation of biologically active bone-like apatite on metals and polymers by a biomimetic process. Thermochim Acta 1996;280:479-490.
56. Heughebaert M, LeGeros RZ, Gineste M, Bonel G. Physico-chemical characterization of deposits associated with HA-ceramics implanted in non-osseous sites. J Biomed Mater Res 1988;23: 257-268.
57. LeGeros RZ, Daculsi G, Orly I, Gregoire M, Heughebaert, Gineste M, Kijkowska R. Formation of carbonate apatite on calcium phosphate materials: Dissolution/precipitation processes. In: Ducheyne P, Kokubo T, Van Bitterswijk (eds). *Bone-Bonding*. Reed Healthcare Communications, The Netherlands, 1992; 201-212.
58. LeGeros RZ, Nery E, Lynch E, Daculsi G. In vivo transformation of biphasic calcium phosphate of varying βTCP/HA ratios: Ultrastructural characterization. Third World Biomaterials Congress, Japan 1988;35.
59. LeGeros RZ, Orly 1, Gregoire M, Daculsi G. Substrate surface dissolution and interfacial biological mineralization. In: Davies JE (ed). The Bone-Biomaterial Interface. Chapter 7. Univ of Toronto Press,1991; 76-89.
60. Urist MR, Silverman BF, Buring K, Dubuc Fl, Rosenberg J. The bone induction principle. Clin Orthop 1967;53:243-283.
61. Chang Y-S, Oka M, Nakamura T, Gu H-O. Bone remodeling around implanted ceramics. J Biomed Mater Res 1996;30:117-124.
62. Kobuki Y, Takita H, Kobayashi D. BMP-induced osteogenesis on the surface of hydroxyapatitte with geometrically feasible and non-feasible structures: Topology of osteogenesis. J Biomed Mater Res 1998;39:190-199.

63. Ripamonti U, Ma S, Reddi AH. The critical role of geometry of porous hydroxyapatite to delivery system induction of bone by osteogenin, a bone morphogenetic protein. Matrix 1992;12: 202-212.
64. Ripamonti, U, Crooks J, Kirbride A. Sintered porous hydroxyapatites with intrinsic osteoinductive activity: Geometric induction of bone formation. South Africa J Science 1999;95:335-343.
65. Toth JM, Lynch KL, A HD. Ceramic induced osteogenesis following subcutaneous implantation of calcium phosphates. Bioceramics 1993;6:9-13.
66. Reddi AH. Morphgenesis and tissue engineering of bone and cartilage: Inductive signals, stem cells and biomimetic biomaterials. Tissue Eng 200;6:351-359.
67. LeNihouhanne D, Daculsi G, Gauthier O, Saffarzadeh A, Delplace S, Pilet P, Layrolle P. Ectopic bone formation by microporous calcium phosphate ceramic particles in sheep muscles. Bone 2005; 36:1086-1093.
68. Kokubo T. Novel biomedical materials based on glasses. In: Shackelford JF (ed). Bioceramics. applications of ceramic and glass materials in medicine. Trans Tech Publications:USA,1999;65-81.
69. Gross UM, Muller-Mai C, Voigt C. Ceravital^{R} bioactive glass ceramics. In: Hench LL, Wilson J (eds). An Introduction to Bioceramics. World Scientific:London, 1993;105-124.
70. Abe Y, Hosonoo H, Tsutsumi S, Shinya A, Yokozuka S. Bioceramics 1988;1: 181-186.
71. LeGeros RZ, Lee Y-K. Synthesis of amorphous calcium phosphates for hard tissue repair using conventional melting technique. J Mat Sci 2004;39: 5577-5579.
72. Moon H-J, Kim H-N, Kim K-M, Choi S-H, Kim C-K, Kim K-D, LeGeros RZ, Lee Y-K. Bone formation in calvaria defects of Sprague-Dawley Rat by transplantation of calcium phosphate glass. J Biomed Mater Res. 2005;74A:497-502.
73. Dressman H. Uber knochenplombierun. Beitr Klin Chir 1892;9:804-810.
74. Mamidwar SS, Ricci JL, Alexander H. Bone regeneration with calcium sulfate-based bone grafts. Inside Dent 2006;Special issue 2:1-8. Roy DM, Linnehan SK. Hydroxyapatite formed from coral-skeletal carbonate by hydrothermal exchange. Nature 1974; 247:220-222.
75. Roy DM, Linnehan SK. Hydroxyapatite formed from coral-skeletal carbonate by hydrothermal exchange. Nature 1974; 247:220-222.
76. Shors EC. The development of coralline porous ceramic bone graft substitutes. In: Laurencin CT (ed). Bone Graft Substitutes. ASTM Mono6, 2003; 271-288.
77. Valentini P, Abensur D, Wenz B. Sinus grafting with porous bone mineral (Bio-Oss) for implant placement: A 5-year study on 15 patients. In J Peridontol Restor Dent 2000;20:245-254.
78. Dard M, Bauer J, Lidendorfer H, Wahlig H, Dingeldein E (1994). Preparation, evaluation, physico-chmiques et biologiques d'une ceramic d'hydroxyapatite issue de l'os bovine. Acta Odont Stomat 1994;185:61-69.
79. Albee FH, Morrison HF. Studies in bone growth. Triple calcium phosphate as a stimulus to osteogenesis. Ann Surg 1920;71:32-36.
80. Nery EB, Lynch KL, Hirthe WM, Mueller KH. Bioceramics implants in surgically produced infrabony defecs. J Periodontol 1975;46:328-339.
81. LeGeros RZ. Variability in βTCP/HA ratios in sintered apatites. J Dent Res 1986;65:292.
82. Daculsi G, Laboux O, Marad O, Weiss P. Current state of the art of biphasic calcium phosphate ceramics. J Mater Sci Mater Med 2003;14:195-200.
83. Jegoux F, Goyenvalle E, Bagot D'arc M, Aguado E, Daculsi G. In vivo performance of composites combining micro-macroporous biphasic calcium phosphate granules and fibrin sealant. Arch Orthop Trauma Surg 2005;125:153-159.
84. Malard O, Guicheux J, Bouler J-M, Gauthier O, de Montreuil CB, Aguado E, Pilet P, LeGeros R, Daculsi G Calcium phosphate scaffold and bone marrow for bone reconstruction in irradiated area: a dog study. Bone 2005:36:323-330.

85. Fujibayashi S, Jitsuhiko S, Tanaka C. Matsushita M, Nakamura T. Lumbar posterolateral fusion with biphasic calcium phosphate ceramic. J Spinal Disord 2001;14:214-221.
86. Schwartz C, Liss P, Jacquemaire B, Lecestre P, Frayssinet P. Biphasic synthetic bone substitute use in orthopaedic and trauma surgery: clinical, radiological and histological results. J Mat Sci Mat Med 1999;10:821-825.
87. Weiss P, Gauthier O, Bouler J-M, Grimaldi G, Daculsi G. InjecTablebone substitute using a hydrophilic polymer. Bone 1999;25:675-705.
88. Wykrota LL, Garrido Ca. Wykrota FHI. Clinical evaluation of biphasic calcium phosphate ceramic used in orthopedic lesions. In: LeGeros RZ, LeGeros JP (eds). Bioceramics 1998;11: 641-644.
89. LeGeros RZ, LeGeros JP. Dense hydroxyapatite. In: Hench LL, Wilson J (eds). An Introduction to Bioceramics. Chapter 9. World Scientific, London, 1993;139-180.
90. Bonfield W. Hydroxyapatite-reinforced polyethylene as an analogous material for bone replacement. In: Ducheyne P, Lemons H (eds). Bioceramics: Materials Characteristics vs. In Vivo Behavior. Ann. NY Acad Sci 1998;523:173-177.
91. Nishikawa T, Masuno K, Tominaga K, Koyama Y. Bone repair analysis in a novel biodegradable hydroxyapatite/collagen composite implanted in bone. Implant Dent 2005;14:252-260.
92. Salgado T, LeGeros JP, Wang J-L. Effect of alumina and apatitic abrasives on Ti alloy substrates. Bioceramics 1998;11:683-686.
93. LeGeros JP, Daculsi G, LeGeros RZ. Tissue response to grit blasted Ti alloy. Proc 25th International Society of Biomaterials.1998.
94. Ishikawa K, Miyamaoto Y, Nagayama M, Asaoka K. Blast coating method: New method of coating titanium surface with hydroxyapatite at room temperature. J Biomed Mater Res (Appl Biomater)1997;38:129-134.
95. Cornell C, Lane J, Chapman M. Multicenter trial of Collagraft™ as bone graft substitute. J Orthop Trauma 1991;5:1-8
96. LeGeros RZ, Chohayeb A, Shulman A. Apatitic calcium phosphates: possible restorative materials. J Dent. Res 1982;61: 343.
97. Brown WE, Chow LC. Dental restorative cement pastes. US patent no. 4518430, 1985.
98. Constanz BR, Ison IC, Fulmer MT, Poser RD, Smith ST, Van Wagner M. Skeletal repair by in situ formation of the mineral phase of bone. Science 1995;267: 1796-1799.
99. Friedman CD, Costantino PD, Takagi S, Chow LC. BoneSource™ Hydroxyapatite cement. A novel biomaterial for craniofacial skeletal tissue engineering and reconstruction. J Biomed Mater Res 1998;43:428-432.
100. Knaack D, Goal MEP. Ailova M, Lee DD. Resorbable calcium phosphate bone substitute. J Biomed Mater Res Appl Biomater 1998;43:399-409.
101. Lee DD. Tofighi A, Aiolova M. α-BSM^R:A biomimetic bone substitute and drug delivery vehicle. Clin Orthop 1999;367(Suppl)S396-S405.
102. Khairoun I, Gauthier O, LeGeros RZ, Daculsi G, Bouler JM. A novel resorbable and injecTablecalcium phosphate cement for bone repair: Compressive strength, porosity and *in vivo* studies. Proc 19th Eur Conf Biomat, Sorrento 2005. (abstract).
103. Geesink RGT. Osteoconductive coatings for total joint arthoplasty. Clin Orhop Rel Res 2002;395:53-65.
104. LeGeros JP, LeGeros RZ, Burgess A, Edwards B, Zitelli J. X-ray diffraction method for the quantitative characterization of calcium phosphate coatings. In: Horowitz E, Parr JE (eds). Characterization and Performance of Calcium Phosphate Coatings for Implants. ASTM STP 1196 American Society for Testing Materials, Philadelphia, 1994; 33-42.
105. Livingstone TL, Daculsi G. Mesenchymal stem cells combined with biphasic calcium phosphate ceramics promote bone regeneration. J Mater Sci Mat Med 2003;14:211-218.

106. Mankani MH, Kuznetsov SA, Fowler B, Kingman A, Robey PG. In vivo bone formation by human bone marrow stromal cells: effect of carrier particle size and shape. Biotech Bioeng 2001;72:96-107.
107. Mastrogiacomo M, Scalglione S, Marinetti R, Docini L, Beltrame F, Cancedda R, Quarto R. Role of scaffold internal structure on in vivo bone formation in macroporous calcium phosphate ceramics. Biomaterials 2006;27:3230-3237.
108. Muraglia MM, Peyrin KV, Rustichelli F, Crovace A, Cancedda R. Tissue engineering of bone: search for a better scaffold. Orthod Craniofac Res 2005;8:277-284.
109. Texiera C, Karkia C, Neweliksky Y, LeGeros RZ. Biphasic calcium phosphate: A scaffold for growth plate chondrocytes. Tissue Eng M 2006 (in press).
110. Bagot D'Arc M, Daculsi G. Micro-macroporous biphasic ceramics and fibrin sealant as a moldable material for bone reconstruction in chronic otitis media surgery. A 15 years experience. J Mater Sci Mater Med 2003;14: 229-231.
111. Ono K, Yamamuro T, Nakamura T, Kokubo T. Apatite-wollastonite containing glass-ceramic-fibrin mixtures as bone defect filler. J Biomed Mater Res 1988;22: 869-885.
112. Dennisen H, van Beck E, Lowik C. Papapoulos S, van dem Hoof A. Ceramic hydroxyapatite implants for the release of bisphosphonate. Bone Miner 1994;25:1223-1234.
113. Seshima H, Yoshinari M, Takemoto S, Hattori M, Kawada E. Inous T, Oda Y. Control of bisphosphate release using hydroxyapatite granules. J Biomed Mater Res Part B. Appl Biomater 2006; 78B:215-221.
114. Korkusuz F, Uchida A, Shinto Y, et al. Experimental implant-related osteomyelitis treated by antibiotic-calcium hydroxyapatite ceramic composites. J Bone Joint Surg 1993;75B: 111-114.
115. Shirtiff ME, Valhoun JH, Mader JT. Experimental osteomylitis treatment with antibiotic-impregnated hydroxyapatite. Clin Orthop Rel Res 2002;401:239-247.
116. McKee M, Schemitsch F, Wild I. Bone substitute with tobramycin heals non-infected non-unions. Orthop Today 2000; 20:1-2.
117. Orsini G, Ricci J, Scarano A, Pecora G, Petrone G, Iezzi G, Piattelli A. Bone-defect healing with calcium sulfate particles and cement: an experimental study in rabbit. J. Biomed Mater Res Part B: Appl Biomater 2004;68B:199-208.
118. Walsh WR, Morberg P, Yu Y, Yang JL, Haggard W. Response of a calcium sulfate bone graft substitute in a confined cancellous defect. Clin Orthop Rel Res 2003;406:228-236.
119. Ozawa M. Experimental study on bone conductivity and absorbability of the pure β-TCP. J Jpn Soc Biomater 1995;13:67-175.
120. Zhang W. Basic research and clinical application of augmented screw fixation with calcium phosphate bone cement for the proximal femoral fractures. PhD thesis, Norman Bethune University of Medical Science, China, 2000.
121. Khairoun I, LeGeros RZ, Daculsi G, et al. Macroporous resorbable and injectible calcium phosphate based cements (MCPC). Provisional patent application no. PCT/US2005/004084 (2005).
122. Guillemin G, Patat J, Fournie J, Chatail M. The use of coral as a bone graft substitute. J Biomed Mater Res 1987;21:557-567.
123. Kenesi C, Vopisin MC, Dhem A. Osteotomie tibiale d'addition interne calee par u coin corail. Chirurgie 1997;122:379-382.
124. Vuola J, Bhling T, Kinnnunen J, Hirvensalo E, Asko-Seljavaara S. Natural coral as bone-defect filling material. J Biomed Mater Res 2000;51:117-122.
125. Gao TJ, Lindholm TS, Kommonen B. The use of a coral composite implant containing bone morphogenetic protein to repair a segmental tibial defect in sheep. Int Orthop 1997;21:194-200.
126. Wilson J, Yii-Urpo A, Risto-Pekka H. Bioactive glasses: clinical applications. In: Hench LL, Wilson J (eds). An Introduction to Bioceramics. World Scientific: London, 1993;63-74.

127. Yamamuro T. A/W glass-ceramic: Clinical applications. In: Hench LL, Wilson J (eds). An Introduction to Bioceramics. World Scientific:London, 1993;89-104.
128. Peltier L. The use of plaster of Paris to fill large defects in bones. Am J. Surg 1959;97:311-315.
129. Kelly CM, Wilkins RM, Biteliis S. The use of a surgical grade calcium sulfate as a bone graft substitute: results of a multicenter trial. Clin Orthop 2000;381: 42-50.
130. Metzger DS, Driskell TD, Paulstrud JR. Tricalcium phosphate ceramic: a resorbable bone implant: Review and current status. J Am Dent Assoc 1982;105:1035-1048.
131. Yamamoto H, Shibata T, Ikeuti M. Calcium phosphate cement injection for osteoporotic vertebral fracture. Clin Orthop Surg 1999;34:435-442.
132. Capello WN, D'Antonio JA, Feinberg JR, Manley MT. Hydroxyapatite coated ítems in younger and older pateints with hip artritis. Clin Orthop Rel Res 2002;405:92-100.
133. Linton JL, Sohn B-VII, Yook J-I, LeGeros RZ. Effects of calcium phosphate ceramic bone graft materials on permanent teeth eruption in beagles. Cleft Palate-Craniofacial J 2002;39:197-207.
134. Sakae T, Ookubo T, LeGeros RZ. Bone formation induced by several carbonate- and fluoride-containing apatite implanted in dog mandibles. Key Engineer Mater 2003;240-242: 395-398.
135. LeGeros JP, Lin S, Mijares D, Dimaano F, LeGeros RZ. Electrochemically deposited calcium phosphate coatings on titanium alloy substrates. Key Engineer Mat 2005;284-286:247-250.
136. Lin S, LeGeros RZ, LeGeros JP. Adherent octacalciumphosphate coating on titanium alloy using a modulated electrochemical deposition method. J Biomed Mater Res 2003;66A:810-828.
137. Rohanizadeh R, LeGeros RZ, Harsono M, Benavid A. Adherent apatite coating on titanium substrate using chemical deposition. J Biomed Mater Res 2005; 72A: 428-438

9

Distraction Osteogenesis of the Orthopedic Skeleton: Basic Principles and Clinical Applications

Mikhail L. Samchukov, Marina R. Makarov, Alexander M. Cherkashin, and John G. Birch

Abstract: Distraction osteogenesis is a unique biologic process of new bone formation between the surfaces of bone segments that are gradually separated by incremental traction. Depending on the anatomic site where the traction is induced, distraction osteogenesis techniques are divided into callotasis (distraction of fracture callus) and physeal distraction (distraction of the bone growth plate). Callotasis, or gradual stretching of the reparative callus forming around osteotomized bone segments, has been utilized as the predominant method of distraction osteogenesis in experimental models and clinical applications.

Although the application of distraction osteogenesis has dramatically increased in the last two decades, it remains one of the most mysterious phenomena of bone biology. Callotasis begins with the development of a reparative callus similar to that observed during bone repair or fracture healing. New bone formation is initiated when a traction force is applied to the bone segments, thereby interrupting the process of fracture healing and placing the callus under tension. As the callus is stretched, new bone is generated parallel to the direction of traction. During this stretching, the soft callus is maintained at the center of the distraction gap while routine fracture healing occurs at the periphery of the regenerate. Therefore, distraction osteogenesis represents a continuum of the individual fracture healing stages that occur simultaneously during the application of tension stress.

Keywords: Distraction osteogenesis, distraction regenerate, physeal distraction, callotasis, Ilizarov.

9.1. Introduction

Distraction osteogenesis gained widespread recognition in the last decade and became the preferred method for correction of limb length inequalities, severe deformities and long bone defects. Distraction osteogenesis is a biological process of new bone formation between the surfaces of bone segments that

Center for Excellence in Limb Lengthening & Reconstruction, Seay Center for Musculoskeletal Research, Texas Scottish Rite Hospital for Children, Dallas, TX

From: *Orthopedic Biology and Medicine: Musculoskeletal Tissue Regeneration, Biological Materials and Methods*
Edited by W. S. Pietrzak © Humana Press, Totowa, NJ

are gradually separated by incremental traction. This process is initiated when a traction force is applied to the bone segments generating a tensional stress within the tissues that joins the divided bone segments, which in turn stimulates new bone formation parallel to the vector of traction. Importantly, a traction force applied to bone segments also creates tension in the surrounding soft tissues, initiating a sequence of adaptive changes termed distraction histogenesis [1, 2, 3].

9.1.1. Brief History and Evolution

Principles of mechanical manipulation of bone segments have been practiced in orthopedics since ancient time, when Hippocrates described the placement of traction forces on broken bones [4]. He used an external apparatus consisting of two leather rings that were connected by four slightly bent rods made from the elastic Cornel tree. The tension applied to the bone segments was controlled by the amount of bending of the rods.

Further evolution of distraction osteogenesis involved the development and integration of traction, bone fixation and osteotomy techniques [5, 6, 7]. The first occurrence of continuous traction for long bone fractures can be traced to the work of de Chauliac in the 14th Century [8], who used a pulley system that consisted of a weight attached to the leg by a cord. Barton, in 1826, is credited with being the first to perform a surgical division of bone, or osteotomy [9]. The development of external skeletal fixation dates from the middle of the 19th Century when Malgaigne constructed an apparatus which was directly attached to bone, thereby allowing direct transmission of a mechanical force to the skeleton [10]. His simple frame was designed to fixate fractures of patella and consisted of two double hooks, which were inserted through the skin into the patellar segments and connected by a screw. Since then, considerable evolution of external skeletal fixation has occurred.

At the turn of the 20th Century, Codivilla [11] combined these techniques to perform the first limb lengthening using external skeletal traction after an oblique osteotomy of the femur. His device utilized a traditional plaster cast placed on the leg and cut in half at the level of the osteotomy. The proximal part of the cast was fastened to a stationary external frame, and the distal part of the cast was connected to a pin inserted through the calcaneus. Elongation was achieved by skeletal traction, applied at the transcalcaneal pin and repeated as often as necessary to achieve the desired result. Later, several surgeons modernized Codivilla's "continuous extension" procedure by modifying the osteotomy technique, distraction protocol, or the device for bone fixation.

A significant contribution in the development of distraction osteogenesis was made by the Russian surgeon Gavriil Ilizarov [1, 2, 12, 13, 14]. In 1951 he designed a new apparatus for bone fixation consisting of two metal rings joined together with three or four threaded rods. Each bone segment was secured to the rings by two thin tensioned wires inserted into the bone at a right angle to each other. He later developed a low energy, subperiosteal osteotomy technique (corticotomy) and a unique protocol for limb lengthening utilizing a five- to seven-day latency period, followed by distraction at a rate of 1 mm per day performed in four increments of 0.25 mm.

Several distraction osteogenesis techniques were developed. Depending on the anatomic site where the tensional stress is induced, these techniques can be divided into 1) callotasis, which means distraction of the fracture callus, and 2) physeal distraction, which is a distraction of the growth plate (Fig. 9.1).

9.1.2. Physeal Distraction

There are two distinct types of physeal distraction (distraction epiphysiolysis and chondrodiatasis), which differ primarily in the rate of distraction across the growth plate [15]. Distraction epiphysiolysis (Fig. 9.1B) involves a relatively rapid rate of bone segment separation usually ranging from 1.0 to 1.5 mm per day. The increased tension at the growth plate produces a fracture of the physis. The subsequent gradual separation of the epiphysis from the metaphysis (~1 mm/day) leads to the replacement of physeal cartilage by trabecular bone [16]. The evidence of new bone formation between gradually separated epiphysis and metaphysis was first experimentally demonstrated in 1958 by Ring [17]. In 1967 Zavialov and Plaskin introduced the term distraction epiphysiolysis and reported the first clinical application of this technique [18].

The second physeal distraction technique, chondrodiatasis, utilizes a very slow rate of bone segment separation (less than 0.5 mm per day). This allows stretching of the growth plate without a fracture (Fig. 9. 1C). Tensional stress developing in a slowly stretched physis intensifies the biosynthetic activity of cartilage cells, resulting in accelerated osteogenesis [16]. Sliedge and Noble, in 1978, first reported the evidence of chondrodiatasis when constant tension was applied across the rabbit's growth plate resulting in a 150 percent growth increase without fracture [19]. A year later, De Bastiani and colleagues [15] introduced the term chondrodiatasis. They demonstrated that slow distraction of the physis at a rate of 0.25 mm twice per day caused cellular hyperplasia without substantial morphological changes. Long-term follow-up indicated

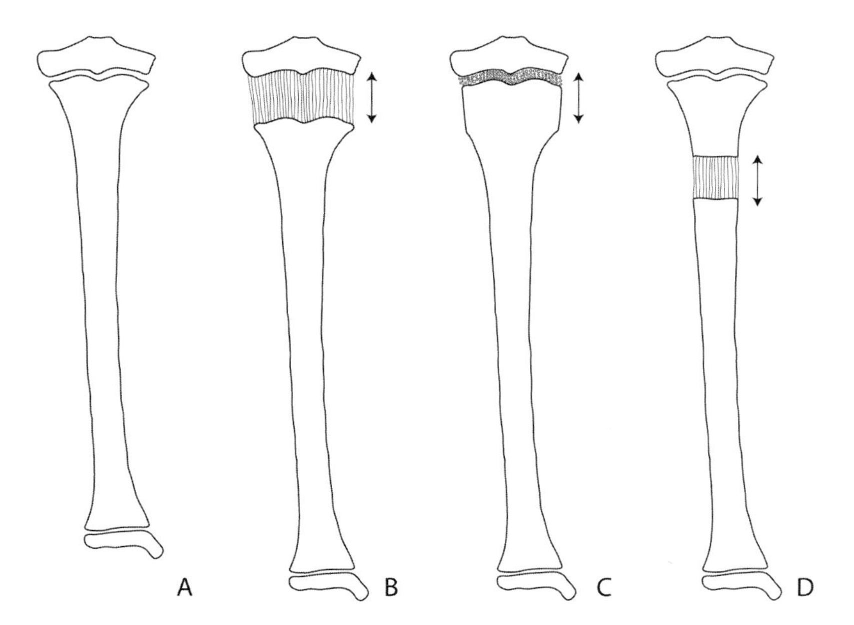

Fig. 9.1 Schematic drawings demonstrating normal tibia (A) and different distraction osteogenesis techniques: distraction epiphysiolysis (B), chondrodiatasis (C) and callotasis (D)

that activity of the cartilage continued during the remaining period of growth, thus preserving the elongation obtained.

Theoretically, physeal distraction osteogenesis offers significant advantages for limb lengthening due to execution of a single stage operative procedure, no soft tissue incision or osteotomy, simulation of “natural” growth, large areas of new bone formation and no additional bone grafts [15, 20, 21, 22]. However, experimental and clinical investigations on physeal distraction have demonstrated a high level of complications which were mainly associated with difficulties in grasping and transfixing very short epiphyseal segments. In addition, the physis was frequently damaged, resulting in premature cessation of growth. As a result, callotasis has been utilized as the predominant method of distraction osteogenesis in experimental models and clinical applications.

9.1.3. Callotasis

Callotasis (Fig. 9.1D) is a gradual stretching of the reparative callus forming around bone segments surgically interrupted by osteotomy [23, 24]. This name was derived from two words – the Latin noun callum (scar tissue between bone segments) and the ancient Greek noun taois (tension or extension). Callotasis begins with the development of a reparative callus between the edges of two bone segments divided by a low energy osteotomy. After the callus has initially formed, a traction force is applied to these bone segments, which gradually pulls them apart. Gradual incremental separation of bone segments places the callus under tensional stress that aligns the newly formed intersegmentary tissues parallel to the direction of traction. After the desired amount of bone lengthening is achieved, the distraction force is discontinued. The newly formed bone (distraction regenerate) then undergoes maturation and remodeling until it becomes undistinguishable from the residual host bone.

9.2. Biologic Basis of New Bone Formation

Clinically (Fig. 9. 2), distraction osteogenesis consists of five sequential periods: 1) osteotomy, 2) latency, 3) distraction, 4) consolidation and 5) remodeling [25]. This same temporal sequence will be followed for describing the biologic mechanisms at work during distraction osteogenesis.

9.2.1. Osteotomy

Distraction osteogenesis begins with an osteotomy (Fig. 9. 2A), which divides a bone into two segments, thereby resulting in a loss of its continuity and mechanical integrity. Discontinuity of a skeletal segment (also referred to as a fracture) triggers an evolutionary process of bone repair known as fracture healing. Traditionally [26, 27], fracture healing has been described as consisting of six sequential stages: 1) impact, 2) induction, 3) inflammation, 4) soft callus, 5) hard callus and 6) remodeling (Fig. 9.3). The stage of impact takes place at the moment of stress and lasts until complete dissipation of energy, which is absorbed by the bone until failure occurs. This is followed by the stage of induction that provides modulation of cells needed for the repair process.

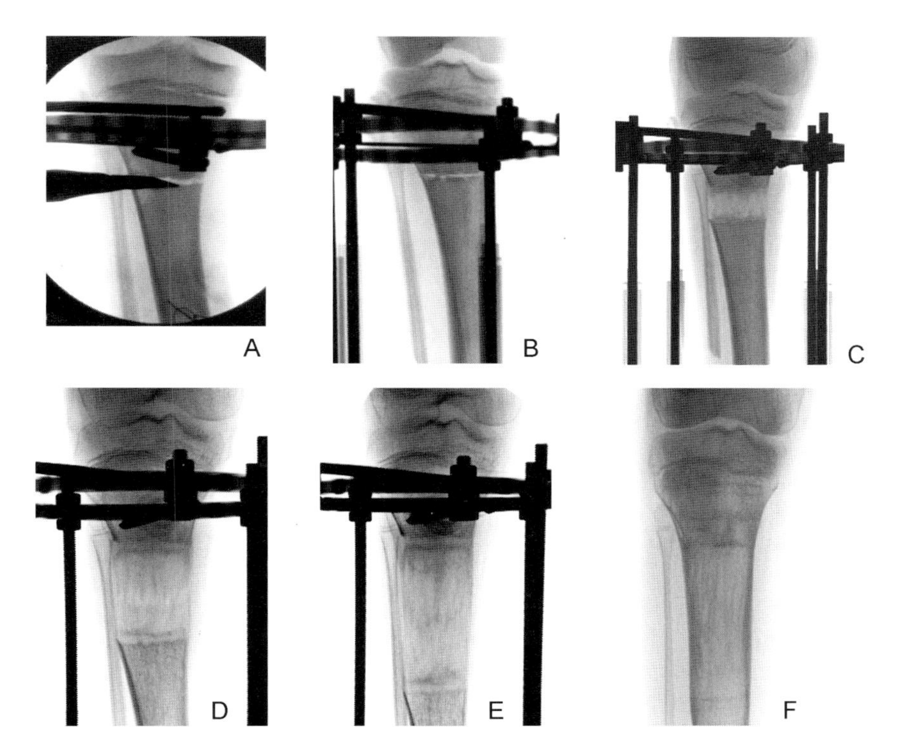

Fig. 9.2 Radiographs of a patient with tibial lengthening demonstrating different clinical stages of distraction osteogenesis: osteotomy (A), latency period (B), distraction period (C, D), consolidation period (E) and remodeling period (F). Note progressive changes in zonal structure of the distraction regenerate

9.2.2. Latency Period

The latency period is the period from bone division to the onset of traction (Fig. 9.2B). This period represents the time allowed for reparative callus formation. The sequence of events occurring during this period (Fig. 9.3) is similar to that seen during the inflammation and soft callus stages of fracture healing [27-29]. Following the surgical separation of a bone into two segments, an ingrowth of capillaries (to restore blood supply) and a tremendous amount of cellular proliferation take place [30]. The stage of inflammation lasts from one to three days, during which time the hematoma surrounding the bone segments is replaced with granulation tissue consisting of inflammatory cells, fibroblasts, collagen and invading capillaries [26, 31, 32].

During the following stage of soft callus that lasts approximately three weeks, capillaries continue to grow [33, 34]. At this time granulation and loose connective tissues are gradually converted to fibrous and cartilaginous tissues [35]. Although callus formation originates principally in the periosteum and endosteum, the formation of cartilaginous tissue occurs more at the periphery of the fracture callus and its amount is variable, being more prominent in animals lower on the evolutionary scale, as well as in areas with excessive movements and low oxygen tension [28].

9.2.3. Distraction Period

During normal fracture healing (Fig. 9.3) the stage of soft callus is followed by the stage of hard callus that typically lasts three to four months. During this period the fibrous and cartilaginous tissues of the soft callus are transformed into woven bone by osteoblasts. This is followed by the final stage of remodeling, when woven bone is slowly remodeled to lamellar bone with gradual reconstitution of the medullary canal [26].

During distraction, however, the normal process of fracture healing is interrupted by the application of gradual traction to the bone segments at the stage of soft callus. This traction progressively separates the bone segments, thereby generating tensional stress in the tissues of the forming soft callus and in the surrounding soft tissues [36]. According to Ilizarov, this tensional stress produces several specific changes in the forming reparative callus that can be characterized as 1) a growth stimulating effect and 2) a shape forming effect [37-40].

The growth stimulating effect of tension activates the biologic elements of the stretched soft callus tissues resulting in 1) increased proliferation of the fibroblastic cell population and 2) prolongation of angiogenesis with increased tissue oxygenation. The shape forming effect of tension alters the phenotypic expression of the fibroblast, which appears as spindle-shaped fibroblast-like cells with hypertrophic intermediate filaments ("distraction" fibroblasts). This shape allows polarization of the fibroblasts, orienting them and their secreted collagen parallel to the axis of distraction (Fig. 9.4). As a result, the fibrous tissue of the soft callus during distraction osteogenesis becomes longitudinally oriented in a direction parallel to the axis of distraction [40-42].

Starting from the second week of distraction, the osteoblasts lay down osteoid tissue on these longitudinally oriented collagen fibers and primary bone trabeculae begin to form. By the end of the second week the osteoid begins to

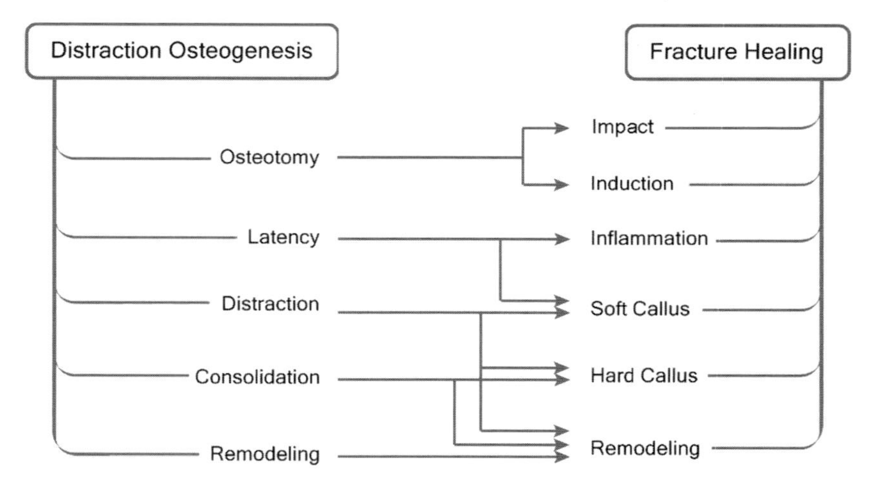

Fig. 9.3 Correlation between clinical stages of distraction osteogenesis and sequential stages of fracture healing. Note overlapping of consecutive fracture healing stages with the individual clinical stages of the distraction osteogenesis after the process of fracture healing is interrupted by the distraction

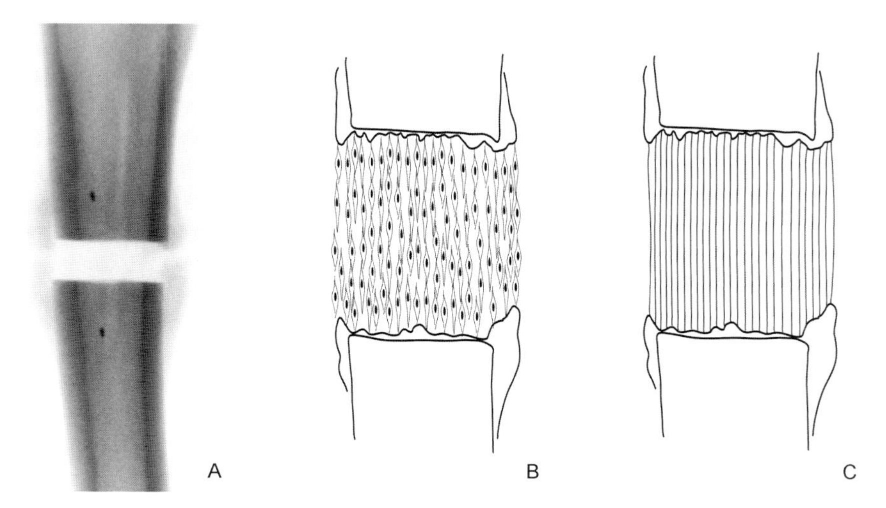

Fig. 9.4 Radiograph of a goat tibia (A) and schematic drawings demonstrating the spindle-shaped fibroblast-like cells (B) and secreted collagen fibers (C) in the distraction gap longitudinally oriented in a direction parallel to the direction of distraction

mineralize [33, 43, 44, 41, 45]. Osteogenesis is initiated at the surfaces of the host bone segments and gradually progress toward the center of the distraction gap.

Since that time the distraction regenerate has a specific three-zonal structure simultaneously representing two stages (soft callus and hard callus) of fracture healing (Figs. 9.2C, and 9.5). In the center, where the influence of tensional stress is maximal, a poorly mineralized, radiolucent fibrous interzone with highly organized longitudinally oriented parallel bundles of collagen and spindle-shaped fibroblast-like cells functions as the center of fibroblast proliferation and fibrous tissue formation [46]. The mixture of fibrous and cartilage tissues within the interzone is suggestive, that during distraction, both membranous and endochondral ossifications play an important role in the process of bone formation [47]. At the periphery of this fibrous interzone, there are two zones of mineralization with longitudinally oriented cylindrical primary trabeculae growing from the surfaces of the host bone segments toward the central interzone [33, 43, 45].

Two major parameters are of critical importance during this period – the rate and rhythm of distraction. The rate of distraction represents the total amount of bone segment movement performed per day, while the rhythm of distraction is the number of increments per day into which the rate of distraction is divided [48].

Bone formation occurs along the vector of tension and is maintained by the growing apices of the primary trabeculae, which remain open during the entire distraction period. These areas, therefore, function as the "growth zone" of the distraction regenerate, providing active osteogenesis throughout the period of distraction [49]. With progression of distraction, two additional radiolucent zones may be evident at the junction of the host bone and the regenerate [50]. In these areas the osteoclasts are removing woven bone tissues and the

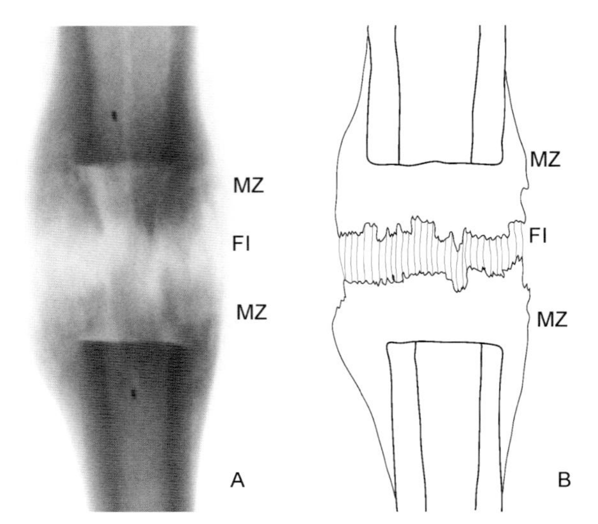

Fig. 9.5 Radiograph of a goat tibia (A) and schematic drawing (B) demonstrating the three-zonal structure of distraction regenerate. Note the radiolucent fibrous interzone (FI) and two radiodense zones of primary trabeculae formation (mineralization zones, MZ) adjacent to the residual host bone segments

initially formed bony scaffold is reinforced by more organized lamellar bone (Fig. 9.2D). This regenerate structure simultaneously represents three stages of fracture healing – the soft callus, hard callus and remodeling stages.

9.2.4. Consolidation Period

The consolidation period is the period between cessation of traction forces and removal of the distraction device. This period represents the time required for complete mineralization of the distraction regenerate. Morphologically, the zonal distribution of the newly formed tissues in the distraction regenerate remains until the end of the distraction period. After distraction ceases, bone trabeculae continue to grow at the center of the regenerate toward each other until overlapping and fusing. The fibrous interzone gradually ossifies and one distinct zone of woven bone completely bridges the gap, indicating a disappearance of the soft callus stage (Fig. 9.2E).

Although the distraction regenerate forms predominantly via direct membranous ossification, isolated islands of cartilage are often observed, suggesting endochondral bone formation [51]. In addition, focal regions of chondrocytes surrounded by a mineralized matrix may be present, suggesting a third (transchondroid) type of bone formation in which cartilage forms, possibly due to decreased oxygen tension, but is then directly transformed into bone, rather than by the traditionally accepted endochondral pathway [52-56].

9.2.5. Remodeling Period

The remodeling period is the period from removal of the distraction device to the application of the full functional loading to the bone segment that contains the distraction regenerate. During this period the zone of primary trabeculae in the center of the regenerate significantly decreases and later is completely resorbed (Fig. 9.2F). As the regenerate matures, the initially formed bony scaffold is reinforced by parallel-fibered and lamellar bone. Both the cortical bone and marrow cavity are restored. Haversian remodeling, representing the last stage of cortical reconstruction, normalizes the bone structure [57, 58]. Usually, it takes a year before the structure of newly formed bony tissue is comparable to that of the preexisting bone.

9.3. Basic Principles of Osteodistraction

Mechanical tension, one of the key signals of morphogenesis during natural bone growth and development, was utilized by Ilizarov as the foundation for his distraction osteogenesis technique. Based on his clinical experience, Ilizarov discovered two biological principles of distraction osteogenesis known as the "Ilizarov Effects" [1-3, 12, 14, 59].

9.3.1. Ilizarov Effects

The first Ilizarov principle is the tension-stress effect on the genesis and growth of tissues. It postulates that gradual traction creates stress that can stimulate and maintain regeneration and active growth of living tissues. Clinically, after distraction, newly formed bone rapidly remodels to conform to the bone's natural structure (Fig. 9.6). The second Ilizarov principle is related to the influence of blood supply and loading on the shape of bones and joints, and theorized that the shape and mass of bones and joints are dependent upon an interaction between mechanical loading and blood supply. For example, if blood supply is inadequate to support normal or increased mechanical loading, then the bone cannot respond favorably, leading to atrophic or degenerative changes. In contrast, if blood supply is adequate to support increased mechanical loading, the bone will demonstrate compensatory hypertrophic changes (Fig. 9.7).

9.3.2. Biological Parameters

The effects of different parameters of osteodistraction on new bone formation were intensively analyzed by Ilizarov in his classic experimental series on dogs [59-61]. The first set of experiments was designed to determine the effect of bone segment fixation stability on the distraction regenerate. Three frame configurations with different bone segment stability of fixation were evaluated: 1) a pair of crossed un-tensioned wires, 2) a pair of crossed tensioned wires and 3) two pairs of crossed tensioned wires (Fig. 9.8). It has been found that stable, but not rigid, fixation of the bone segment with preserved axial micromotion provided by two crossed tensioned wires (configuration B) generates primarily direct membranous bone formation in the distraction gap. In cases with either insufficient fixation (configuration A) or too rigid fixation (configuration C), new bone formed through cartilaginous tissues resulted in fibrous nonunion. Functional use of the limb in an external fixator stimulates callus formation and ossification of the bone regenerate.

To determine the relative importance of the preservation of osteogenic tissues during osteotomy on new bone formation during distraction, different degrees of periosteum, nutrient artery and bone marrow damage were analyzed. The results demonstrated that periosteum, bone marrow and the nutrient

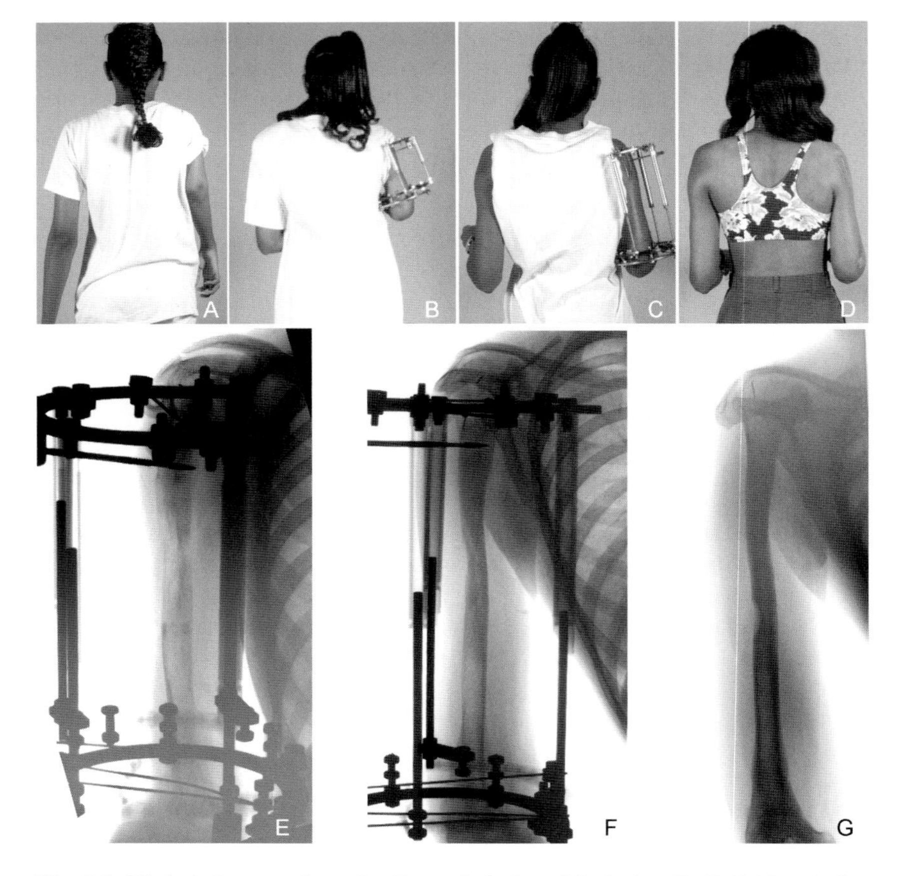

Fig. 9.6 Clinical photographs and radiographs before (A), during (B, C, E, F) and after (D, G) 14.5 cm of humeral lengthening in a 14-year-old girl with right upper extremity brachial plexus palsy

artery are all important for new bone formation. Research also demonstrated that lower-power osteotomy with maximum preservation of osteogenic tissues and periosteal/endosteal blood supply, as well as an adequate duration of the latency period, resulted in enhanced new bone formation in cases undergoing limb lengthening and deformity correction via distraction osteogenesis.

To investigate the effect of the direction of distraction on the orientation of newly formed bone, bone regenerates formed via longitudinal versus transverse (relative to anatomical bone segment axis) distraction were compared. In both cases the bone regenerate within distraction gap was always formed along the vector of applied traction emphasizing the critical importance of the precisely calculated direction of distraction in cases of limb reconstruction via distraction osteogenesis.

The influence of the rate and rhythm of distraction on formation of regenerate bone was also studied. The results of those studies proved that regenerate bone formation depends upon both the rate and rhythm of distraction. The optimal rate of distraction appears to be 1 mm per day (Fig. 9.9A). If the rate of distraction is less than 0.5 mm per day, the bone may consolidate prematurely (Fig. 9.9B). If the rate of distraction is more than 1.5 mm per day, local ischemia in

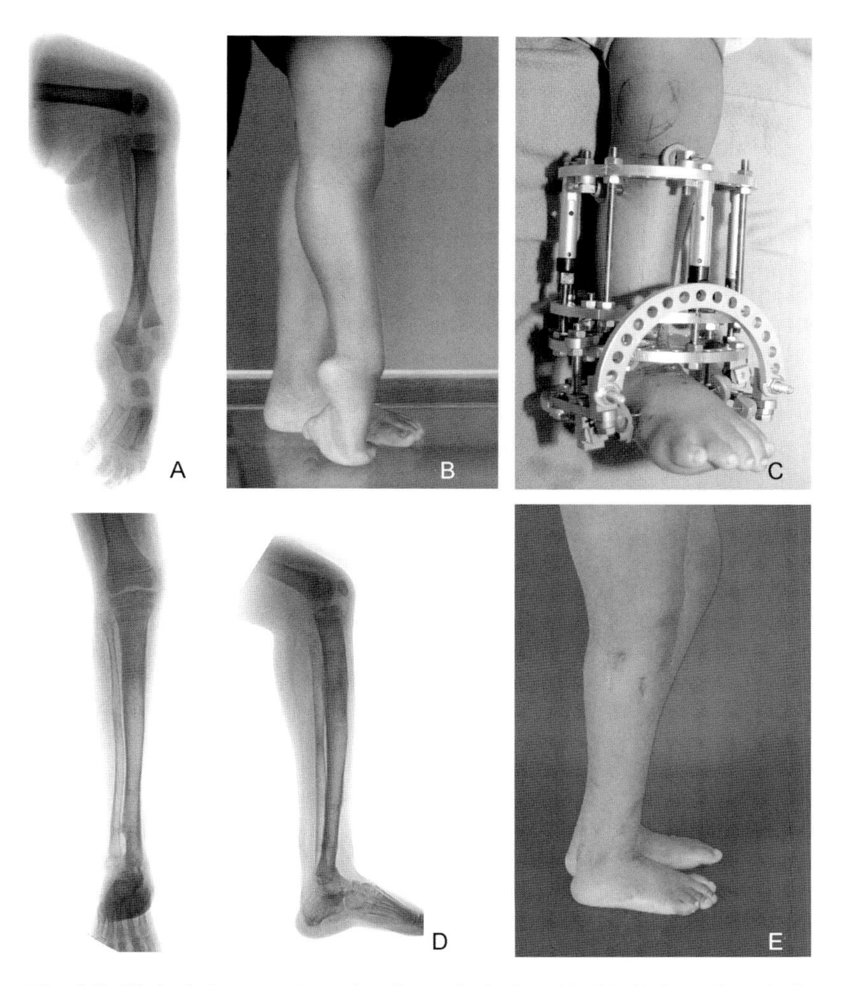

Fig. 9.7 Clinical photographs and radiographs before (A, B), during (C) and after (D, E) 4.5 cm of tibial lengthening and foot reconstruction in a six-year-old girl with Type IV right tibial hemimelia, leg length discrepancy and fixed 70 degrees of equinus contracture with tibiotalar joint subluxation

the interzone and delayed ossification or pseudoarthrosis may result (Fig. 9.9C). The results also proved that more frequent rhythms of distraction led to more favorable regenerate formation and caused less soft tissue problems. Therefore, special distraction mechanisms were developed to obtain a high frequency rhythm close to continuous traction.

9.3.3. Biomechanical Parameters

The successful application of the distraction osteogenesis technique is equally dependent on biologic and biomechanical factors. The biomechanical parameters of osteodistraction can be divided into several categories, including extrinsic or fixator-related factors, intrinsic or tissue-related factors and factors related to distraction device and distraction vector orientation [62-66].

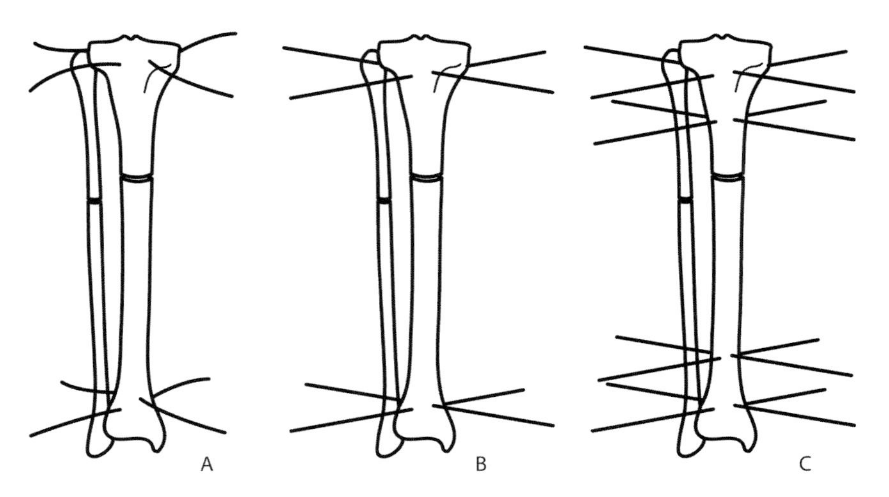

Fig. 9.8 Schematic drawings demonstrating frame configurations with a pair of crossed un-tensioned wires (A), a pair of crossed tensioned wires (B), and two pairs of crossed tensioned wires (C) to determine the effect of bone segment fixation stability on the distraction regenerate

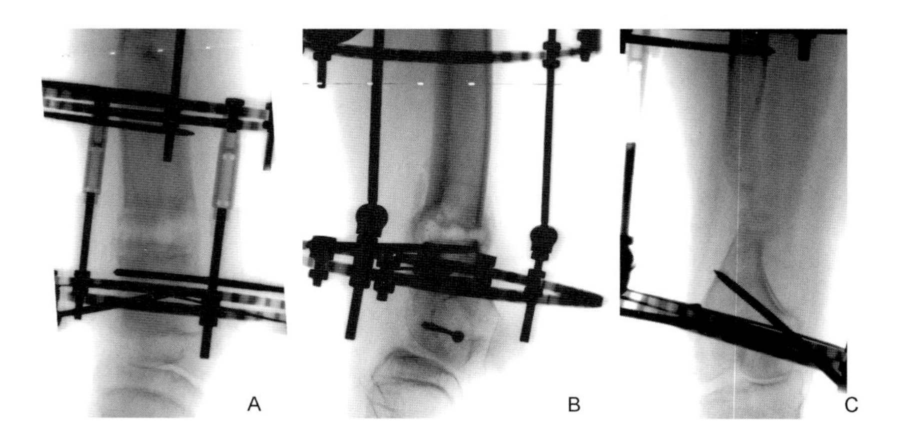

Fig. 9.9 Radiographs during femoral lengthening demonstrating normal (A), hypertrophic (B), and hypotrophic (C) forms of the distraction regenerate

Numerous extrinsic parameters affect the mechanical integrity of the distraction device, which in turn influences the stability of bone fixation. These parameters include the number, length and diameter of fixation pins, the configuration of ring block constructs, the rigidity of the distraction mechanism, and material properties of the device.

There are several intrinsic parameters affecting the biomechanical behavior of the external fixator and the quality of the forming distraction regenerate. Those parameters include the geometric shape, cross sectional area and density of the distracted bone segments, the length of the distraction regenerate, and the tension of the soft tissue envelope including skin, fascia, nerves, muscles, tendons and ligaments. Another critically important biomechanical parameter of distraction osteogenesis is the orientation of the distraction device and the resulting distraction vector relative to the anatomic axis and mechanical axis of the bone segments, and desired direction of distraction.

9.4. Conclusions

Distraction osteogenesis is a unique biological process of new bone formation under the influence of traction forces. Until it is interrupted by traction forces, new bone formation during distraction osteogenesis is similar to that observed during fracture healing. The application of incremental traction to the soft callus aligns the developing interfragmentary tissues parallel to the axis of distraction. Tension stress provides an environment that maintains the soft callus at the center of the distraction gap, while it allows the progression of routine fracture healing at the periphery of the regenerate. Therefore, distraction osteogenesis represents a continuum of individual stages that, because of tensile force application, occur simultaneously rather than sequentially, as during fracture healing.

9.5. Future Trends and Needs

We have been distracting bones of the human skeleton since the late 1800s, albeit in a rudimentary fashion. Over this 100-plus year history, many pivotal events have taken place to bring us to the current state of the art. As we become more comfortable with the mere application of this exciting technique, we will most certainly begin to find more novel uses for it, as well as different iterations of previous uses.

The future development of distraction osteogenesis will almost certainly establish a more complete understanding of the biology of new bone formation under the influence of gradual traction. Major trends will include: 1) a more detailed description of the effect of gradual bony distraction on the surrounding soft tissues, 2) refinement of distraction protocols, 3) modification of osteotomy techniques, 4) further improvement of distraction devices, 5) enhancement of regenerate maturation with pharmacological agents, such as growth factors and cytokines and 6) development of new techniques to monitor distraction regenerate formation and remodeling. In the end, the uses and applications of distraction osteogenesis in treating both simple and complex deformities of the human skeleton are restricted neither by the mechanical configurations of the distraction device nor by the biologic capacity of the human body, but are actually only limited by the boundaries of our imagination.

References

1. Ilizarov GA. The tension-stress effect on the genesis and growth of tissues: Part I. The influence of stability of fixation and soft-tissue preservation. Clin Orthop 1989;238:249-281.
2. Ilizarov GA. The tension-stress effect on the genesis and growth of tissues: Part II. The influence of the rate and frequency of distraction. Clin Orthop 1989;239: 263-285.

3. Ilizarov GA. Clinical application of the tension-stress effect for limb lengthening. Clin Orthop 1990;250:8-26.
4. Peltier LF. External skeletal fixation for the treatment of fractures. In: Peltier LF, ed. Fractures. A History and Iconography of their Treatment, San Francisco: Norman Publishing, 1990:183-196.
5. Wiedemann M. Callus distraction: a new method? A historical review of limb lengthening. Clin Orthop 1996;327:291-304.
6. Cope JB, Samchukov ML, Cherkashin AM. Historical development and evolution of craniofacial distraction osteogenesis. In: Samchukov ML, Cope JB, Cherkashin AM, editors. Craniofacial Distraction Osteogenesis, St. Louis: Mosby-Year Book, Inc., 2001:3-17.
7. Paterson D. Leg-lengthening procedures. A historical review. Clin Orthop 1990;250:27-33.
8. Peltier LF. A brief history of traction. J Bone Joint Surg 1968;50-A:1603-1617.
9. Barton JR. On the treatment of anchylosis by the formation of artificial joints. N Am Med Surg J 1827;3:279-292.
10. Malgaigne JF. Traite des fractures et des luxations. Parise: JB Bailliere, 1847.
11. Codivilla A. On the means of lengthening in the lower limbs, the muscles, and tissues, which are shortened through deformity. Am J Orthop Surg 1905;2:353-369.
12. Ilizarov GA. The principles of the Ilizarov method. Bull Hosp Joint Dis Orthop Inst 1988;48:1-11.
13. Ilizarov GA, Soybelman LM. Some clinical and experimental data concerning lengthening of lower extremities. Exp Khir Anestesiol 1969;14:27-32.
14. Ilizarov GA. Some possibilities with our method for treating damage to and disorders of locomotor apparatus. J Craniofac Surg 1995;6:352-354.
15. De Bastiani G, Aldegheri R, Renzi-Brivio L, Trivella G. Limb lengthening by distraction of the epiphyseal plate. A comparison of two techniques in rabbit. J Bone Joint Surg 1986;68-B:545-548.
16. Aldegheri R, Trivella G, Lavini FM. Epiphyseal distraction. Chondrodiatasis. Clin Orthop 1989;241:117-127.
17. Ring PA. Experimental bone lengthening by epiphyseal distraction. Br J Surg 1958;46:169-173.
18. Zavialov PV, Plaskin JT. Elongation of crural bones in children using a method of distraction epiphysiolysis. Vestn Khir 1967;103:67-70.
19. Sledge CB, Noble J. Experimental limb lengthening by epiphyseal distraction. Clin Orthop 1978;136:111-119.
20. Peltonen JI, Alitalo I, Karaharju EO, Helio H. Distraction of the growth plate. Experiments in pigs and sheep. Acta Orthop Scand 1984;55:359-362.
21. De Pablos J, Jr., Villas C, Canadell J. Bone lengthening by physeal distraction. An experimental study. Int Orthop 1986;10:163-170.
22. De Pablos J, Jr., Canadell J. Experimental physeal distraction in immature sheep. Clin Orthop 1990;250:73-80.
23. Murray JH, Fitch RD. Distraction histogenesis: Principles and indications. J Am Acad Orthop Surg 1996;4:317-327.
24. Gantous A, Phillips JH, Catton P, Holmberg D. Distraction osteogenesis in the irradiated canine mandible. Plast Reconstr Surg 1994;93:164-168.
25. Samchukov ML, Cope JB, Cherkashin AM. Introduction to Distraction Osteogenesis. In: Samchukov ML, Cope JB, Cherkashin AM, editors. Craniofacial Distraction Osteogenesis, St. Louis: Mosby-Year Book, Inc., 2001:xxvii-xxxvi.
26. Brighton CT. Principles of fracture healing. In: Instructional Course Lectures, Rosemont, IL: American Academy of Orthopaedic Surgeons, 1984:60-82.
27. Frost HM. The biology of fracture healing. An overview for clinicians. Part I. Clin Orthop 1989;248:283-293.
28. Schenk RK, Hunziker EB. Histologic and ultrastructural features of fracture healing. In: Brighton CT, Friedlaender GE, Lane JM, editors. Bone Formation and Repair, Rosemont, IL: American Academy of Orthopaedic Surgeons, 1994:117-146.

29. Landry PS, Marino AA, Sadasivan KK, Albright JA. Bone injury response. An animal model for testing theories of regulation, Clin Orthop 1996;332:260-273.
30. McKibbin B. The biology of fracture healing in long bones. J Bone Joint Surg 1978;60-B:150-162.
31. Andrew JG, Andrew SM, Freemont AJ, Marsh DR. Inflammatory cells in normal human fracture healing. Acta Orthop Scand 1994;65:462-466.
32. Hulth A. Current concepts of fracture healing. Clin Orthop 1989;249:265-284.
33. Irianov YM. Spatial organization of a microcirculatory bed in distraction bone regenerates. Genij Ortopedii 1996;1:14-18.
34. Irianov YM. Peculiarities of angiogenesis in distraction regenerates. Genij Ortopedii 1996;2-3:132.
35. Postacchini F, Gumina S, Perugia D, De Marino C. Early fracture callus in the diaphysis of human long bones. Clin Orthop 1995;310:218-228.
36. Delloye C, Delefortrie G, Coutelier L, Vincent A. Bone regenerate formation in cortical bone during distraction lengthening. An experimental study. Clin Orthop 1990;250:34-42.
37. Kallio TJ, Vauhkonen MV, Peltonen JI, Karaharju EO. Early bone matrix formation during distraction. A biochemical study in sheep. Acta Orthop Scand 1994;65:467-471.
38. Holbein O, Neidlinger-Wilke C, Suger G, et al. Ilizarov callus distraction produces systemic bone cell mitogens. J Orthop Res 1995;13:629-638.
39. Mosheiff R, Cordey J, Rahn BA, et al. The vascular supply to bone in distraction osteoneogenesis: An experimental study. J Bone Joint Surg 1996;78-B:497-498.
40. Asonova SN. Morphogenesis mechanisms of limb connective tissue structure in the condition of gradual distraction. Genij Ortopedii 1996;2-3:124.
41. Aronson J, Harrison BH, Stewart CL, Harp JH, Jr. The histology of distraction osteogenesis using different external fixators. Clin Orthop 1989;241:106-116.
42. Aronson J. Experimental assessment of bone regenerate quality during distraction osteogenesis. In: Brighton CT, Friedlaender GE, Lane JM, editors. Bone Formation and Repair, Rosemont, IL: American Academy of Orthopaedic Surgeons, 1994: 441-463.
43. Irianov YM. Scanning electron microscopy of distraction regenerate. Genij Ortopedii 1996;2-3:132.
44. Maffulli N. Callotasis lengthening: A review of some technical aspects. Bull Hosp Joint Dis Orthop Inst 1996;54:249-254.
45. Schenk RK, Gachter A. Histology of distraction osteogenesis. In: Brighton CT, Friedlaender GE, Lane JM, editors. Bone Formation and Repair, Rosemont: American Academy of Orthopaedic Surgeons, 1994:387-394.
46. Yasui N, Kojimoto H, Sasaki K, et al. Factors affecting callus distraction in limb lengthening. Clin Orthop 1993;293:55-60.
47. Waanders NA, Senunas LE, Steen H, et al. Bone formation in distraction osteogenesis. Histologic and immunohistochemical findings. In: Proceedings of 40th Annual Meeting of the Orthopedic Research Society, New Orleans, Louisiana, February 20-24, 1994:231.
48. Samchukov ML, Cherkashin AM, Cope JB. Distraction osteogenesis: Origins and evolution. In: McNamara JAJr, Trotman CA, editors. Distraction Osteogenesis and Tissue Engineering, Ann Arbor: Center for Human Growth and Development, University of Michigan, 1998:1-35.
49. Aronson J, Good B, Stewart CL, et al. Preliminary studies of mineralization during distraction osteogenesis. Clin Orthop 1990:250:43-49.
50. Samchukov ML, Cherkashin AM, Cope JB. Distraction osteogenesis: History and biologic basis of new bone formation. In: Lynch SE, Genco RJ, Marx RE, editors. Tissue Engineering: Applications in Maxillofacial Surgery and Periodontics, Carol Stream: Quintessence Publishing Co., 1998:131-146.
51. Windhager R, Tsuboyama T, Siegl H, et al. Effect of bone cylinder length on distraction osteogenesis in the rabbit tibia. J Orthop Res 1995;13:620-628.

52. Yasui N, Sato M, Ochi T, et al. Three modes of ossification during distraction osteogenesis in the rat. J Bone Joint Surg 1997;79-B:824-830.
53. Sawaki Y, Heggie ACC. The vascular change during and after mandibular distraction. In: Diner PA, Vasquez MP, editors. 2nd International Congress on Cranial and Facial Bone Distraction Processes, Bologna: Monduzzi Editore, 1999:23-27.
54. Li G, Simpson AH, Triffitt JT. The role of chondrocytes in intramembranous and endochondral ossification during distraction osteogenesis in the rabbit. Calc Tiss Int 1999;64:310-317.
55. Samchukov ML, Cope JB, Cherkashin AM, Harper RH. Tissue maturation during distraction osteogenesis in bone of different embryonic origins. In: Book of Abstracts. International Congress on Cranial and Facial Bone Distraction Processes, Paris, France, 1997:Paper 004.
56. Bassett CAL, Herrman I. Influence of oxygen concentration and mechanical factors on differentiation of connective tissue *in vitro*. Nature 1961;190:460.
57. Tajana GF, Morandi M, Zembo MM. The structure and development of osteogenetic repair tissue according to Ilizarov technique in man. Characterization of extracellular matrix. Orthop 1989;12:515-523.
58. Saleh M, Stubbs DA, Street RJ, et al. Histologic analysis of human lengthened bone. J Pediatr Orthop 1993;2:16-21.
59. Ilizarov GA. Transosseous Osteosynthesis – Theoretical and Clinical Aspects of the Regeneration and Growth of Tissues. New York: Springer-Verlag, 1992:1-800.
60. Frankel VH, Gold G, Golyakhovsky V. The Ilizarov technique. Bull Hosp Joint Dis Orthop Inst 1988;48:17-27.
61. Shevtsov VI. Professor G.A. Ilizarov's contribution to the method of transosseous osteosynthesis. Bull Hosp Joint Dis Orthop Inst 1997;56:11-15.
62. Kummer FJ. Technical note: Evaluation of new Ilizarov rings. Bull Hosp Joint Dis Orthop Inst 1990; 50:88-90.
63. Orbay GO, Kummer FJ, Frankel VN. The effect of wire configuration on the stability of the Ilizarov external fixator. Clin Orthop 1992;279:299-302.
64. Calhoun JH, Li F, Bauford WL, et al. Rigidity of half-pins for the Ilizarov external fixator. Bull Hosp Joint Dis Orthop Inst 1992;52:21-26.
65. Podolsky A, Chao EYS. Mechanical performance of Ilizarov circular external fixators in comparison with other external fixators. Clin Orthop 1993;293:61-70.
66. Bronson D, Samchukov M, Birch J, Browne R, Ashman R. Stability of external circular fixation: a multi-variable biomechanical analysis. Clin Biomech 1998;13:441-448.

10

Distraction Osteogenesis of the Facial Skeleton

Robert J. Havlik

Abstract: Distraction osteogenesis of the facial skeleton has provided both a powerful tool to those who are interested in studying the biology of bone and has added a powerful technique to the armamentarium of surgeons who treat facial disfigurement. The application of bone distraction to the facial skeleton has been largely derived from prior work in the lower extremity, and the fundamental biologic concepts of distraction osteogenesis must be thoroughly understood before the extension of this work to the facial skeleton can be consistently applied successfully. Bone distraction initiates a complex biologic process that induces biosynthetic pathways to form additional soft tissue and bone. The application of this principle to the facial skeleton must also take into consideration specific characteristics of the face and its anatomy. Surgeons traditionally view the face in three separate domains: 1) the upper face – from the eyes to the top of the head, 2) the mid-face – from the upper teeth to the eyes, and 3) the lower face – from the lower teeth to the neck. Each of these three domains of the facial skeleton has its specific biological requirements and constraints, and each domain requires different considerations for fixation of bone devices and for the design of linkage systems. In its most elementary form, the bone distraction device must meet two essential criteria: 1) provide rigid fixation in three dimensions of the bone on either side of the bone osteotomy site (or distraction gap) and 2) provide for a linkage system that will allow the two bone components to separate gradually at a set rate (usually approximately one millimeter per day). This chapter will briefly review the fundamental biology of distraction osteogenesis, review its development in each of the three facial domains and review the inherent biological constraints and requirements of each of these areas.

Keywords: Bone, face, distraction osteogenesis, craniofacial, surgery.

Division of Plastic Surgery, Indiana University School of Medicine, Indianapolis, IN

From: *Orthopedic Biology and Medicine: Musculoskeletal Tissue Regeneration, Biological Materials and Methods*
Edited by W. S. Pietrzak © Humana Press, Totowa, NJ

10.1. Introduction

Distraction osteogenesis was developed as a technique to treat the clinical problem of leg length discrepancy. Codivilla's first reported attempts at limb lengthening were made nearly 100 years ago [1]. Following these initial reports, the influential Italian orthopedic surgeon Putti reported his work with the "osteon," a pin fixed, spring loaded device that expanded a femoral osteotomy site. This device used a single pin proximal and distal to the femoral osteotomy site, and consequently lacked adequate stability [2]. Putti's influence led to large numbers of patients being treated, large numbers of treatment failures and, consequently, a large number of crippled patients [3]. Despite the fact that Abbot recognized that two points of bone fixation were necessary proximal and distal to the osteotomy site to control rotation of the bone fragments and provide enough stability to allow bony healing to occur in the early 1930s, this early experience with bone distraction was so unfavorable (could be described as 'catastrophic') that the technique was essentially banished from mainstream use in Western medicine to the edges of the earth [3]. Instead, Western orthopedists adopted the alternative of Phemister's contribution of ablation of the growth plate of the "normal" leg to correct leg length discrepancy problems.

Fortunately, at the "edge of the earth" in Siberia, USSR, Ilizarov began his great work with distraction osteogenesis. He performed thousands of animal experiments and demonstrated both the power of distraction osteogenesis and the essential biologic principles for its successful application [4, 7]. He also demonstrated its successful application in humans, and provided care through a major orthopedic hospital dedicated primarily to lower extremity distraction osteogenesis in Siberia. In order to understand the principles of distraction osteogenesis, it is first necessary to understand the basic elements of bone healing.

10.2. Fundamentals of Bone Healing

In the ideal state, the discontinuity between bone ends is created by a fine diamond saw with strict attention to limiting thermal energy during the osteotomy, and close attention to avoiding injury to the surrounding soft tissue. The osteotomy is performed in a young animal with an excellent blood supply and an excellent supply of osteoblastic progenitor cells [8]. The osteotomy site is immobilized by rigid fixation, completely eliminating motion between the abutting ends of the bone fragments. In this artificial situation bone healing will occur by a process known as "direct bone healing." In those sites where bone is directly touching, "contact healing" will occur [9]. Within the cortical bone disrupted by the osteotomy, the Haversian canals will differentiate into osteoclastic cutting cones. These osteoclastic cutting cones are larger in diameter than the Haversian canals and contain both the blood vessels and the osteoblasts and osteoclasts. The osteoclasts in the apex of the cutting cone bore across the site of osteotomy by resorbing bone (Fig. 10.1). They traverse the osteotomy site and bore through the bone on the contralateral side and re-establish vascular continuity with the Haversian canals on the opposite side. In the "wake," or defect, created by this large osteoclastic cutting cone, the osteoblasts that line the lateral aspects of the cutting cones synthesize new bone and fill in the walls of the channel created by the larger head of the cutting cone. This leads to bone

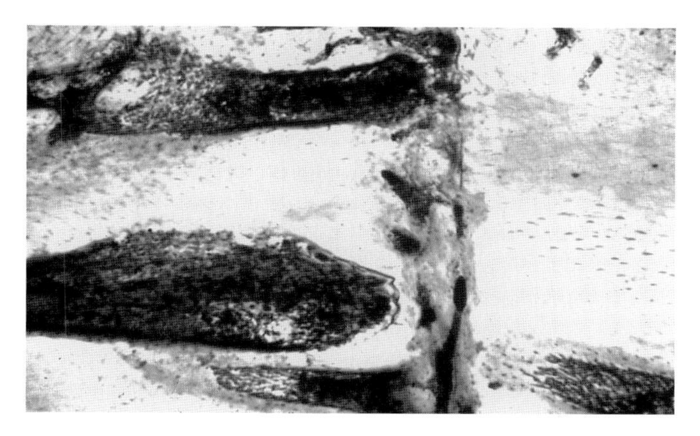

Fig. 10.1 Osteoclastic cutting cone with increased diameter of head as it is actively "drilling" through bone by dissolving bone (*photo courtesy of Synthes U.S.A.)*

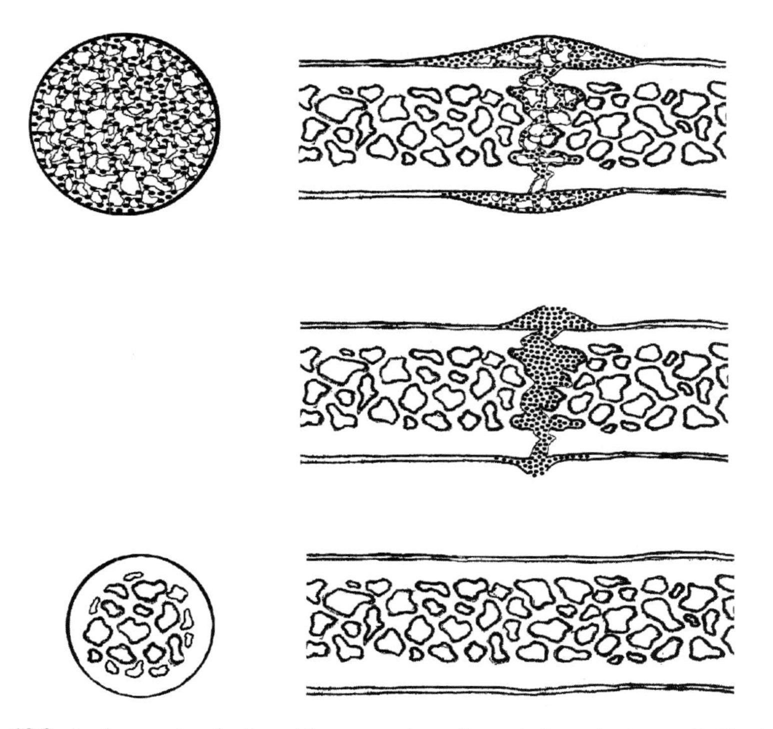

Fig. 10.2 As these osteoclastic cutting cones bore through the osteotomy site/fracture gap, they lay down new bone in a lamellar fashion along the walls of the vascular channel. As this happens at many sites through the cross section of the bone, bony integrity and, consequently, strength are re-established. Illustration courtesy of Min Li, M.D

bridging across the discontinuity between the bones and the re-establishment of structural integrity (Fig. 10.2).

The above description of 'direct' bone healing only occurs in tightly controlled experimental conditions. It is seldom the case after operative osteotomy and virtually never the case after traumatic injury, simply because the gaps between the bone ends cannot be approximated as accurately. The gap between the bone ends will be filled with "osteoid," an intermediary tissue consisting of fibroblasts, osteoblasts and vascular tissue similar to the composition of 'granulation tissue' in open wounds. If there is a favorable blood supply and the presence of appropriate numbers of osteoprogenitor cells, with sufficiently rigid fixation, this "osteoid" tissue will undergo progressive differentiation to form bone and reconstitute structural integrity through the process of osteoclastic cutting cones boring through the "osteoid." In a clinical situation in which there is sufficient blood supply and a sufficient number of osteoprogenitor cells, the critical balance is the degree of fixation relative to the forces and loads applied to the fragmentary gap which will tend to cause displacement of the bone ends [8, 10]. If fixation is insufficient, there will be a progressive deposition of fibrous tissue. This creates a proliferation of bone 'callus.' The callus will tend to stabilize the bone fragment ends. If the callus stabilization is adequate, the fibrous tissue will differentiate into bone. If it is not adequate, it is likely that cartilage will be formed in the gap between the bone ends, which will result in a nonunion. The osteoclastic cutting cones cannot bore through cartilage. The exact cause for cartilage formation is uncertain. With persistent motion in the fragmentary gap, there may be an inability to form adequate vascularity to support the healing process. Caplan has shown in the past that the vascularity can influence the path of differentiation of the osteoprogenitor cells to form bone or cartilage [8, 10-12]. Indeed, Caplan feels that the "definitive discriminator" in the differentiation of mesenchymal stem cells into either chondrocytes or osteoblasts is the degree of vascularity present [11]. This finding can be combined with the need for interfragmentary stability. Similar to the situation in skin grafting, if there is a lateral shear force present between the graft and its bed during the time of revascularization of the skin graft, neovascularization of the graft will be disrupted and the skin graft will die. If there is lateral shear force present in the bone fragmentary gap, vascularity will be compromised. The mesenchymal stem cells may then differentiate into cartilage and a nonunion may be the final result [10, 11].

10.3. Fundamentals of Distraction Osteogenesis

Distraction osteogenesis is essentially a technique to control the microcosm of the gap between the ends of the bone in the osteotomy site. The truly amazing fact is that Ilizarov's work on bone healing and distraction osteogenesis was being carried on in isolation in Siberia with the thoroughness, precision and accuracy of Western science before these mechanisms of bone healing were completely elucidated by Western scientists [4.7], the technique of distraction osteogenesis specifically controls the microcosm of the distraction gap so that the cellular machinery induced to heal the bone defect is perpetuated in its stimulated state as the distance between the ends of the bone are slowly increased and the bone is lengthened. In an elegant and classic set of experiments, Ilizarov used the canine hindlimb as a model to illustrate the importance of rigidity in a bone distraction gap (Fig. 10.3) [4, 7]. The distraction gap is, of course, analogous to the fragmentary gap in an osteotomy or fracture line. Ilizarov used five separate groups of animals and provided progressively more rigid fixation at the bone distraction gap in each animal. In the first group of animals he performed an open osteotomy and used a single circular fixation ring on either side of the osteotomy [7]. Bony stability was provided by a Kirschner wire strung from one side of the ring, passing through the

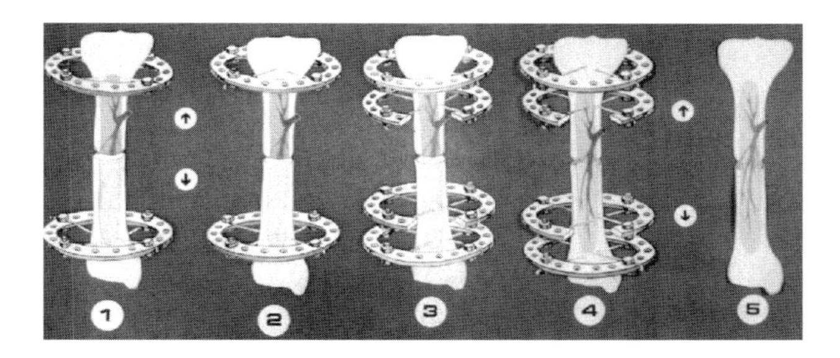

Fig. 10.3 Ilizarov's classic and elegant series of experiments illustrating the effect of progressively rigid fixation on bone formation and healing. Illustration #1 is a single ring fixator on each side of the osteotomy gap with cross wires placed through the bone. Illustration #2 is a single ring fixator on each side of the osteotomy gap with cross wires placed through the bone and tensioned with a pulling force by an external device, thereby increasing the rigidity of the wire, and hence the fixation system. Illustration #3 shows two ring fixators on each side of the osteotomy gap with cross wires placed through the bone and tensioned with force by an external device. Illustration #4 shows two ring fixators on each side of the osteotomy gap with cross wires placed through the bone and tensioned with a force by an external device, and an incomplete osteotomy, or "corticotomy" through the bone, preserving the integrity of the medullary cavity blood supply. Fixation in Illustration #5 is identical to #3 and #4, but the corticotomy was done through a closed approach with preservation of the nutrient artery. Illustration used with permission from Ilizarov G (1992) *The transosseous synthesis: Theoretical and clinical aspects of regeneration and the growth of tissue*. Springer-Verlag, Berlin

soft tissue and bone, to the other side of the ring. One pair of these transfixion wires was used in each fragment of bone and they were oriented in a crossed fashion. In the second group of animals a single circular fixation ring was placed on either side of the osteotomy. Similar to group one, one pair of crossed Kirschner wires was placed through each bone fragment. Unlike group one, the wires in the second group were tightened by applying tension on the transfixion wires, increasing their rigidity and hence, fixator stability. This reduced the mobility of the bone fragments. In the third group of dogs, a total of four circular fixation rings were used, with two rings on either side of the distraction gap. Each ring had one pair of tensioned and crossed Kirschner wires. In the fourth group of dogs, the fixator was identical to group three, but the bone was cut with an open osteotomy and one-third of the cross sectional area of the bone marrow was preserved. In group five, further preservation of the soft tissues was performed by using a closed technique for the bone fracture, preserving the nutrient artery. In all groups distraction of the bone ends was performed at a rate of one-half millimeter per day, followed by an appropriate period of bony consolidation. In each group animals were sacrificed immediately after osteotomy and at seven days, 14 days, 21 days, 28 days, six weeks, two months, three months, four months and six months after osteotomy.

In this model the first group showed considerable mobility between the bone ends and there was minimal osteogenesis. The distraction gap at 14 days was largely filled with fibrous tissue and large islands of cartilage (Fig. 10.4a). In the second group of dogs, with the single pair of tension loaded Kirschner wires in each bone fragment, stability and bone formation increased substantially. The upper and lower portions of the gap were filled "with cone shaped segments of regenerated osseous tissue separated by a fibrocartilagenous layer" (Fig. 10. 4b). The third group of dogs, with two fixation rings and two pairs of tensioned wires on either side of the distraction gap, showed a high level of osteogenic activity, with the connective tissue fibers and osseous trabeculae showing a longitudinal orientation in the distraction gap. Some of these animals had already shown a fusion of the regenerate bone in the distraction gap to the cortical plate of the bone end (Fig. 10.4c). In group four and group five, which had similar fixation to group three, but enhanced preservation of the soft tissue and vascularity, osteogenesis was even more profound. This occurred to such a degree that the animals in group

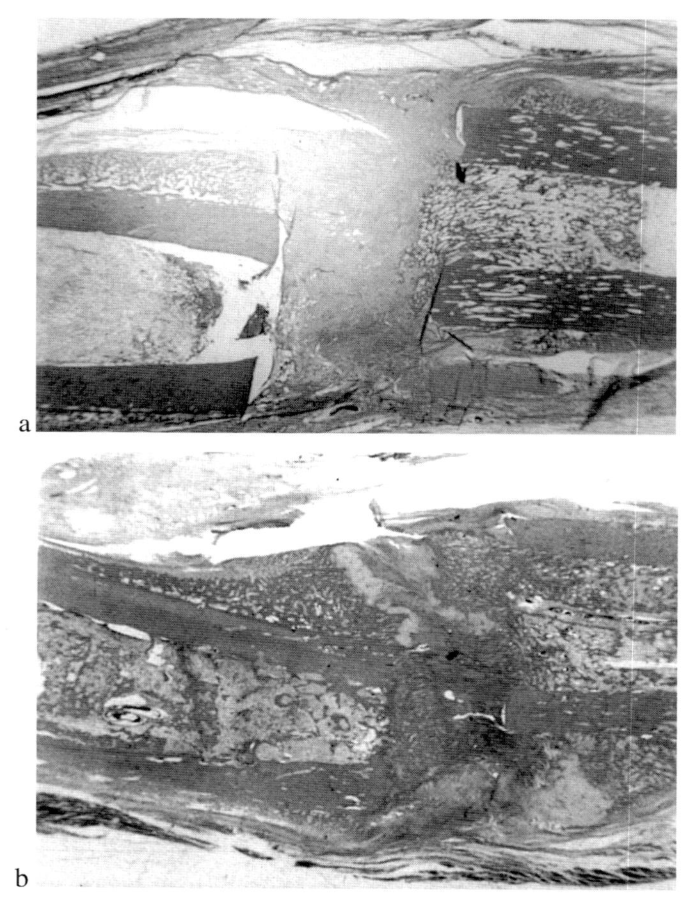

Fig. 10.4 Photomicrographs showing results of longitudinal distraction of 0.5 mm/day in four stages (0.125 mm Q6h). All animals were sacrificed on day #14. Fig. 10.4a shows results in group #1 with a single ring fixator. The distraction gap is filled with poorly differentiated connective tissue with a few islands of cartilage. In Fig. 10.4b, illustrating the results in group #2 with a single ring fixator, but with rigidity increased due to tension applied to the wires, there are small cone shaped segments of regenerated bone attached to each bone fragment, separated by a fibrocartilagenous layer. In Fig. 10.4c, with two rings on either side of the osteotomy, the distraction gap contains regenerated osseous tissue with longitudinal trabeculae. In Fig. 10.4d, osteogenesis has overtaken distraction and consolidated the bone prematurely. Reproduced with permission from Ilizarov G (1992) *The transosseous synthesis: Theoretical and clinical aspects of regeneration and the growth of tissue*. Springer-Verlag, Berlin

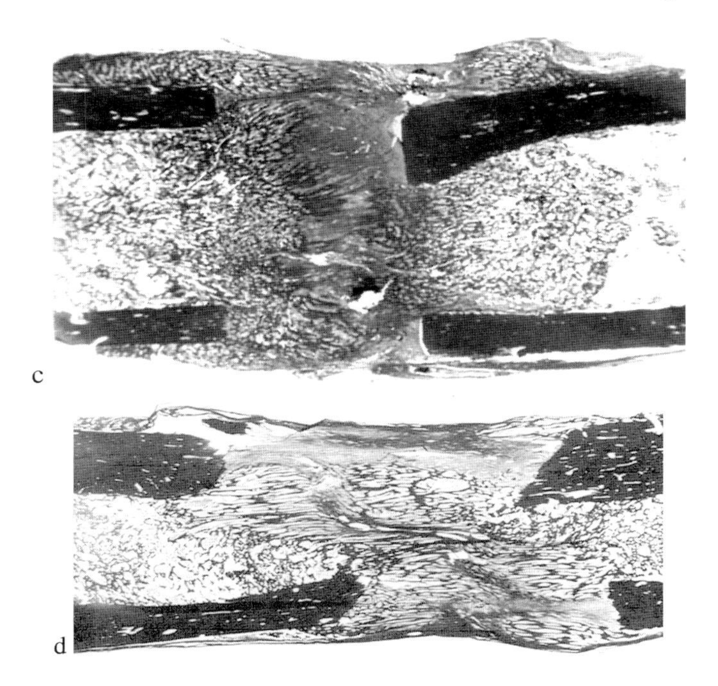

Fig. 10.4 (continued)

five could not be distracted at one-half millimeter per day. These animals would heal and consolidate their bone at this distraction rate. It was necessary to distract them at a much faster rate of 1.5 to 1.6 millimeters per day to overcome the intense osteogenesis present (Fig. 10.4d). This study elegantly demonstrates the impact of rigidity on bone healing. Furthermore, it also illustrates that, with increased lateral shear at the fragmentary gap, minimal bone is formed, but extensive cartilage is produced. Ilizarov carefully differentiates the effect of motion in an axial orientation parallel to the axis of the long bones from lateral shear stress. He feels that axial micromotion, parallel to the bone ends, is beneficial to bone healing, whereas lateral shear stress is severely detrimental to bone healing. The neovascularization of the osteotomy gap is critically dependent upon adequate immobilization against lateral shear stress, similar to the absolute requirement for immobilization during the neovascularization of skin grafts from the recipient beds.

This experiment, combined with other extensive basic science and clinical experiments, allowed Ilizarov to elucidate several principles to optimize the results in distraction osteogenesis that essentially control the microcosm of the gap between the ends of the bone. First, the bone fixation must provide for absolute stability against lateral shear stress (perpendicular to the axis of bone distraction) across the bone distraction gap. Secondly, the surgical technique should be precise and minimize the disruption of soft tissue and intraosseous blood supply. Third, the distraction frame should provide for a mechanism to allow for separation (lengthening) of the bone ends by approximately one millimeter per day. Finally, a "delay" of three to five days is necessary prior to the onset of distraction to allow for the initiation of blood vessel growth into the gap between the bone ends. Strict adherence to these principles allowed Ilizarov to establish success in the laboratory and in clinical practice, and allowed him to establish the "Law of Tension Stress," which states: "Living Tissue, when subjected to slow steady traction, becomes metabolically activated in both the biosynthetic and proliferative pathways, a phenomenon dependent upon both vascularity and functional use" [7].

10.4. Distraction Osteogenesis in the Facial Skeleton

The application of distraction osteogenesis in the facial skeleton has largely occurred since the early 1990s. McCarthy and his collaborators at New York University extended Ilizarov's work to the facial skeleton through elegant experiments in the canine model and the subsequent application of these techniques and principles in humans [13-17]. The facial skeleton has several advantages in relation to the load bearing axial skeleton, including excellent blood supply to support the process of distraction osteogenesis and a relatively low force-load profile. However, it also has several special considerations and several anatomical pitfalls that are unique to the facial skeleton. These must be fully understood in order to appreciate the complexity of distraction osteogenesis in the facial skeleton.

Distraction osteogenesis can move each of the skeletal components of the face in any of the three dimensions. In addition, the application to the facial skeleton in the growing child must consider the fourth dimension of time and growth. Facial distraction frequently may be performed as early as the first week of life for breathing obstruction due to a hypoplastic mandible, but also may be performed in adulthood for facial asymmetries. The timing of surgery and its interplay with and impact upon growth becomes the fourth dimension for consideration and planning. Surgeons view the face as composed of three separate domains: 1) the upper face – from the eyes to the top of the head, 2) the mid-face – from the upper teeth to the eyes and 3) the lower face – from the lower teeth to the neck. The adaptation of distraction osteogenesis to the face involves completely different considerations in each domain. The anatomical considerations are substantively different for each domain and these differences have driven the development of distinctly different types of distraction hardware. Adaptation to each domain of the face requires complete and novel conceptualization of the bone distraction appliance as a device to allow for rigid fixation to each bony component on each side of the osteotomy, and a linkage system to control the gap between the ends of the bone. The lower face's skeletal component is the mandible, and the mandible is the most similar to other "long" bones or axial skeletal components because it is tubular and has a marrow filled center. It is also the area where distraction osteogenesis was first applied in the facial skeleton, so we will begin a discussion of specific applications with this domain.

10.5. Distraction Osteogenesis in the Lower Facial Skeleton - Mandible

Snyder first described distraction osteogenesis of the mandible in 1973, prior to the "discovery" and popularization of Ilizarov's work in Western medicine [18]. However, McCarthy and colleagues must be credited with recognizing the power of these principles and techniques within the facial skeleton, and the early developmental and clinical work that brought this field to fruition for clinical applications in the face [13-17]. The mandible is the most common site of distraction osteogenesis in the head and neck, accounting for greater than two-thirds of all facial distraction osteogenesis procedures in a recent review [19].

While the mandible is very similar to the long bones of the axial skeleton in its tubular nature, there are several specific aspects which merit consideration. First, the mandible's location within the head and neck makes the surgical approach and fixation somewhat problematic. The ramus and body of the mandible are located within the posterior face, beneath the posterior cheek (Fig. 10.5), and the surgical approach for osteotomy and fixation must contend with the presence of the facial nerve within the soft tissue of the cheek. This motor nerve arises as a single nerve trunk from the stylomastoid foramen at the base of the skull behind the ear, and then branches into five main trunks which provide control for the majority of facial movement for that side of the face. Injury leads to readily appreciable asymmetry in facial movement. The surgical approach can safely be performed either from inferiorly through an incision parallel to the lower border of the mandible (Risdon incision) (Fig. 10.5), through an approach from inside the mouth (a 'trans-oral' approach), or directly through the cheek with placement of pins and an external distraction device. Although this latter approach was initially used

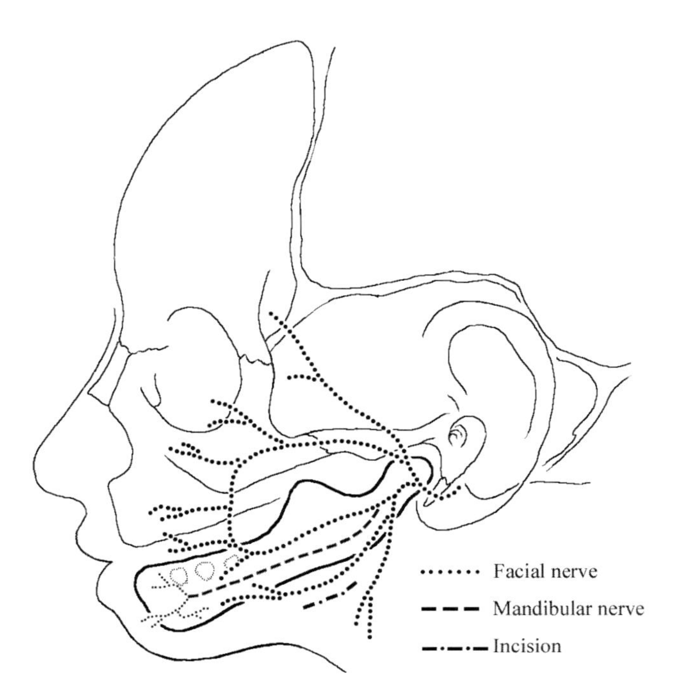

Fig. 10.5 Illustration of anatomy of cheek and posterior face, depicting the relevant anatomical structures – mandibular body and ramus, inferior alveolar nerve and facial nerve. The Risdon incision is depicted in classic location, two centimeters below the body of the mandible. Illustration courtesy of Min Li, M.D

frequently in distraction osteogenesis, the significant limitation of the facial scars has made it less desirable. Secondly, following incision and exposure, the positioning of the distraction device should be assessed. This will allow guidance to establish the site of the osteotomy. Third, the bone osteotomy must be precisely placed so that it minimizes the possibility of injury to the inferior alveolar nerve. This nerve lies contained within the medullary cavity of the mandible and provides sensibility to the teeth within the mandible and to the lower lip. This consideration of an intramedullary nerve does not exist in the application of distraction to the extremities. The osteotomy can be designed so that it lies posterior to the nerve (Fig. 10.6), or an incomplete osteotomy, known as a 'corticotomy,' can be performed to minimize the risk of nerve injury. In addition, the dental follicles and teeth themselves are at risk for injury. The mandible is packed full of teeth, particularly in the infant and child where there exist both deciduous and permanent dental follicles. In this latter case, the entire body of the mandible is packed with discrete dental follicles that are programmed to generate teeth. The position of the osteotomy and the site of pin or screw placement must consider this issue. Following the completion of the osteotomy, the distraction device can then be applied directly on the surface of the bone with osseous screws, an 'internal distractor,' or pins can be placed percutaneously through the skin of the cheek with the body of the distractor positioned outside the cheek, an 'external distractor.' Unlike the extremities where percutaneous "through and through" whole pins must be used, this cannot be easily applied in the face, and the distraction device is usually applied internally with screws directly to the surface of the bone, or with percutaneous "half-pins" that exit the external surface of the mandibular ramus and pass through the cheek skin. Finally, the lower jaw is extremely sensitive to

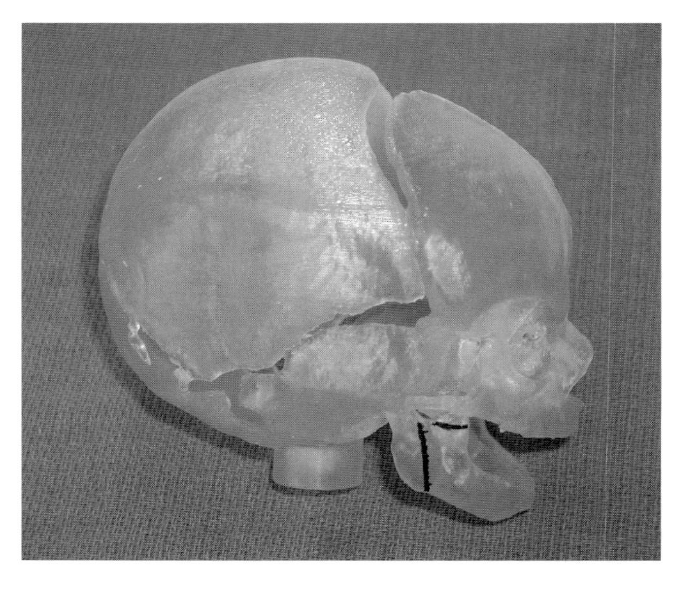

Fig. 10.6 Location of vertical ramus osteotomy posterior to course of inferior alveolar nerve, and associated coronoid resection

malposition and malocclusion (inappropriate alignment of the upper and lower jaws during mastication). The presence of a seed or other foreign body within one's teeth is a reminder of this exquisite relationship. Despite this location within the face, the diminutive size of the skeletal components, and the several vital structures that traverse this area, a comprehensive review of the experience using distraction osteogenesis revealed that the incidence of injury to these vital structures has been in the range of 5 to 6 percent [19].

There are many disorders in which distraction osteogenesis has proven to be an effective treatment in the facial skeleton. These disorders of mandibular hypoplasia include Pierre Robin Sequence, hemifacial microsomia, craniofacial microsomia, Nager's syndrome, Treacher Collins syndrome and other craniofacial syndromes. Pierre Robin sequence is characterized by the triad of a hypoplastic mandible, glossoptosis (the tongue falling backwards in the mouth) and ventilatory obstruction [20]. In addition, this anomaly is frequently associated with a cleft of the palate. The ventilatory obstruction is particularly problematic within the first six months of life, and can lead to death. Treatment options include tracheostomy, suturing the lip and tongue together (lip-tongue adhesion) [21], or distraction lengthening the mandible by distraction osteogenesis [22]. Some controversy about the use of mandibular distraction osteogenesis does exist, because the mandible in these Pierre Robin infants does undergo some degree of "catch-up" growth, and opponents argue that a "permanent" technique such as distraction osteogenesis of the mandible may not be optimal for a potentially time-limited problem. Therefore, distraction osteogenesis in Pierre Robin sequence patients is most often limited to those children with severe enough compromise in breathing that they will require either a tracheostomy or a jaw lengthening procedure. Despite the often small size of the infant and the correspondingly small size of the mandible, the technique has proven reliable in providing a solution to these complex problems [23-27]. While the longer term implications for dental development are currently not well defined, distraction osteogenesis can be technically performed with little perioperative morbidity.

For craniofacial microsomia, hemifacial microsomia, Nager's syndrome and Treacher Collins syndrome, the classification of mandibular hypoplasia first proposed by Pruzansky in 1969 [28], and its modification by Kaban and Mulliken in 1980 [29], has proven to be quite useful, and now has potentially even greater significance since it has direct implications for guiding therapy (Fig. 10.7). Class I mandibles have a normal overall shape of the mandible, but a diminution in size. Class IIA mandibles have moderate hypoplasia of the mandible with hypoplasia of the ramus and condyle of the mandible, but the condyle and temperomandibular (TMJ) joint are present and adequately positioned to provide stability in mandibular opening with the contralateral joint. Class IIB mandibles are characterized by profound hypoplasia of the mandibular ramus and the absence of a functional TMJ joint. Class III mandibles have virtually no mandibular ramus and the mandible ends behind the dental elements. Although different surgical treatment approaches to mandibular hypoplasia do exist, the Class I mandibles often are best treated with conventional orthognathic surgery, or may respond solely to orthodontics. Some Class IIA mandibles will often be amenable to conventional orthognathic surgery, while the more severely afflicted Class IIA and IIB mandibles will benefit from distraction osteogenesis. Class III mandibles have very limited

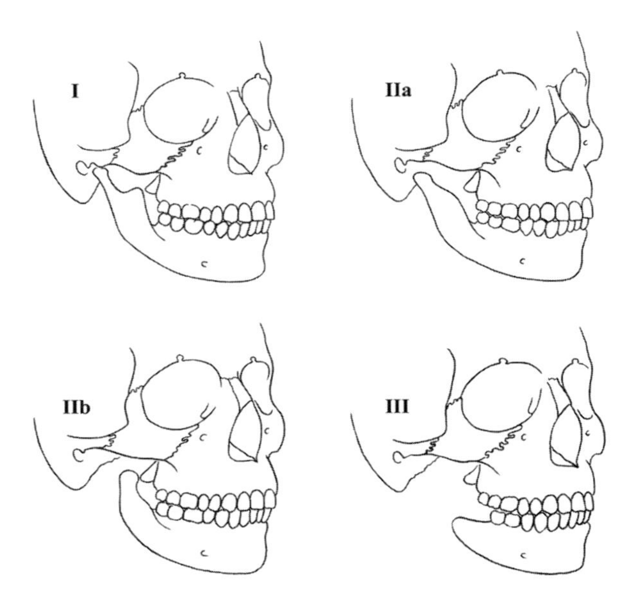

Fig. 10.7 Illustration of classification system for mandibular hypoplasia, based upon classification described by Pruzansky and expanded by Kaban and Mulliken. Illustration courtesy of Min Li, M.D

bone present behind the dentition, and so are not amenable to osteotomy and distraction osteogenesis and require mandible reconstruction with a composite costochondral graft to re-establish facial structure and correct the deficiency on posterior facial height. It should be noted that in treating the more complex mandibulofacial dysostosis syndromes such as Nager's and Treacher Collins syndromes, there may be a tendency for the mandible to undergo a slight relapse [30].

Technical considerations discussed earlier include the presence of facial nerve, the inferior alveolar nerve and the dental elements. In addition, the fact that the mandible is hypoplastic must be considered, since both the ramus and the body of the mandible are small and are, therefore, more difficult to control. In fact, distraction osteogenesis may be performed during the first week of life, in infants that weigh only 1 kilogram. The internal distractors are affixed through small shelf-like footplates (Fig. 10.8) and secured to the bone with screws, while the external distractors are affixed with pins (Fig. 10.9). The technical difficulty in this surgery can be appreciated by considering the small hypoplastic ramus, the small body of the mandible and the distractor form three independent elements after the bone is cut, and these three elements must be simultaneously controlled to allow for the precise application and alignment of the distraction device in the appropriate vector of lengthening relative to the face.

The author's preference is to perform a transverse incision parallel to the body of the mandible (Risdon incision) extending deep to the platysma

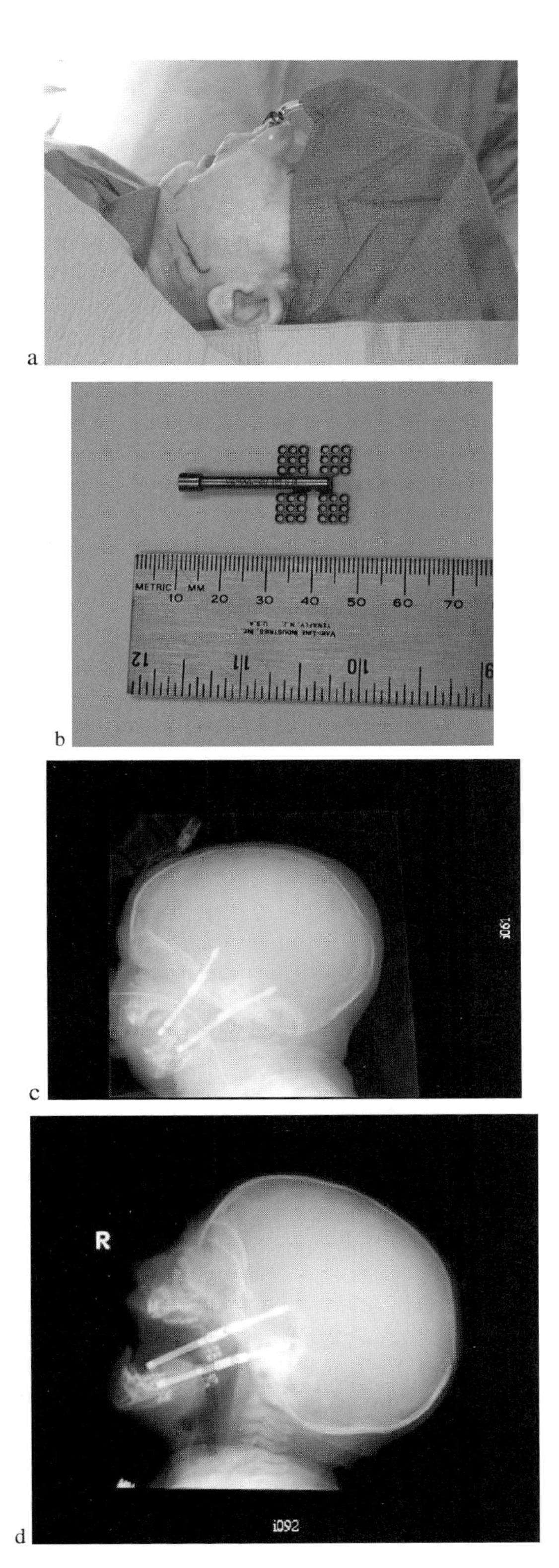

Fig. 10.8 Mandibular distraction in child with Pierre Robin sequence, ventilatory obstruction and mandibular hypoplasia. 10.8a) Intra-op positioning; 10.8b) Titanium micro-distraction device; 10.8c) Post-op radiographs prior to the start of distraction – note the position of the footplates; 10.8d) Post-op radiographs upon completion of distraction

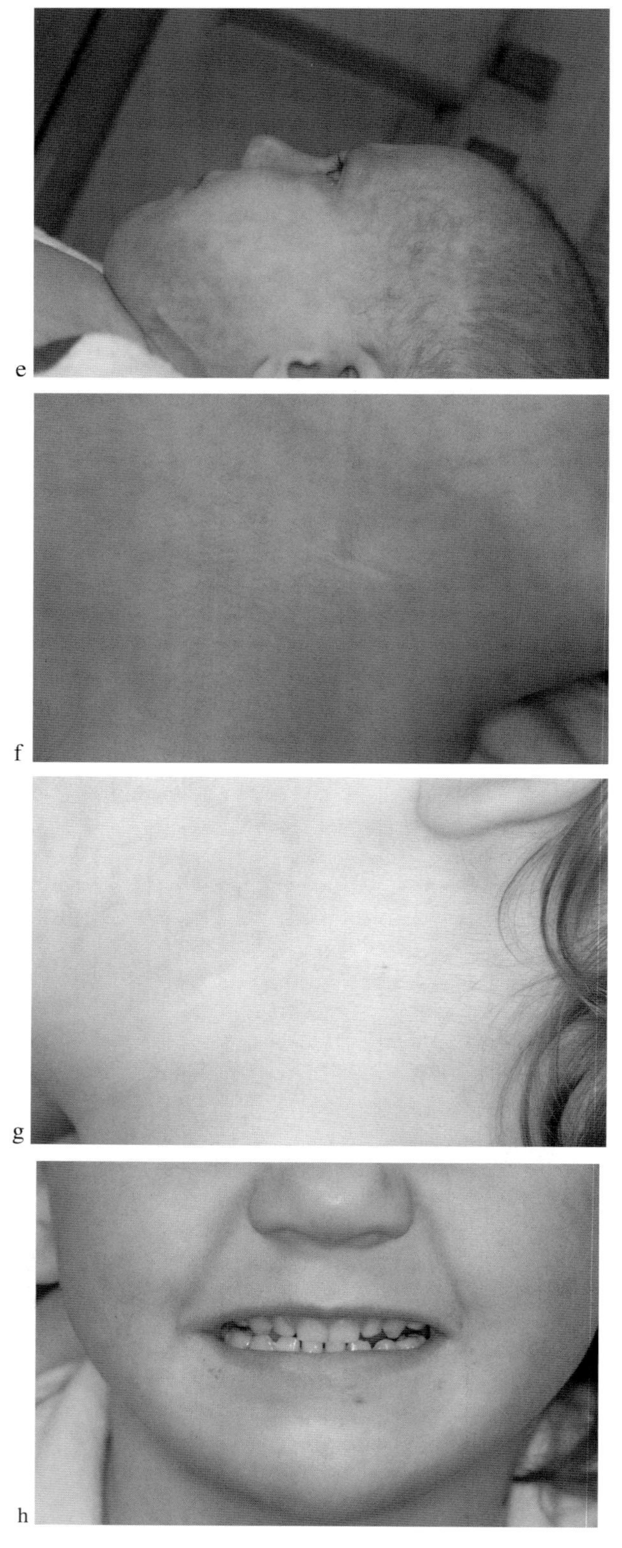

Fig. 10.8 (continued) – note the expansion of distance between the footplates of the distraction device and the large expansion in the airway space; 10.8e) Immediate post-op following removal of distraction devices, note incision healing; 10.8f, 10.8g) scars of neck well healed at two years post- distraction; 10.8h) Dental occlusion at 30 months of age

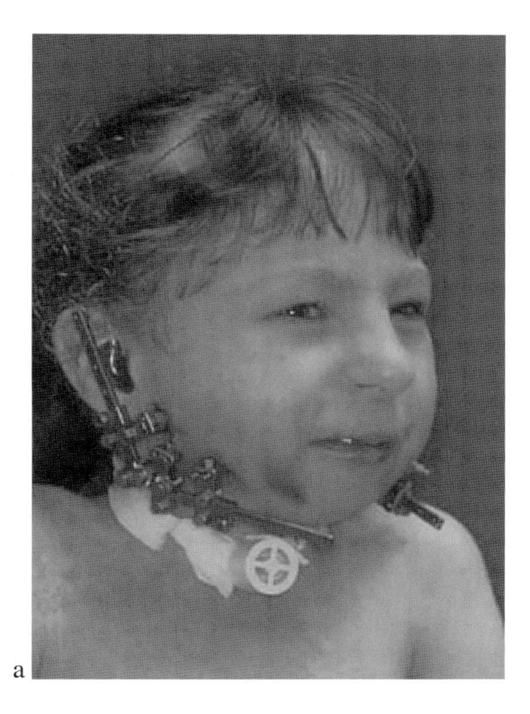

a

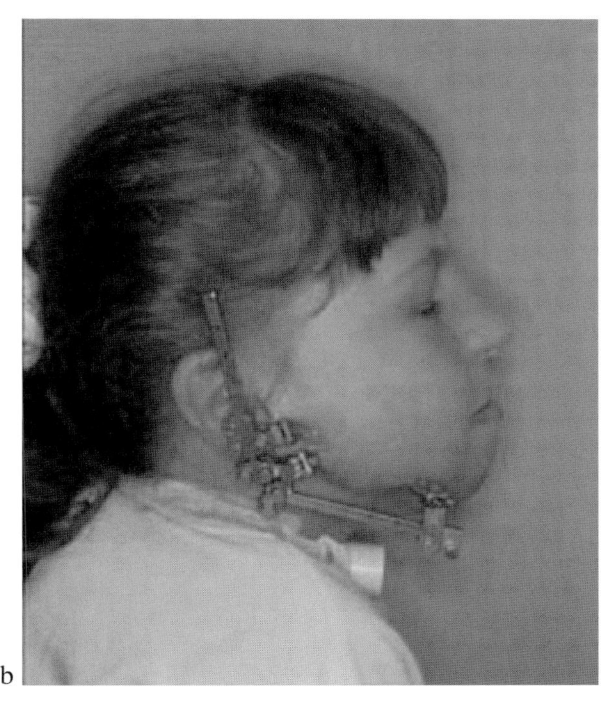

b

Fig. 10.9 Pin fixed mandibular distraction device placed at six years of age. 10.9a) At the initiation of distraction; 10.9b) At the completion of distraction; 10.9c) Two years post-operatively. The scar with the external device/percutaneous pin method, where the pins pass through the cheek skin, is generally less favorable than the Risdon technique, but the device allows for multiangular distraction

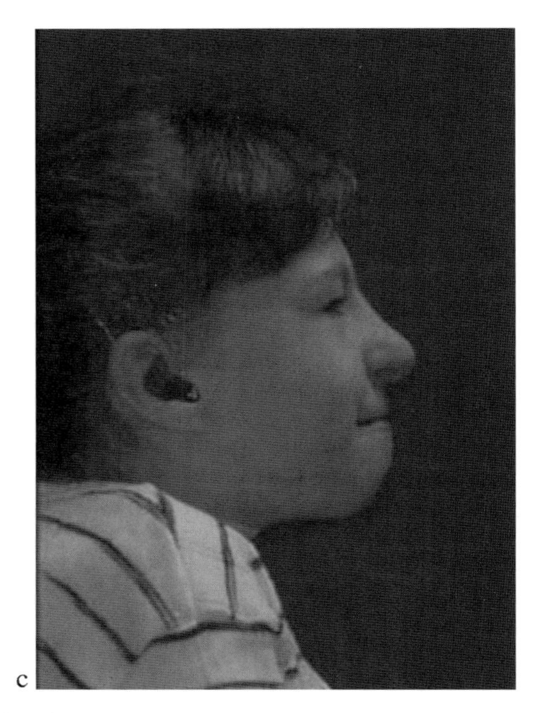

c

Fig. 10.9 (continued)

muscle, elevate the soft tissue off of the side of the mandible, and perform a vertical cut through the ramus of the mandible, posterior to the dentition and the inferior alveolar nerve (Fig. 10.8a). The device (titanium microdistractor) is then affixed to the body of the mandible along its inferior border, and to the posterior portion of the ramus in any position to allow for the proper alignment and vector of distraction. The latency period prior to the beginning of the actual process of bone distraction is three to four days after surgery, and distraction is carried out according to Ilizarov's protocol of one millimeter per day advancement [4]. Distraction is continued until the lower jaw is advanced such that the alveolus in infants (gum line) or dentition of the lower jaw lies just in front of the upper alveolus or dentition (usually 15 to 20 mm advancement). The consolidation period for bony healing then requires approximately six to eight weeks. A second surgery to remove the device is performed approximately three months after the initial surgery.

Distraction osteogenesis has become the preferred technique for the treatment of many disorders with mandibular hypoplasia. In general, these applications include "large-scale" movements for which conventional jaw surgery is not well suited and prone to relapse. Refinements of the distraction process include the development of a multi-axial, multi-angular distractor by McCarthy and colleagues [14]. Burstein and colleagues have recently reported an innovative approach using a distraction appliance that is dissolvable, so that a second surgery for removal is not necessary [31, 32].

10.6. Distraction Osteogenesis in the Middle Facial Skeleton – Maxilla and Zygoma

The midface is defined as the area between and including the lower orbits and the upper dentition. Surgical advancement of the midface can be performed to address midfacial deficiencies with occlusal abnormalities of the dentition; improve the prominence of the eyes due to maxillary hypoplasia (ocular proptosis); improve facial aesthetics by improving the relationship between the forehead, the zygoma, the eye and the mandible, and improve the airway. The surgical procedures commonly employed include the LeFort I osteotomy, the LeFort III osteotomy, or the monobloc advancement (Figs. 10.10, 10.11 and 10.12). If the problem lies solely at the level of the dental occlusion, then a LeFort I osteotomy and advancement is likely all that is needed. The LeFort I osteotomy can be performed through a trans-oral approach, by the use of an incision behind the upper lip. The LeFort I requires the surgeon to perform osteotomies through the maxillary and nasal walls, followed by separation of the maxilla and palatine bones from the pterygoid plates at the pterygo-maxillary fissure.

If orbital/ocular issues such as ocular proptosis and ocular exposure are problematic and need to be addressed, as is frequently the case in syndromic craniofacial dysostoses such as Apert's syndrome, Crouzon's syndrome, Saethre-Chotzen syndrome and Pfeifffer's syndrome, then the LeFort III osteotomy or monobloc osteotomy is necessary (Figs. 10.11, 10.12). These procedures typically require a scalp incision and reflection of the forehead with a circumferential dissection of the orbital contents (eye and ocular muscles) from the surrounding bone of the orbit. In the LeFort III the bone is cut just below the nasofrontal junction and the cribiform plate that separates the brain from the nasal cavity. The bone cut then extends down the medial wall of the orbit, and across the orbital floor to the inferior orbital fissure. In addition, the bone is cut through the lateral orbital rim, extending down to the inferior orbital fissure. Craniofacial separation is then performed at the junction between the pterygoid plates and the maxilla – the pterygo-maxillary junction. In a monobloc osteotomy, a frontal craniotomy is performed and the bone between the eye and the brain (orbital roof) is cut, and this cut is continued down the medial and lateral orbital walls, and across the orbital floor, essentially creating a circumferential cut through each orbit (Fig. 10.12). The osteotomies through the orbits are connected to each other anterior to the cribiform plate, the bone

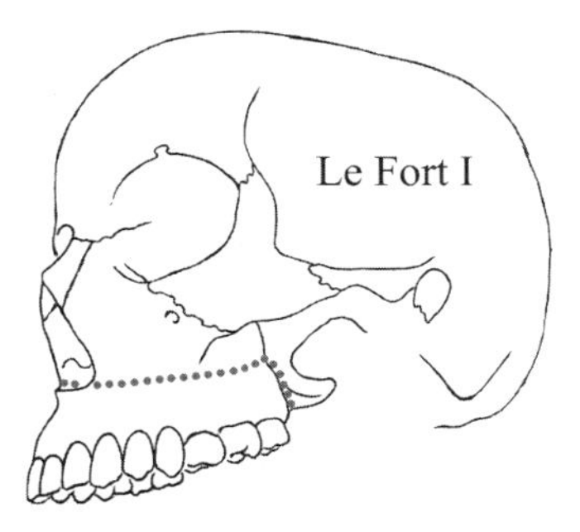

Fig. 10.10 Illustration of Le Fort I osteotomy, with bone cut depicted a typical lower midfacial site. Separation between the skull base and the maxilla occurs at the pterygo-maxillary fissure *(illustration courtesy of Min Li, M.D.)*

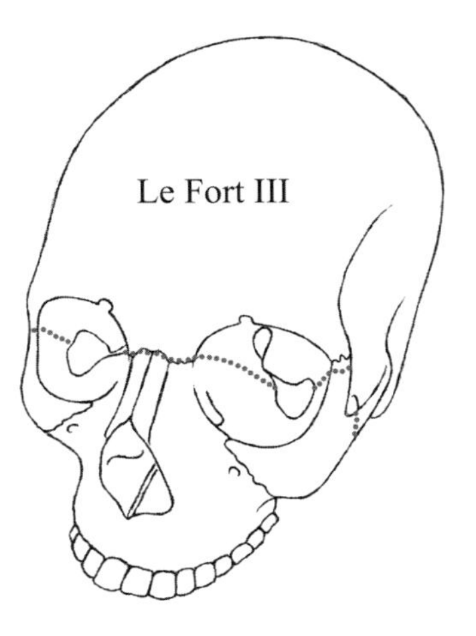

Fig. 10.11 Illustration of a subcranial Le Fort III osteotomy, with bone cut depicted across the nasofrontal junction and the orbital floors, in addition to the lateral orbital wall and the zygomatic arch. Separation between the skull base and the maxilla occurs at the pterygo-maxillary fissure. Illustration courtesy of Min Li, M.D.

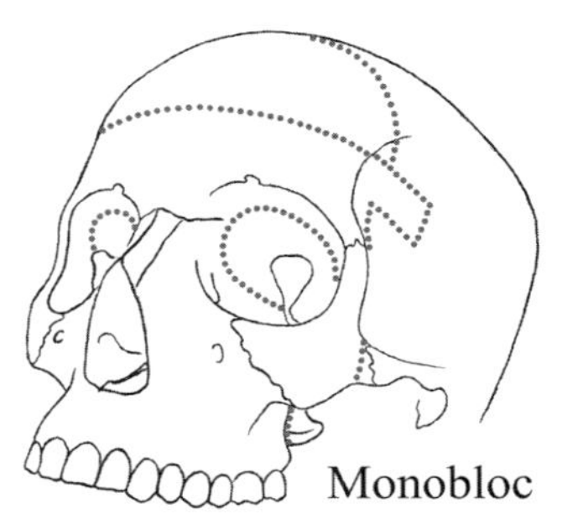

Fig. 10.12 Illustration of a "monobloc" osteotomy, with bone cut depicted across the forehead and circumferentially around the orbital walls and across the zygomatic arch. In addition, the bone cut traverses the anterior cranial base in front of the cribiform bone. Separation between the skull base and the maxilla occurs at the pterygo-maxillary fissure. Illustration courtesy of Min Li, M.D.

that separates the brain from the nasal cavity. The midface is then separated by craniofacial separation at the junction between the pterygoid plates and the maxilla – the pterygo-maxillary junction.

In conventional jaw surgery – at either the LeFort I, the LeFort III or the monobloc level – it is often difficult to obtain larger scale advancements of greater than 10 millimeters [33, 34]. While several authors do report stability with large scale advancement [35-37], concern exists regarding stability with consistently large scale advancements and the possibility of relapse [33, 38, 39]. Although plates and screws and "rigid" fixation are employed, the potential for "relapse" of the advancement obtained at surgery does exist in larger scale advancements, particularly in patients with scarring from prior cleft surgery. This may occur through constant pressure and osteolysis at the screw-bone interface. Therefore, distraction osteogenesis has been applied in those situations requiring larger scale corrections at the LeFort I [40, 41], LeFort III [38, 42] and monobloc [43-45] levels.

The technical issues in midface distraction osteogenesis are many, and of considerable significance. First, the bone that is being distracted is lamellar. It is not tubular, and there is no medullary cavity. Second, unlike previous areas of the body in which distraction osteogenesis has been applied, the distraction gap does not consist of a single site, but is complex and actually has multiple osteotomy sites throughout the entire midface, whether a LeFort I, a LeFort III or a monobloc advancement. Third, the bone on either side of the osteotomy and distraction gap is irregular in shape and contour, and different hardware may be necessary to provide optimal fixation to the bone for each side of the distraction gap. For example, optimal bone fixation requires a different approach for the cranium than the face following craniofacial separation. Similarly, the linkage system that is responsible for driving the distraction components apart by one millimeter per day also deserves special consideration as a linkage between two potentially non-similar bone fixation devices.

Three primary approaches to midfacial distraction have been used to date –two utilizing internal devices and a third using an external approach. The initial description of midfacial distraction by Chin and Toth [34, 40] utilized an internal straight screw driven appliance. This threaded device is mounted perpendicular to the facial plane, with footplates attached to the zygoma and the maxilla, and the lower midface was slowly advanced. Cohen and colleagues described an internal distraction device based upon an orthodontist jackscrew [46]. This device was placed in the temporal area and secured to the body of the zygoma. Advancement occurred by turning a cable that exited remotely.

Difficulties with these internal devices exist with some of the subpopulations with midfacial hypoplasia that have been treated with the LeFort III and monobloc osteotomies using these internal devices. It is well-known that the maxillary-zygomatic junction (or suture) is inherently unstable in many of the facial dysostoses [33]. This has led to dissociation and separation of the body of the zygoma from the maxilla during advancement, and also led to the development of a transverse facial concavity, or "dish-face," in place of the aesthetically pleasing transverse facial convexity. It is of critical importance that the distraction process maintains a transverse facial convexity and also corrects the vertical facial concavity in these syndromic patients for optimal facial aesthetics. If the distraction is performed at the monobloc level instead of the LeFort III level, stability is often maintained due to force loading through the rigidity of the supraorbital bar, or 'bandeau,' thereby significantly bypassing the instability of the maxillary-zygomatic suture. In addition, another significant limitation with current internal distraction devices is that the distraction vector is "set" at the time of surgery and cannot be adjusted as the facial advancement occurs. Several solutions for these inherent problems have been advanced [33], but for many surgeons, these limitations have led to a preference of external distraction devices over the internal devices in the midface.

The external device was first adapted for distraction osteogenesis by Polley and Figueroa [41, 43] and can be used for either the LeFort I, Lefort III or monobloc levels. This device consists of an external frame made of lightweight aluminum that is supported on the skull by percutaneous "pins" in the manner of a neurosurgical "halo." These pins are supported on the lateral aspect of the skull with either three or four pins per side. The frame is discontinuous posteriorly and extends around the anterior three-quarters of the skull. Anteriorly, a vertical carbon fiber rod extends inferiorly in front of the face, and this rod serves as a post for supporting the screw driven distraction frames. Either one or two cross-members are supported by the vertical bar, and these cross-members serve as the fixation point for screw driven distraction points (Fig. 10.13). This entire frame serves as one site of bone fixation to the skull.

The second site of bone fixation can be either to a metallic appliance fixed to the maxillary dentition [41], to a dental borne appliance that is also attached to the facial skeleton [38] or to a dental device that is wired circumferentially around the palate [42]. The linkage system between the midface and the halo, attached to the skull, is provided by surgical stainless steel wire. Although this is not truly a "rigid" linkage system between the points of bone fixation (the midface and the skull), it can be considered functionally rigid since the "floating" midface following osteotomy is always under considerable tension from the anterior pull of the wires. This has been proven clinically to reliably lead to lamellar bone formation at the level of the pterygomaxillary junction [39]. In addition, unlike internal distractors where the vector of the distraction advancement is set at the time of device placement, the external device allows adjustment of the distraction vector in all three dimensions as the distraction proceeds, allowing the process to be "fine-tuned" as distraction proceeds (Figs. 10.13d, 10.13e).

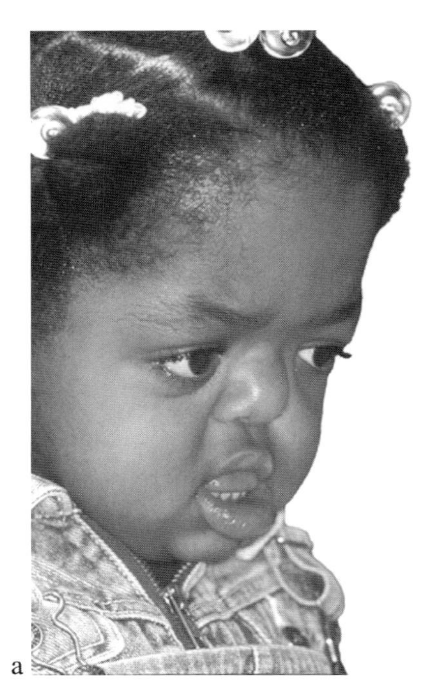

Fig. 10.13 Photographs and illustration of midfacial distraction osteogenesis at LeFort III level. 10.13a) Hypoplastic midface characteristic of Apert's syndrome; 10.13b) Acrylic dental splint fabricated with indwelling metallic tubes for distraction process; 10.13c) Illustration of distraction splint in place. It is essential to note that the illustration is drawn for clarity. In practice, there is an additional pair of wires that passes through the acrylic splint (one on each side) and passes through the soft palate and encircles the hard palate to provide rigid attachment of the acrylic splint to the dentition; 10.13d) Distraction halo and splint in place in mid-distraction; 10.13e) Following completion of distraction, note improvement in cranio-orbital-midfacial relationships, as well as occlusal relationship

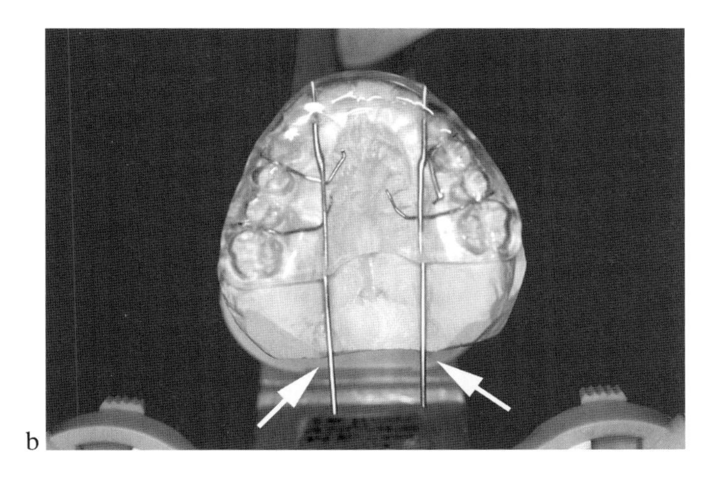

b

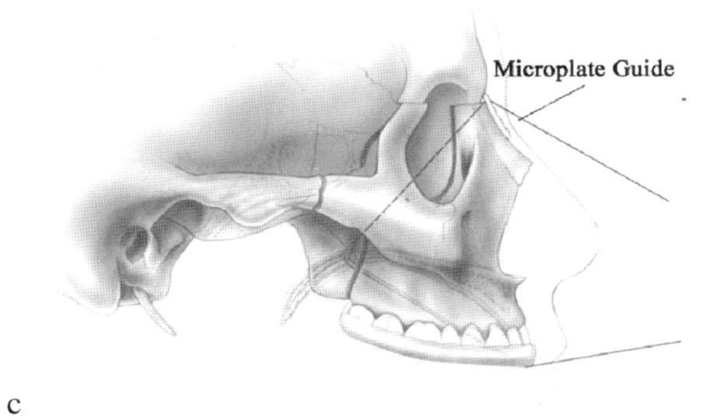

c

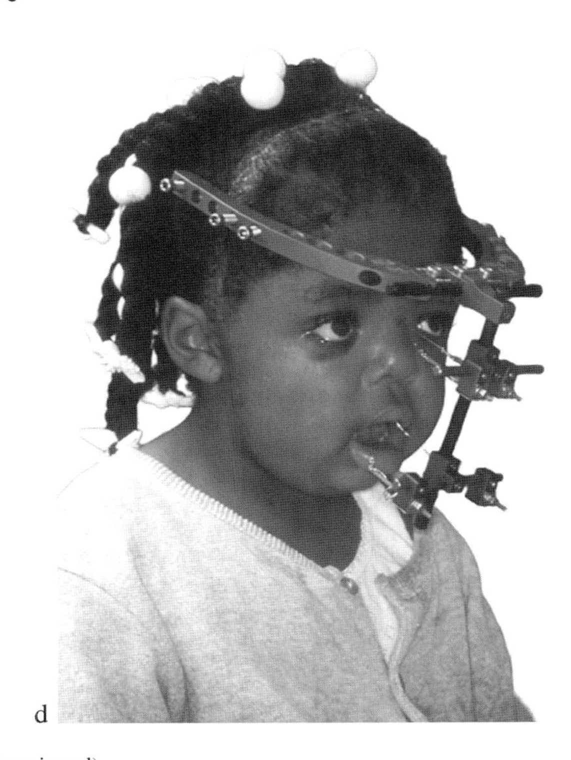

d

Fig. 10.13 (continued)

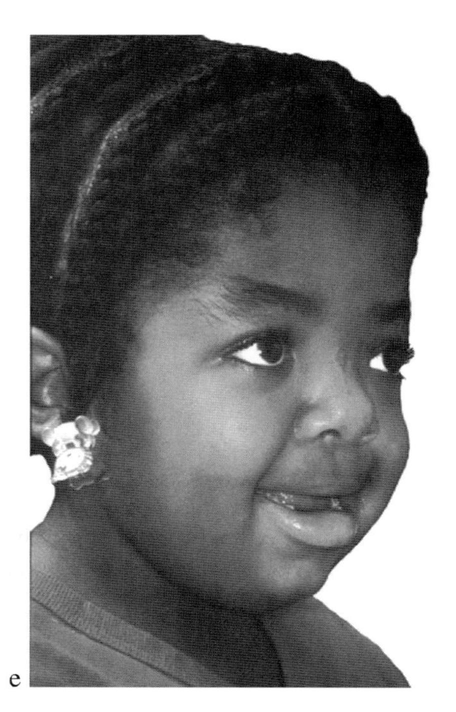

e

Fig. 10.13 (continued)

10.7. Distraction Osteogenesis in the Upper Facial Skeleton – Frontal Bones and Upper Orbit

The upper facial skeleton consists of the frontal bones of the skull. These bones have a complex architecture that is responsible for the forehead and the upper orbital architecture. The frontal bones also show changes with age. In late childhood (5-8 years), the frontal sinus ducts invade the frontal bones and create the frontal sinuses. The frontal bones are routinely divided by surgeons into upper and lower frontal components, primarily because in most conventional surgical procedures a transverse osteotomy is performed through the frontal bones 10 to 15 millimeters above the upper rim of the orbit to allow direct visualization of the anterior cranial base and the roof of the orbit, and to allow for safe and direct surgical approach to these anatomical areas. The lower frontal bone is known as the brow, the supraorbital bar or the "bandeau."

The frontal bones are frequently involved in both "simple" synostosis (premature coronal and metopic suture closure) as well as the more complex faciocraniosynostoses such as Apert's, Crouzon's, Sethre-Chotzen, etc. The vast majority of these cases are successfully managed by conventional surgical approaches and rigid fixation of the bone fragments using either resorbable or metallic plate and screw fixation devices. The advancements and reconstructions obtained by conventional surgery have proven to be reliable and reasonably stable.

The success of conventional surgical approaches to manage the upper face and upper orbit has led to a limited need and, consequently, a limited use of distraction osteogenesis of the frontal bones. This is reflected in the data from a survey of the clinical utilization of distraction osteogenesis by craniofacial and oral and maxillofacial surgeons performed by Mofid, et al. [19] that showed that less than 1 percent of surgeries involved distraction osteogenesis in the upper face and orbit, compared with 27 percent in the midface and 71 percent in the mandible. Although this survey was performed over five years ago, there is little to suggest that the relative use of the techniques in the three separate facial domains has recently changed significantly. The only minor exception to this is when the supraorbital bar is utilized with the midface as a "monobloc" for midfacial advancement, and even in this application, utilization is limited.

The anatomic considerations in the cranial vault include a very low load demand profile and cortical bone that is derived from membranous origin. During maturation at four to six years of age, the majority of the bone in the skull (from temporal crest to temporal crest) will develop an inner and outer cortical plate with an intervening diploic space of medullary-type bone.

Several different technologies have been advocated for use in the cranial vault, including small screw driven appliances similar to the midfacial devices [44, 45], as well as large metal springs [47]. Like the midface, application of the screw driven device requires a percutaneous activation cable [44, 46]. There have been no large series of experience with these devices. Lauritzen, et al. first reported experience with the large implantable spring technique in 1998, and they have since reported favorable results in a series of 10 patients with bicoronal synostosis treated with this technique in 2001 [47]. Methodologically, the technique does not follow the Ilizarov principle of screw driven distraction of the bone fragments at a fixed length per day, and this should be noted [7]. Further experience with this technique is necessary before it can be widely recommended.

10.8. Conclusions

Distraction osteogenesis has been established as a safe and effective modality for the treatment of facial anomalies in patients of all ages. The principles and the technique provide a powerful tool for the treatment of those problems that were previously treated with limited effectiveness by conventional methods. The application of distraction osteogenesis to the three domains of the facial skeleton requires an appreciation of both the specific anatomical considerations that are present at each site, and the utilization of a device of optimal design and configuration for that specific domain of the face. One size does not fit all. The refinement in both technique and hardware utilizing these principles that has occurred in the past 15 years is substantial. As the technique continues to evolve and expand into new applications, further refinement will be required for the hardware components necessary to meet new challenges.

References

1. Codivilla A, On the means of lengthening in the lower limbs, the muscles and tissues which are shortened through deformity. Am. J. Orthoped. Surg., 1905;2: 353–358.

2. Putti V, The operative lengthening of the femur. JAMA, 1921;77: 934–935.
3. Moseley CF, Leg lengthening: The historical perspective. Orthop Clin North Am, 1991. 22: p. 555-561.
4. Ilizarov GA, Clinical application of the tension-stress effect for limb lengthening. Clin Orthop, 1992;250:8-26.
5. Ilizarov GA, The tension-stress effect on the genesis and growth of tissues. Part I: The influence of stability of fixation and soft-tissue preservation. Clin Orthop, 1989;238:249-281.
6. Ilizarov GA, The tension-stress effect on the genesis and growth of tissues. Part II: The influence of the rate and frequency of distraction. Clin Orthop, 1989;239: 263-285.
7. Ilizarov GA, The transosseous synthesis: Theoretical and clinical aspects of regeneration and the growth of tissue. 1992, Berlin: Springer-Verlag.
8. Caplan AI, The mesengenic process. Clinics in Plastic Surgery, 1994;21: 429-435
9. Schenck R, Histology of fracture repair and non-union. AO/ASIF Instructional Course Bulletin. Davos:AO/ASIF, 1978.
10. Bruder SP, Fink DJ, and Caplan AI, Mesenchymal stem cells in bone development, bone repair, and skeletal regeneration therapy. J Cell Biochem, 1994;56:283-294.
11. Caplan, A., *Mesenchymal stem cells*. Journal of Orthopedic Research, 1991. 9: p. 641-50.
12. Caplan AI, Bone development. Ciba Foundation Symposium, 1993. 136: p. 3-21.
13. McCarthy JG, Schreiber J, Karp N, Thorne CH, Grayson BH, Lengthening of the human mandible by gradual distraction. Plast Reconstr Surg, 1992;89: 1-8.
14. McCarthy JG, Williams JK, Grayson BH, Crombie JS, Controlled multi-planar distraction of the mandible: Device development and clinical application. J Craniofac Surg, 1998;9:322-329.
15. McCarthy JG, Stelnicki EJ, Mehrara BJ, Longaker MT, Distraction osteogenesis of the craniofacial skeleton. Plast Reconstr Surg, 2001;107: 1812-1827.
16. McCarthy JG, Katzen JT, Hopper R, Grayson BH, The first decade of mandibular distraction: Lessons we have learned. Plast Reconstr Surg, 2002;110:1704-1713.
17. Karp NS, Thorne CH, McCarthy JG, Sissons HA, Bone lengthening in the craniofacial skeleton, Ann Plast Surg, 1990;24: 231-237.
18. Snyder CC, Levine GA, Swanson HM, Browne EZ, Mandibuar lengthening by gradual distraction:preliminary report. Plast Reconstr Surg., 1973;51:506-508.
19. Mofid MM., Manson PN, Robertson BC, Tufaro AP, Elias JJ, Vander Kolk CA, Craniofacial distraction osteogenesis: A review of 3278 cases. Plast Reconstr Surg, 2001;108:1103-1114.
20. Robin P, Glossoptosis due to atresia and hypotrophy of the mandible. Am J Dis. Child, 1934;48: 541-end page.
21. Randall P, The Robin sequence: Micrognathia and glossoptosis with airway obstruction, in Plastic Surgery, J. McCarthy, Editor. 1990, W.B.Saunders: Philadelphia. p. 3123-34.
22. Denny AD, Talisman R, Hanson PR, Recinos RF, Mandibular distraction osteogenesis in very young patients to correct airway obstruction. Plast Reconstr Surg, 2001;108:302-311.
23. Singhal V. Mandibular distraction osteogenesis in preventing tracheostomy in children with upper airway obstruction secondary to micrognathia. in ASPS/PSEF/ ASMS 71st Annual Meeting. 2002. San Antono, TX.
24. Denny AD, Distraction osteogenesis in Pierre Robin neonates with airway obstruction. Clin in Plast Surg, 2004;31:221-229.
25. Denny A, Amm C, New technique for airway correction in neonates with severe Pierre Robin sequence. J Pediatr, 2005;147: 97-101.
26. Denny A, Kalantarian B, Mandibular distraction in neonates: a strategy to avoid tracheostomy. Plast Reconstr Surg, 2002;109:896-904.

27. Singhal V, Neonatal internal mandibular distraction osteogenesis for upper airway management in Pierre Robin and other syndromic infants - Short term follow-up in American Association of Plastic Surgeons - 85th Annual Meeting. 2006. Hilton Head, SC.
28. Pruzansky S, Not all dwarfed mandibles are alike. Birth Defects, 1969;5(2):120-129.
29. Kaban LB, M. Moses MH, Mulliken JB, Surgical corrections of hemifacial microsomia in the growing child. Plast Reconstr Surg, 1980;82: 9-19.
30. Stelnicki EJ, Lin WY, Lee C, Grayson BH, McCArthy JG, Long-term outcome study of bilateral mandibular distraction: A comparison of Treacher Collins and Nager syndromes to other types of micrognathia. Plast Reconstr Surg, 2002;109: 1819-1825.
31. Burstein FD, Williams JK, Hudgins R, Graham L, Teague G, Paschal M, Simms C, Single stage craniofacial distraction using resorbable devices. J Craniofac surg 2002;13:776-782.
32. Burstein FD, Williams JK Mandibular distraction osteogenesis in Pierre Robin sequence: Application of a new internal single stage resorbable device. Plast Reconstr Surg, 2005;115: p. 61-67.
33. Gosain AK, Santoro TD, Havlik RJ, Cohen SR, Holmes RE, Midface distraction following LeFort III and monobloc osteotomies: Problems and solutions. Plast Reconstr Surg, 2002;109:1797-1808.
34. Chin M, Toth BA, LeFort III advancement with gradual distraction using internal devices. Plast Reconstr Surg, 1997;100:819-830.
35. Phillips JH, George AK, Thompson B, LeFort III osteotomy or distraction osteogenesis imperfecta: Your choice. Plast Reconstr Surg, 2006;117:1255-1260.
36. McCarthy JG, La Trenta GS, Breitbart AS, Grayson BH, Bookstein FL, The LeFort III advancement osteotomy in the child under 7 years of age. Plast Reconstr Surg, 1990;86:633-646.
37. Kaban LB, Conover M, Mulliken JB, Midface position after LeFort III advancment: a long-term follow-up study, Cleft Palate J, 1986;3(Supp.1):75-77.
38. Fearon JA The LeFort III osteotomy: To distract or not to distract? Plast Reconstr Surg, 2001;107:1091-1103.
39. Figueroa AA, Polley JW, Friede H, Ko EW, Long term stablity after maxillary advancement with distraction osteogenesis using a rigid external distraction device in cleft maxillary deformties. Plast Reconstr Surg, 2004;114:1382-1392.
40. Chin M, Toth BA, Distraction osteogenesis in maxillofacial surgery using internal devices. Review of five cases. J Oral Maxillofac Surg, 1996;54:45-53.
41. Polley JW, Figueroa AA, Management of severe maxillary deficiency in childhood and adolescence through distraction osteogenesis with an external adjustable rigid distraction device J Craniofac Surg, 1997;8: 181-185.
42. Havlik RJ, Seelinger MJ, Fashemo DV, Hathaway R, "Cat's Cradle" midfacial fixation distraction osteogenesis after LeFort III osteotomy. J Craniofac Surg, 2004;15:946-952.
43. Polley JW, Figueroa AA, Charbel FT, Berkowitz R, Reisberg D, Cohen M, Monobloc craniomaxillofacial distraction osteogenes in a newborn with severe craniofacial synpstosis: A preliminary report. J Craniofac Surg, 1995;6:421-423.
44. Cohen SR, Boydston W, Burstein FD, Hudgins R, Monobloc distraction osteogenesis during infancy: Report of a case and presentation of a new device. Plast Reconstr Surg, 1998;101:1919-1924.
45. Arnaud E, Marchac D, Reniern D, Reduction of Morbidity of Frontofacial Monobloc Advancement by Osteodistraction. Plast Reconstr Surg., In Press.
46. Cohen SR, Rutrick RE, Burstein FD, Distraction osteogenesis in the human craniofacial skeleton: Initial experience with new distraction system. J Craniofac Surg., 1995;6:368-374.

47. Gewalli F, da Silva Guimaraes-Ferreira JP, Sahlin P, et al, Long-term follow-up of dynamic cranioplasty for brachycephaly – non-syndromic bicoronal synostosis. Scand J Plast Reconstr Surg Hand Surg, 2001;35:157-164.

11

Bone Morphogenetic Proteins and Other Bone Growth Factors

Barbara D. Boyan[1], Ramsey C. Kinney[1], Kimberly Singh[1], Joseph K. Williams[2], Yolanda Cillo[3], and Zvi Schwartz[1,4]

Abstract: Dr. Marshall Urist's discovery of the osteoinductive properties of bone morphogenetic proteins (BMPs) nearly 40 years ago marked the beginning of a new era in bone biology that has bridged the gap from bench to bedside. BMPs have the potential to greatly advance the fields of orthopaedic, oral/maxillofacial and craniofacial plastic surgery, as well as dentistry. Numerous BMPs have now been identified; of these, recombinant human BMP-2 and BMP-7 (OP-1) are the best characterized. These BMPs exert their effects via serine/threonine receptor-activated Smad signaling. Mutations that alter BMP regulation at the cellular level have been shown to result in various skeletal disorders. Animal studies in which BMPs are tested in sites that would otherwise not support bone formation have demonstrated the osteoinductive properties of several of the BMPs, and studies assessing the use of BMPs in orthotopic sites have provided great insight into optimal BMP delivery methods. Currently, BMP-2 and BMP-7 are approved for specific human orthopaedic applications. It is becoming clear that clinical use of BMPs requires application-specific testing to determine correct dosing and delivery kinetics. Autologous growth and angiogenic factors are also being explored for use in orthopaedics and will also likely play important roles in enhancing BMP delivery. Long-term effects, especially in developing bone, will need to be probed before BMP treatment can be expanded to more general clinical use. Bone morphogenetic proteins have great clinical potential; however, further investigations into their applied biology are necessary for safe and effective therapeutic applications.

Keywords: Bone morphogenetic protein, bone growth factors, orthopaedic surgery.

[1]Institute of Bioengineering and Bioscience, Georgia Institute of Technology, Atlanta, GA
[2]Craniofacial Plastic Surgery, Children's Healthcare of Atlanta, Atlanta, GA
[3]Medtronic, Inc., Memphis, TN
[4]Hebrew University Hadassah Faculty of Dental Medicine, Jerusalem, Israel

From: *Orthopedic Biology and Medicine: Musculoskeletal Tissue Regeneration, Biological Materials and Methods.*
Edited by W. S. Pietrzak © Humana Press, Totowa, NJ

11.1. Introduction

The principle of osteoinductivity was first described by Marshall Urist in 1965 when he demonstrated that demineralized bone matrix (DBM) had the ability to induce formation of mature bone ossicles in tissues that would otherwise not form bone [1]. Dr. Urist recognized the importance of this finding and hypothesized that at least part of the osteoinductivity was due to proteins released from the demineralized bone. He coined the term "bone morphogenetic protein" in 1977 [2] because protein extracts of the demineralized bone caused formation of the new bone ossicle by a process very similar to embryonic bone development. Subsequent studies showed that mesenchymal cells were recruited to the demineralized bone surface (Fig. 11.1). These cells differentiated into chondroblasts, which synthesized and ultimately calcified a Type II collagen/sulfated proteoglycan-rich extracellular matrix. Once calcification occurred the tissue was invaded by blood vessels, bringing osteoprogenitor cells to the implant site. These cells differentiated into secretory osteoblasts and formed bone on the calcified cartilage scaffold via endochondral ossification. Moreover, the cartilage was replaced by haematopoietic marrow, typical of marrow formation within the developing embryonic bone. Implantation of isolated BMPs initiates a similar cascade of events (Fig. 11.2).

Over the ensuing years, Dr. Urist inspired many scientists to investigate the proteins responsible for osteoinduction. Because the BMPs were difficult to extract from bone matrix, their route to commercialization was frustrating at best. Dr. Urist and his colleagues were able to show that there were multiple potential BMPs, as well as natural inhibitors to their activity within the bone extracts [3], but it was not until the advent of molecular technology that it was possible to definitively isolate and purify individual BMPs and to study their cellular and molecular actions. The first presentation of the genetically derived sequence for BMP was 23 years after the original description of the osteoinductive property of demineralized bone [4].

We now know that BMPs are a family of glycoproteins involved in tissue morphogenesis that are highly conserved genetically in mammals. BMPs are

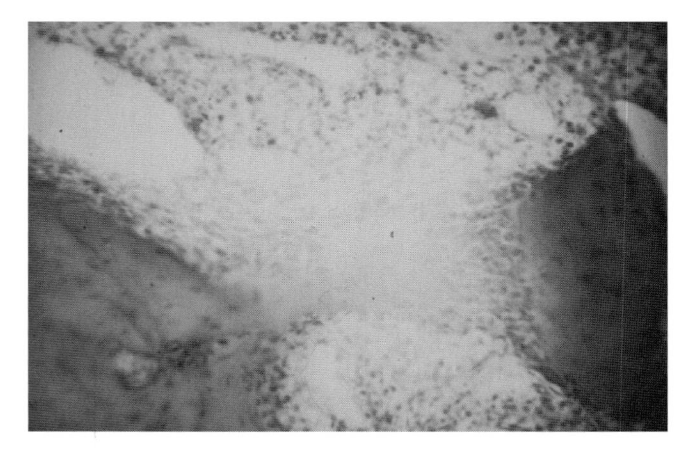

Fig. 11.1 BMP-2 causes delineation of mesenchymal cells into secretory osteoblasts *in vivo* (Courtesy of Prof. Philip Boyne, Loma Linda University). Note the influx of stem cells in the center of the section and their differentiation into osteoblast cells in the periphery

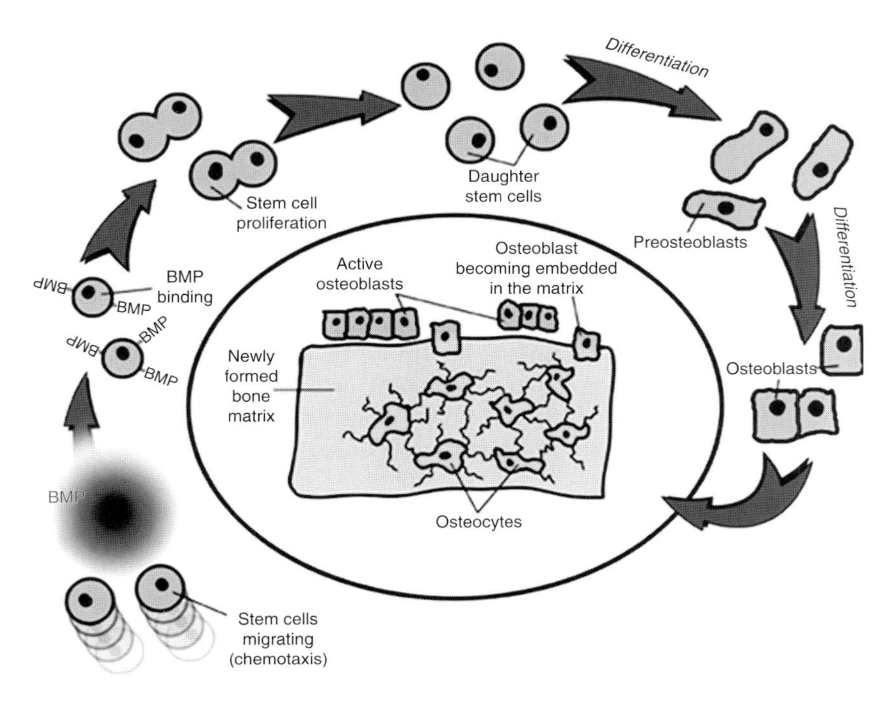

Fig. 11.2 BMP-2 acts on multipotent mesenchymal cells, inducing them to enter the osteoblast lineage, forming new bone. BMP-2 acts as a morphogen, inducing lineage commitment by first attracting stem cells towards target site. After BMP-2 binding, the stem cells begin to proliferate and differentiate into osteoblast precursors, which ultimately leads to new bone formation by osteoblasts and to their differentiation into osteocytes (Courtesy of Medtronic, Inc.)

produced by many cell types and they serve both autocrine and paracrine functions, not only during embryogenesis but also throughout the life of the animal. While they are particularly important during tissue regeneration, the BMPs also modulate normal cell differentiation and maturation, as described below. These proteins hold great promise in the repair of surgical defects caused by trauma, congenital defects, deformities and potentially following tumor resection.

11.2. Basic Science

More than 15 BMP family members have been identified and characterized (see [5–8]for reviews). These proteins share a number of features that have been conserved through evolution, indicating their importance to embryologic development and tissue homeostasis. As members of the TGF-β family, many of the BMPs possess a cysteine-knot motif [9]. The family name was defined by the ability of Urist's original purified protein to induce bone formation [1], but studies of transgenic and knockout mice, and animals and humans with naturally occurring mutations in BMPs and related genes, have shown that BMP signaling plays roles in many other organ systems, including heart, kidney, brain and cartilage. The convention of numbering BMPs evolved as a consequence of the initial cloning of four BMP genes based on the amino acid sequence of Urist's original protein [4]. BMP-1, which is not a member of the TGF-β1 family, is homologous to the decapentaplegic protein from Drosophila and has metalloproteinase activity [10]. BMP-2 is the Urist protein. BMP-3 was identified by Hari Reddi's group based on the purification of a protein from bone matrix that he termed "osteogenin" [11], and what is now known as BMP-7 was based on purification of another protein termed "osteogenic protein-1" (OP-1) [12–13]. Other BMPs were either identified through molecular technology or were isolated from tissues and found to possess homology with the earlier forms of BMP.

As a direct consequence of commercialization, scientists had access to recombinant forms of BMP-2 and BMP-7 and, for this reason, much of what we know about how BMPs function at the cellular level has resulted from studies using these two proteins. Activation of subtypes I and II serine/threonine kinase receptors initiates BMP-2 signaling [14] (Fig. 11.3). These receptors form a heterotetrameric-activated complex consisting of four type I and II receptor subunits [15]. Smad proteins play a central role in relaying the BMP signal from the receptor to target genes in the nucleus. Binding of BMP-2 to its receptor results in phosphorylation of Smads 1, 5 and 8 [16]. The phosphorylated Smads interact with Smad4, and this complex travels to the nucleus where it interacts with other transcription factors such as Runx2 as in osteoblasts [17].

BMP signaling is tightly regulated in a number of ways. Cells that produce BMPs also produce binding proteins that inhibit its ability to interact with its receptor. BMPs are stored in the extracellular matrix in latent form via binding

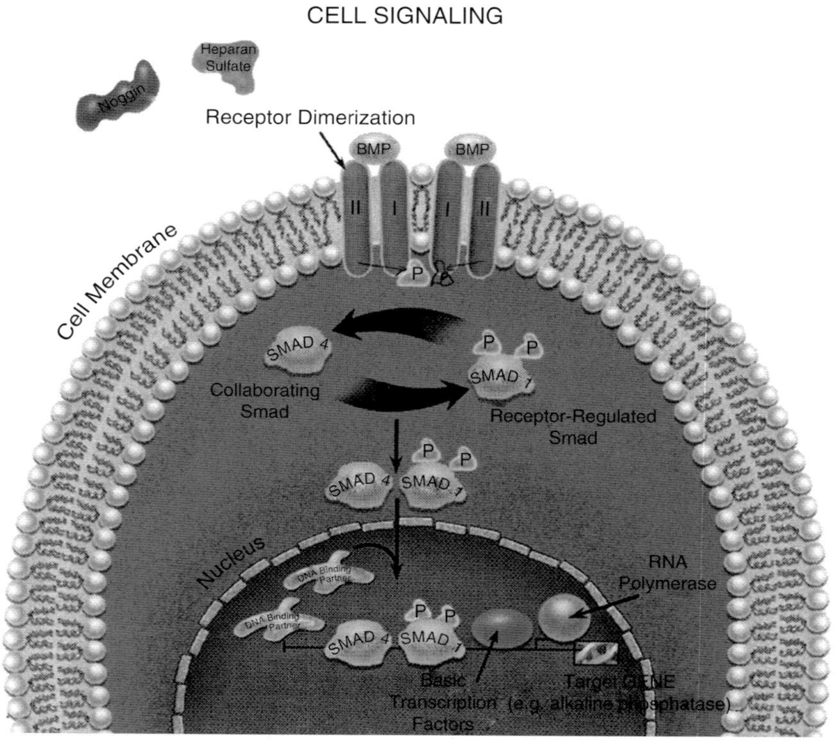

Fig. 11.3 Mechanism of BMP-2 signaling in osteoblast-like cells. BMPs bind to cell surface type I and II serine/theonine receptors. This activated receptor complex induces Smad signaling and phosphorylation whereby the Smad1 and Smad4 complex is translocated to the nucleus where it interacts with specific transcription factors for target gene production (Courtesy of Medtronic, Inc.)

proteins; unbound BMPs are rapidly degraded by extracellular proteases, further limiting their bioavailability [4]. Other proteins prevent the ability of BMPs to interact with their receptors. For example, noggin, chordin and other cysteine knot-containing BMP antagonists bind with BMP-2, 4 and 7 and block BMP signaling [18]. Within the cell, Smad6 competes for Smads 1, 5 and 8, preventing binding to Smad4, and translocation to the nucleus [19]. Ubiquitination of Smads via Smurf1 is another mechanism for downregulating response to BMPs [20].

Control of BMP availability and signaling is of critical importance to BMP-sensitive cells. Interestingly, overexpression of noggin in mature osteoblasts causes osteoporosis in mice [21]and overexpression of Smad6 in chondrocytes causes delays in chondrocyte differentiation and maturation [22]. Mutations of BMP inhibitors such as sclerostin are associated with a number of human disorders affecting the skeleton [23]. As a result, the development of BMPs for clinical use has been complex and has required extensive cell biology to provide a basis for designing appropriate delivery vehicles and dosage.

11.3. Review of Preclinical Studies

Preclinical studies have shown that BMPs can be used in various therapeutic interventions in orthopaedics including bone defects, fracture nonunions and spinal fusions. Early studies addressed the ability of individual BMPs to induce bone formation. The assay most commonly used was a variation on the model first described by Urist [24–25]. In this assay demineralized bone powders or isolated BMP-containing protein extracts were implanted intramuscularly in immunocompetent mice, rats and rabbits. Implant sites were then examined by plane X-ray to determine if bone formation had occurred. The format of the assay was formalized by Reddi, et al. [26–27] by demonstrating that the events involved followed a regular and highly reproducible time course. As the field became more sophisticated and individual proteins were tested independently, the assay also became more sophisticated. Immunocompromised mice and rats were used to eliminate the confounding variable of any potential immune response. It also became clear that X-ray alone was not a reliable end point because materials could become calcified and present as positive when, in fact, new bone formation had not occurred [8]. The results of these studies confirmed that BMPs were osteoinductive, but not necessarily to the same degree, and not all members of the family [29].

Two of the BMPs – BMP-2 (INFUSE® Bone Graft, Medtronic, Inc., Memphis, TN) and BMP-7 (OP-1®, Stryker Biotechnology, Kalamazoo, MI) – were under clinical development and were made available to academic scientists. The resulting experiments supported the osteoinductive properties of BMPs, but at the same time they revealed important issues that influenced the clinical development of both of these proteins. One of the major concerns in the preclinical development process was how to best deliver the factor. As noted above, BMPs are rapidly cleared from implant sites. When produced by cells as part of their autocrine and paracrine signaling pathways, the levels of available active protein are tightly regulated. The method of delivery had to take these problems into consideration. The Urist team developed polymeric implants for delivery of BMPs to orthotopic sites [30]. Purified BMPs were dried onto the surfaces of the polymeric scaffolds and then implanted at nonunion sites or in large bone defects, both in animal models and in human patients [31]. In a study examining treatment of chronic nonunions in dogs, Heckman, et al. incorporated purified canine BMPs into polylactic acid foams and showed successful union could be achieved [32]. However, when they used guanidine-HCl extracted bovine bone as a scaffold material, the isolated BMPs could not successfully override the inflammatory response to the implant [33]. These studies and others like them clearly demonstrated that the properties of the carrier were critical in determining the potential for clinical effectiveness.

A number of alternative carriers were suggested and tested, including demineralized bone matrix [34], polylactide co-glycolide foams [35], bovine extracellular matrix components [36–37] and composites containing calcium phosphate particles [38]. It became evident that loading capacity and release kinetics were both important variables. In addition, carriers were not equally effective at all sites. For example, when OP-1 was used with bovine collagen in tooth pulp chambers in preclinical studies, dentinogenesis was induced [39–43]. However, initial clinical studies suggested that the normal inflammatory response associated with positive bone formation intramuscularly resulted in swelling and pain in the enclosed root canal. There was also concern that any one BMP by itself would not be as effective as the natural cocktail of BMPs that could be isolated from demineralized bone. Although partially purified BMPs were effective with respect to osteoinduction, attempts to commercialize these cocktails met with frustration as relatively little was known about the identities of the many proteins that could be isolated, and there was concern that donor variability or host immune responses would be problematic [43].

Gene therapy was used as an an alternative approach, based on the hypothesis that osteoblasts or osteoprogenitor cells would then produce increased levels of a specific BMP, but in the presence of its normal regulatory companions [44–46]. While this was successful in animal models, however, it has not yet proven to be a viable commercial approach. Moreover, BMPs diffusing from an implant site can induce heterotopic bone formation; this is also the case if mesenchymal cells overexpress BMPs in non-bony sites [47].

To circumvent the delivery vehicle problem, initial studies using the genetically produced BMPs did not use a physically implantable carrier. This proved effective in some applications. In preclinical studies using a critical size segmental defect to model treatment of nonunions in humans [48], BMP-7 was injected at the time the defect was created. However, when OP-1 was used in a collagen carrier to treat nonunions in humans, the delivery method was not as effective [49].

There are a number of reasons that the preclinical and clinical studies may have differed in their outcomes. It may have been due, in part, to the very real differences between an acute defect in a rat or dog, and a chronic nonunion in humans. Other factors may have played roles as well. The quality of the healing response in acute defects and chronic nonunions differs considerably, and the types of cells that repopulate the site following resection may also differ [50]. In addition, BMP is rapidly cleared from the implant site, reducing its availability. If BMP-sensitive cells were not present at the time the BMP was present, new bone formation may not have been induced. These early studies clearly demonstrated that if a carrier was to be used, it needed to deliver BMPs at an appropriate dose and at an appropriate time.

Preclinical studies also revealed another confounding variable, the need to increase BMP dose with movement up the phylogenetic tree (Table 11.1).

Table 11.1 Effective dosing of BMP-2 differs among species as shown by the increase in BMP-2 dosage and healing time as the size of the animal increases

Species Time	BMP-2 Concentration (mg/mL)	Healing
Rat	0.01–0.05	2–3 wks
Rabbit	0.2–0.4	3–4 wks
Dog	0.75	6–8 wks
Monkey	0.75–1.5	3–6 mo
Human	1.5	6–12 mo

Martin, Boden, et al., *J. Spinal Disorders*, 1999

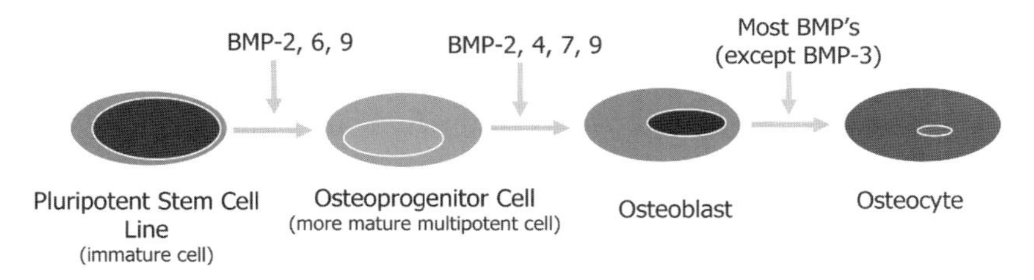

Fig. 11.4 BMPs act at different points in the osteoblast lineage. Pluripotent mesenchymal stem cells are induced to become multipotent osteoprogenitor stem cells by BMPs-2, -6 and -9. Further differentiation into mature osteoblasts is achieved by exposure of these cells to BMPs -2, -4, -7 and -9 before becoming mature osteocytes via additional exposure to BMPs (Adapted from Cheng, et al., *JBJS* 2003; 85:1544–1552; Courtesy of Prof. Philip Boyne)

Early studies using mice and rats underestimated the dose needed for effectiveness in rabbits, and studies using rabbits did not predict doses needed for canines, nonhuman primates or humans. Exactly why this is so is not yet well understood. It may be related, in part, to the requirement for an appropriate dose to be present when cells expressing BMP receptors and a competent signaling apparatus are present. Mice and rats exhibit more rapid healing responses than are seen in higher level animals. In addition, laboratory studies use younger animals to limit costs, but human clinical studies are performed in older subjects. It has been known for some time that the osteoinductivity of demineralized bone varies with the age of donor animal [51] or human [52], and with the age of the recipient animal. The concentration of BMP-2 in bone also decreases with age [53], and bone healing is slower in older humans due to reduced numbers of mesenchymal stem cells [54].

This may also help explain differences in response to BMP-2 or BMP-7 in various clinical applications. BMP-2 acts on multipotent mesenchymal stem cells (Fig. 11.4), inducing them to differentiate into chondrocytes or osteoblasts depending on treatment site and environmental factors such as oxygen tension. Recently, we also found that effectiveness of BMP-2 *in vitro* depends on the substrate used to culture the cells (Boyan, et al., unpublished). Human mesenchymal stem cells exhibit greater osteoblastic differentiation when grown on calcium phosphate surfaces than on tissue culture polystyrene, suggesting that osteoblastic differentiation may be enhanced when an osteoconductive material is used in an orthotopic site.

BMP-7 appears to act on cells further along the osteochondral cascade [55] (Fig. 11.4). Once osteogenesis is initiated, both BMP-2 and BMP-7 act on the differentiating osteoblasts, but at different points in the lineage. Thus, different carriers with different release kinetics are needed for optimal delivery of these factors.

11.4. Clinical Review

Recombinant forms of human BMP-2 and human BMP-7 (OP-1) are now approved for use in orthopaedics in the United States, but for different applications. Recombinant human BMP-2 (rhBMP-2) is approved for use in spinal anterior interbody fusions, and for acute open tibia fractures when delivered on an absorbable collagen sponge (INFUSE® Bone Graft, Medtronic, Inc., Memphis, TN). Recombinant human BMP-7 (rhBMP-7; OP-1®, Stryker Biotech, Kalamazoo, MI) has been approved via a humanitarian device exemption (HDE) for use in chronic nonunions as an alternative to autograft in recalcitrant bone nonunions where alternative treatments have failed, and in revision posterolateral spine fusions in compromised patients. In both of these indications for use, a criterion is that autograft is not available. Although each of these approvals were based on pre-market approval studies that demonstrate safety, only the INFUSE® Bone Graft approvals demonstrated effectiveness in two separate pre-market approval studies (PMAs).

11.4.1. Spinal Fusion

The first BMP to receive an approval for use in spinal fusion procedures was rhBMP-2 INFUSE® Bone Graft, which became commercially available in July 2002. The initial approval for use with the LT-CAGE® Lumbar Tapered Fusion Device (Medtronic, Memphis, TN) was given based on data from a large IDE/PMA study involving 279 patients receiving INFUSE® Bone Graft, and 143 receiving iliac crest autograft for one level anterior lumbar interbody fusion in which INFUSE® Bone Graft was found to be equivalent to autogenous iliac crest bone graft.

Multiple clinical studies, including the above study, were combined into an integrated analysis evaluating 679 patients in which 277 patients had cages placed with INFUSE® Bone Graft, and 402 had cages with iliac crest autograft [56]. In this analysis the patients who received INFUSE® Bone Graft had statistically significantly superior outcomes with regard to blood loss, length of hospital stay, re-operation rate, median time to return to work and fusion rates at six, 12 and 24 months. In addition, at three, six, 12 and 24 months, the Oswestry Disability Index scores and the Physical Component Scores and Pain Index of the SF-36 scale showed statistically significant improvement of outcomes in the INFUSE® Bone Graft group, compared to the group receiving autograft.

Since the original approval in 2002 the FDA has expanded the INFUSE® Bone Graft approved indications to include use with an INTERFIX Cage and to include spinal levels L2-S1. Additional publications report the use of INFUSE® Bone Graft with stand-alone allograft bone dowels [57] and other allograft bone constructs [58], in cervical fusion [59–61], in stand-alone posterior lumbar interbody fusions [62] and in transforaminal lumbar interbody fusion [63–64].

In the more challenging posterolateral fusion model, neither commercially available BMP has yet definitively shown effectiveness and received full marketing approval. The published data on OP-1 in this indication were on small numbers of patients with successful fusion rates of 55 percent (11/20), 50 percent (5/10) and 74 percent (14/19), compared to autograft fusion rates of 40 percent (4/10), 45 percent (historical control) and 60 percent (6/10) [65–67]. Another small prospective randomized study carried out in Japan [68] evaluated the use of OP-1 Putty for posterolateral lumbar fusion using pedicle screw fixation, compared to local autograft with hydroxyapatite-tricalcium phosphate (HA-TCP) granules. Radiographic fusion rates at one year postoperatively showed that seven of nine OP-1 patients, and nine of 10 autograft patients appeared fused. The hardware was then surgically removed and biopsy specimens were taken from the fusion mass in the 16 patients who appeared healed. Histologic examination revealed that although all patients had macroscopic new bone formation, only four of seven OP-1, and seven of nine of the local autograft/HA-TCP group had attained solid fusion.

Current reports on the use of INFUSE® Bone Graft in posterolateral fusion have no data from a randomized clinical trial. A pilot posterolateral study evaluating the use of INFUSE® Bone Graft supplemented with MasterGraft™ Ceramic granules (Medtronic, Memphis, TN) has completed enrollment and all patients have attained one year follow-up. There are also reports on the use of an investigational rhBMP-2 product that uses a different carrier to deliver the rhBMP-2, in this case, a collagen sponge carrier with ceramic granules imbedded within it. A different concentration of rhBMP-2 (2.0 mg/ml) is used with this carrier. Early results from one study site reporting six and 12 month follow-up from this study report a solid bilateral fusion in 26 of 37 receiving rhBMP-2 at six months, and 30 of 37 patients receiving rhBMP-2 at 12 months, compared to six of 35 receiving autograft at six months, and 15 of 35 receiving iliac crest autograft at 12 months [69]. Another study on the two year follow-up from this study combining data on 98 patients from two study sites, reported a fusion rate in the iliac crest bone graft group of 73 percent, compared to an 88 percent fusion rate in the rhBMP-2/compression resistant matrix group. Other studies have described the use of INFUSE® Bone Graft combined with iliac crest autograft [70]and in adult deformity [71]. At this time the FDA is reviewing data on both OP-1 and the new rhBMP-2 product, AMPLIFY™ Matrix or rhBMP-2 Matrix, for posterolateral spine applications.

11.4.2. Acute Long Bone Fracture

INFUSE® Bone Graft has been shown to be efficacious for use in treatment of open tibial fractures. The BESTT study is a large, 450-patient trial in which all patients received standard surgical treatment of closed intramedullary rodding and appropriate wound care with the study group of 148 patients having INFUSE® Bone Graft placed at the time of wound closure [72]. There was a 44 percent reduction in risk of failure (i.e., secondary intervention because of delayed union), significantly faster fracture healing ($p = 0.0022$) and significantly fewer invasive interventions (i.e., less requirement for bone grafting and nail exchange; $p = 0.0264$), compared to the control group who received treatment with standard of care. The investigational group also had significantly fewer hardware failures ($p = 0.0174$), fewer infections (Gustilo type III) (p = 0.0219) and improved wound healing (83 percent, compared to 65 percent at six weeks) than the control group. This study did not include fractures with areas of measurable cortical defect.

This clinical effectiveness was further established in a recent publication combining the above study with a concurrent prospective, randomized, multicenter clinical study designed to evaluate the use of rhBMP-2 to treat open tibial fractures [73]. This study was a 60-patient trial conducted in the United States that was carried out at the same time as the BESTT study. The raw patient data results of these trials were analyzed and reported together with additional subgroup analysis assessing the clinical outcomes for type-III open and for reamed intramedullary nail groups. This subgroup analysis included just those patients receiving the 1.5 mg/cc concentration of rhBMP-2 currently approved by the FDA (INFUSE® Bone Graft, Medtronic, Memphis, TN). The first subgroup consisted of 131 patients with Gustilo-Anderson type-IIIA or IIIB, and the second subgroup consisted of 113 patients treated with reamed intramedullary nails. A total of 169 patients were included in the control and investigational groups. Both studies used identical designs and measures.

In the subgroup analysis there was a reduction in the number of patients treated with rhBMP-2 who required secondary autologous bone grafting procedures to treat delayed or nonunions. Just 2 percent of the group that received INFUSE® Bone Graft required secondary bone grafting, compared to 20 percent in the control group. The authors calculated this to be a 90 percent reduction in relative risk for bone graft need and also reported a significant reduction in the number of invasive secondary interventions when INFUSE® Bone Graft was used (e.g., bone grafting, fibular osteotomy, exchange nailing) with a risk reduction of 68 percent. It was reported that fracture healing was also attained sooner in the patients receiving INFUSE® Bone Graft (average 95.1 days), compared to the control group (126.6 days).

There was no significant difference observed between the control and the INFUSE® Bone Graft group, in the subgroup treated with reamed intramedullary rods, although healing time, both clinically and radiographically, was slightly shorter in the INFUSE® Bone Graft group. This group included type I through type III B fractures. The lack of significance was believed to be due, in part, to a lack of sufficient power in this subgroup.

Although not approved for use in fractures with bone loss, a recent publication reports the results of a prospective FDA-approved IDE study evaluating the use of INFUSE® Bone Graft with freeze-dried cancellous allograft bone chips to treat diaphyseal tibial shaft fractures with substantial bone loss from 1 cm to 5 cm [74]. The allograft chips were implanted within the defect, and the INFUSE® Bone Graft was applied as an onlay around the defect site. The control group was treated with iliac crest autograft. In all patients these procedures were staged reconstructions as part of the admitting treatment plan. Eighty-seven percent (87 percent; 13/15) of the patients treated with INFUSE Bone Graft healed without further surgery, compared to 67 percent (10/15) of those treated with autograft.

OP-1 has been evaluated for use in open tibia fractures in a Canadian study completed by the Canadian Orthopaedic Trauma Society that was prospective and randomized [75]. Although these data were presented as a poster, they have not yet been published. This study evaluated 124 fractures: 62 controls that received tibial nails with wound care and 62 that received OP-1 at the time of wound closure (<7 days after injury). The primary end point for evaluation was radiographic evidence of healing and clinical follow-up at six months and rate of secondary intervention. Follow-up reported in the poster did not clearly indicate if all patients were included in the analysis. It was reported that 17 patients with standard of care required secondary intervention, compared to eight in the group that received OP-1. There was a trend towards improved functional outcome. The poster did not report the independent radiographic assessments or even clinician's assessment of radiographic rate or occurrence of fracture healing; only the number of secondary interventions which were required on an unspecified number of patients.

11.4.3. Chronic Nonunion

No BMP has yet been found to be judged effective for use in chronic non-unions based on equivalence to or superiority over controls treated with autograft. OP-1 has been studied for this indication in an FDA-approved prospective randomized clinical IDE trial evaluating 122 patients with 124 tibial nonunions [49]. At the primary end point of nine months following treatment, 81 percent of the OP-1 ($n=63$) and 85 percent of the autograft group ($n=61$) were judged healed by clinical criteria. By radiographic criteria, 75 percent of the OP-1 group and 84 percent of the autograft group were judged healed. It was reported that there was no statistical difference between the groups with continued levels of success throughout two years of observation ($p = 0.939$). In 90 percent of patients enrolled in the study, an exchange nailing was carried out at the time of the bone graft placement (OP-1 or iliac crest autograft).

Recombinant hBMP-2 has not been studied in a randomized prospective FDA-approved IDE clinical trial in this indication. Non-randomized data were presented at the 2006 Orthopaedic Trauma Association annual meeting in 2006 [76–78].

11.5. Future Trends and Needs

11.5.1. BMPs

At present the doses required for clinical effectiveness are relatively large when one considers that the concentration of BMPs in bone is less than $20\,\mu g/kg$ [6]. Producing the needed quantities of protein at a price that makes it readily accessible for the many potential uses in musculoskeletal care has been problematic. Even when one considers that BMPs reduce or even eliminate the need for bone graft, either autologous or allogeneic, the cost savings may not justify the expense for some of these procedures. In addition, although there is no evidence to suggest that there will be any long-term effects associated with use of recombinant BMPs, it is not yet known whether the large doses will have downstream consequences that we cannot now predict. For example, while there is no evidence that BMP-2 is toxic, overuse and overdosing were contributing factors to the edema that has been associated with BMP-2 use in some applications in the cervical spine [60–61]. It is possible that development of alternative delivery methods may be beneficial, but there are significant costs, as well as time factors, associated with this as any new carrier would require a large FDA IDE study. New carriers could include vehicles that will reduce the amount of protein, as well as vehicles that ensure delivery at appropriate times in the regenerative process. It is also important that we continue to study the complex biology of this powerful group of morphogens. We do not have sufficient knowledge to predict all of the negative outcomes that can result with BMP use; we do not know if or how it can be used in skeletally immature patients, and we do not have sufficient information to know whether repeated use of one or more BMPs can affect fetal development or immune response.

11.5.2. Other Growth Factors

Recombinant human BMPs are not the only approach for improving musculoskeletal tissue repair and regeneration. An alternative approach is to take advantage of the extractability of BMPs from demineralized bone. Why demineralization of bone makes the material osteoinductive is not well understood. It is believed that removal of mineral exposes BMPs stored in the extracellular matrix to mesenchymal cells at the implant site. Some of these BMPs may leach from the demineralized bone, but other material-dependent features may play roles as well. Regardless of the mechanism(s), BMPs can be isolated from demineralized bone using chaotropic agents, concentrated, and then used clinically. These natural BMP cocktails have been developed using bovine bone as the source [79]and more recent data was presented at the Orthopaedic Research Society using human demineralized bone [80].

While these natural BMP cocktails that are extracted from demineralized bone matrix show promise for clinical use in a variety of applications, they are cleared for use by the FDA through the 510K pathway as bone void fillers. The 510K pathway does not require a randomized prospective clinical trial, as is required for the recombinant proteins, nor does it require a clinical trial or clinical data, and it usually relies on animal studies for market release. Comparison of these natural cocktails, which have not been extensively studied in clinical trials, to the recombinant proteins which have, should be undertaken with caution until long-term clinical trial data are available.

One area of development is based on factors that are normally present during wound healing. When an injury occurs platelets release factors within the clot that stimulate mesenchymal cell recruitment and proliferation, reduce inflammation and stimulate angiogenesis [81–82] (Fig. 11.5). These include TGF-βs, platelet-derived growth factors (PDGF), insulin-like growth factor (IGF), vascular endothelial growth factors (VEGF) and fibroblast growth factor-2 (FGF-2). Interestingly, BMPs are also present within the clot [83]. This naturally occurring cocktail can be isolated and concentrated during surgery, suggesting that the patient's own platelet-rich plasma (PRP) could be used as a stimulator of bone formation.

A variety of methods are now commercially available for preparing PRP and a similar material termed "autologous growth factors," which is PRP plus the white blood cell buffy coat obtained during PRP preparation. Clinical outcomes using PRP have not been as hoped, however. When used in oral and maxillofacial surgery applications, PRP appears to be more effective, but thus far, it has not proven to be so in orthopaedic applications (see [84–85] for reviews). One reason for this may be that orthopaedic surgeons often use PRP with bone graft and recent studies show that it inhibits the osteoinductive properties of demineralized bone matrix [86–87], as well as osteogenic effects of BMPs on osteoblast-like cells *in vitro* [88]. While PRP has not been successful

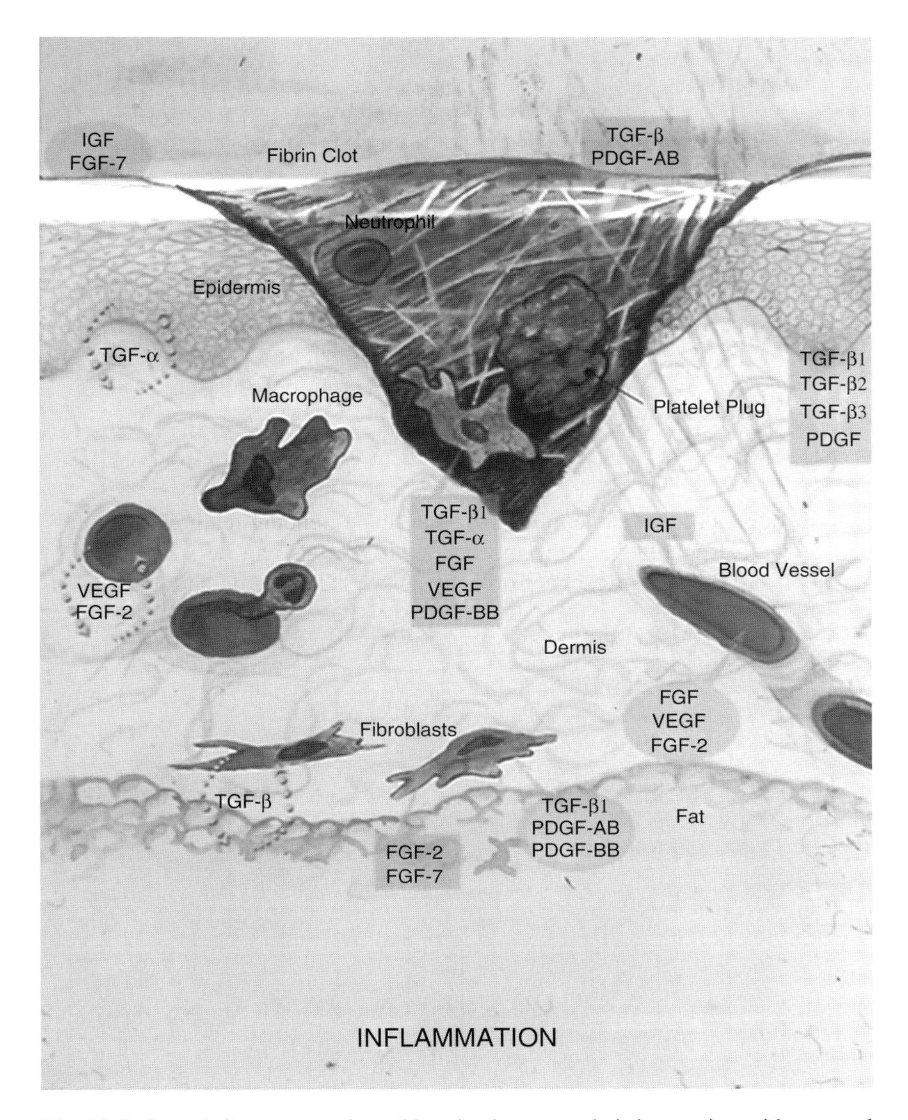

Fig. 11.5 Growth factors are released by platelets upon their interaction with exposed tissue in the wound site and contribute to local production of inflammatory markers (Courtesy of Prof. Philip Boyne). Platelets are among the first cell responders to tissue injury and form a hemostatic platelet plug. Platelets release factors within the clot that stimulate mesenchymal cell recruitment and proliferation, reduce inflammation and stimulate angiogenesis through the production of TGF-βs, platelet-derived growth factors (PDGF), insulin-like growth factor (IGF), vascular endothelial growth factors (VEGF) and fibroblast growth factor-2 (FGF-2)

as an adjunct in spinal fusion, it may prove useful in trauma. Recent studies examining the use of PRP in segmental defects indicate that it may stimulate angiogenesis, potentially leading to improved osteogenesis [89]. However, others have shown that PRP had no effect on bone formation in the same model [90]. The most likely reason for these differences in reported effects is that PRP varies considerably by donor [91].

Another approach is to use specific components of platelet releasate to enhance healing with the understanding that, although they are not osteoinductive, they may potentiate the normal healing process. Some of these factors are themselves members of the TGF-β superfamily, including TGF-β1, TGF-β3, and the growth/differentiation factors (GDFs) [92]. There is potential for these factors to enhance fibrogenesis, however, depending on dose and release kinetics. For example, TGF-β1 induces mesenchymal stem cells to differentiate into chondrocytes and is used for this purpose in tissue engineering applications [93]. When it is used *in vivo* in chondral defects, chondrogenesis is enhanced [94], but when it is used in acute bone wounds, cartilage formation does not occur; instead TGF-β1 increases mesenchymal cell proliferation and increases Type I collagen production. Thus, the site of application is a critical variable when selecting any of the growth factors for use in a musculoskeletal application.

PDGF formulated with a beta tricalcium phosphate carrier is used as a bone graft material in oral applications [95] and is under development for use in orthopaedic applications. Its primary mode of action is to increase proliferation of multipotent mesenchymal cells; thus, when it is used in a well vascularized site like bone, it may increase the supply of progenitor cells for subsequent action by differentiation signals within the local environment. As is the case with many of the growth factors, PDGF also acts on cells already committed to a musculoskeletal lineage. Studies examining the effects of PDGF on committed cartilage cells showed that the number of cells was increased without altering the ability of the cells to produce extracellular matrix rich in sulfated proteoglycans [96]. If doses were small and exposure times short, the cells retained their chondrocyte phenotype. However, at higher concentrations and longer exposure times, fibrogenesis resulted. When demineralized bone matrix was implanted with PDGF, a dose-dependent decrease in osteoinductivity was observed [86]. Both of these studies demonstrate the need for determining optimal dose *in vitro* and *in vivo* for factors of this type. More is not always better.

Vascularization is essential for bone healing and, for this reason, factors that stimulate angiogenesis are particularly intriguing as biological adjuncts to therapy. Again, dose, delivery vehicle and release kinetics are important variables. VEGF has been the most studied angiogenic factor. It induces endothelial differentiation and formation of blood vessels at the site of implantation, but for reasons that are not well understood, these small capillaries are not stable over time [97–98]. FGF-2 is also angiogenic and has been used to stimulate osteogenesis [99–100]; however, the format in which it is used is critical and not all carriers deliver FGF-2 effectively [101]. As is the case for all of the factors discussed here, FGF-2 is pleiotropic in its effects [102], and its clinical effectiveness may depend on other factors present at the implantation site.

While not growth factors in the classic sense, specific sequences of extracellular proteins may also have growth factor-like activities. There is an increasing awareness that structural proteins in the extracellular matrix can directly regulate cell activity in a growth factor-like manner. Because these amino acid motifs can be produced synthetically, they are attractive from a commercial point of view. Examples include peptide sequences in osteopontin [103] and in collagen [104], which are constituents of the bone extracellular matrix. Similarly, sequences within components of the clot or haematoma have been investigated for their potential in musculoskeletal therapies. An example is thrombin peptide 508 (TP508, Chrysalin®, OrthoLogic Corp, Tempe, AZ), which has been shown in preclinical studies to accelerate fracture healing by increasing the callus mass [105].

Finally, comment should be made about biophysical strategies that stimulate growth factor production locally. For the most part, acute bone defects will heal if the fracture ends are well apposed and stability is maintained. In some cases healing can be helped using bone growth stimulators, even if nonunion has become established. For many years the mechanisms by which biophysical stimulation exerted its effects were not understood. More recently it has become clear that they function by stimulating release of growth factors locally. For example, pulsed electromagnetic fields (PEMF) cause a rapid increase in BMP-2 mRNA in osteoblasts [106]. *In vitro* studies using human nonunion cells, human and rat osteoblasts [107] and rat chondrocytes [108], and *in vivo* studies using demineralized bone-induced bone formation as a model [109], show that PEMF increases production of TGF-β1 (see [110] for a review). Electric fields also increase IGF-1 production as well as expression of receptors for IGF-1 in osteoblasts. Similarly, ultrasound signals modulate growth factor expression [111].

11.6. Conclusions

This chapter shows that growth factors can be successfully used to treat musculoskeletal defects. In the United States only a limited number of factors are approved for use, and in a limited number of applications. While it is evident that these factors have potential far beyond their current approvals, there are many caveats that must be heeded. Dose, delivery vehicle and release kinetics are specific to each site and may also vary depending on the desired outcome at a site. Growth factors have many effects, some of which we do not yet know, and outcomes may be unpredictable. For these reasons, careful preclinical studies are essential. However, the differences in how species respond to these factors are confounding, necessitating the need for well controlled clinical studies before reaching conclusions. Single proteins are a first step, but we must remember that, in normal biology, these proteins do not exist independently of their binding proteins and natural inhibitors or of other factors that can modulate the intensity of their effects. We must eventually move to combinations of factors to best meet the specific requirements for each application.

Acknowledgements: The authors thank Professor Philip Boyne, Professor Emeritus, Loma Linda University, and Medtronic, Inc. for their generous gifts of graphics to support this paper. We acknowledge the support of Children's Healthcare of Atlanta, the Georgia Tech/Emory Center for the Engineering of Living Tissues, NIH, NSF and the Plastic Surgery Education Foundation for their support.

References

1. Urist MR. Bone: formation by autoinduction. Science 1965;150(698):893–9.
2. Urist MR, Mikulski AJ, Nakagawa M, Yen K. A bone matrix calcification-initiator noncollagenous protein. Am J Physiol 1977;232(3):C115–27.
3. Urist MR, Lietze A, Mizutani H, et al. A bovine low molecular weight bone morphogenetic protein (BMP) fraction. Clin Orthop Relat Res 1982(162):219–32.
4. Wozney JM, Rosen V, Celeste AJ, et al. Novel regulators of bone formation: molecular clones and activities. Science 1988;242(4885):1528–34.
5. Wozney JM. The bone morphogenetic protein family and osteogenesis. Mol Reprod Dev 1992;32(2):160–7.
6. Wozney JM. Bone morphogenetic proteins. Prog Growth Factor Res 1989;1(4):267–80.
7. Reddi AH. Bone and cartilage differentiation. Curr Opin Genet Dev 1994;4(5):737–44.
8. Chen D, Zhao M, Mundy GR. Bone morphogenetic proteins. Growth Factors 2004;22(4):233–41.
9. Scheufler C, Sebald W, Hulsmeyer M. Crystal structure of human bone morphogenetic protein-2 at 2.7 A resolution. J Mol Biol 1999;287(1):103–15.
10. Shimell MJ, Ferguson EL, Childs SR, O'Connor MB. The Drosophila dorsal-ventral patterning gene tolloid is related to human bone morphogenetic protein 1. Cell 1991;67(3):469–81.
11. Sampath TK, Muthukumaran N, Reddi AH. Isolation of osteogenin, an extracellular matrix-associated, bone-inductive protein, by heparin affinity chromatography. Proc Natl Acad Sci U S A 1987;84(20):7109–13.
12. Ozkaynak E, Rueger DC, Drier EA, et al. OP-1 cDNA encodes an osteogenic protein in the TGF-beta family. Embo J 1990;9(7):2085–93.
13. Sampath TK, Coughlin JE, Whetstone RM, et al. Bovine osteogenic protein is composed of dimers of OP-1 and BMP-2A, two members of the transforming growth factor-beta superfamily. J Biol Chem 1990;265(22):13198–205.
14. Koenig BB, Cook JS, Wolsing DH, et al. Characterization and cloning of a receptor for BMP-2 and BMP-4 from NIH 3T3 cells. Mol Cell Biol 1994;14(9):5961–74.
15. Moustakas A, Heldin CH. From mono- to oligo-Smads: the heart of the matter in TGF-beta signal transduction. Genes Dev 2002;16(15):1867–71.
16. Chen Y, Bhushan A, Vale W. Smad8 mediates the signaling of the ALK-2 [corrected] receptor serine kinase. Proc Natl Acad Sci U S A 1997;94(24):12938–43.
17. Zhao M, Qiao M, Oyajobi BO, Mundy GR, Chen D. E3 ubiquitin ligase Smurf1 mediates core-binding factor alpha1/Runx2 degradation and plays a specific role in osteoblast differentiation. J Biol Chem 2003;278(30):27939–44.
18. Reddi AH. Interplay between bone morphogenetic proteins and cognate binding proteins in bone and cartilage development: noggin, chordin and DAN. Arthritis Res 2001;3(1):1–5.
19. Wrana JL, Attisano L. The Smad pathway. Cytokine Growth Factor Rev 2000;11(1–2):5–13.
20. Ebisawa T, Fukuchi M, Murakami G, et al. Smurf1 interacts with transforming growth factor-beta type I receptor through Smad7 and induces receptor degradation. J Biol Chem 2001;276(16):12477–80.
21. Wu XB, Li Y, Schneider A, et al. Impaired osteoblastic differentiation, reduced bone formation, and severe osteoporosis in noggin-overexpressing mice. J Clin Invest 2003;112(6):924–34.
22. Horiki M, Imamura T, Okamoto M, et al. Smad6/Smurf1 overexpression in cartilage delays chondrocyte hypertrophy and causes dwarfism with osteopenia. J Cell Biol 2004;165(3):433–45.
23. van Bezooijen RL, Roelen BA, Visser A, et al. Sclerostin is an osteocyte-expressed negative regulator of bone formation, but not a classical BMP antagonist. J Exp Med 2004;199(6):805–14.

24. Yeomans JD, Urist MR. Bone induction by decalcified dentine implanted into oral, osseous and muscle tissues. Arch Oral Biol 1967;12(8):999–1008.
25. Urist MR, Jurist JM, Jr., Dubuc FL, Strates BS. Quantitation of new bone formation in intramuscular implants of bone matrix in rabbits. Clin Orthop Relat Res 1970;68:279–93.
26. Huggins C, Wiseman S, Reddi AH. Transformation of fibroblasts by allogeneic and xenogeneic transplants of demineralized tooth and bone. J Exp Med 1970;132(6):1250–8.
27. Reddi AH, Huggins C. Biochemical sequences in the transformation of normal fibroblasts in adolescent rats. Proc Natl Acad Sci U S A 1972;69(6):1601–5.
28. Carnes DL, Jr., De La Fontaine J, Cochran DL, et al. Evaluation of 2 novel approaches for assessing the ability of demineralized freeze-dried bone allograft to induce new bone formation. J Periodontol 1999;70(4):353–63.
29. Helm GA, Sheehan JM, Sheehan JP, et al. Utilization of type I collagen gel, demineralized bone matrix, and bone morphogenetic protein-2 to enhance autologous bone lumbar spinal fusion. J Neurosurg 1997;86(1):93–100.
30. Urist MR, Nilsson O, Rasmussen J, et al. Bone regeneration under the influence of a bone morphogenetic protein (BMP) beta tricalcium phosphate (TCP) composite in skull trephine defects in dogs. Clin Orthop Relat Res 1987(214):295–304.
31. Johnson EE, Urist MR, Finerman GA. Resistant nonunions and partial or complete segmental defects of long bones. Treatment with implants of a composite of human bone morphogenetic protein (BMP) and autolyzed, antigen-extracted, allogeneic (AAA) bone. Clin Orthop Relat Res 1992(277):229–37.
32. Heckman JD, Ingram AJ, Loyd RD, Luck JV, Jr., Mayer PW. Nonunion treatment with pulsed electromagnetic fields. Clin Orthop Relat Res 1981(161):58–66.
33. Heckman JD, Ehler W, Brooks BP, et al. Bone morphogenetic protein but not transforming growth factor-beta enhances bone formation in canine diaphyseal nonunions implanted with a biodegradable composite polymer. J Bone Joint Surg Am 1999;81(12):1717–29.
34. Reddi AH, Cunningham NS. Initiation and promotion of bone differentiation by bone morphogenetic proteins. J Bone Miner Res 1993;8 Suppl 2:S499–502.
35. Boyan BD, Lohmann CH, Somers A, et al. Potential of porous poly-D,L-lactide-co-glycolide particles as a carrier for recombinant human bone morphogenetic protein-2 during osteoinduction in vivo. J Biomed Mater Res 1999;46(1):51–9.
36. Ogawa Y, Schmidt DK, Nathan RM, et al. Bovine bone activin enhances bone morphogenetic protein-induced ectopic bone formation. J Biol Chem 1992;267(20):14233–7.
37. Sampath TK, Maliakal JC, Hauschka PV, et al. Recombinant human osteogenic protein-1 (hOP-1) induces new bone formation in vivo with a specific activity comparable with natural bovine osteogenic protein and stimulates osteoblast proliferation and differentiation in vitro. J Biol Chem 1992;267(28):20352–62.
38. Hotz G, Herr G. Bone substitute with osteoinductive biomaterials–current and future clinical applications. Int J Oral Maxillofac Surg 1994;23(6 Pt 2):413–7.
39. Nakashima M. Induction of dentine in amputated pulp of dogs by recombinant human bone morphogenetic proteins-2 and -4 with collagen matrix. Arch Oral Biol 1994;39(12):1085–9.
40. Rutherford B, Fitzgerald M. A new biological approach to vital pulp therapy. Crit Rev Oral Biol Med 1995;6(3):218–29.
41. Rutherford B, Spangberg L, Tucker M, Charette M. Transdentinal stimulation of reparative dentine formation by osteogenic protein-1 in monkeys. Arch Oral Biol 1995;40(7):681–3.
42. Rutherford RB, Wahle J, Tucker M, Rueger D, Charette M. Induction of reparative dentine formation in monkeys by recombinant human osteogenic protein-1. Arch Oral Biol 1993;38(7):571–6.

43. Six N, Lasfargues JJ, Goldberg M. Differential repair responses in the coronal and radicular areas of the exposed rat molar pulp induced by recombinant human bone morphogenetic protein 7 (osteogenic protein 1). Arch Oral Biol 2002;47(3):177–87.
44. Lieberman JR, Le LQ, Wu L, et al. Regional gene therapy with a BMP-2-producing murine stromal cell line induces heterotopic and orthotopic bone formation in rodents. J Orthop Res 1998;16(3):330–9.
45. Musgrave DS, Bosch P, Ghivizzani S, Robbins PD, Evans CH, Huard J. Adenovirus-mediated direct gene therapy with bone morphogenetic protein-2 produces bone. Bone 1999;24(6):541–7.
46. Riew KD, Wright NM, Cheng S, Avioli LV, Lou J. Induction of bone formation using a recombinant adenoviral vector carrying the human BMP-2 gene in a rabbit spinal fusion model. Calcif Tissue Int 1998;63(4):357–60.
47. Kawai M, Bessho K, Maruyama H, Miyazaki J, Yamamoto T. Simultaneous gene transfer of bone morphogenetic protein (BMP) -2 and BMP-7 by in vivo electroporation induces rapid bone formation and BMP-4 expression. BMC Musculoskelet Disord 2006;7:62.
48. Cook SD. Preclinical and clinical evaluation of osteogenic protein-1 (BMP-7) in bony sites. Orthopedics 1999;22(7):669–71.
49. Friedlaender GE, Perry CR, Cole JD, et al. Osteogenic protein-1 (bone morphogenetic protein-7) in the treatment of tibial nonunions. J Bone Joint Surg Am 2001;83-A Suppl 1(Pt 2):S151–8.
50. Boyan BD, Caplan AI, Heckman JD, Lennon DP, Ehler W, Schwartz Z. Osteochondral progenitor cells in acute and chronic canine nonunions. J Orthop Res 1999;17(2):246–55.
51. Syftestad GT, Urist MR. Bone aging. Clin Orthop Relat Res 1982(162):288–97.
52. Schwartz Z, Somers A, Mellonig JT, et al. Ability of commercial demineralized freeze-dried bone allograft to induce new bone formation is dependent on donor age but not gender. J Periodontol 1998;69(4):470–8.
53. Honsawek S, Powers RM, Wolfinbarger L. Extractable bone morphogenetic protein and correlation with induced new bone formation in an in vivo assay in the athymic mouse model. Cell Tissue Bank 2005;6(1):13–23.
54. Srouji S, Livne E. Bone marrow stem cells and biological scaffold for bone repair in aging and disease. Mech Ageing Dev 2005;126(2):281–7.
55. Knutsen R, Wergedal JE, Sampath TK, Baylink DJ, Mohan S. Osteogenic protein-1 stimulates proliferation and differentiation of human bone cells in vitro. Biochem Biophys Res Commun 1993;194(3):1352–8.
56. Burkus JK, Heim SE, Gornet MF, Zdeblick TA. Is INFUSE bone graft superior to autograft bone? An integrated analysis of clinical trials using the LT-CAGE lumbar tapered fusion device. J Spinal Disord Tech 2003;16(2):113–22.
57. Burkus JK, Sandhu HS, Gornet MF, Longley MC. Use of rhBMP-2 in combination with structural cortical allografts: clinical and radiographic outcomes in anterior lumbar spinal surgery. J Bone Joint Surg Am 2005;87(6):1205–12.
58. Pradhan BB, Bae HW, Dawson EG, Patel VV, Delamarter RB. Graft resorption with the use of bone morphogenetic protein: lessons from anterior lumbar interbody fusion using femoral ring allografts and recombinant human bone morphogenetic protein-2. Spine 2006;31(10):E277–84.
59. Baskin DS, Ryan P, Sonntag V, Westmark R, Widmayer MA. A prospective, randomized, controlled cervical fusion study using recombinant human bone morphogenetic protein-2 with the CORNERSTONE-SR allograft ring and the ATLANTIS anterior cervical plate. Spine 2003;28(12):1219–25; discussion 25.
60. Boakye M, Mummaneni PV, Garrett M, Rodts G, Haid R. Anterior cervical discectomy and fusion involving a polyetheretherketone spacer and bone morphogenetic protein. J Neurosurg Spine 2005;2(5):521–5.

61. Shields LB, Raque GH, Glassman SD, et al. Adverse effects associated with high-dose recombinant human bone morphogenetic protein-2 use in anterior cervical spine fusion. Spine 2006;31(5):542–7.
62. Haid RW, Jr., Branch CL, Jr., Alexander JT, Burkus JK. Posterior lumbar interbody fusion using recombinant human bone morphogenetic protein type 2 with cylindrical interbody cages. Spine J 2004;4(5):527–38; discussion 38–9.
63. Schwender JD, Holly LT, Rouben DP, Foley KT. Minimally invasive transforaminal lumbar interbody fusion (TLIF): technical feasibility and initial results. J Spinal Disord Tech 2005;18 Suppl:S1–6.
64. Villavicencio AT, Burneikiene S, Nelson EL, Bulsara KR, Favors M, Thramann J. Safety of transforaminal lumbar interbody fusion and intervertebral recombinant human bone morphogenetic protein-2. J Neurosurg Spine 2005;3(6):436–43.
65. Vaccaro AR, Anderson DG, Patel T, et al. Comparison of OP-1 Putty (rhBMP-7) to iliac crest autograft for posterolateral lumbar arthrodesis: a minimum 2-year follow-up pilot study. Spine 2005;30(24):2709–16.
66. Vaccaro AR, Patel T, Fischgrund J, et al. A 2-year follow-up pilot study evaluating the safety and efficacy of op-1 putty (rhbmp-7) as an adjunct to iliac crest autograft in posterolateral lumbar fusions. Eur Spine J 2005;14(7):623–9.
67. Vaccaro AR, Patel T, Fischgrund J, et al. A pilot study evaluating the safety and efficacy of OP-1 Putty (rhBMP-7) as a replacement for iliac crest autograft in posterolateral lumbar arthrodesis for degenerative spondylolisthesis. Spine 2004;29(17):1885–92.
68. Kanayama M, Hashimoto T, Shigenobu K, Yamane S, Bauer TW, Togawa D. A prospective randomized study of posterolateral lumbar fusion using osteogenic protein-1 (OP-1) versus local autograft with ceramic bone substitute: emphasis of surgical exploration and histologic assessment. Spine 2006;31(10):1067–74.
69. Glassman SD, Dimar JR, Carreon LY, Campbell MJ, Puno RM, Johnson JR. Initial fusion rates with recombinant human bone morphogenetic protein-2/compression resistant matrix and a hydroxyapatite and tricalcium phosphate/collagen carrier in posterolateral spinal fusion. Spine 2005;30(15):1694–8.
70. Singh K, Smucker JD, Boden SD. Use of recombinant human bone morphogenetic protein-2 as an adjunct in posterolateral lumbar spine fusion: a prospective CT-scan analysis at one and two years. J Spinal Disord Tech 2006;19(6):416–23.
71. Luhmann SJ, Bridwell KH, Cheng I, Imamura T, Lenke LG, Schootman M. Use of bone morphogenetic protein-2 for adult spinal deformity. Spine 2005;30(17 Suppl):S110–7.
72. Govender S, Csimma C, Genant HK, et al. Recombinant human bone morphogenetic protein-2 for treatment of open tibial fractures: a prospective, controlled, randomized study of four hundred and fifty patients. J Bone Joint Surg Am 2002;84-A(12):2123–34.
73. Swiontkowski MF, Aro HT, Donell S, et al. Recombinant human bone morphogenetic protein-2 in open tibial fractures. A subgroup analysis of data combined from two prospective randomized studies. J Bone Joint Surg Am 2006;88(6):1258–65.
74. Jones AL, Bucholz RW, Bosse MJ, et al. Recombinant human BMP-2 and allograft compared with autogenous bone graft for reconstruction of diaphyseal tibial fractures with cortical defects. A randomized, controlled trial. J Bone Joint Surg Am 2006;88(7):1431–41.
75. McKee MD, Schemirsch EH, Waddel JP, et al. The effect of human recombinant bone morphogenic protein (rhBMP-7) on the healing of open tibial shaft fractures: results of a multi-center, prospective, randomized clinical trial. In: Orthopaedic Tramua Association, Paper #45; 2002; 2002.
76. Cole JD, Nguyen S. Review of healing with rhBMP-2/ACS use in the Medicare-aged population. In: Orthopaedic Trauma Association, Poster #102; 2006; 2006.
77. Hicks BD. BMP-2 and its use in nonunions and malunions. In: Orthopaedic Trauma Association, Poster #27; 2006; 2006.

78. Jones CB, Ringler JR, Enders TJ. Clinical outcomes for long-bone nonunions implanted with bone morphogenetic protein. In: Orthopaedic Trauma Association, Poster #30; 2006; 2006.
79. Hu ZM, Peel SA, Sandor GK, Clokie CM. The osteoinductive activity of bone morphogenetic protein (BMP) purified by repeated extracts of bovine bone. Growth Factors 2004;22(1):29–33.
80. Kay JF, Khaliq SK, King E, Murray SS, Brochman EJ. Amounts of BMP-2, BMP-4, BMP-7 and TGF-B1 contained in DBM particles and DBM extract. In: Orthopaedic Research Society, Paper #1724; 2006; 2006.
81. Carano RA, Filvaroff EH. Angiogenesis and bone repair. Drug Discov Today 2003;8(21):980–9.
82. Simpson AH, Mills L, Noble B. The role of growth factors and related agents in accelerating fracture healing. J Bone Joint Surg Br 2006;88(6):701–5.
83. Zhang Z, Lu S, Wang J. [Distribution and effectiveness of endogenic bone morphogenetic protein (BMP) in bone defect]. Zhonghua Wai Ke Za Zhi 1996;34(10):596–8.
84. Grageda E. Platelet-rich plasma and bone graft materials: a review and a standardized research protocol. Implant Dent 2004;13(4):301–9.
85. Roukis TS, Zgonis T, Tiernan B. Autologous platelet-rich plasma for wound and osseous healing: a review of the literature and commercially available products. Adv Ther 2006;23(2):218–37.
86. Ranly DM, McMillan J, Keller T, et al. Platelet-derived growth factor inhibits demineralized bone matrix-induced intramuscular cartilage and bone formation. A study of immunocompromised mice. J Bone Joint Surg Am 2005;87(9):2052–64.
87. Thorwarth M, Wehrhan F, Schultze-Mosgau S, Wiltfang J, Schlegel KA. PRP modulates expression of bone matrix proteins in vivo without long-term effects on bone formation. Bone 2006;38(1):30–40.
88. Gruber R, Kandler B, Fischer MB, Watzek G. Osteogenic differentiation induced by bone morphogenetic proteins can be suppressed by platelet-released supernatant in vitro. Clin Oral Implants Res 2006;17(2):188–93.
89. Rai B, Oest ME, Dupont KM, Ho KH, Teoh SH, Guldberg RE. Combination of platelet-rich plasma with polycaprolactone-tricalcium phosphate scaffolds for segmental bone defect repair. J Biomed Mater Res A 2007.
90. Sarkar MR, Augat P, Shefelbine SJ, et al. Bone formation in a long bone defect model using a platelet-rich plasma-loaded collagen scaffold. Biomaterials 2006;27(9):1817–23.
91. Ranly DM, Lohmann CH, Andreacchio D, Boyan BD, Schwartz Z. Platelet-rich plasma inhibits demineralized bone matrix-induced bone formation in nude mice. J Bone Joint Surg Am 2007;89(1):139–47.
92. Vladimirov BS, Dimitrov SA. Growth factors–importance and possibilities for enhancement of the healing process in bone fractures. Folia Med (Plovdiv) 2004;46(2):11–7.
93. Chen CW, Tsai YH, Deng WP, et al. Type I and II collagen regulation of chondrogenic differentiation by mesenchymal progenitor cells. J Orthop Res 2005;23(2):446–53.
94. Hunziker EB, Driesang IM, Morris EA. Chondrogenesis in cartilage repair is induced by members of the transforming growth factor-beta superfamily. Clin Orthop Relat Res 2001(391 Suppl):S171–81.
95. McGuire MK, Kao RT, Nevins M, Lynch SE. rhPDGF-BB promotes healing of periodontal defects: 24-month clinical and radiographic observations. Int J Periodontics Restorative Dent 2006;26(3):223–31.
96. Schmidt MB, Chen EH, Lynch SE. A review of the effects of insulin-like growth factor and platelet derived growth factor on in vivo cartilage healing and repair. Osteoarthritis Cartilage 2006;14(5):403–12.
97. Coultas L, Chawengsaksophak K, Rossant J. Endothelial cells and VEGF in vascular development. Nature 2005;438(7070):937–45.

98. Yancopoulos GD, Davis S, Gale NW, Rudge JS, Wiegand SJ, Holash J. Vascular-specific growth factors and blood vessel formation. Nature 2000;407(6801):242–8.
99. Nakamae A, Sunagawa T, Ishida O, et al. Acceleration of surgical angiogenesis in necrotic bone with a single injection of fibroblast growth factor-2 (FGF-2). J Orthop Res 2004;22(3):509–13.
100. Rabie AB, Lu M. Basic fibroblast growth factor up-regulates the expression of vascular endothelial growth factor during healing of allogeneic bone graft. Arch Oral Biol 2004;49(12):1025–33.
101. Niedhart C, Maus U, Miltner O, Graber HG, Niethard FU, Siebert CH. The effect of basic fibroblast growth factor on bone regeneration when released from a novel in situ setting tricalcium phosphate cement. J Biomed Mater Res A 2004;69(4):680–5.
102. Botta M, Manetti F, Corelli F. Fibroblast growth factors and their inhibitors. Curr Pharm Des 2000;6(18):1897–924.
103. McKee MD, Nanci A. Osteopontin at mineralized tissue interfaces in bone, teeth, and osseointegrated implants: ultrastructural distribution and implications for mineralized tissue formation, turnover, and repair. Microsc Res Tech 1996;33(2):141–64.
104. Green J, Schotland S, Stauber DJ, Kleeman CR, Clemens TL. Cell-matrix interaction in bone: type I collagen modulates signal transduction in osteoblast-like cells. Am J Physiol 1995;268(5 Pt 1):C1090–103.
105. Wang H, Li X, Tomin E, et al. Thrombin peptide (TP508) promotes fracture repair by up-regulating inflammatory mediators, early growth factors, and increasing angiogenesis. J Orthop Res 2005;23(3):671–9.
106. Bodamyali T, Bhatt B, Hughes FJ, et al. Pulsed electromagnetic fields simultaneously induce osteogenesis and upregulate transcription of bone morphogenetic proteins 2 and 4 in rat osteoblasts in vitro. Biochem Biophys Res Commun 1998;250(2):458–61.
107. Lohmann CH, Schwartz Z, Liu Y, et al. Pulsed electromagnetic fields affect phenotype and connexin 43 protein expression in MLO-Y4 osteocyte-like cells and ROS 17/2.8 osteoblast-like cells. J Orthop Res 2003;21(2):326–34.
108. Lohmann CH, Boyan BD, Simon BJ, Schwartz Z. Pulsed electromagnetic fields have direct effects on growth plate chondrocytes. Osteologie 2005;14(4):185–94.
109. Aaron RK, Ciombor DM. Acceleration of experimental endochondral ossification by biophysical stimulation of the progenitor cell pool. J Orthop Res 1996;14(4):582–9.
110. Aaron RK, Boyan BD, Ciombor DM, Schwartz Z, Simon BJ. Stimulation of growth factor synthesis by electric and electromagnetic fields. Clin Orthop Relat Res 2004(419):30–7.
111. Harle J, Mayia F, Olsen I, Salih V. Effects of ultrasound on transforming growth factor-beta genes in bone cells. Eur Cell Mater 2005;10:70–6; discussion 6.

12

Biological Approaches to Spinal Fusion

Andrew K. Simpson, Peter G. Whang, and Jonathan N. Grauer

Abstract: Bone grafting procedures are frequently performed for spinal applications in an attempt to promote successful arthrodesis. Autograft remains the gold standard grafting material. However, due to relatively limited supply and the morbidity associated with procurement of autograft, there has been a great deal of interest in developing alternative bone graft materials. Allograft and ceramic preparations are osteoconductive matrices that support bone formation, but these materials exhibit minimal osteoinductive potential. Recent research efforts have focused specifically on osteoinductive substances such as demineralized bone matrices, recombinant human bone morphogenetic proteins and autologous bone marrow aspirates. Since none of these materials deliver all of the elements required for bone formation when implanted alone, composite grafts, consisting of osteoinductive factors combined with an osteoconductive carrier, may prove to be more effective in stimulating spinal fusion than any single graft substitute.

Keywords: Spinal fusion, bone graft substitute, osteoconductive matrix, demineralized bone matrix, bone morphogenetic protein.

12.1. Introduction

Arthrodesis of the spine is a common surgical procedure which may represent the treatment of choice for a variety of pathologies, including degenerative conditions, deformity, trauma or instability. By eliminating the motion between diseased motion segments, spinal fusion may serve to decrease pain, maintain alignment and protect the neural elements. While several different surgical techniques have been developed to gain access to the spinal column and neural elements, in the majority of cases the spine is exposed using either

---

Department of Orthopaedics and Rehabilitation, Yale University School of Medicine, New Haven, CT

From: *Orthopedic Biology and Medicine: Musculoskeletal Tissue Regeneration, Biological Materials and Methods.*
Edited by W. S. Pietrzak © Humana Press, Totowa, NJ

an anterior or a posterior approach. A particular surgical approach is generally selected based on the specific location of the pathology, but other factors such as surgeon preference or the status of the surrounding tissues may also determine which strategy is employed.

Similar to the treatment of a fracture, once a spine has been prepared for arthrodesis, it is typically immobilized in some fashion to minimize micromotion and promote bony healing. Immobilization of the spine may either be accomplished through external bracing or by the introduction of internal fixation, a technique which has become increasingly popular among spine surgeons. A variety of spinal instrumentation systems are currently available, ranging from anterior cervical plates to posterior pedicle screws. While internal fixation will temporarily increase the rigidity of the spinal segment to facilitate fusion, these constructs will fatigue and eventually fail over time, if biological fusion is not achieved. The development of a failed fusion, also known as a pseudarthrosis, is dependent on multiple local and host factors, as well as the properties of the bone graft material that is implanted.

The gold standard graft material for spinal fusion is still autologous iliac crest bone graft. Unfortunately, the supply of autograft is limited and the harvesting of bone from the iliac crest is an invasive procedure which is associated with significant morbidity. As a result there has been a great deal of interest in developing materials that may be used as supplements or even alternatives to autogenous bone graft. This chapter will discuss the biological processes underlying spinal fusion and the mechanisms by which these graft materials serve to stimulate a successful arthrodesis.

12.2. The Biology of Spinal Fusion

Spinal fusion consists of a tightly regulated series of molecular and cellular events that are dependant upon the biological and biomechanical conditions of the host, as well as the presence of the three components required for bone formation: mesenchymal stem cells with osteogenic potential, osteoinductive factors that may bring about the differentiation of these osteoblastic cells, and an osteoconductive scaffold to support new bone formation. Since the efficacy of bone graft material is largely dictated by the local fusion environment, a thorough understanding of the different surgical techniques and approaches available for inducing fusion is essential for identifying the optimal graft option for a specific spinal application.

A posterolateral fusion is the most common type of arthrodesis performed in the lumbar spine. Decortication of the posterior surfaces of the spine in conjunction with placement of an appropriate bone graft substance results in the formation of bridging bone across adjacent transverse processes. These fusions are often stabilized with supplementary instrumentation, usually consisting of segmental pedicle screw fixation. The biomechanical environment of the posterolateral spine is unique in that the motion segment is subject to tensile forces rather than compression, making it more challenging to obtain a solid intertransverse fusion. For this reason the graft material used to enhance bony fusion of the posterior elements does not need to provide any significant structural support.

Multiple prospective studies have reported noninstrumented fusion rates in the posterolateral lumbar spine to be between 40 and 60 percent [1, 2]. Due to these suboptimal results, posterolateral fusions are usually supplemented with transpedicular internal fixation to provide immediate structural support prior to the development of solid arthrodesis. Zdeblick demonstrated that the use of pedicle screw instrumentation in the lumbar spine generated higher fusion rates, compared to either semi-rigid fixation or uninstrumented constructs [3]. In a more recent clinical series assessing instrumented posterolateral lumbar fusions, the rate of successful arthrodesis approached 90 percent [4].

Because posterolateral fusions do not address any pathology affecting the anterior spinal column, other strategies are utilized to manage anterior structural deficiencies. Interbody fusions involving the anterior vertebral column tend to exhibit higher fusion rates compared to posterolateral fusions, primarily because of the differences between the relative surface areas and biomechanical forces characteristic of the anterior and posterior regions of the spine [5]. Interbody fusions ideally comprise the entire extent of the intervertebral space so that decortication of the cartilaginous end plates generates a significantly greater surface area of cancellous bone than that observed posterolaterally between adjacent transverse processes. Unlike the posterior spine, the anterior vertebral column is under compression, which is more conducive to new bone growth than the distraction forces experienced by the posterior elements. Thus, any bone graft material inserted in the intervertebral space must have sufficient biomechanical properties to withstand these substantial loads; alternatively, graft substances may also be placed within a structural device such as a cage or dowel.

In the lumbar spine these interbody procedures may be performed anteriorly (ALIF), posteriorly (PLIF) or through a transforaminal approach (TLIF). In all of these clinical scenarios, the disc material is excised and the resultant defect must be reconstructed with some type of graft material. Circumferential lumbar fusions using adjunctive posterior transpedicular instrumentation may also increase the rigidity of these segments even more, reducing graft subsidence and giving rise to even higher arthrodesis rates [6]. While internal fixation is clearly beneficial in the thoracolumbar spine, studies evaluating the results of anterior cervical interbody fusions have consistently reported success rates of 90 percent or greater for both instrumented and uninstrumented constructs [7–10].

For both posterolateral and interbody procedures, the manner in which the local environment is prepared for fusion may significantly influence arthrodesis rates and clinical outcomes. As with fracture healing, spinal fusion is initiated by the influx of inflammatory mediators and osteoprogenitor cells through the vascular supply of the surrounding tissues. The surgeon may augment the vascularity of the fusion site by minimizing trauma to adjacent anatomic structures during the exposure, removing any scar tissue from the operative field, and denuding the cartilaginous end plates within the disc space and the cortical bone of the posterior elements. In particular, proper decortication is critically important because the bleeding cancellous surfaces serve as the primary source of osteogenic cells to support the formation of new bone [11].

There are also a myriad of systemic factors which may compromise a patient's osteogenic potential, mainly by affecting the local blood supply or the subsequent inflammatory response. For example, it is well established that individuals who smoke will demonstrate higher rates of pseudoarthrosis because tobacco use is known to interfere with bone metabolism and regeneration [12–15]. Similarly, nonsteroidal anti-inflammatory medications and other drugs that attenuate the systemic inflammatory cascade have also been shown to inhibit new bone formation [16, 17]. Einhorn, et al. demonstrated that even the nutritional status of a patient can influence bone healing [18]. Collectively, these findings indicate that spinal fusion is a complex process that is affected by all of these considerations: the type and location of the arthrodesis, the use of instrumentation, proper fusion bed preparation and any number of local and systemic host factors.

To stimulate bone formation and decrease the risk of developing a pseudarthrosis, nearly all spinal fusions incorporate some form of bone graft material, whose biological and biomechanical properties will inevitably play a role in the ability of the surgeon to achieve a solid arthrodesis. Autologous corticocancellous bone is the most widely used graft substance for promoting spinal fusion because it is the only single material that contributes all of the elements involved in bone regeneration (i.e., osteogenic cells, osteoinductive signaling molecules and an osteoconductive matrix). However, as discussed earlier, autograft is only available in limited quantities and often requires a separate incision and a more extensive surgical dissection; moreover, the harvesting of autogenous bone from the iliac crest may also give rise to numerous postoperative complications such as infection, hematoma, fracture, neurovascular injury and intractable pain [19, 20]. In an attempt to avoid this significant morbidity, a variety of biologically active materials have been developed as potential alternatives to iliac crest autograft for spinal fusion; examples of contemporary graft options include allograft and other osteoconductive scaffolds, demineralized bone matrices, recombinant osteoinductive proteins and other autologous blood and bone marrow products.

12.3. Allograft and Synthetic Osteoconductive Materials

Second only to blood, allogeneic bone is one of the most commonly transplanted tissues among humans, and has been used successfully for spinal fusion as well as other orthopaedic applications [21]. Once it is harvested from a human cadaver, allograft bone is generally processed either by freezing or freeze-drying (lyophilization) to decrease its antigenicity, eradicate any infectious agents and preserve the grafts for long-term storage. Unlike autogenous bone, allografts may elicit a host immune reaction which has been shown to be related to delayed graft incorporation and inferior biomechanical properties of the fusion mass [22]. The degree of histocompatibility mismatch is in part dependant upon the methods by which these tissues are prepared; freeze-drying reduces allograft antigenicity more than freezing, but upon rehydration, these lyophilized grafts may demonstrate inferior material properties [23, 24]. Allografts are osteoconductive and may possess limited osteoinductive potential, but this material is not considered to be osteogenic, because donor osteoprogenitor cells are removed during tissue processing.

The efficacy of allograft for spinal fusion is largely determined by the location where it is placed within the spine. When nonstructural allograft bone is placed under tension, as in the posterior spine, it incorporates at a slower rate than autograft and leads to lower rates of arthrodesis when used alone [25, 26]. Thus, for posterior spinal applications, allograft is generally employed as a bone graft extender rather than a true substitute for autograft. The exception to this is in the pediatric scoliosis population, where allograft appears to be a reasonable alternative to autograft for posterolateral fusions. In these patients, the use of allograft resulted in similar rates of arthrodesis compared to autograft, with far less morbidity [27–29].

While in the majority of clinical scenarios autogenous bone is preferable to allograft for promoting posterolateral fusions, the implantation of structural allografts in the anterior column is associated with relatively high fusion rates, both in the cervical and the thoracolumbar regions of the spine [30, 31]. The superior outcomes achieved with the use of allograft for interbody fusions are believed to be due to the improved graft remodeling and incorporation that occurs when this material is placed in the more physiologic state of compression.

Another potential alternative to autograft for spinal fusion is a synthetic osteoconductive scaffold, such as ceramic. Ceramics lack any osteoinductive or osteogenic capabilities, and for this reason these products are best used as bone graft extenders and may not function effectively as stand-alone graft materials. An inherent disadvantage of ceramics is that they are brittle and relatively weak. When ceramics are introduced into the anterior spinal column, where they are subject to significant compressive loads, these products must be protected with internal fixation until bone ingrowth occurs [31]. Like allograft, ceramics are also inferior to autogenous bone when placed under tension, as in the posterior spine [32]. There is some evidence that combining these osteoconductive matrices with other biologically active materials (e.g., demineralized bone matrices or osteoinductive growth factors) to form a composite graft may lead to increased amounts of bone formation [33, 34].

12.4. Demineralized Bone Matrices

Demineralized bone matrices (DBMs) are also derived from cadaveric bone and, therefore, comprise a specialized class of allograft tissue. The donor bone is decalcified by acid extraction, giving rise to a composite of Type I collagen and noncollagenous proteins, including low concentrations of bone morphogenetic proteins (BMPs) and other constitutively expressed growth factors [31]. Because of their relatively poor biomechanical properties, DBMs are frequently combined with some type of an osteoconductive carrier or structural graft when they are employed for spinal fusion applications.

Since numerous DBM products are currently commercially available, all of which appear to exhibit significant variability in their osteoinductive activities, it has been difficult to definitively establish the efficacy of this graft material for inducing spinal fusion; however, the results of the initial preclinical studies performed using animals have certainly been encouraging. DBMs have been used successfully as autograft extenders in both rabbit and canine models [35, 36]. In addition, a composite graft consisting of DBM and allograft bone significantly improved the arthrodesis rates in rabbits, compared to those observed with allograft alone. A DBM gel has also been shown to be as effective as autogenous bone graft for stimulating posterolateral fusions in rabbits [37]. In this same study different combinations of these graft materials were assessed and the highest fusion rates were obtained when the DBM and autograft were combined in a 3:1 ratio.

There continues to be a paucity of controlled, randomized clinical trials evaluating the use of DBMs in humans. In a series by An, et al. 77 patients underwent one, two or three level noninstrumented anterior cervical discectomy and fusion procedures, using either freeze-dried structural allografts filled with a DBM or autogenous iliac crest bone graft alone [38]. At a minimum of one year follow-up, fusion rates of 54 percent and 74 percent were observed in the allograft/DBM and autograft groups, respectively. This inferior fusion rate, in conjunction with the higher rate of graft subsidence noted in the allograft/DBM cohort, led the authors to recommend autograft for these types of anterior cervical fusions. In contrast, another study involving 50 subjects who had all been managed with lumbar interbody fusions reported a 96 percent success rate following implantation of titanium mesh cages packed with a DBM and a coralline hydroxyapatite carrier [39].

It is important to emphasize that the various DBM preparations may have disparate osteoinductive potentials, which seems to be related to the absolute quantity as well as the specific composition of the BMPs actually present in each preparation [40]. Furthermore, it has also been suggested that the consistency of each DBM, which is primarily influenced by the carrier material within which it is suspended, may also affect its osteoinductivity. Lee, et al. compared the osteoinductive properties of multiple commercially available DBM products in the posteriolateral spines of athymic rats [41]. In this study the fusion rates ranged from 0 percent to 80 percent, indicating that there is a great deal of variability between the osteoinductive potencies of different DBM formulations.

12.5. Bone Morphogenetic Proteins and Osteoinductive Growth Factors

Many bone graft materials like allograft and the DBMs contain physiologic concentrations of osteoinductive signaling proteins. Utilizing recombinant gene technology, however, large quantities of a single growth factor are now able to be produced in a purified form. The efficacy of recombinant human bone morphogenetic proteins (rhBMPs), including rhBMP-2 and rhBMP-7 (also known as osteogenic protein-1, or OP-1), has already been established in a number of randomized, controlled clinical studies, resulting in the approval of these products for specific clinical indications [42–44].

The osteoinductive capacity of rhOP-1 for posterolateral spinal fusion has been clearly documented in both rabbits [45, 46] and dogs [47], with reported arthrodesis rates of 100 percent and 72 percent, respectively. In a sheep model of interbody fusion, the use of rhOP-1 was associated with significantly greater bone formation than a combination of autograft and a hydroxyapatite scaffold [48].

As part of a multicenter, randomized, prospective, controlled clinical trial, Vaccaro, et al. compared rhOP-1 putty to autogenous iliac crest bone graft for posterolateral lumbar arthrodesis [1]. The authors observed greater clinical improvement and increased fusion rates among the patients treated with rhOP-1, compared to the autograft control group. Based on the favorable results of this pilot study, rhOP-1 has recently been approved by the United States Food and Drug Administration (FDA) for revision posterolateral lumbar fusions.

Similar success has also been achieved in animals using rhBMP-2 as a substitute for autogenous bone. Boden, et al. inserted titanium cages containing rhBMP-2 and a collagen carrier in an attempt to induce anterior lumbar interbody fusions in rhesus monkeys [49]. At 24 months the rhBMP-2 animals exhibited a 100 percent fusion rate. The authors also demonstrated that animals receiving higher concentrations of rhBMP-2 produced bone at a faster rate and generated fusion masses of greater density. Moreover, these results confirmed that a solid arthrodesis could be acquired through a minimally invasive laparoscopic approach. In another preclinical study, biomechanical testing of sheep interbody fusion constructs revealed that spines implanted with rhBMP-2 exhibited greater stiffness than those treated with autograft [50]. Even in the posterolateral spine, which is generally considered to be a more challenging environment for arthrodesis, Sandhu, et al. reported a 100 percent fusion rate using rhBMP-2 in a canine model [51].

Clinical studies evaluating rhBMP-2 in humans have suggested that this osteoinductive protein may represent a viable bone graft substitute for both interbody and posterolateral fusion applications. In one large prospective, randomized trial involving 279 patients with lumbar degenerative disc disease who underwent anterior lumbar interbody fusion (ALIF) with tapered cages filled with either rhBMP-2 or autogenous bone, the fusion rate of the rhBMP-2 cohort was higher than that of the autograft controls (94.5 percent versus 88.7 percent, respectively) at 24 months [44]. In addition, 5.9 percent of the control group experienced adverse events related to their bone grafting procedures and 32 percent reported persistent donor site pain at the time of final follow-up. The efficacy of rhBMP-2 for stimulating posterolateral spinal fusion was examined in another prospective, randomized clinical trial in which rhBMP-2 was again compared to autogenous bone, both with and without pedicle screw instrumentation [52]. In this series all of the subjects receiving rhBMP-2 demonstrated radiographic evidence of a solid arthrodesis, regardless of whether or not supplementary internal fixation was employed; the radiographic fusion rate of the patients managed with autograft and instrumentation was only 40 percent. As a result of these studies the combination of rhBMP-2 and an absorbable collagen sponge (INFUSE®, Medtronic Sofamor Danek, Memphis, TN) has been approved by the FDA for use with threaded fusion devices in the anterior lumbar spine as a treatment for degenerative disc disease.

Other osteoinductive proteins such as BMP-9, GDF-5 and LMP-1 have recently been identified and are currently subjects of active research. BMP-9 has been shown to induce spinal fusion in rodents when delivered via gene therapy [53]. Recombinant human growth and differentiation factor-5 (rhGDF-5) placed in an osteoconductive matrix gave rise to arthrodesis rates comparable to those obtained with autograft in a sheep model of posterolateral fusion [54]. LIM mineralization protein-1 (LMP-1) is another osteoinductive growth factor which potentiates the cellular response to exogenous BMPs [55]. In a series of gene therapy experiments bone marrow cells transfected with the DNA encoding LMP-1 proved to be extremely effective for promoting posterolateral arthrodesis in rodents, with a fusion rate of 100 percent [56]. It is anticipated that as the molecular and cellular mechanisms underlying these novel osteoinductive signaling proteins continue to be elucidated, they may eventually be available for use in humans as alternatives to autogenous bone for spinal fusion and other orthopaedic applications.

There are a number of different options for the delivery of these osteoinductive substances. At this time these soluble factors are typically retained within some type of osteoconductive scaffold to restrict their diffusion away from the fusion site, but most of these carriers require the administration of supraphysiologic doses of these proteins. In response to the limitations of these existing systems, gene therapy techniques are being developed that may allow for the sustained local release of these molecules at more physiologic levels, resulting in a more potent osteoinductive signal to the surrounding tissues [57]. However, the safety and efficacy of gene therapy approaches have not yet been definitively established, to justify its widespread implementation among humans.

12.6. Autologous Bone Marrow and Stem Cells

Autologous bone marrow represents another source of osteogenic cells and osteoinductive proteins for spinal fusion. One of the advantages of this technique is that the morbidity resulting from the aspiration of bone marrow is significantly less than that associated with the procurement of iliac crest autograft, and the addition of this material to an osteoconductive matrix produces a composite graft that may serve as an effective substitute for autogenous bone. In one study autologous bone marrow aspirates were found to significantly increase the rate of arthrodesis when used as a graft extender in a rabbit model of posterolateral fusion. However, unfractionated bone marrow has only moderate osteogenic potential because, even in healthy adults, it has been estimated that approximately one out of every 50,000 nucleated bone marrow cells is capable of undergoing differentiation into an osteoblast [58]. For this reason attempts have been made to increase the effective concentration of osteoprogenitor cells in these aspirates through the application of selective retention technology, or by expanding the number of these mesenchymal stem cells(MSCs) in culture [59]. As these bone grafting strategies continue to evolve, further studies are necessary to define the role of this material as either a bone graft extender or as a true alternative to autogenous bone for spinal fusion [60].

12.7. Future Trends and Needs

Significant research efforts remain focused on the isolation and development of bone graft supplements and alternatives. Although there is much interest and commercialization in motion sparing technologies, fusion remains the gold standard treatment option for many clinical scenarios.

At the present time osteoinductive proteins have received the majority of focus. These proteins are proving to be a powerful means of inducing fusion. Nonetheless, site specific indications and the importance of dose and carrier continue to be revealed.

Osteoconductive matrices continue to be evaluated, both as bone graft supplements as well as carriers for osteoinductive molecules. Allograft has long been the most commonly used osteoconductive graft material in the United States; however, there are many factors which make synthetic alternatives increasingly more appealing, including safety and availability.

Isolating osteogenic cells such as osteoblasts and MSCs from autograft intraoperatively remains a challenge technically and logistically. However, adaptation of methods utilized in the laboratory may make intraoperative harvesting of osteogenic cells, and subsequent clonal expansion, a possibility in the coming years.

With future efforts focused on the development of novel materials and spinal fusion technologies, we can expect to see a concurrent increase in our understanding of the molecular and cellular events that occur during spinal fusion. Elucidating these basic principles will allow further advance in the field of spinal fusion, and potentially lead to identification of novel molecules and materials to aid in fusion.

12.8. Conclusion

The development of bone graft alternatives has progressed rapidly over recent years, with several options now available for various clinical applications. Iliac crest autograft is still recognized as the gold standard graft material for spinal fusion because it is the only substance that contains osteogenic cells, osteoinductive growth factors and an osteoconductive matrix. Since no single method provides all the elements necessary for bone formation, it is likely that composite grafts, consisting of multiple biologically active materials implanted together, may enhance spinal fusion in a synergistic fashion. With further advances in the understanding of the intricate cascade of molecular and cellular events underlying spinal fusion, these bone grafting techniques continue to be refined. Additional studies are clearly warranted to corroborate the safety, efficacy and cost-effectiveness of the existing techniques, as well as to evaluate novel approaches such as gene therapy. Nevertheless, it is critical to recognize that the success of these surgical procedures remains dependent upon the basic principles essential to achieving a solid arthrodesis: optimizing the biological environment by selecting the appropriate bone graft material, maintaining biomechanical stability, meticulous preparation of the fusion bed and proper patient selection.

References

1. Vaccaro AR, Anderson DG, Patel T, et al. Comparison of OP-1 Putty (rhBMP-7) to iliac crest autograft for posterolateral lumbar arthrodesis: a minimum 2-year follow-up pilot study. Spine 2005;30:2709–16.
2. Vaccaro AR, Patel T, Fischgrund J, et al. A pilot study evaluating the safety and efficacy of OP-1 Putty (rhBMP-7) as a replacement for iliac crest autograft in posterolateral lumbar arthrodesis for degenerative spondylolisthesis. Spine 2004;29:1885–92.
3. Zdeblick TA. A prospective, randomized study of lumbar fusion. Preliminary results. Spine 1993;18:983–91.
4. Chen WJ, Tsai TT, Chen LH, et al. The fusion rate of calcium sulfate with local autograft bone compared with autologous iliac bone graft for instrumented short-segment spinal fusion. Spine 2005;30:2293–7.
5. Sandhu HS, Grewal HS, Parvataneni H. Bone grafting for spinal fusion. Orthop Clin North Am 1999;30:685–98.
6. Madan SS, Harley JM, Boeree NR. Anterior lumbar interbody fusion: does stable anterior fixation matter? Eur Spine J 2003;12:386–92.
7. Mutoh N, Shinomiya K, Furuya K, et al. Pseudarthrosis and delayed union after anterior cervical fusion. Int Orthop 1993;17:286–9.

8. Gore DR, Sepic SB. Anterior cervical fusion for degenerated or protruded discs. A review of one hundred forty-six patients. Spine 1984;9:667–71.
9. Samartzis D, Shen FH, Lyon C, et al. Does rigid instrumentation increase the fusion rate in one-level anterior cervical discectomy and fusion? Spine J 2004;4:636–43.
10. Connolly PJ, Esses SI, Kostuik JP. Anterior cervical fusion: outcome analysis of patients fused with and without anterior cervical plates. J Spinal Disord 1996;9:202–6.
11. Urist M. Bone and Bone Transplants. Philadelphia: WB Saunders, 1980.
12. Brown CW, Orme TJ, Richardson HD. The rate of pseudarthrosis (surgical nonunion) in patients who are smokers and patients who are nonsmokers: a comparison study. Spine 1986;11:942–3.
13. Hollo I, Gergely I, Boross M. Smoking results in calcitonin resistance. JAMA 1977;237:2470.
14. Kwiatkowski TC, Hanley EN, Jr., Ramp WK. Cigarette smoking and its orthopedic consequences. Am J Orthop 1996;25:590–7.
15. de Vernejoul MC, Bielakoff J, Herve M, et al. Evidence for defective osteoblastic function. A role for alcohol and tobacco consumption in osteoporosis in middle-aged men. Clin Orthop Relat Res 1983:107–15.
16. Nilsson OS, Bauer HC, Brosjo O, et al. Influence of indomethacin on induced heterotopic bone formation in rats. Importance of length of treatment and of age. Clin Orthop Relat Res 1986:239–45.
17. Deguchi M, Rapoff AJ, Zdeblick TA. Posterolateral fusion for isthmic spondylolisthesis in adults: analysis of fusion rate and clinical results. J Spinal Disord 1998;11:459–64.
18. Einhorn TA, Bonnarens F, Burstein AH. The contributions of dietary protein and mineral to the healing of experimental fractures. A biomechanical study. J Bone Joint Surg Am 1986;68:1389–95.
19. Arrington ED, Smith WJ, Chambers HG, et al. Complications of iliac crest bone graft harvesting. Clin Orthop Relat Res 1996;329:300–9.
20. Banwart JC, Asher MA, Hassanein RS. Iliac crest bone graft harvest donor site morbidity. A statistical evaluation. Spine 1995;20:1055–60.
21. Prolo DJ, Rodrigo JJ. Contemporary bone graft physiology and surgery. Clin Orthop Relat Res 1985:322–42.
22. Stevenson S, Li XQ, Martin B. The fate of cancellous and cortical bone after transplantation of fresh and frozen tissue-antigen-matched and mismatched osteochondral allografts in dogs. J Bone Joint Surg Am 1991;73:1143–56.
23. Hamer AJ, Strachan JR, Black MM, et al. Biochemical properties of cortical allograft bone using a new method of bone strength measurement. A comparison of fresh, fresh-frozen and irradiated bone. J Bone Joint Surg Br 1996;78:363–8.
24. Pelker RR, Friedlaender GE, Markham TC. Biomechanical properties of bone allografts. Clin Orthop Relat Res 1983;174:54–7.
25. Jorgenson SS, Lowe TG, France J, et al. A prospective analysis of autograft versus allograft in posterolateral lumbar fusion in the same patient. A minimum of 1-year follow-up in 144 patients. Spine 1994;19:2048–53.
26. Nugent PJ, Dawson EG. Intertransverse process lumbar arthrodesis with allogeneic fresh-frozen bone graft. Clin Orthop Relat Res 1993;287:107–11.
27. Blanco JS, Sears CJ. Allograft bone use during instrumentation and fusion in the treatment of adolescent idiopathic scoliosis. Spine 1997;22:1338–42.
28. Dodd CA, Fergusson CM, Freedman L, et al. Allograft versus autograft bone in scoliosis surgery. J Bone Joint Surg Br 1988;70:431–4.
29. Jones KC, Andrish J, Kuivila T, et al. Radiographic outcomes using freeze-dried cancellous allograft bone for posterior spinal fusion in pediatric idiopathic scoliosis. J Pediatr Orthop 2002;22:285–9.
30. Malloy KM, Hilibrand AS. Autograft versus allograft in degenerative cervical disease. Clin Orthop Relat Res 2002;394:27–38.

31. Vaccaro AR, Chiba K, Heller JG, et al. Bone grafting alternatives in spinal surgery. Spine J 2002;2:206–15.
32. Bucholz RW, Carlton A, Holmes RE. Hydroxyapatite and tricalcium phosphate bone graft substitutes. Orthop Clin North Am 1987;18:323–34.
33. Damien CJ, Parsons JR, Prewett AB, et al. Effect of demineralized bone matrix on bone growth within a porous HA material: a histologic and histometric study. J Biomater Appl 1995;9:275–88.
34. Kania RE, Meunier A, Hamadouche M, et al. Addition of fibrin sealant to ceramic promotes bone repair: long-term study in rabbit femoral defect model. J Biomed Mater Res 1998;43:38–45.
35. Frenkel SR, Moskovich R, Spivak J, et al. Demineralized bone matrix. Enhancement of spinal fusion. Spine 1993;18:1634–9.
36. Martin GJ, Jr., Boden SD, Titus L, et al. New formulations of demineralized bone matrix as a more effective graft alternative in experimental posterolateral lumbar spine arthrodesis. Spine 1999;24:637–45.
37. Morone MA, Boden SD. Experimental posterolateral lumbar spinal fusion with a demineralized bone matrix gel. Spine 1998;23:159–67.
38. An HS, Simpson JM, Glover JM, et al. Comparison between allograft plus demineralized bone matrix versus autograft in anterior cervical fusion. A prospective multicenter study. Spine 1995;20:2211–6.
39. Thalgott JS, Giuffre JM, Klezl Z, et al. Anterior lumbar interbody fusion with titanium mesh cages, coralline hydroxyapatite, and demineralized bone matrix as part of a circumferential fusion. Spine J 2002;2:63–9.
40. Peterson B, Whang PG, Iglesias R, et al. Osteoinductivity of commercially available demineralized bone matrix. Preparations in a spine fusion model. J Bone Joint Surg Am 2004;86-A:2243–50.
41. Lee YP, Jo M, Luna M, et al. The efficacy of different commercially available demineralized bone matrix substances in an athymic rat model. J Spinal Disord Tech 2005;18:439–44.
42. Friedlaender GE, Perry CR, Cole JD, et al. Osteogenic protein-1 (bone morphogenetic protein-7) in the treatment of tibial nonunions. J Bone Joint Surg Am 2001;83-A Suppl 1:S151–8.
43. Govender S, Csimma C, Genant HK, et al. Recombinant human bone morphogenetic protein-2 for treatment of open tibial fractures: a prospective, controlled, randomized study of four hundred and fifty patients. J Bone Joint Surg Am 2002;84-A:2123–34.
44. Burkus JK, Gornet MF, Dickman CA, et al. Anterior lumbar interbody fusion using rhBMP-2 with tapered interbody cages. J Spinal Disord Tech 2002;15:337–49.
45. Grauer JN, Patel TC, Erulkar JS, et al. 2000 Young Investigator Research Award winner. Evaluation of OP-1 as a graft substitute for intertransverse process lumbar fusion. Spine 2001;26:127–33.
46. Patel TC, Erulkar JS, Grauer JN, et al. Osteogenic protein-1 overcomes the inhibitory effect of nicotine on posterolateral lumbar fusion. Spine 2001;26:1656–61.
47. Cunningham BW, Shimamoto N, Sefter JC, et al. Osseointegration of autograft versus osteogenic protein-1 in posterolateral spinal arthrodesis: emphasis on the comparative mechanisms of bone induction. Spine J 2002;2:11–24.
48. Blattert TR, Delling G, Dalal PS, et al. Successful transpedicular lumbar interbody fusion by means of a composite of osteogenic protein-1 (rhBMP-7) and hydroxyapatite carrier: a comparison with autograft and hydroxyapatite in the sheep spine. Spine 2002;27:2697–705.
49. Boden SD, Martin GJ, Jr., Horton WC, et al. Laparoscopic anterior spinal arthrodesis with rhBMP-2 in a titanium interbody threaded cage. J Spinal Disord 1998;11:95–101.
50. Sandhu HS, Toth JM, Diwan AD, et al. Histologic evaluation of the efficacy of rhBMP-2 compared with autograft bone in sheep spinal anterior interbody fusion. Spine 2002;27:567–75.

51. Sandhu HS, Kanim LE, Kabo JM, et al. Evaluation of rhBMP-2 with an OPLA carrier in a canine posterolateral (transverse process) spinal fusion model. Spine 1995;20:2669–82.
52. Boden SD, Kang J, Sandhu H, et al. Use of recombinant human bone morphogenetic protein-2 to achieve posterolateral lumbar spine fusion in humans: a prospective, randomized clinical pilot trial: 2002 Volvo Award in clinical studies. Spine 2002;27:2662–73.
53. Helm GA, Alden TD, Beres EJ, et al. Use of bone morphogenetic protein-9 gene therapy to induce spinal arthrodesis in the rodent. J Neurosurg 2000;92:191–6.
54. Jahng TA, Fu TS, Cunningham BW, et al. Endoscopic instrumented posterolateral lumbar fusion with Healos and recombinant human growth/differentiation factor-5. Neurosurgery 2004;54:171–80; discussion 80–1.
55. Sangadala S, Boden SD, Viggeswarapu M, et al. LIM mineralization protein-1 potentiates bone morphogenetic protein responsiveness via a novel interaction with Smurf1 resulting in decreased ubiquitination of Smads. J Biol Chem 2006;281:17212–9.
56. Boden SD, Titus L, Hair G, et al. Lumbar spine fusion by local gene therapy with a cDNA encoding a novel osteoinductive protein (LMP-1). Spine 1998;23:2486–92.
57. Ludwig SC, Boden SD. Osteoinductive bone graft substitutes for spinal fusion: a basic science summary. Orthop Clin North Am 1999;30:635–45.
58. Burwell RG. The function of bone marrow in the incorporation of a bone graft. Clin Orthop Relat Res 1985;200:125–41.
59. Curylo LJ, Johnstone B, Petersilge CA, et al. Augmentation of spinal arthrodesis with autologous bone marrow in a rabbit posterolateral spine fusion model. Spine 1999;24:434–8; discussion 8–9.
60. Muschler GF, Matsukura Y, Nitto H, et al. Selective retention of bone marrow-derived cells to enhance spinal fusion. Clin Orthop Relat Res 2005;432:242–51.

13

Electrical Bone Stimulation

Josh Simon and Bruce Simon

Abstract: Delayed unions and nonunions of long bone fractures are common complications encountered in orthopaedic medicine. Five to 10 percent (300,000 to 600,000) of the 6 million fractures occurring annually in the United States develop some form of compromised union, amounting to an estimated economic loss of $3 billion to $6 billion annually. Electrical stimulation modalities have been employed for decades to promote the healing of delayed unions and nonunions. Although the positive clinical benefits of these treatments have been widely reported, electrical stimulation was largely regarded as a "black box" technology. Today, the black box can be replaced with a mechanism of action. This chapter compiles a basic mechanism of action for the effects of electrical stimulation on bone healing. In short, electrical stimulation up-regulates production of mRNA from DNA, which leads to up-regulated expression of growth factors that are beneficial to the bone healing cascade. Stimulation of cells by these growth factors causes them to proliferate and differentiate, and these events lead to better callus formation, mineralization and vascularization, which in turn provide a better clinical outcome in the form of a faster healing rate, or any healing rate at all, in an area that would not normally heal on its own.

Keywords: Electrical stimulation, bone stimulator, EBI, nonunion, delayed union, bone healing, growth factor, osteoinduction.

13.1. Introduction

Delayed unions and nonunions of long bone fractures are common complications encountered in orthopaedic medicine. Five to 10 percent (300,000 to 600,000) of the 6 million fractures occurring annually in the United States develop some form of compromised union, amounting to an estimated economic loss

Biomet Osteobiologics, Parsippany, NJ

From: *Orthopedic Biology and Medicine: Musculoskeletal Tissue Regeneration, Biological Materials and Methods.*
Edited by W. S. Pietrzak © Humana Press, Totowa, NJ

of $3 billion to $6 billion annually [1–2]. Numerous treatment modalities have been designed to combat fracture nonunions including, but not limited to, internal and external fixation devices, bone grafts, bone substitutes, biologics like platelet extracts and bone morphogenetic proteins, and biophysical stimulation including ultrasound and electrical stimulation.

Electrical stimulation modalities have been employed for decades to promote bone healing. Although the positive clinical benefits of these treatments have been widely reported, electrical stimulation was largely regarded as a "black box" technology. Physicians understood that applying one of these devices to a patient could produce a faster bone healing rate, or any healing rate at all in cases where the patient's natural osseous healing processes have ceased. However, the mechanistic events set in motion by the treatment were poorly understood. Recent literature has elucidated pieces of the overall mechanism of action, mitigating the black box status afforded to electrical stimulation. This chapter aims to present that mechanism and its basic biological and chemical sequence of events compiled from the literature. A substantial body of clinical evidence demonstrates safety and efficacy. This information is also compiled and reviewed.

13.2. Basic Science – Mechanism of Action

Initial observations of bone tissue's electric properties in the 1950s and 1960s gave rise to the development of electrical stimulation for use in bone healing applications [3–8]. When placed under mechanical strain, bone generates electric fields. Electronegative potentials form in areas of compression and electropositive potentials form in areas of tension. It is thought that these endogenous strain-related electric fields may form the basis by which bone remodels in response to mechanical stimuli (i.e., Wolff's Law). Specifically, bone structure adjusts to prevailing mechanical loads by remodeling to accommodate the applied forces. Bony sites which experience stress will undergo bone formation and remodeling, while sites that do not experience mechanical stress will be more likely to undergo bone resorption. Formation and resorption are correlated with the dominant charge in the area. Electronegative regions trigger cells to form bone, while bone resorption occurs in the electropositive regions. Strain-related electrical potentials in bone arise partly from the piezoelectric properties of the mineral matrix and partly from the electrokinetic effects of streaming potentials (i.e., the fluidic movement of ions within the bone structure). A second method by which bone naturally generates electric fields is in response to injuries. This type of field is not unique to bone, in fact, and can be detected in soft tissue injuries as well. These potentials are called injury potentials. Finally, biopotential or growth potential denotes the third method by which bone generates electric fields. Growth potential is formed in areas of rapid bone formation such as at the growth plates of developing skeletal structures [9]. Both injury potentials and growth potentials are metabolically driven processes.

For reasons that are not fully understood, these natural bone potentials sometimes cease to function. The shutting down of naturally occurring electric potentials in bone may be one of several factors contributing towards nonunion. Hypothetically, simulating the effects of these endogenous electric fields on bone cell activities with electrical stimulation devices will produce a therapeutic effect on healing. Several types of electrical stimulation devices are in use for this purpose. They include inductive coupling (IC) devices

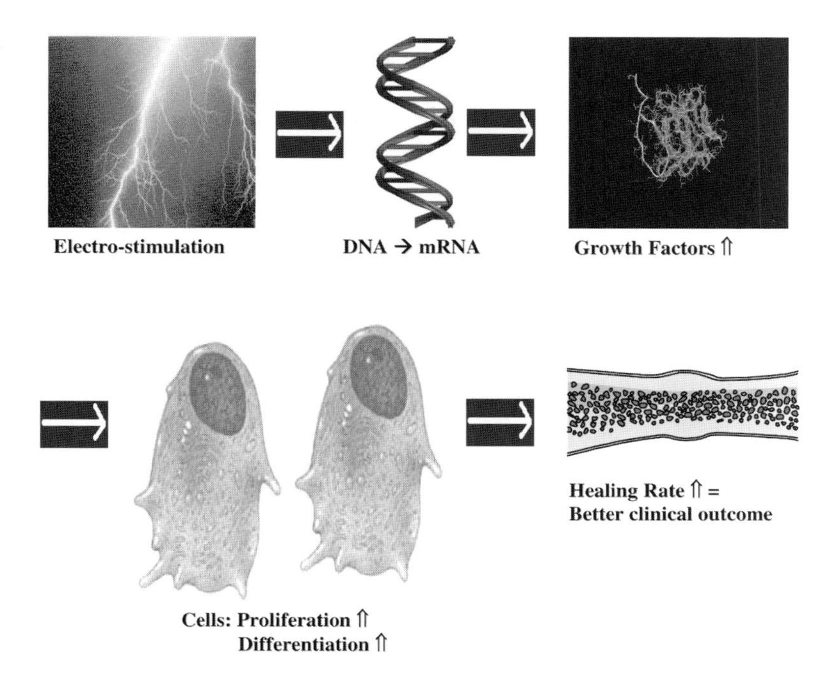

Fig. 13.1 General Mechanism of Action for Electrical Stimulation. Upon treatment with electrical stimulation, a DNA event upregulates production of certain mRNAs which code for growth factors. These growth factors enter the tissue matrix and trigger proliferation and differentiation of cells via autocrine and paracrine action. On a macroscopic level, these events produce larger bone callus and vascularization at the site, which leads to a better clinical outcome in the form of a faster healing rate, or any healing rate at all in the case of nonunions, which, by definition, never heal

such as pulsed electromagnetic fields (PEMF) and combined magnetic fields (CMF), direct current (DC), and capacitive coupling (CC).

It is helpful to review the mechanism of action for electrical stimulation from the perspective of different levels (Fig. 13.1). Ultimately, the clinical level is of most concern. Physicians require their patients to recover from injury in the shortest possible time with the fewest complications and the least cost. The information reviewed later in this chapter portrays the clinical aspects of fracture healing and electrical stimulation. However, clinical studies alone do not explain why these devices work. Study of the mechanism of action begins with scientific data on animals. Understanding the effects of electrical stimulation at the animal level allows for further explanation on the cellular and tissue levels. Below these levels lie the key growth factors that operate under the influence of electrical stimulation, and since growth factors are protein compounds produced by mRNA, understanding the mechanism for these treatments requires knowledge of their effects at the mRNA and DNA levels. Descriptions of the mechanism of action for each of the three modalities is given with attention to these functional and interrelated levels of action.

2.1. Inductive Coupling

IC stimulation is a noninvasive technology consisting of one or two external coils connected to a signal generator (Fig. 13.2). The coils are constructed

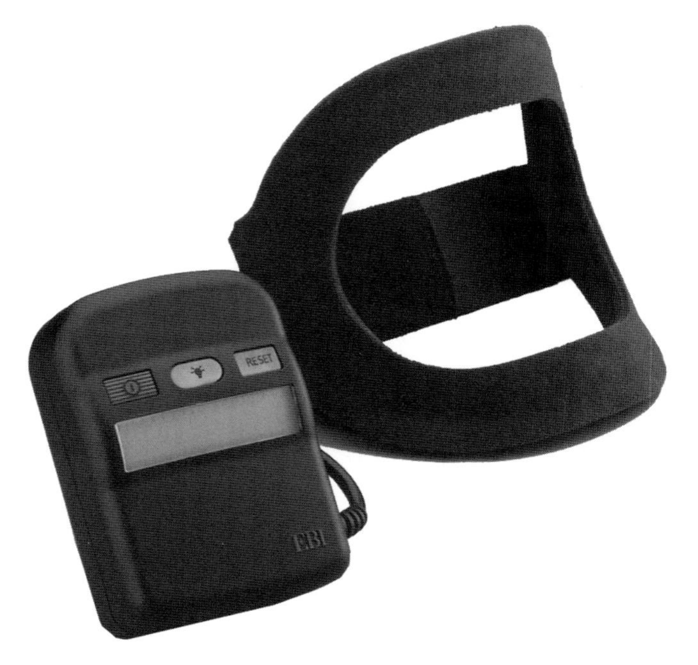

Fig. 13.2 EBI Bone Healing System. A coil, seen on the right, noninvasively delivers pulsed electromagnetic fields which are generated by the small box on the left

from long wires of conducting material which are placed noninvasively over the fracture site. Upon electrification, the coils produce a sinusoidal or pulsed magnetic field over the affected area that induces a secondary electric field in the bone and tissues. The concept is similar to an electrical generator, where a magnetic field is moved over a conductor, producing an electric current in response. Non-ferromagnetic objects, such as fracture casts, allow the magnetic field to penetrate through to the bone defect site without attenuation.

IC signals vary in types of pulse (single pulse or pulsed burst with frequencies typically ranging from 1 to 100 bursts/second), amplitudes, waveform configurations and time-varying magnetic fields of 0.1 to 20G. The literature contains studies on a wide array of different IC pulses, and biological response varies with the specific parameters of the signals. In short, scientific and clinical studies conducted on one pulse type do not apply directly for all pulse types. Clinical therapies currently available that are based on the IC technology are PEMF and CMF. PEMF produces a magnetic field made up of repetitive pulsed burst or single pulsed signals. CMF delivers an alternating magnetic field superimposed on a static field.

13.2.1.1. Preclinical Animal Studies

In animals IC has produced benefits at various stages of bone healing. Anatomical and histological studies report that PEMF stimulates the healing of canine nonunions [10–11], lupine osteotomies [12–13], and fresh fractures in rats [14–15] and dogs [16–17]. Angiogenesis and increased vascularization during the early stages of healing have also been observed [18–20].

Additionally, PEMF has been shown to augment endochondral ossification through upregulation of matrix molecules in the healing callus and stimulation of the progenitor cell pool at the fracture site [21–24]. During late stage callus maturation, the rate of healing, mineral apposition rate and ultimate torsional strength and stiffness at eight to 10 weeks were significantly greater than untreated controls in dogs [25]. PEMF treatment has also shown efficacy in unconventional cases of bone healing, such as in the distraction [26–28], but not consolidation [29] phases of distraction osteogenesis, and in the presence of hydroxyapatite implants [30–31], and porous ceramic scaffolds [32].

Data from animal sources points to the utility of IC, but it only describes the surface of the mechanism, i.e. the end result. To better understand the mechanism of action, IC's effects on individual cells and tissues must be explored.

13.2.1.2. Cell and Tissue Studies

Cellular studies on IC indicate increased osteoblastic proliferation and differentiation [21–22, 33], modulation of bone and cartilage cell matrix production [13, 23, 34] and inhibition of osteoclastic resorption [35–40]. These phenomena may be the basis of *in vivo* results described above. Enhanced cellular proliferation and differentiation typically lead to enhanced callus formation and maturation at the various stages of bone healing.

In turn, these cellular events may be due to regulation of growth factors associated with IC treatment [18–19, 34, 41–50], and the alteration of gene expression of proteins, cytokine signaling, various membrane functions and the modulation of transmembrane signaling by altering the density and distribution of receptor populations [37, 51–76]. Specifically, PEMF causes bone to increase calcium uptake and renders it insensitive to parathyroid hormone (PTH) [37, 72] by inhibiting the accumulation of cyclic-Adenosine Monophosphate (cAMP) naturally associated with PTH stimulation [57–58] and the expression of PTH receptors on the cell surface [70]. Similar cAMP inhibition has been reported in fibroblastic cells [65]. CMF has also been shown to increase calcium uptake by osteoblasts *in vitro* [66]. Calcium ions play a direct role in mineralization of bone, and they mediate interactions between cell surface receptors, antibodies, hormones and even neurotransmitters [52, 71]. These activities at the surfaces of bone cells play directly into manipulation of bone healing through amplification of signal transduction pathways [55–56], which eventually go on to modulate mRNA and DNA synthesis. Moreover, calcium release from intracellular stores is also a key metabolic driving force for cellular activity under the action of PEMF [56, 74]. A study by Farndale, et. al. suggests that ionic transport of extracellular ions through the cell membrane is not affected over a short-term timescale in red blood cells or epithelial cells [64]. Therefore, the action of PEMF on calcium uptake and eventual cellular proliferation and differentiation may be principally due to effects on endothelial cells, osteoblasts and osteoclasts.

Concomitant with cellular membrane and ionic transport events, IC up-regulates growth factor production for certain molecules relevant to bone healing. Preceding the production of these agents, which are usually proteins, is the transcription of precursor mRNA. The synthesis of mRNA for multiple growth factors, such as Bone Morphogenetic Protein (BMP) 2 and BMP-4, is increased by PEMF stimulation [77] (see Table 13.1), and

Table 13.1 Upregulation of growth factors with IC stimulation

Reference	Modality	Model	Outcome
Nagai and Ota [79]	PEMF	Osteoblasts	↑ BMP-2, -4 mRNA
Yajima, et al. [80]	PEMF	Osteoblasts	↑ BMP-4, -5, -7 mRNA
Bodamyali, et al. [77]	PEMF	Osteoblasts	↑ BMP-2, -4 mRNA, ↑ proliferation
Aaron, et al. [34]	PEMF	*In vivo* Endochondral Ossification	↑ TGF-β1, ↑ differentiation
Aaron, et al. [244]	PEMF	*In vivo* Endochondral Ossification	↑ TGF-β1 mRNA, ↑ differentiation, ↑ protein
Lohmann, et al. [48]	PEMF	MG63 Osteoblasts	↑ TGF-β1, ↑ differentiation
Lohmann, et al. [49]	PEMF	MLO-Y4 Osteoblast-like cells	↑ TGF-β1, ↑ PGE_2
Guerkov, et al. [46]	PEMF	Human nonunion cells	↑ TGF-β1
Fitzsimmons, et. al. [45]	CMF	TE-85 Osteoblasts	↑ IGF-2, ↑ proliferation
Ryaby, et al. [50]	CMF	Osteoblasts	↑ IGF-2
Tepper, et al. [19]	PEMF	Endothelial cells	↑ FGF-2, ↑ FGF-2 mRNA, ↑ proliferation

the resultant growth factors may then act on cells in the surrounding area through autocrine and paracrine action [41]. Electric and electromagnetic fields can produce a sustained upregulation of growth factors that enhances, but does not disorganize, endochondral bone formation [78]. Moreover, resultant upregulation of mRNA for BMP-2 and -4 might be related to, and possibly mediate, the bone inductive effect of PEMF [79]. Maximal increases in BMP -4, -5 and -7 are seen after 24 hours of exposure to PEMF treatment *in vitro* [80], and expression of BMP -4, and -7 in rat osteoblasts *in vivo* is coincident with bone induction [77]. Upregulation of mRNA expression and protein synthesis for TGF-β1 are coincident with increased cellular matrix synthesis and gene expression [34]. This upregulation was observed in a consistent and uniform dose dependent manner correlated with exposure time and amplitude. Notably, the pattern of TGF-β1 expression was unchanged through the developmental sequence, indicating that PEMF stimulation up-regulates and enhances, but does not disorganize, chondrogenesis, endochondral ossification and the natural physiological expression of TGF-β1. Further exploration by Aaron, et. al. indicates that PEMF stimulation of chondrogenesis may be modulated by TGF-β1 [34].

Within the nucleus, mRNA production originates with transcription. To modulate this process, IC must ultimately affect DNA either directly or indirectly. Data on upregulation of transcription implies this connection to DNA. Recent studies on IC stimulation's effects on DNA shed light on this stage of the mechanism of action. The basis for interaction between DNA and electromagnetic fields may be due to field-charge interactions with the electrons in the DNA [81]. Assuming that electron affinity is a measure of electron density at a DNA base pair, theoretical calculations indicate that repulsive forces generated by electromagnetic fields are greatest in DNA sequences rich in cytosine (C) and thymine (T) nucleotides [82–83]. If these areas are more likely to come apart, they may be more amenable to transcription. Alternatively or concurrently, IC may affect the protein structures associated with DNA, such as histones and transcription factors. By making DNA available for easier transcription, a gene's expression could be up-regulated. For example, short-term exposure to PEMF was reported to increase c-fos and c-myc gene expression in TE-85 osteoblasts [63]. Upregulation of these genes was linked to modified expression of transcription factor AP-1 [78, 84].

13.2.1.3. Consolidated Mechanism of Action

Taken in whole, the information on IC gives clues to the main flow of the mechanism of action for bone healing. For certain PEMF signals, a set of possible trigger effects on DNA causes increased mRNA transcription. Increased production of mRNA leads to regulation of growth factors, which affect cells through autocrine and paracrine action. Cellular effects from growth factors are wide and varied, but break down generally into the categories of differentiation and proliferation triggers. Concurrently, changes in cell surface characteristics lead to changes in intracellular pathways that may eventually also amplify DNA events that feed forward into increased cellular proliferation and differentiation. Overall, increased cellular proliferation and differentiation typically lead to enhanced callus formation and maturation, which typically lead to better radiographic and, oftentimes, better clinical outcomes.

13.2.2. Capacitive Coupling

CC stimulation noninvasively generates electric fields in tissues. Electrodes with conductive gel are placed on the skin over the bone defect site (Fig. 13.3). They are then connected to an external alternating current (AC) signal generator, which delivers a current of about 5 mA (Root Mean Square) and 1 to 10 Volts peak to peak. Frequencies in the literature typically range from 20 to 200 kHz, and the frequency of the clinically marketed device (Orthopak™ 2 Bone Growth Stimulator, Biomet, Inc., Parsippany, NJ) is 60 kHz. The resultant local voltage gradient in the tissue is about 1 to 100 mV/cm [85].

13.2.2.1. Preclinical Animal Studies

Efficacy of CC stimulation for orthopaedic use has been observed with *in vivo* models for bone healing [86–89], and osteoporosis [87, 90–92]. Results from Brighton, et al. indicate successful rabbit growth plate stimulation to statistically significant accelerated growth in a capacitively coupled electrical field. Moreover, a dose-response effect was noted among the amplitudes in the study [86]. In diaphyseal bone increased mineralization and callus formation have been shown in fresh fractures [85], and in delayed unions [89]. Similarly to the data given for IC, animal data for CC points to its utility, but it only describes the surface of the mechanism, i.e., the end result. CC's effects on individual cells elucidate more of the mechanism of action.

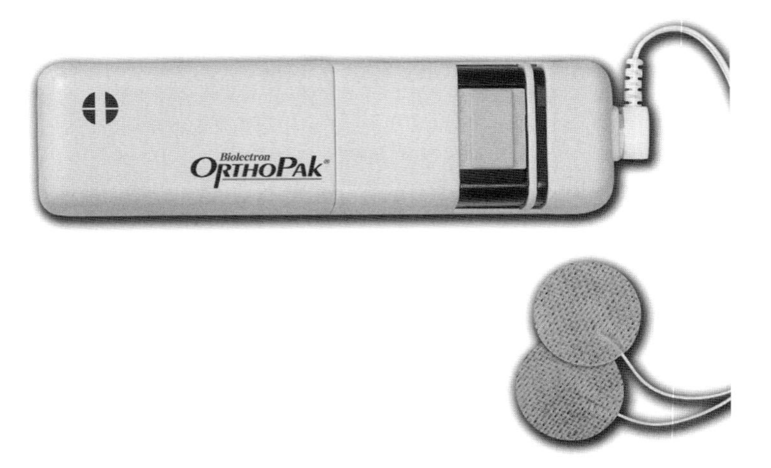

Fig. 13.3 OrthoPak Capacitive Coupling Device. Two small electrodes affixed noninvasively near the site of injury deliver an oscillating electric field which is generated by a four ounce power pack

13.2.2.2. Cell and Tissue Studies

In vitro studies on CC stimulation investigated the roles of signal field strength, pulse pattern and duty cycle on cell function [93]. Similar to that of IC, CC efficacy varies with signal parameters [93] and duration of treatment [56, 78]. At sine-wave frequencies of 60 kHz, CC stimulation reportedly increases *in vitro* proliferation of osteoblasts [93–95], and chondrocytes [96–98]. A dose-response to CC stimulation was described by Brighton, et al. [56]. MC3T3-E1 osteoblast-like cell cultures were exposed to CC stimulation for zero, 30 minutes, two hours, six hours and 24 hours. Proliferation increased with increasing treatment time.

Examination of CC's influence on cellular proliferation and bone formation at the biochemical level reveals transmembrane calcium (Ca^{2+}) translocation via voltage-gated calcium channels as a key step in the mechanism of action [56, 99]. Using rat calvarial bone cells and MC3T3-E1 osteoblasts, Lorich, et al. investigated the biochemical pathway mediating the response of bone cells to capacitive coupling stimulation [99]. Cells were cultured and treated with a capacitively coupled 60 kHz sine wave signal or inactive device. Signal transduction inhibitors, such as verapamil and W-7, were administered to block specific biochemical pathways involving voltage-gated Ca^{2+} channels and the Ca^{2+}-calmodulin pathway. Effects on cellular proliferation and PGE_2 production were analyzed. Results showed that the biochemical pathways mediating the response of bone cells to CC stimulation involve extracellular Ca^{2+} translocation via voltage-gated calcium channels, activation of phospholipase A_2 and a subsequent increase in PGE_2. Increases in cytosolic Ca^{2+} and its reaction with calmodulin also led to amplification of a wide array of enzymatic pathways, pumps and target proteins, leading to enhanced cell proliferation. The inositol phosphate pathway does not play a role in CC stimulated cell responses [99–100].

Interactions between the Ca^{2+}-calmodulin pathway and growth factor synthesis under the action of CC stimulation have also been found. These interactions also seem linked to cellular proliferation [101]. Using MC3T3-E1 osteoblastic cultures with signal transduction inhibitors and TGF-β_1 antibodies, it was reported that CC stimulation promotes synthesis of TGF-β_1 via the calcium-calmodulin pathway [101].

The role of other growth factors in the mechanism of action of CC stimulation has also been investigated. The effect of CC stimulation on the expression of factors related to bone formation was investigated using an animal model first described by Morone, et al. [102]. Posterolateral intertransverse process fusions were performed bilaterally at L4-L5 with autograft on rabbits. Experimental rabbits received CC stimulation and were evaluated against unstimulated control rabbits. Results indicated that CC stimulation up-regulates specific temporal and spatial gene expressions of BMP-2, BMP-6 and TGF-β_1 [103–104]. Similar to growth factor upregulation with IC stimulation, CC was found to enhance but not disorganize the natural physiological expression of these growth factors. At 21 days two of three rabbits in this study had unilateral fusions in the CC-treated group, compared to one of three rabbits in the control group. By 28 days CC-treated rabbits had one bilateral fusion and two unilateral fusions, in contrast to two of three rabbits in the control group with unilateral fusions. None of the rabbits in the control group achieved bilateral fusions.

Upregulation of growth factors with CC treatment is a significant part of the mechanism of action leading to proliferation and differentiation of cells involved in the bone healing process. Cells exhibiting up-regulated growth factor production will spur activity within surrounding tissue through autocrine and paracrine action. To elucidate the deeper mechanism of action behind CC requires study of the source of growth factor upregulation, which is essentially protein production: mRNA. Capacitively coupled electric fields have been reported to increase production of IGF-2 mRNA [95]. More recently, Zhuang, et al. reported increased production of TGF-β_1 mRNA under CC stimulation [101]. In this study mRNA production was linked to the Ca^{2+}-calmodulin pathway. To date, the most recent study of up-regulated transcription for growth factor production reports consistent increased synthesis of BMP -2, -4, -5, -6 and -7 mRNA's [105]. This study also showed the optimal CC frequency was 60 kHz, 20 mV/cm at a 50 percent duty cycle for a duration of 24 hours, which is equivalent to the signal used clinically.

Increased transcription of mRNA implies direct and indirect effects of CC stimulation on DNA. A few studies note these effects [56, 93, 97, 100, 106–107]. DNA synthesis in cartilage cells is increased by exposure to oscillating electric fields [106], and [3H]thymidine incorporation is increased in articular chondrocytes under CC influence [107]. Similar [3H]thymidine incorporation results were obtained in bovine growth plate chondrocytes [97]. In bone cells proliferative effects attributed to CC stimulation also coincide with increased DNA synthesis [56, 93, 100]. Again, these effects are linked with translocation of Ca^{2+} ions and the Ca^{2+}-calmodulin pathway.

13.2.2.3. Consolidated Mechanism of Action

Mechanistic data on CC stimulation presented here gives clues to the main flow of the mechanism of action for bone healing. Initiatory trigger effects on DNA that lead to increased mRNA transcription are not fully understood at this time. Increased production of mRNA has been reported, and this phenomena leads to upregulation of growth factors, which affect cells through autocrine and paracrine action. Cellular effects from growth factors are wide and varied, but break down generally into the categories of differentiation and proliferation triggers. These growth factor effects have been closely tied to changes in intracellular pathways, such as the Ca^{2+}-calmodulin pathway which is known to eventually amplify DNA events that feed forward into more cellular proliferation and possibly differentiation. A major contrast between the mechanisms of action for IC and CC is that CC is known to act through translocation of extracellular calcium through the cell membrane. IC stimulation relies on intracellular stores of calcium to activate the same pathways. Overall, increased cellular proliferation and differentiation typically lead to enhanced callus formation and maturation, which typically lead to better radiographic and better clinical outcomes.

13.2.3. Direct Current

Direct Current (DC) stimulators are implantable devices comprised of one or more titanium electrodes (cathodes) connected to a platinum-plated power supply (anode) (Fig. 13.4). The device is surgically implanted with the cathode placed at the fracture site and the anode in the soft tissue. Upon contact with body tissues and fluids, the circuit between the cathode and anode is completed and a local electric current is produced at the fracture site. The currents investigated typically range from 5 to 100 μA [108].

13.2.3.1. Preclinical Animal Studies

Numerous animal studies detail the effects of DC stimulation on bone repair. Early studies in rats indicated that DC stimulation had beneficial effects on the healing of fractures [109–111], but the mechanism was not known at that time. Fibular osteotomies in rats treated with implantable DC stimulation also showed significantly improved macroscopic, radiologic and histopathologic parameters over controls [112]. During the same decade, DC stimulation data

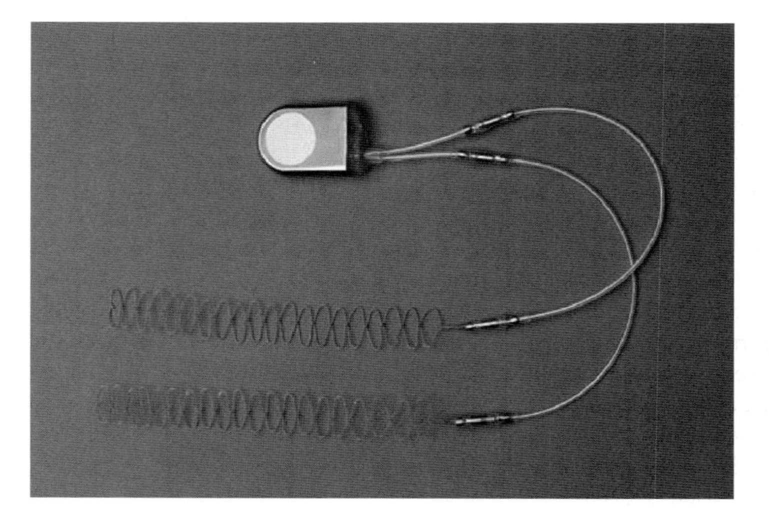

Fig. 13.4 SpF Direct Current Stimulator. This implantable stimulator delivers a constant electric current generated from a platinum-plated battery pack which acts as the anode for the circuit. The cathode wires are placed into a bony site, and current begins to flow through the area after the incision is closed and the unit is submersed in body fluids

on rabbits indicated general benefits to bone healing [113–115] and increased endosteal and periosteal callus formation [116]. Similar results were reported soon after in a lupine delayed fibular union model [117]. One rabbit study observed no significant increase in rabbit fibular osteotomy healing, but the same study went on to show efficacy in human nonunions for the same device [118]. Use of DC stimulation with intramedullary electrodes [119–120] and divided titanium bone chambers [121] showed that active healing of the bone at the metal-bone interface proceeded long after the normal time accounted for by reactive bone formation. When a similar study using movable k-wires in the medulary canal was conducted, however, it was noted that micromotion of the wires could confound the analysis of causality for new bone growth in the canal [122]. A later study repeated this model and showed that bone formation under the influence of DC stimulation was much more likely in an area of active cells, like those found near a fracture or in bone marrow [123]. In other rabbit studies improvements in healing using DC stimulation were noted for growth plate cartilage [124], physeal cartilage [125], patellar ligament [126] and macroscopic angiogenesis [127]. Notably in rabbit spine fusions, the combined use of coralline hydroxyapatite scaffolds with DC stimulation performed equally to autograft treatment [128–129]. Efficacy in spine fusions for this model was also found to increase with increasing microcurrent [130], but increased DC current was unable to produce fusion in the presence of poor bone graft materials, such as calcium sulfate, even though it still increased the nominal growth that occurred regardless [131]. Canine delayed union models reveal benefits for DC stimulation in tibial [132–134], radial [135] and ulnar [136] defects. Macroscopic observations in radial defects showed that DC stimulation brought about increases in bone density and was likely to affect early events in the fracture healing sequence [137–138]. Efficacy of DC stimulation was also reported for canine spine fusions [139–140]. Compelling evidence for a dose-response with increasing current density (i.e., microamperage per unit length of cathode) was reported in canine spine fusions [141]. Coupled with similar dose response data in rabbits, it was determined that increasing DC microamperage or decreasing overall cathode length can maximize benefits of DC stimulation's bone healing qualities, if the cathode wires are constructed from titanium. Increasing amperage about 20 μA with stainless steel cathode wires produces tissue necrosis [114]. All current commercially available DC stimulators use titanium leads for this reason. The upper limit of the dose-response curve for titanium lead wires is unknown, but it is thought that it could be as high as 500 μA. Similarly, DC stimulation was shown to be efficacious as an adjunct to interbody spinal fusions in sheep, with increasing success for higher microcurrents from 60 μA to 100 μA, which was the highest current evaluated [142]. Increased efficacy with higher current density was also seen in a primate model for anterior lumbar interbody fusions (ALIF) which employed DC stimulation in conjunction with titanium cages [143].

General efficacy of DC stimulation in animals as a result of increased bone formation, angiogenesis and callus formation points to activities on the cellular and tissue levels. All of these events typically lead to better bone formation, which can be translated to possible efficacy in humans. Further detail into the mechanism of action for DC stimulation is given by *in vitro* studies on cell and tissue behavior.

13.2.3.2. Cell and Tissue Studies

Cellular studies with DC stimulation show that electrochemical reactions at the cathode lower local oxygen concentration and increase pH [144–147]. These electrochemical reactions in animals have been linked to improved bone healing [87, 148]. The primary faradic reaction is: $O_2 + 2H_2O + 4e^- \rightarrow 4OH^-$. Electrons from the cathode reduce water and oxygen to produce hydroxyl ions. Reduction in oxygen concentration and an increase in pH due to increased concentration of hydroxyl ions promote chondrogenesis and endochondral ossification. Metabolically active cells located in the growth plate follow a predominantly anaerobic metabolic pathway. Relatively low oxygen concentration is found at the bone-cartilage junction in the growth plate [149], in areas of new bone formation and in fracture calluses [150–152], and has been shown to promote bone growth [153–155]. Increased pH is found in areas of calcification at the growth plate [156] and sites of active bone fracture healing [157], where it is linked to facilitated mineral deposition during fracture repair [158]. Increased pH also inhibits proliferation of osteoclasts and subsequent resorption of bone [159–160], and stimulates osteoblastic activity [160], thus resulting in increased bone formation.

A mouse culture model was used to investigate the effects of DC and resultant faradic products on bone remodeling [145]. Explanted mouse calvarial cultures were treated with DC in isolation from faradic products, DC with faradic products or DC with faradic products and hydrogen peroxide scavenger. Control samples consisted of calvariae in culture that were exposed to parathyroid hormone (PTH) treatment as a positive control or to elevated media pH, or to salt bridges and electrodes with no current or no treatment at all. Results showed a net calcium efflux into the medium, which was an indication of bone resorption activity. DC electric fields alone were observed to enhance calcium uptake, and greater uptake was observed with DC and faradic products together at the cathode. Hydroxyl ions increased at the cathode, resulting in increased local pH.

A second faradic product generated at the cathode was hydrogen peroxide (H_2O_2). This compound accelerates bone remodeling through stimulation of bone resorption and possibly the differentiation of osteoclasts [161]. As the bony surface becomes pitted by resorption, osteoblasts deposit new bone. H_2O_2 has also been found to stimulate macrophages to release Vascular Endothelial Growth Factor (VEGF) [162], an angiogenic growth factor that plays a role in fracture healing.

The mechanism of action behind DC stimulation is not fully explained by changes in local pH and oxygen tension. It has also been found to involve the upregulation of a number of osteoinductive growth factors [104]. Posterolateral intertransverse process spine fusions with autograft were performed bilaterally on rabbits and treated either with or without DC stimulation. Outcomes revealed that all rabbits in the DC-treated group had fused bilaterally at 21 days, compared to two unilateral and no bilateral fusions in the control group. At 28 days the DC-treated group again had 100 percent bilateral fusions versus two unilateral fusions and one bilateral fusion in the control group. Analysis on specific temporal and spatial gene expression of growth factors within the fusion mass, specifically BMP-2, 6 and 7, showed that DC stimulation up-regulated, but did not disorganize, mRNA expression of the proteins [104, 163].

13.2.3.3. Consolidated Mechanism of Action

When known aspects of DC's effects on bone healing are compiled, a basic mechanistic picture emerges. To date, the literature lacks information on how DC stimulation prompts DNA synthesis. However, the proliferative effects of DC on cells are known, and imply increased DNA synthesis under the action of DC. Likely causes for increased DNA synthesis are intracellular pathways up-regulated by faradic products and growth factor influence at the cell surface. As with the mechanisms for IC and CC, these effects could markedly increase the action of transcription factors and histones which modulate DNA synthesis and transcription. Increased production of mRNA for important osteoinductive growth factors due to DC stimulation has been reported. Upregulation of mRNA expression for multiple growth factors, such as BMPs, may lead to increased expression of the corresponding protein growth factors. Growth factor expression by cells leads to wider tissue stimulation through autocrine and paracrine action. Overall, increased cellular proliferation and differentiation due to growth factor influence typically lead to enhanced callus formation and maturation, which typically lead to better radiographic and better clinical outcomes.

13.3. Clinical Science

Treating fractures with electrical stimulation came into widespread clinical usage in the late 1970s. The majority of published clinical studies focus on nonunions, though numerous other orthopaedic and soft tissue applications have been studied. Current therapies approved for clinical use are 1) noninvasive PEMF and CMF, which are based on IC technology, 2) implantable DC stimulation and 3) noninvasive CC stimulation.

13.3.1. Inductive Coupling

In addition to nonunions and fractures, positive results using PEMF have also been reported for scaphoid nonunion [164–168], knee arthrodesis [169], congenital pseudarthrosis of the tibia [170–174], Jones fractures [175–176], relief of pain and stiffness in osteoarthritis [177–180] and osteonecrosis of the femoral head [181–188]. A multicenter study on the use of PEMF reported treatment of 1,007 ununited fractures and 71 failed arthrodesis [189]. Ninety percent of nonunions in the study had durations of over nine months. The overall success rate was 77 percent, and the success rate for tibial nonunions alone was 82 percent. For patients in the United States the study reported that those with infected nonunions had a success rate of 72 percent. Success rates were not correlated with presence of metallic implants and the duration of nonunion. A comprehensive retrospective review of the effectiveness of PEMF in enhancing healing of delayed nonunions [190] revealed that PEMF's effectiveness increases with the number of revision surgeries, and that PEMF is effective in increasing union rates for closed fractures. Of the 44 studies evaluated in the review, 28 explored PEMF-treated tibial nonunions and reported an overall success rate of 81 percent, ranging from 13 percent to 100 percent. Another study of 127 delayed and nonunions of the tibial diaphysis showed an 87 percent success rate with PEMF [191]. Median healing time was 5.2 months. Results of a tibial nonunion study employing PEMF showed a success rate of 64 percent of 149 patients with a mean time after injury of 2.5 years. Among the successes, 85 percent healed within three to six months of treatment [192].

Prospective, randomized, double-blind, placebo-controlled clinical trials are a highly stringent form of evaluation in clinical science. This format produces more reliable results than uncontrolled and/or retrospective studies and meta-analyses. There are five such controlled studies for PEMF. Borsalino, et al. conducted double-blind placebo-controlled prospective analysis of 31 femoral intertrochanteric osteotomies involving degenerative joint disease of the hip [177, 193]. Patients were treated for eight hours per day for three months with either active or placebo PEMF devices. Statistically significant improvements in healing including higher bone density (41 percent) and trabecular bridging (64 percent) were seen in the treated group, compared to the control group. A second placebo-controlled double-blind randomized trial investigating PEMF's effects on tibial delayed unions [194] studied 45 patients with moderate to severe diaphyseal tibia fractures with delayed unions. Fracture ages ranged from 16 to 32 weeks post-injury and were randomized to active or placebo stimulator treatment for 12 hours per day over 12 weeks. An orthopaedic surgeon and a radiologist independently carried out blinded clinical and radiographic assessments of the data. Both clinical and radiographic evaluations showed increased healing in fractures treated with PEMF. Unions were observed in nine of 20 patients (45 percent) with active devices, compared to three of 22 patients (14 percent) with placebo devices. Radiographic unions were observed in five patients in the PEMF-treated group, progress toward radiographic union in another five and no progress in 10. The placebo group showed union only in one patient, progress toward union in one and no progress in 23 patients. Statistical analysis revealed significance between the treatment groups, thereby pointing to the efficacy of PEMF stimulation in tibial delayed unions. Another placebo-controlled prospective evaluation of 40 tibial osteotomies for degenerative arthrosis was reported by Mammi, et al [195]. Bony bridging in greater than 50 percent of the osteotomy site at 60 days after osteotomy was evident in 72.2 percent (13/18) of the patients. For placebo controls, 26.3 percent (five of 19 patients) achieved this level of bony bridging. In another randomized, double-blinded study of tibial nonunions, Parnell and Simonis similarly observed increased success rates with PEMF [196]. Finally, the use of PEMF for enhancement of tibial nonunion healing with external fixation was evaluated a decade later in 34 consecutive patients [197]. After six months of follow-up patients were evaluated for clinical and radiographic union. By chance, there was an imbalance in smoking habit between the two groups. Union rate in the smoker subgroup was 75 percent (6/8) in the active PEMF group, compared to 46 percent (6/13) for the placebo group. PEMF-treated non-smokers had 100 percent (10/10) union rate, compared to 67 percent (2/3) in the placebo group. In total, 24 of 34 patients progressed to bony union.

For CMF, clinical studies are fewer in number. They report on the treatment of fracture nonunions [198] and spine fusions [199]. A retrospective uncontrolled study with CMF reported positive success for 20 patients with 23 extremity nonunions ranging from three months to three years in duration. Fifty percent of the osteotomy sites underwent two or more surgical procedures prior to treatment [198]. For primary noninstrumented posterolateral spine fusions, a randomized, double-blind, placebo-controlled trial indicated that

64 percent of patients with CMF treatment healed at nine months, compared with 43 percent of patients with placebo devices. Stratification of the results according to gender revealed fusion in 67 percent of CMF-treated females, compared with 35 percent of those with placebo devices and no statistically significant effect of the active device in the male study population [199].

13.3.2. Capacitive Coupling

CC has also been investigated in double-blind studies. Efficacy of CC on long bone nonunions, defined by greater than nine months after injury, was evaluated. Patients received treatment with active or placebo devices for 24 hours per day for a maximum of six months. Six of 10 patients in the CC-treated group had a mean healing time of 21 weeks, compared to no unions in 11 patients in the placebo group [200]. Another prospective double-blind, placebo-controlled trial evaluated efficacy of CC treatment in lumbar spine fusions in 179 patients [201]. Fusion success rates were 84.7 percent for the active patients and 64.9 percent for the placebo patients, and the results were highly statistically significant. Best results were achieved when CC stimulation was used in conjunction with internal spinal fixation.

Successful treatment of 22 recalcitrant nonunions was reported by Brighton, et al. [202–203]. Recalcitrance was determined by failure to heal after either previous bone grafting or another type of electrical stimulation or both. Seventeen of the nonunions (77.3 percent) achieved solid osseous union after an average of 22.5 weeks of CC treatment. Osteomyelitis, presence of metallic internal-fixation devices, extent of recalcitrance or full weight bearing on the extremity in a cast did not affect success rates in this study. Two other separate studies also found that osteomyelitis was not a factor that affected CC efficacy [204–205]. CC treatment of the lower extremities also showed positive results for stress fractures in athletes [206]. Twenty-one athletes with 25 lower limb stress fractures consisting of navicular, second and fifth metatarsal, fibula, tibia and talus were treated. After 52 days, 22 fractures were healed, one was not healed and two were improved.

A retrospective meta-analysis using a logistic regression model compared the efficacy of capacitive coupling, direct current and bone grafting in treating tibial nonunions [207]. Healing rates, risk factors and success rates were compared in 271 tibial nonunions of average duration of 23.5 months. Risk factors included duration of nonunion, prior bone graft surgery, prior electrical stimulation, open fracture, osteomyelitis, comminuted or oblique fracture and atrophic nonunion. Analysis indicated comparable rates between the three treatment methods when no risk factors were present. As the number of risk factors increased, efficacy decreased. Bone graft surgery was found to yield the worse healing rate if a nonunion had previously been treated unsuccessfully with bone graft surgery. In the presence of atrophic nonunion, CC did not fare as well as DC in this study.

13.3.3. Direct Current

The general consensus is that double-blind studies with placebo implant devices are unethical in humans, and that is why there are no reports of double-blind placebo-controlled clinical studies with DC stimulators. Most clinical studies evaluate these devices against some standard of care instead of dummy controls.

For bone defects of appendages and extremities, implantable DC technology has been reported to produce union success rates of 70 to 90 percent [108] of cases. A study by Paterson, et al. evaluated efficacy of DC stimulation in 84 patients with delayed and nonunion tibial fractures in a large multicenter study [208]. Clinical and radiographical results indicated an overall success rate of 86 percent, with an average time to union of 16 weeks. A 10-year clinical and roentgenographic follow-up assessment on the patients from this trial was later conducted [209]. The authors located 38 patients from the original study. All fractures from the DC stimulation group remained united with signs of normal bone remodeling, and no adverse affects were reported among the participants. This 10-year evaluation exhibits long-term safety and efficacy of DC stimulation in treating delayed and nonunions. In another multicenter study success rates of 78 percent of 258 were seen in patients treated with DC stimulation [210–211]. DC stimulation efficacy has also been observed in the treatment of nonunion in the foot [212], avascular necrosis of the talus [213], patients requiring foot or ankle arthrodesis due to arthritis [214–215], failed fusions [216–217], Charcot osteoarthropathy [212], slow healing fracture and tendon injury [215], tibia congenital pseudarthrosis [218–224] and avascular necrosis of the femoral head [225–227].

Successful use of DC stimulation in lumbar spine fusion was first reported by Dwyer in 1974 [228–229]. In this study 11 out of 12 patients with lumbosacral fusions showed evidence of osteogenesis and metaplastic fusion. Later, similar results in patients with secondary lumbosacral fusions were reported [230]. A review of DC spine trials in the 1970s by Kane, et al. [216] reports a prospective randomized controlled trial series on "difficult patients," i.e., patients with one or more previous failed fusions, a grade II or worse spondylolisthesis, a multiple-level fusion or the presence of another high risk factor such as obesity. Radiographic fusion assessed by blinded independent radiologists was achieved in 15 of 28 control patients (54 percent), compared with 25 of 31 DC-treated patients (81 percent). DC stimulation has also been successfully employed for enhancement of lumbar interbody fusion [231]. Fusion rates in this study were significantly higher in stimulated patients (93 percent versus 75 percent). Compelling evidence of DC efficacy was most prominent in high risk groups such as smokers (92 percent versus 71 percent), and those with no internal fixation (91 percent versus 65 percent) and L4–L5 fusions (91 percent versus 59 percent). Some of these lumbar spine fusion studies have been included in retrospective reviews as well [232–233]. By the mid-1990s, DC stimulation was suggested for use as a critical component of lumbar spine fusion repair [234]. Further investigation of DC stimulation for spine fusion in patients with high risk factors was reported a year later. Particularly, multi-level spine fusions infer a significant degree of risk in the form of typically lower fusion rates. A prospective trial explored the effects of DC stimulation on multi-level procedures [235]. Among 118 DC-stimulated patients, the overall fusion success rate was 91.5 percent. Out of 90 two-level procedures fusion rate was 93 percent. Among 22 three-level procedures fusion rate was 91 percent. Eighty-five patients (72 percent) had no pain after treatment. 27 patients (23 percent) had mild pain occasionally, and six patients (5 percent) had some degree of moderate pain. Concomitant with risk factors, the already high fusion rates associated with spine hardware were further increased when used in conjunction with DC stimulation [236]. Ninety-six percent of patients with stimulation had solid fusion versus 85 percent fusion in patients who did not have stimulation. Several later studies continued to evaluate the effects of DC stimulation on smokers in conjunction with spine instrumentation [237], and in conjunction with other risk factors [238–243]. In total, the studies express the utility of DC stimulation for improving fusion rates in high risk patients both with and without instrumentation.

13.4. Future Trends and Needs

Electrical stimulation technology has come a long way from its early days of black box theory, but with any scientific or clinical pursuit, the discovery of answers produces more questions. The presently known correlations that exist between treatment with electrical stimulation and upregulation of growth factors have two limitations that can be resolved with further research: 1) most of the correlations have been proven in animals only, and 2) the number of growth factors that are known to be up-regulated by electrical stimulation are only part of the entire larger mechanism, and they do not give complete account of the treatments' effects. It is not only likely that similar growth factor correlations occur in humans, it is also probable that the expression of far more growth factors that are as yet unstudied can be influenced by electrical stimulation. Future studies can uncover these effects in both humans and animals.

From a clinical perspective, the applications for electrical stimulation are expected to increase, especially in areas where a single growth factor is not enough to produce healing, like osteoarthritis. Applications for diabetic foot ulcers and wound healing are also being researched.

13.5. Conclusion

This chapter presented the mechanism of action for three electrical stimulation modalities, and their basic biological and chemical sequences of events compiled from the literature. Additionally, a substantial body of compiled clinical evidence was presented to demonstrate safety and efficacy. Preclinical and clinical evidence and their interactions have great importance in forming a substantive picture of the usefulness of electrostimulation therapies. Understanding the mechanism of action allows for maximization of clinical data usage. Indeed, the clinical stage of healing is the ultimate step of the mechanism of action, which begins with invisible DNA and charge interactions, and cascades up to visible outcomes.

References

1. Praemer A, Furner S, Rice D. Musculoskeletal Conditions in the United States. Park Ridge, IL: American Academy of Orthopaedic Surgeons; 1992.
2. Praemer A, Furner S, Rice D. Musculoskeletal Conditions in the United States. 2nd ed. Rosemont, IL: American Academy of Orthopaedic Surgeons; 1999.
3. Bassett C. Electrical effects in bone. Sci Am 1965;213(4):18–25.
4. Bassett C, Pawluck R, Becker R. Effects of electric currents on bone formation in vivo. Nature 1964;204:652–4.
5. Bassett C, Becker R. Generation of electric potentials by bone in response to mechanical stress. Science 1962;137:1063–4.

6. Fukada E, Yasuda I. On the piezoelectric effect of bone. J Phy Soc Japan 1957;12:1158.
7. Downey M. Bone growth stimulators: Current concepts. In: Podiatry Management Magazine; 2005.
8. Yasuda I. On the piezoelectric property of bone. J Jpn Orthop Surg Soc 1954;28:267–79.
9. Rubinacci A, De Ponti A, Shipley A, Samaja M, Karplus E, Jaffe L. Bicarbonate dependence of ion current in damaged bone. Calcif Tissue Int 1996;58:423–8.
10. Enzler M, Sumner-Smith G, Waelchli-Suter C, Perren S. Treatment of nonuniting osteotomies with pulsating electromagnetic fields. A controlled animal experiment. Clin Orthop 1984;187:272–6.
11. Enzler MA, Waelchli-Suter C, Perren SM. [Prevention of pseudarthrosis using magnetic stimulation? Experimental demonstration of Bassett's method on beagles]. Unfallheilkunde 1980;83(5):188–94.
12. de Haas WG, Lazarovici MA, Morrison DM. The effect of low frequency magnetic fields on the healing of the osteotomized rabbit radius. Clinical Orthopaedics & Related Research 1979(145):245–51.
13. Fredericks D, Nepola J, Baker J, Abbott J, Simon B. Effects of pulsed electromagnetic fields on bone healing in a rabbit tibial osteotomy model. J Orthop Trauma 2000;14(2):93–100.
14. Leisner S, Shahar R, Aizenberg I, Lichovsky D, Levin-Harrus T. The effect of short-duration, high-intensity electromagnetic pulses on fresh ulnar fractures in rats. J Vet Med 2002;49(1):33–7.
15. Sarker AB, Nashimuddin AN, Islam KM, et al. Effect of PEMF on fresh fracture-healing in rat tibia. Bangladesh Medical Research Council Bulletin 1993;19(3):103–12.
16. Bassett CA, Hess K. Synergistic effects of pulsed electromagnetic fields (PEMFs) and fresh canine cancellous bone grafts. In: Orthop Trans; 1984; 1984. p. 341.
17. Olmstead M, Ost P, Hohn R. The effect of pulsing electromagnetic fields on bone healing in fresh canine tibial fractures. Parsippany: EBI; 1984.
18. Yen-Patton G, Patton W, Beer D, Jacobson B. Endothelial cell response to pulsed electromagnetic fields: stimulation of growth rate and angiogenesis in vitro. J Cell Physiol 1988;134(1):37–46.
19. Tepper O, Callaghan M, Chang E, et al. Electromagnetic fields increase in vitro and in vivo angiogenesis through endothelial release of FGF-2. FASEB J 2004;18(11):1231–3.
20. Greenough C. The effects of pulsed electromagnetic fields on blood vessel growth in the rabbit ear chamber. J Orthop Res 1992;10(2):256–62.
21. Aaron R, Ciombor D. Acceleration of experimental endochondral ossification by biophysical stimulation of the progenitor cell pool. J Orthop Res 1996;14(4):582–9.
22. Aaron R, Ciombor D, Jolly G. Stimulation of experimental endochondral ossification by low-energy pulsing electromagnetic fields. J Bone Miner Res 1989;4(2):227–33.
23. Ciombor D, Lester G, Aaron R, Neame P, Caterson B. Low frequency EMF regulates chondrocyte differentiation and expression of matrix proteins. J Orthop Res 2002;20(1):40–50.
24. Grace K, Revell W, Brookes M. The effects of pulsed electromagnetism on fresh fracture healing: osteochondral repair in the rat femoral groove. Orthopedics 1998;21(3):297–302.
25. Inoue N, Ohnishi I, Chen D, Deitz L, Schwardt J, Chao E. Effect of pulsed electromagnetic fields (PEMF) on late-phase osteotomy gap healing in a canine tibial model. J Orthop Res 2002;20(5):1106–14.
26. van Roermund P, ter Haar Romeny B, Hoekstra A, et al. Bone growth and remodeling after distraction epiphysiolysis of the proximal tibia of the rabbit. Effect of electromagnetic stimulation. Clin Orthop 1991;266(304–312).

27. Fredericks D, Piehl D, Baker J, Abbott J, Nepola J. Effects of pulsed electromagnetic field stimulation on distraction osteogenesis in the rabbit tibial leg lengthening model. J Ped Orthop 2003;23(4):478–83.
28. Fredericks D, Abbott J, Nepola J. The effects of pulsed electromagnetic field (PEMF) stimulation on distraction osteogenesis in the rabbit tibial leg-lengthening model. In: Eleventh Annual Meeting of The Orthopaedic Trauma Association; September 29 - October 1; Tampa, FL: Orthopaedic Trauma Association; 1995. p. 48.
29. Talylor K, Inoue N, Rafiee B, Tis J, McHale K. Effect of pulsed electromagnetic fields on maturation of regenerate bone in a rabbit limb lengthening model. J Orthop Res 2006;24(1):2–10.
30. Fini M, Cadossi R, Cane V, et al. The effect of pulsed electromagnetic fields on the osteointegration of hydroxyapatite implants in cancellous bone: a morphologic and microstructural in vivo study. J Orthop Res 2002;20(4):756–63.
31. Fini M, Giavaresi G, Giardino R, Cavani F, Cadossi R. Histomorphometric and mechanical analysis of the hydroxyapatite-bone interface after electromagnetic stimulation: an experimental study in rabbits. J Bone Joint Surg 2006;88(1):123–8.
32. Shimizu T, Zerwekh J, Videman T, et al. Bone ingrowth into porous calcium phosphate ceramics: influence of pulsing electromagnetic field. J Orthop Res 1988;6(2):248–58.
33. Aaron R, Ciombor D. Interim report on the effects of the osteoarthritis signal in human osteoarthritic cartilage in organ culture. Unpublished Report Generated for EBI, LP 1996.
34. Aaron R, Wang S, Ciombor D. Upregulation of basal TGFbeta1 levels by EMF coincident with chondrogenesis–implications for skeletal repair and tissue engineering. J Orthop Res 2002;20(2):233–40.
35. Chang K, Hong-Shong Chang W, Yu Y, Shih C. Pulsed electromagnetic field stimulation of bone marrow cells derived from ovariectomized rats affects osteoclast formation and local factor production. Bioelectromagnetics 2004;25(2):134–41.
36. Chang K, Chang W, Wu M, Shih C. Effects of different intensities of extremely low frequency pulsed electromagnetic fields on formation of osteoclast-like cells. Bioelectromagnetics 2003;24(6):431–9.
37. Spadaro J, Bergstrom W. In vivo and in vitro effects of a pulsed electromagnetic field on net calcium flux in rat calvarial bone. Calcif Tissue Int 2002;70(6):496–502.
38. Chang K, Chang W, Huanga S, Huanga S, Shih C. Pulsed electromagnetic fields stimulation affects osteoclast formation by modulation of osteoprotegerin, RANK ligand and macrophage colony-stimulating factor. J Orthop Res 2005;23(6):1308–14.
39. Shankar V, Simon B, Bax C, et al. Effects of electromagnetic stimulation on the functional responsiveness of isolated rat osteoclasts. J Cell Physiol 1998;176(3):537–44.
40. De Ponti A, Villa I, Boniforti F, Rubinacci A. Ionic currents at the growth plate of intact bone: Occurrence and ionic dependence. Electro Magnetobiology 1996;15(1):37–48.
41. Aaron R, Boyan B, Ciombor D, Schwartz Z, Simon B. Stimulation of growth factor synthesis by electric and electromagnetic fields. Clin Orthop 2004;419:30–7.
42. Aaron R, Ciombor D. Synergistic effects of growth factors and pulsed fields on proteoglycan synthesis in articular cartilage. J Cell Biol 1991;115:448A.
43. Fitzsimmons R, Ryaby J, Magee F, Baylink D. IGF-II receptor number is increased in TE-85 osteosarcoma cells by combined magnetic fields. J Bone Miner Res 1995;10(5):812–9.
44. Fitzsimmons RJ, Baylink DJ. Growth factors and electromagnetic fields in bone. Clin Plast Surg 1994;21(3):401–6.
45. Fitzsimmons RJ, Ryaby JT, Mohan S, Magee FP, Baylink DJ. Combined magnetic fields increase insulin-like growth factor-II in TE-85 human osteosarcoma bone cell cultures. Endocrinology 1995;136(7):3100–6.

46. Guerkov H, Lohmann C, Liu Y, et al. Pulsed electromagnetic fields increase growth factor release by nonunion cells. Clin Orthop 2001;384:265–79.
47. Kubota K, Yoshimura N, Yokota M, Fitzsimmons RJ, Wikesjo ME. Overview of effects of electrical stimulation on osteogenesis and alveolar bone. J Periodontol 1995;66(1):2–6.
48. Lohmann C, Schwartz Z, Liu Y, et al. Pulsed electromagnetic field stimulation of MG63 osteoblast-like cells affects differentiation and local factor production. J Orthop Res 2000;184(4):637–46.
49. Lohmann C, Schwartz Z, Liu Y, et al. Pulsed electromagnetic field stimulation of MLO-Y4 osteocyte-like cells enhances PGE2 and TGF-BETA 1 production. J Orthop Res 2003;21(2):326–34.
50. Ryaby J, Fitzsimmons R, Khin N, Baylink D. The role of insulin-like growth factor II in magnetic field regulation of bone formation. Bioelectrochem Bioenerg 1994;35:87–91.
51. Aaron R, Ciombor D, Bolander M. Modulation of gene expression in experimental endochondral ossification by pusling electromagnetic fields. In: Transactions of the Bioelectrical Repair and Growth Society; Cleveland, OH; 1989.
52. Adey WR. Biological effects of electromagnetic fields. Journal of Cellular Biochemistry 1993;51(4):410–6.
53. Blank M, Findl E. Mechanistic Approaches to Interactions of Electric and Electromagnetic Fields with Living Systems. New York: Plenum Press; 1987.
54. Blank M, Soo L. Na, K-ATPase activity as a model for the effects of EMF on cells. In: Blank M, ed. Proceedings of the First World Congress for Electricity and Magnetism in Biology and Medicine. San Francisco: San Francisco Press; 1990.
55. Bond J, Weyth N. Membranes, electromagnetic fields, and critical phenomena. In: Blank M, Findl E, eds. Mechanistic Approaches to Interactions of Elecrtric and Electromagnetic Fields with Living Systems. New York: Plenum Press; 1987.
56. Brighton C, Wang W, Seldes R, Zhang G, Pollack S. Signal transduction in electrically stimulated bone cells. J Bone Joint Surg 2001;83-A(10):1514–23.
57. Cain CD, Adey WR, Luben RA. Evidence that pulsed electromagnetic fields inhibit coupling of adenylate cyclase by parathyroid hormone in bone cells. J Bone Miner Res 1987;2(5):437–41.
58. Cain CD, Donato N, Byus C, Adey WR, Luben RA. Pulsed electromagnetic field modifies cAMP metabolism and ornithine decarboxylase activity in primary bone cells. In: IEE International Conference on Electromagnetic Fields in Medicine and Biology; 1985; London; 1985. p. 9.
59. Chiabrera A, Bianco B, Moggia E, Kaufman J. Zeeman-Stark modeling of the RF EMF interaction with ligand binding. Bioelectromagnetics 2000;21:312–24.
60. Chiabrera A, Grattarola M, Viviani R. Interaction between electromagnetic fields and cells: microelectrophoretic effect on ligands and surface receptors. Bioelectromagnetics 1984;5(2):173–91.
61. Cossarizza A, Angioni S, Petraglia F, et al. Exposure to low frequency pulsed electromagnetic fields increases interleukin-1 and interleukin-6 production by human peripheral blood mononuclear cells. Experimental Cell Research 1993;204(2): 385–7.
62. Cossarizza A, Monti D, Bersani F, et al. Extremely low frequency pulsed electromagnetic fields increase interleukin-2 (IL-2) utilization and IL-2 receptor expression in mitogen-stimulated human lymphocytes from old subjects. FEBS Letters 1989;248(1–2):141–4.
63. De Mattei M, Gagliano N, Moscheni C, et al. Changes in polyamines, c-myc and c-fos gene expression in osteoblast-like cells exposed to pulsed electromagnetic fields. Bioelectromagnetics 2005;26(3):207–14.
64. Farndale RW, Maroudas A, Marsland TP. Effects of low-amplitude pulsed magnetic fields on cellular ion transport. Bioelectromagnetics 1987;8(2):119–34.

65. Farndale RW, Murray JC. The action of pulsed magnetic fields on cyclic AMP levels in cultured fibroblasts. Biochim Biophys Acta 1986;881(1):46–53.
66. Fitzsimmons RJ, Ryaby JT, Magee FP, Baylink DJ. Combined magnetic fields increased net calcium flux in bone cells. Calcif Tissue Int 1994;55(5):376–80.
67. Goodman E, Greenebaum B, Marron M, Carrick K. Effects of intermittent electromagnetic fields on mitosis and respiration. J Bioelectricity 1984;3:57.
68. Goodman E, Sharpe P, Greenebaum B, Marron M. Pulsed magnetic fields alter the cell surface. FEBS Letters 1986;199(2):275–8.
69. Karabakhtsian R, Broude N, Shalts N, Kochlatyi S, Goodman R, Henderson A. Calcium is necessary in the cell response to EM fields. FEBS Letters 1994;349(1):1–6.
70. Luben RA. Gene expression of parathyroid hormone (PTH) receptors and functionally related antigens in bone cells: desensitization with hormones and electromagnetic fields (EF). In: Transactions of the Bioelectrical Repair and Growth Society; Washington, DC; 1988. p. 20.
71. Luben RA. Effects of low-energy electromagnetic fields (pulsed and DC) on membrane signal transduction processes in biological systems. Health Physics 1991;61(1):15–28.
72. Luben RA, Cain CD, Chen M, Rosen D, Adey WR. Effects of electromagnetic stimuli on bone and bone cells in vitro: inhibition of responses to parathyroid hormone by low-energy low-frequency fields. Proc Natl Acad Sci USA 1982;79:4180.
73. McLeod BR, Liboff AR, Smith SD. Electromagnetic gating in ion channels. J Theor Biol 1992;158(1):15–31.
74. Satake T. [Effect of pulsed electromagnetic fields (PEMF) on osteoblast-like cells. Alterations of intracellular Ca2+]. Kanagawa Shigaku 1990;24(4):692–701.
75. Smith O, Goodman E, Greenebaum B, Tipnis P. An increase in the negative surface charge of U937 cells exposed to a pulsed magnetic field. Bioelectromagnetics 1991;12(3):197–202.
76. Varani K, Gessi S, Merighi S, et al. Effect of low frequency electromagnetic fields on A2A adenosine receptors in human neutrophils. Brit J Pharmacol 2002;136(1):57–66.
77. Bodamyali T, Bhatt B, Hughes F, et al. Pulsed electromagnetic fields simultaneously induce osteogenesis and upregulate transcription of bone morphogenetic proteins 2 and 4 in rat osteoblasts in vitro. Biochem Biophys Res Commun 1998;250(2):458–61.
78. Aaron R, Ciombor DM, Wang S, Simon B. Clinical Biophysics: The Promotion of Skeletal Repair by Physical Forces. Ann NY Acad Sci 2006;1068:513–31.
79. Nagai M, Ota M. Pulsating electromagnetic field stimulates mRNA expression of bone morphogenetic protein-2 and -4. J Dent Res 1994;73(10):1601–5.
80. Yajima A, Ochi M, Hirose Y. Effects of pulsing electromagnetic fields on gene expression of bone morphogenetic proteins in human osteoblastic cell line in vitro. J Bone Miner Res 1996;11(Suppl 1):381.
81. Blank M, Goodman R. Electromagnetic fields may act directly on DNA. J Cell Biochem 1999;75(3):369–74.
82. Blank M, Goodman R. Electromagnetic initiation of transcription at specific DNA sites. J Cell Biochem 2001;81(4):689–92.
83. Blank M, Goodman R. Initial interactions in electromagnetic field-induced biosynthesis. J Cell Physiol 2004;199(3):359–63.
84. Jin M, Blank M, Goodman R. ERK1/2 phosphorylation, induced by electromagnetic fields, diminishes during neoplastic transformation. J Cell Biochem 2000;78(3):371–9.
85. Black J. Electrical Stimulation: Its Role in Growth, Repair, and Remodelling of the Musculoskeletal System. New York: Praeger; 1986.
86. Brighton C, Pfeffer G, Pollack S. In vivo growth plate stimulation in various capacitively coupled electrical fields. J Orthop Res 1983;1(1):42–9.
87. Black J, Balligand M, Nunamaker D, Brighton C. Electrical stimulation of fresh fractures: Faradic stimulation of tibial osteotomies in the dog. In: 31st Annual Meeting of the Orthopeadic Research Society; Las Vegas, NV: Orthopaedic Research Society; 1985. p. 29.

88. Chang W, Hwang I, Liu H. Enhancement of fracture healing by specific pulsed capacitively-coupled electric field stimulation. Front Med Biol Eng 1991;3(1):57–64.
89. Rijal K, Kashimoto O, Sakurai M. Effect of capacitively coupled electric fields on an experimental model of delayed union of fracture. J Orthop Res 1994;12(2):262–7.
90. Carter EJ, Vresilovic E, Pollack S, Brighton C. Field distributions in vertebral bodies of the rat during electrical stimulation: a parametric study. IEEE Trans Biomed Eng 1989;36(3):333–45.
91. Brighton C, Luessenhop C, Pollack S, Steinberg D, Petrik M, Kaplan F. Treatment of castration-induced osteoporosis by a capacitively coupled electrical signal in rat vertebrae. J Bone Joint Surg Am 1989;71(2):228–36.
92. Leussenhop C, Brighton C, Pollack S. Treatement of castration-induced osteoporosis with a 60 kHz capacitively coupled electrical signal. In: Transactions of the Bioelectrical Repair and Growth Society; Toronto, Canada; 1987. p. 80.
93. Brighton C, Okereke E, Pollack S, Clark C. In vitro bone-cell response to a capacitively coupled electrical field. The role of field strength, pulse pattern, and duty cycle. Clin Orthop 1992;285:255–62.
94. Fitzsimmons R, Farley J, Adey W, Baylink D. Frequency dependence of increased cell proliferation, in vitro, in exposures to a low-amplitude, low-frequency electric field: evidence for dependence on increased mitogen activity released into culture medium. J Cell Phys 1989;139(3):586–91.
95. Fitzsimmons R, Strong D, Mohan S, Baylink D. Low-amplitude, low-frequency electric field-stimulated bone cell proliferation may in part be mediated by increased IGF-II release. J Cell Physiol 1992;150(1):84–9.
96. Armstrong P, Brighton C, Star A. Capacitively coupled electrical stimulation of bovine growth plate chondrocytes grown in pellet form. J Orthop Res 1988;6(2):265–71.
97. Brighton C, Jensen L, Pollack S, Tolin B, Clark C. Proliferative and synthetic response of bovine growth plate chondrocytes to various capacitively coupled electrical fields. J Orthop Res 1989;7(5):759–65.
98. Brighton C. The semi-invasive method of treating nonunion with direct current. Orthop Clin North Amer 1984;15(1):33–45.
99. Lorich D, Brighton C, Gupta R, et al. Biochemical pathway mediating the response of bone cells to capacitive coupling. Clin Orthop 1998;350:246–56.
100. Brighton C, Fisher JJ, Levine S, et al. The biochemical pathway mediating the proliferative response of bone cells to a mechanical stimulus. J Bone Joint Surg Am 1996;78(9):1337–47.
101. Zhuang H, Wang W, Seldes R, Tahernia A, Fan H, Brighton C. Electrical stimulation induces the level of TGF-beta1 mRNA in osteoblastic cells by a mechanism involving calcium/calmodulin pathway. Biochem Biophys Res Commun 1997;237(2):225–9.
102. Morone M, Boden S, Hair G, et al. Gene expression during autograft lumbar spine fusion and the effect of bone morphogenetic protein 2. Clin Orthop 1998(352):252–65.
103. Gan J, Fredericks D, Glazer P. Direct current and capacitive coupling electrical stimulation upregulates osteopromotive factors for spinal fusions. Harv Med J 2004;6:57–9.
104. Fredericks D, Peterson E, Bobst J, Glazer P, Nepola J, Simon B. Effects of direct current electrical stimulation on expression of BMP-2,4,6,7, bFGF, VEGF, TGF-beta, ALK2, and ALK3 in a rabbit posterolateral spine fusion model. In: North American Spine Society; October 26th - October 30th; Chicago, IL; 2004.
105. Wang Z, Clark C, Brighton C. Up-regulation of bone morphogenetic proteins in cultured murine bone cells with use of specific electric fields. J Bone Joint Surg 2006;88(5):1053–65.

106. Rodan G, Bourret L, Norton L. DNA synthesis in cartilage cells is stimulated by oscillating electric fields. Science 1978;199(4329):690–2.
107. Brighton C, Unger A, Stambough J. In vitro growth of bovine articular cartilage chondrocytes in various capacitively coupled electrical fields. J Orthop Res 1984;2(1):15–22.
108. Black J. Methods for stimulating tissues. In: Electrical Stimulation: Its role in growth, repair, and remodelling of the musculoskeletal system. New York, NY: Praeger; 1987:85–101.
109. Spadaro J, Becker R. Function of implanted cathodes in electrode-induced bone growth. Med Biol Eng Comput 1979;17(6):769–75.
110. Inoue S, Ohashi T, Yasuda I, Fukada E. Electret induced callus formation in the rat. Clin Orthop 1977(124):57–8.
111. Treharne R, Brighton C, Korostoff E, Pollack S. Application of direct current in vitro fetal rat tibiae. In: 22nd Annual Meeting of the Orthopaedic Research Society; New Orleans, LA: Orthopaedic Research Society; 1976. p. 113.
112. Zorlu U, Tercan M, Ozyazgan I, et al. Comparative study of the effect of ultrasound and electrostimulation on bone healing in rats. Am J Phys Med Rehabil 1998;77(5):427–32.
113. Lavine L, Lustrin I, Shamos M, Moss M. The influence of electric current on bone regeneration in vivo. Acta Orthop Scandinav 1971;42(4):305–14.
114. Friedenberg Z, Zemsky L, Pollis R, Brighton C. The response of non-traumatized bone to direct current. J Bone Joint Surg Am 1974;56(5):1023–30.
115. Stefan S, Sansen W, Mulier J. Experimental study on the electrical impedance of bone and the effect of direct current on the healing of fractures. Clin Orthop 1976;120:264–7.
116. Weigert M, Werhahn C. The influence of electric potentials on plated bones. Clin Orthop 1977;124:20–30.
117. Petersson C, Johnell O. Electrical stimulation of osteogenesis in delayed union of the rabbit fibula. Arch Orthop Trauma Surg 1983;101(4):247–50.
118. Kleczynski S. Electrical stimulation to promote the union of fractures. Int Orthop 1988;12(1):83–7.
119. Esterhai J, Friedenberg Z, Brighton C, Black J. Temporal course of bone formation in response to constant direct current stimulation. J Orthop Res 1985;3(2):137–9.
120. Brighton C, Hunt R. Ultrastructure of electrically induced osteogenesis in the rabbit medullary canal. J Orthop Res 1986;4:27–36.
121. Buch F, Albrektsson T, Herbst E. The bone growth chamber for quantification of electrically induced osteogenesis. J Orthop Res 1986;4(2):194–203.
122. Spadaro J, Albanese S, Chase S. Bone formation near direct current electrodes with and without motion. J Orthop Res 1992;10(25):729–38.
123. Yonemori K, Matsunaga S, Ishidou Y, Maeda S, Yoshida H. Early effects of electrical stimulation on osteogenesis. Bone 1996;19(2):173–80.
124. Sato O, Akai M. Effect of direct-current stimulation on the growth plate. In vivo study with rabbits. Arch Orthop Trauma Surg 1989;109:9–13.
125. Takei N, Akai M. Effect of direct current stimulation on triradiate physeal cartilage. In vivo study in young rabbits. Arch Orthop Trauma Surg 1993;112(4):159–62.
126. Akai M, Oda H, Shirasaki Y, Tateishi T. Electrical stimulation of ligament healing. An experimental study of the patellar ligament of rabbits. Clin Orthop 1988;235:296–301.
127. Nannmark U, Buch F, Albrektsson T. Influence of direct currents on bone vascular supply. Scand J Plast Reconstr Surg Hand Surg 1988;22(2):113–5.
128. Bozic K, Glazer P, Zurakowski D, Simon B, Hayes W, Lipson S. The effect of coralline hydroxyapatite and direct current electrical stimulation in spinal fusion: A rabbit model. In: Combined Orthopaedic Research Societies Meeting; September Hamamatsu, Japan; 1998.

129. Bozic K, Glazer P, Zurakowski D, Simon B, Lipson S, Hayes W. In vivo evaluation of coralline hydroxyapatite and direct current electrical stimulation in lumbar spinal fusion. Spine 1999;24(20):2127–33.
130. France J, Norman T, Santrock R, McGrath B, Simon B. The efficacy of direct current stimulation for lumbar intertransverse process fusions in an animal model. Spine 2001;26(9):1002–8.
131. Glazer P, Spencer U, Alkalay R, Schwardt J. In vivo evaluation of calcium sulfate as a bone graft substitute for lumbar spinal fusion. Spine J 2001;1(6):395–401.
132. Paterson D, Carter R, Maxwell G, Hillier T, Ludbrook J, Savage J. Electrical bone-growth stimulation in an experimental model of delayed union. Lancet 1977;1(8025):1278–81.
133. Paterson D, Hillier T, Carter R, Ludbrook J, Maxwell G, Savage J. Experiemtnal delayed union of the dog tibia and its use in assessing the effect of an electrical bone growth stimulator. Clin Orthop 1977;128:340–50.
134. Harrington D, Walter J, Walter T, Chen T, Bodamer W, Black D. The efficacy of electrical stimulation on experimentally induced nonunion fracture of the canine tibia. Trans Bioelec Repair and Growth Soc 1982;2:84.
135. Fuentes A, Marcondes de Souza J, Valeri V, Mascarenhas S. Experimental model of electric stimulation of pseudarthrosis healing. Clin Orthop 1984(183):267–75.
136. Jacobs R, Luethi U, Dueland R, Perren S. Electrical stimulation of experimental nonunions. Clin Orthop 1981(161):146–53.
137. Chakkalakal D, Lippiello L, Shindell R, Connolly J. Electrophysiology of direct current stimulation of fracture healing in canine radius. IEEE Trans Biomed Eng 1990;37(11):1048–58.
138. Chakkalakal D, Lippiello L, Wilson R, Shindell R, Connolly J. Mineral and matrix contributions to rigidity in fracture healing. J Biomech 1990;23(5):425–34.
139. Kahanovitz N, Arnoczky S, Hulse D, Shires P. The effect of postoperative electromagnetic pulsing on canine posterior spinal fusions. Spine 1984;9(3):273–9.
140. Kahanovitz N, Arnoczky S. The efficacy of direct current electrical stimulation to enhance canine spinal fusions. Clin Orthop 1990;251:295–9.
141. Dejardin L, Kahanovitz N, Arnoczky S, Simon B. The effect of varied electrical current densities on lumbar spinal fusions in dogs. Spine J 2001;1(5):341–7.
142. Toth J, Seim Hr, Schwardt J, Humphrey W, Wallskog J, Turner A. Direct current electrical stimulation increases the fusion rate of spinal fusion cages. Spine 2000;25(20):2580–7.
143. Cook S, Patron L, Christakis P, Bailey K, Banta C, Glazer P. Direct current stimulation of titanium interbody fusion devices in primates. Spine J 2004;4(3):300–11.
144. Baranowski T, Black J. The mechanism of faradic stimulation of osteogenesis. In: Blank M, Findl E, eds. Mechanistic Approaches to Interactions of Electric and Electromagnetic Fields with Living Systems. New York: Plenum Press; 1987:399.
145. Bodamyali T, Kanczler J, Simon B, Blake D, Stevens C. Effect of faradic products on direct current-stimulated calvarial organ culture calcium levels. Biochem Biophys Res Commun 1999;264(3):657–61.
146. Wang Q, Shizhen Z, Xie Y, Zhengqun Z, Yang G. Electrochemical reactions during constant DC current stimulation: An in vitro experiment with cultured rat calvarial cells. Electro Magnetobiology 1995;14(1):31–40.
147. Wang Q, Zhong S, Ouyang J, et al. Osteogenesis of electrically stimulated bone cells mediated in part by calcium ions. Clin Orthop 1998;348:259–68.
148. Urban M, Brighton C, Black J. Dose-response relationship for faradic stimulation of osteogenesis in the rabbit tibia by use of a single-strand platinum cathode. In: Electromagnetics in Biology and Medicine. San Francisco, CA; 1991:199–206.
149. Brighton C, Heppenstall R. Oxygen tension in zones of the epiphyseal plate, the metaphysis and diaphysis. An in vitro and in vivo study in rats and rabbits. J Bone Joint Surg Am 1971;53(4):719–28.

150. Brighton C, Krebs A. Oxygen tension of nonunion of fractured femurs in the rabbit. Surg Gyn Obstet 1972;135(3):379–85.
151. Brighton C, Krebs A. Oxygen tension of healing fractures in the rabbit. J Bone Joint Surg Am 1972;54(2):323–32.
152. Heppenstall R, Grislis G, Hunt T. Tissue gas tensions and oxygen consumption in healing bone defects. Clin Orthop 1977;106:357–65.
153. Bassett C, Hermann I. Influence of oxygen concentration and mechanical factors on differentiation of connective tissues in vitro. Nature 1961;190:460–1.
154. Brighton C, Ray R, Soble L, Kuettner K. In vitro epiphyseal-plate growth in various oxygen tensions. J Bone Joint Surg Am 1969;51(7):1383–96.
155. Brighton C, Adler S, Black J, Itada N, Friedenberg Z. Cathodic oxygen consumption and electrically induced osteogenesis. Clin Orthop 1975;107:277–82.
156. Howell D, Pita J, Marquez J, Madruga J. Partition of calcium, phosphate, and protein in the fluid phase aspirated at calcifying sites in epiphyseal cartilage. J Clin Invest 1968;47(5):1121–32.
157. Richards D, Brookes M. Osteogenesis and the pH of the osseous circulation. Calcif Tissue Res 1968;2(Suppl 1):93.
158. Chakkalakal D, Mashoof A, Novak J, Strates B, McGuire M. Mineralization and pH relationships in healing skeletal defects grafted with demineralized bone matrix. J Biomed Mater Res 1994;28(12):1439–43.
159. Arnett T, Spowage M. Modulation of the resorptive activity of rat osteoclasts by small changes in extracellular pH near the physiological range. Bone 1996;18(3):277–9.
160. Bushinsky D. Metabolic alkalosis decreases bone calcium efflux by suppressing osteoclasts and stimulating osteoblasts. Am J Physiol 1996;271(1 Pt 2):216–22.
161. Steinbeck M, Kim J, Trudeau M, Hauschka P, Karnovsky M. Involvement of hydrogen peroxide in the differentiation of clonal HD-11EM cells into osteoclast-like cells. J Cell Phys 1998;176(3):574–87.
162. Cho M, Hunt T, Hussain M. Hydrogen peroxide stimulates macrophage vascular endothelial growth factor release. Am J Physiol Heart Circ Physiol 2001;280(5): H2357–63.
163. Petersen E, Fredericks D, Bobst J, Nepola J, Simon B. Effects of direct current electrical stimulation on expression of BMP 2, 4, 6, 7, bFGF, VEGF, and ALK2 receptor in a rabbit posteriolateral spine fusion model. In: Bioelectromagnetics Society Meeting; June 22–27; Maui, HI; 2003.
164. Dunn A, Rush G. Electrical stimulation in treatment of delayed union and nonunion of fractures and osteotomies. South Med J 1984;77(12):1530–4.
165. Frykman G, Taleisnik J, Peters G, et al. Treatment of nonunited scaphoid fractures by pulsed electromagnetic field and cast. J Hand Surg [Am] 1986;11(3):344–9.
166. Adams B, Frykman G, Taleisnik J. Treatment of scaphoid nonunion with casting and pulsed electromagnetic fields: a study continuation. J Hand Surg [Am] 1992;17(5):910–4.
167. Melone CJ, Pess G. Treatment of scaphoid pseudarthroses with bone grafting and pulsing electromagnetic fields: American Academy of Orthopedic Surgeons; 1986.
168. Beckenbaugh R. Noninvasive pulsed electromagnetic stimulation in the treatment of scaphoid nonunions. In: 31st Annual Meeting of the Orthopaedic Research Society; Las Vegas, NV: Orthopaedic Research Society; 1985.
169. Bigliani L, Rosenwasser M, Caulo N, Schink M, Bassett C. The use of pulsing electromagnetic fields to achieve arthrodesis of the knee following failed total knee arthroplasty. A preliminary report. J Bone Joint Surg Am 1983;65(4):480–5.
170. Bassett C, Caulo N, Kort J. Congenital "pseudarthroses" of the tibia: treatment with pulsing electromagnetic fields. Clin Orthop 1981;154:136–48.
171. Fontanesi G, Giancecchi F, Rotini R, Cadossi R. Treatment of delayed union and pseudarthrosis by low frequency pulsing electromagnetic stimulation. Study of 35 cases. Ital J Orthop Traumatol 1983;9(3):305–18.

172. Fontanesi G, Dalmonte A, Rinaldi, et al. The effect of low frequency pulsing electromagnetic fields for the treatment of congenital and acquired pseudarthrosis. J Bioelectricity 1984;3:55.
173. Bassett C, Schink-Ascani M. Long-term pulsed electromagnetic field (PEMF) results in congenital pseudarthrosis. Calcif Tissue Int 1991;49(3):216–20.
174. Ito H, Shirai Y, Gembun Y. A case of congenital pseudarthrosis of the tibia treated with pulsing electromagnetic fields. 17-year follow-up. J Nippon Med School 2000;67(3):198–201.
175. Holmes G. The treatment of delayed unions and nonunions of the proximal fifth metatarsal with pulsed electromagnetic fields. In: 24th Meeting of the American Orthopaedic Foot and Ankle Society; July; Coeur D'Alene, France; 1994.
176. Holmes G. The treatment of delayed unions and nonunions of the proximal fifth metatarsal with pulsed electromagnetic fields. Foot Ankle Int 1994;15(10):552–6.
177. Borsalino G, Fornaciari F, Rocchi R, Bettati E, Ulohogilan S, Bagnacani M. PEMF stimulation of femoral head bone remodelling after osteotomy in osteoarthritis patients: A double-blind study. In: Bioelectric Repair and Growth Society; Utrecht, The Netherlands; 1986.
178. Sutbeyaz S, Sezer N, Koseoglu B. The effect of pulsed electromagnetic fields in the treatment of cervical osteoarthritis: a randomized, double-blind, sham-controlled trial. Rheumatol Int 2005;26(4):320–4.
179. Thamsborg G, Florescu A, Oturai P, Fallentin E, Tritsaris K, Dissing S. Treatment of knee osteoarthritis with pulsed electromagnetic fields: a randomized, double-blind, placebo-controlled study. Osteoarthritis Cartilage 2005;13(7):575–81.
180. Fischer G, Pelka R, Barovic J. Adjuvant treatment of knee osteoarthritis with weak pulsing magnetic fields. Results of a placebo-controlled trial prospective clinical trial. Z Orthop Ihre Grenzgeb 2005;143(5):544–50.
181. Bassett C, Schink-Ascani M, Lewis S. Effects of pulsed electromagnetic fields on Steinberg ratings of femoral head osteonecrosis. Clin Orthop 1989;246:172–85.
182. Aaron R, Lennox D, Bunce G, Ebert T. The conservative treatement of osteonecrosis of the femoral head. Clin Orthop 1989;249:209–18.
183. Seber S, Omeroglu H, Cetinkanat H, Kose N. [The efficacy of pulsed electromagnetic fields used alone in the treatment of femoral head osteonecrosis: a report of two cases]. [Turkish]. Acta Orthopaedica et Traumatologica Turcica 2003;37(5):410–3.
184. Bassett CA, Schink M, Mitchell S. Treatement of osteonecrosis of the hip with specific, pulsed electromagnetic fields (PEMFs), a preliminary clinical report. In: Arlet J, Ficat R, Hungerforg D, eds. Bone Circulation. Baltimore: Williams & Wilkins; 1984.
185. Aaron R, Ciombor D. Treatment of osteonecrosis of the femoral head with pulsed external magnetic fields. Ann NY Acad Sci 1985;435:367.
186. Aaron R, Lennox D, Bunce G, Ebert T. The conservative treatment of osteonecrosis of the femoral head. A comparison of pulsed electromagnetic fields and core decompression. Trans Bioelectr Repair Growth Soc 1988;8:24.
187. Rosenberg A, Barden R, Galante J. The use of pulsed electromagnetic fields in the treatment of femoral head osteonecrosis. Trans Bioelectr Repair Growth Soc 1987;7:92.
188. Eftekhar N, Schink-Ascani M, Mitchell S, Bassett C. Osteonecrosis of the femoral head treated by pulsed electromagnetic fields (PEMFs): a preliminary report. In: Hungerford D, ed. The Hip. St. Louis, MO; 1983:306–30.
189. Bassett C, Mitchell S, Gaston S. Pulsing electromagnetic field treatment in ununited fractures and failed arthrodeses. JAMA 1982;247(5):623–8.
190. Gossling H, Bernstein R, Abbott J. Treatment of ununited tibial fractures: a comparison of surgery and pulsed electromagnetic fields (PEMF). Orthopedics 1992;15(6):711–9.
191. Bassett C, Mitchell S, Gaston S. Treatment of ununited tibial diaphyseal fractures with pulsing electromagnetic fields. J Bone Joint Surg Am 1981;63(4):511–23.

192. Heckman JD, Ingram AJ, Loyd RD, Luck JV, Jr., Mayer PW. Nonunion treatment with pulsed electromagnetic fields. Clinical Orthopaedics & Related Research 1981(161):58–66.
193. Borsalino G, Bagnacani M, Bettati E, et al. Electrical stimulation of human femoral intertrochanteric osteotomies. Double-blind study. Clin Orthop 1988;237:256–63.
194. Sharrard W. A double-blind trial of pulsed electromagnetic fields for delayed union of tibial fractures. J Bone Joint Surg Br 1990;72(3):347–55.
195. Mammi GI, Rocchi R, Cadossi R, Massari L, Traina GC. The electrical stimulation of tibial osteotomies. Double-blind study. Clinical Orthopaedics & Related Research 1993(288):246–53.
196. Parnell E, Simonis R. The effect of electrical stimulation in the treatment of nonunion of tibial fractures. J Bone Joint Surg Br 1991;73B(Suppl):S178.
197. Simonis R, Parnell E, Ray P, Peacock J. Electrical treatment of tibial nonunion: a prospective, randomised, double-blind trial. Injury 2003;34(5):357–62.
198. Longo 3rd J. Successful treatment of recalcitrant nonunions with combined magnetic field stimulation. Surg Technol Int 1997;6:397–403.
199. Linovitz R, Pathria M, Bernhardt M, et al. Combined magnetic fields accelerate and increase spine fusion: a double-blind, randomized, placebo controlled study. Spine 2002;27(13):1383–9.
200. Scott G, King J. A prospective, double-blind trial of electrical capacitive coupling in the treatment of nonunion of long bones. J Bone Joint Surg Am 1994;76(6):820–6.
201. Goodwin C, Brighton C, Guyer R, Johnson J, Light K, Yuan H. A double-blind study of capacitively coupled electrical stimulation as an adjunct to lumbar spinal fusions. Spine 1999;24(13):1349–56.
202. Brighton C, Pollack S. Treatment of nonunion of the tibia with a capacitively coupled electrical field. J Trauma 1984;24(2):153–5.
203. Brighton C, Pollack S. Treatment of recalcitrant nonunion with a capacitively coupled electrical field. A preliminary report. J Bone Joint Surg 1985;67-A(4):577–85.
204. Abeed RI, Naseer M, Abel EW. Capacitively coupled electrical stimulation treatment: results from patients with failed long bone fracture unions. J Orthop Trauma 1998;12(7):510–3.
205. Zamora-Navas N, Borras V, Antelo L, Saras A, Pena R. Electrical stimulation of bone nonunion with the presence of a gap. Acta Orthop Belg 1995;61(3):169–76.
206. Benazzo F, Mosconi M, Beccarisi G, Galli U. Use of capacitive coupled electric fields in stress fractures in athletes. Clin Orthop 1995;310:145–9.
207. Brighton C, Shaman P, Heppenstall R, Esterhai JJ, Pollack S, Friedenberg Z. Tibial nonunion treated with direct current, capacitive coupling, or bone graft. Clin Orthop 1995;321:223–34.
208. Paterson D, Lewis G, Cass C. Treatment of delayed union and nonunion with an implanted direct current stimulator. Clin Orthop 1980;184:117–28.
209. Cundy P, Paterson D. A ten-year review of treatment of delayed union and nonunion with an implanted bone growth stimulator. Clin Orthop 1990;259:216–22.
210. Bassett C, Mitchell S, Norton L, Caulo N, Gaston S. Electromagnetic repairs of nonunion. In: Brighton C, Black J, Pollack S, eds. Electrical Properties of Bone & Cartilage. New York: Grune and Stratton; 1979:605–30.
211. Brighton C. The treatment of nonunions with electricity. J Bone Joint Surg Am 1981;63(5):847–51.
212. Cohen M, Roman A, Lovins J. Totally implanted direct current stimulator as treatment for a nonunion in the foot. J Foot Ankle Surg 1993;32(4):375–81.
213. Janis L, Krawetz L, Wagner S. Ankle and subtalar fusion utilizing a tricortical bone graft, bone stimulator, and external fixator after avascular necrosis of the talus. J Foot Ankle Surg 1996;35(2):120–6.
214. Midis N, Conti S. Revision ankle arthrodesis. Foot and Ankle Int 2000;23(3):243–7.

215. Reynolds J. The use of implantable direct current stimulation in bone grafted foot and ankle arthrodesis. In: Mid- American Orthopaedic Association; April; Hilton Head, SC: Mid- American Orthopaedic Association; 1997.
216. Kane W. Direct current electrical bone growth stimulation for spinal fusion. Spine 1988;13(3):363–5.
217. Welch W, Willis S, Gerszten P. Implantable direct current stimulation in para-axial cervical arthrodesis. Adv Ther 2004;21(6):389–400.
218. Baker J, Cain T, Tullos H. Intramedullary fixation for congenital pseudarthrosis of the tibia. J Bone Joint Surg 1992;74-A(2):169–78.
219. Brighton C, Friedenberg Z, Zemsky L, Pollis P. Direct-current stimulation of nonunion and congenital pseudarthrosis. Exploration of its clinical application. J Bone Joint Surg Am 1975;57(3):368–77.
220. Lavine L, Lustrin I, Shamos M. Treatment of congenital pseudarthrosis of the tibia with direct current. Clin Orthop 1977;124:69–74.
221. Paterson D, Lewis G, Cass C. Treatment of congenital pseudarthrosis of the tibia with direct current stimulation. Clin Orthop 1980;148:129–35.
222. Paterson D, Simonis R. Electrical stimulation in the treatment of congenital pseudarthrosis of the tibia. Trans Bioelec Repair and Growth Soc 1983;3:2.
223. Paterson D. Treatment of nonunion with a constant direct current: a totally implantable system. Orthop Clin North Am 1984;15(1):47–59.
224. Paterson D, Simonis R. Electrical stimulation in the treatment of congenital pseudarthrosis of the tibia. J Bone Joint Surg 1985;67-B(3):454–62.
225. Steinberg M, Brighton C, Hayken G, Tooze S, Steinberg D. Early results in the treatment of avascular necrosis of the femoral head with electrical stimulation. Orthop Clin North Am 1984;15(1):163–75.
226. Steinberg M, Brighton C, Steinberg D, Tooze S, Hayken G. Treatment of avascular necrosis of the femoral head by a combination of bone grafting, decompression, and electrical stimulation. Clin Orthop 1984;186:137–53.
227. Steinberg M, Brighton C, Corces A, et al. Osteonecrosis of the femoral head. Clin Orthop 1989;249:199–208.
228. Dwyer A. The use of electrical current stimulation in spinal fusion. Orthop Clin North Am 1975;6(1):265–73.
229. Dwyer A. Direct current stimulation in spinal fusion. Med J Aust 1974;1:73–5.
230. Kane W. The use of supplementary electronic bone growth in primary and secondary lumbo sacral fusions. In: Brighton C, Black J, Pollack S, eds. In Electrical Properties of Bone & Cartilage. New York: Grune & Stratton; 1979:563–6.
231. Meril A. Direct current stimulation of allograft in anterior and posterior lumbar interbody fusions. Spine 1994;19(21):2393–8.
232. Pettine K. A retrospective controlled study of implantable direct current stimulation in lumbar spinal fusion. In: North American Spine Society; October 18–21; Washington, DC; 1995.
233. Kant A. An analysis of the effect of electrical stimulation as an adjunct to lumbar spinal fusion: A retrospective controlled study of implantable direct current stimulation in lumbar spine fusion. In: North American Spine Society; October 18–21; Washington, DC; 1995.
234. Kahanovitz N, Pashos C. The Role of Direct Current in the Critical Pathway for Lumbar Spinal Fusion. J Care Manag 1996;2(6):2–8.
235. Tejano N, Puno R, Ignacio J. The use of implantable direct current stimulation in multilevel spinal fusion without instrumentation. A prospective clinical and radiographic evaluation with long-term follow-up. Spine 1996;21(16):1904–8.
236. Rogozinski A, Rogozinski C. Efficacy of implanted bone growth stimulation in instrumented lumbosacral spinal fusion. Spine 1996;21(21):2479–83.
237. Banco R, Grottkau B, Cicerchia D, Banco S, Cowan S. A randomized preliminary trial to determine the effect of DC stimulation on instrumented fusion in smokers.

In: Joint Session CNS/AANS- Disorders of the Spine and Peripheral Nerves; 1997; Newport Beach, CA; 1997.
238. Kucharzyk D. A controlled prospective outcome study of implantable electrical stimulation with spinal instrumentation in a high-risk spinal fusion population. Spine 1999;24(5):465–8.
239. Ortman B. Use of implantable DC stimulation in elderly spine fusion patients. In: Mid-America Orthopedic Association; April; Hilton Head Island, SC; 1997.
240. Ortman B. Comparison of spinal fusion patients and outcomes by age. In: Joint Session CNS/AANS- Disorders of the Spine and Peripheral Nerves; February; Newport Beach, CA; 1997.
241. Kucharzyk D. The role of electrical stimulation with spinal instrumentation. In: Joint Session CNS/AANS- Disorders of the Spine and Peripheral Nerves; February; Newport Beach, CA; 1997.
242. Kane W, Czop S. An analysis of risk factors affecting posterolateral spinal fusion success with implantable direct current stimulation. In: Joint Session CNS/AANS- Disorders of the Spine and Peripheral Nerves; Newport Beach, CA; 1997.
243. Birney T. A retrospective review of patient outcomes using internal fixation and implantable direct current stimulation in lumbar spinal fusion. In: Mid-America Orthopedic Association; Hilton-Head Island, NC; 1997.
244. Aaron R, Ciombor D, Keeping H, Wang S, Capuano A, Polk C. Power frequency fields promote cell differentiation coincident with an increase in transforming growth factor-beta(1) expression. Bioelectromagnetics 1999;20(7):453–8.

Color Plates

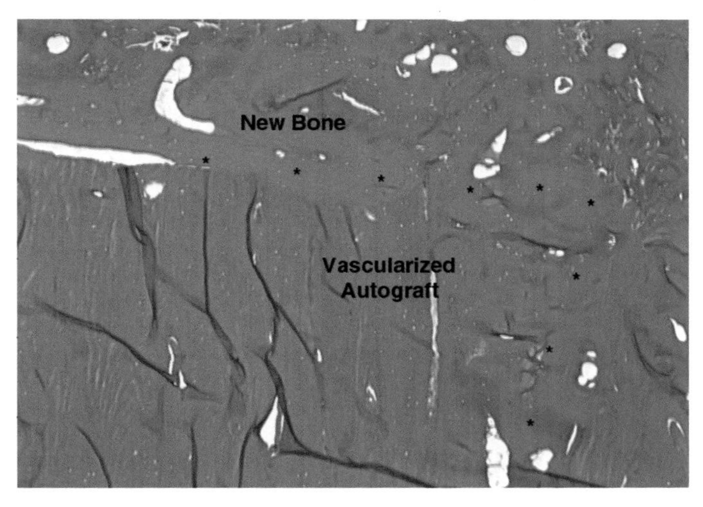

Fig. 4.1 A vascularized fibular autograft used to treat osteonecrosis of the femoral head is shown. Most of the graft is viable one year after implantation, and it has provided an osteoconductive surface for a few areas of new bone formation. The (*) symbols mark the interface between cortical autograft and new bone that has formed in the femoral head

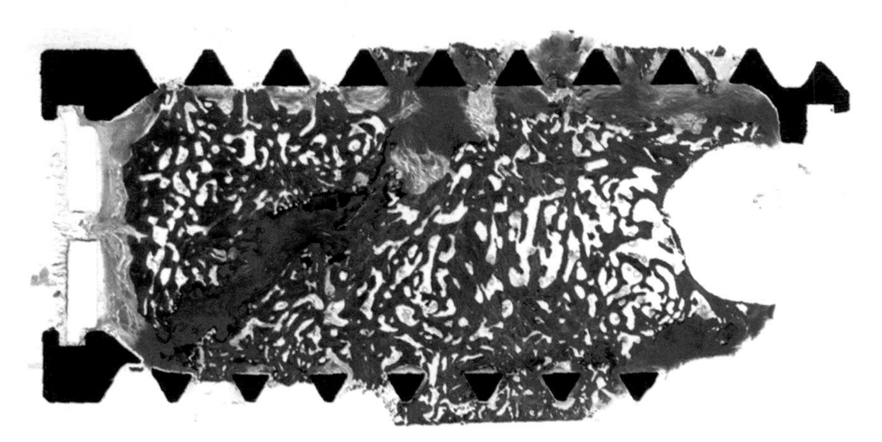

Fig. 4.2 The photomicrograph of histological sections through the center of a clinically failed intervertebral body fusion cage shows incorporated iliac crest autograft

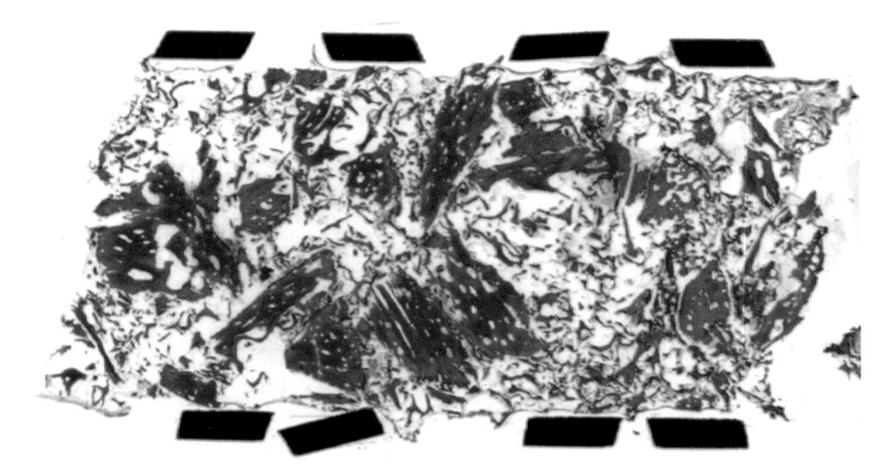

Fig. 4.3 The lower-magnification photomicrograph shows unincorporated iliac crest autograft in a Harms cage that had been used for cervical fusion, but failed shortly after insertion. Although this case was not clinically successful, it illustrates an appropriate combination of cortical and cancellous bone fragments prepared from iliac crest

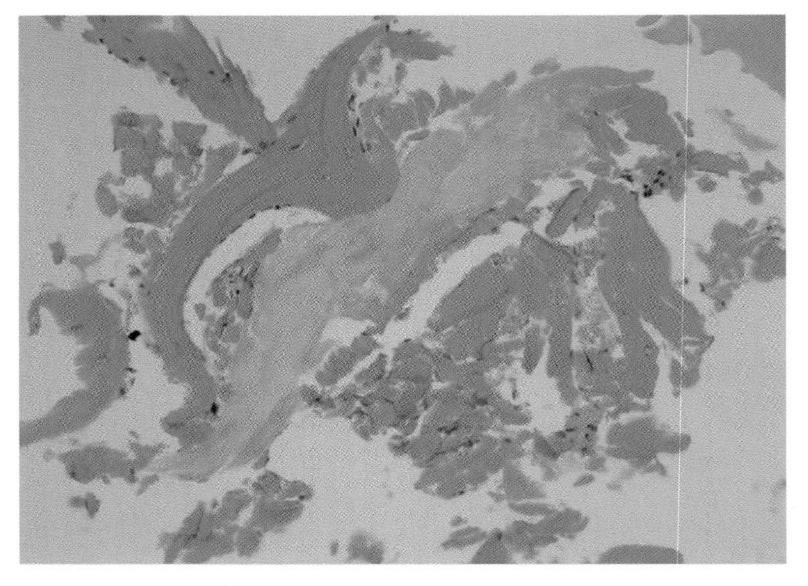

Fig. 4.4 The decalcified section of the shavings of one preparation of locally harvested autograft shows shavings of cancellous bone, almost completely devoid of cells. Fibrous tissue, hyaline cartilage and fibrocartilage were also present in this preparation

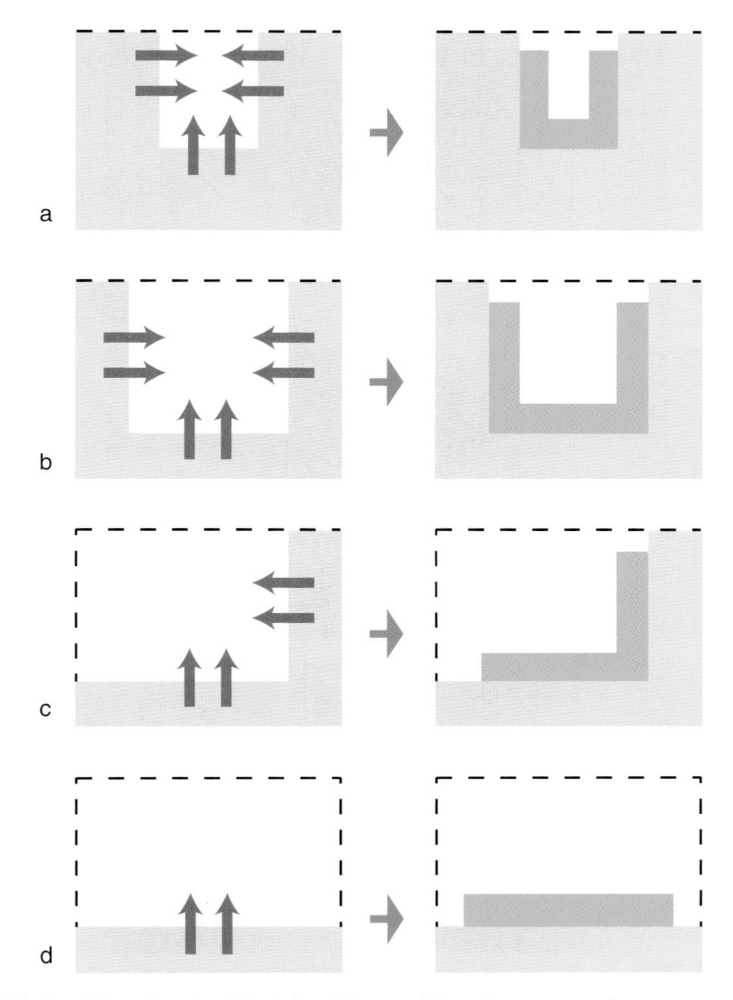

Fig. 7.3 Small/smaller (a) critical size defects subjected to regenerative treatment (e.g., covered with a membrane: dotted line) will heal with larger amounts of bone in terms of percent of defect fill than large/larger (b) critical size defects subjected to the same treatment during the same amount of time. Similarly, a 3-wall defect (b) subjected to regenerative treatment will present more bone fill than a 2- wall (c) or 1-wall (d) defect subjected to the same regenerative treatment during the same period of time

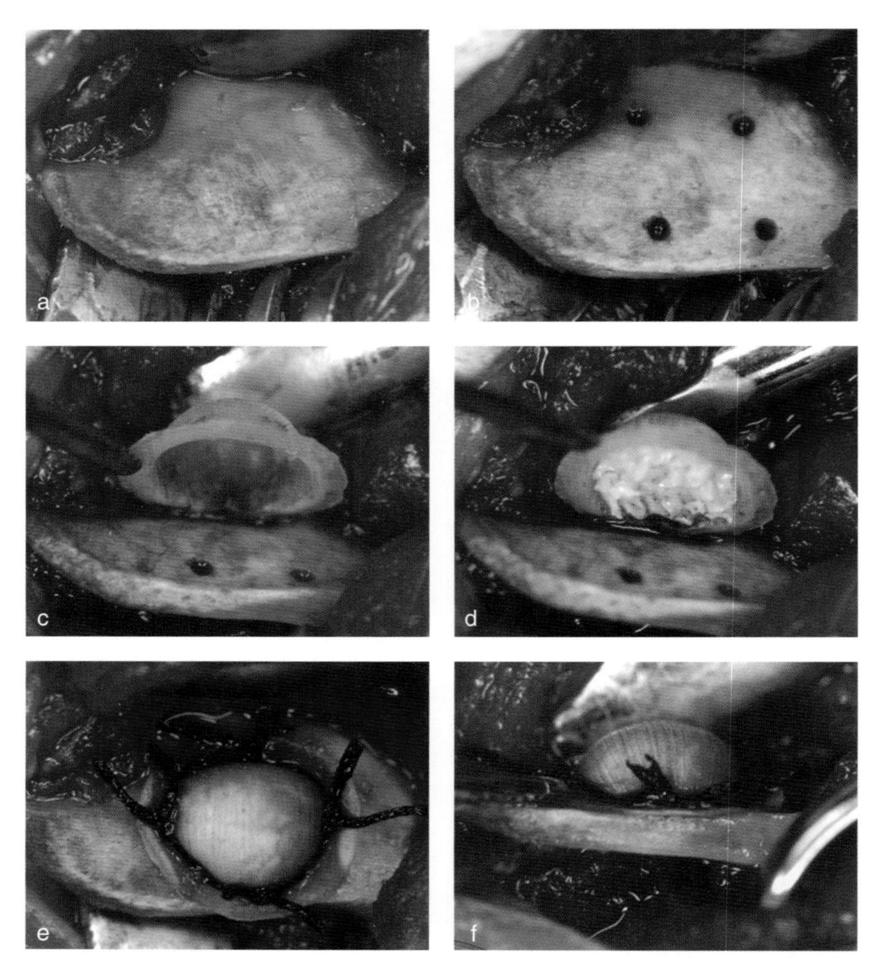

Fig. 7.4 The mandibular ramus is exposed (a) and four holes are drilled (b). A Teflon capsule is then placed and may be either left empty to serve as control (c) or be filled with biomaterial under testing (e.g., DBB) (d). The capsule is stabilized by means of sutures passing through the collar of the capsule and the holes in the ramus (e), and thus a tight adaptation of the capsule onto the bone surface can be achieved (f)

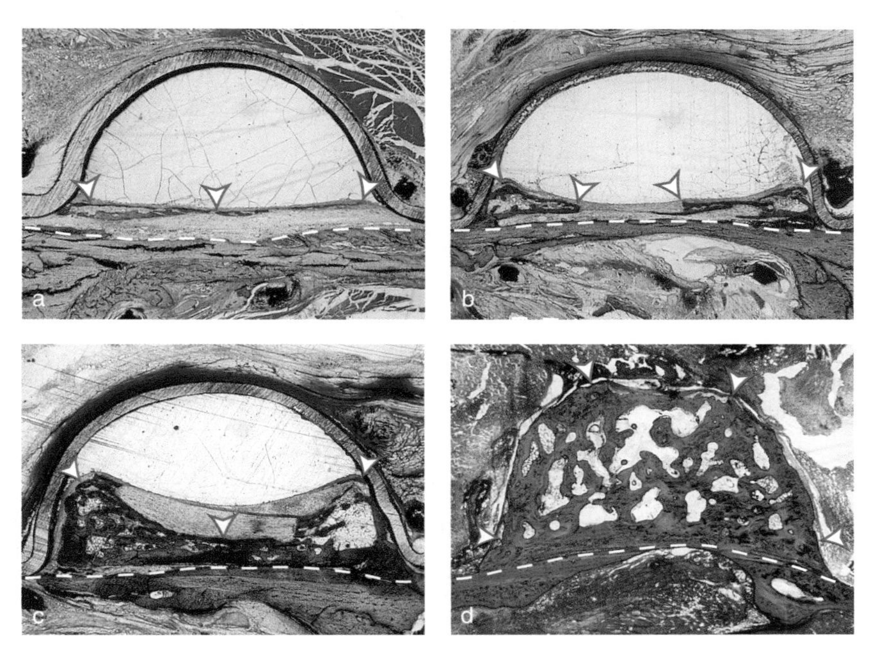

Fig. 7.5 In originally empty capsules bone formation (arrowheads) can be observed already after one month of healing (a), and increasing amounts of new bone are formed after two (b) and four months (c), until 12 months (d) where the capsules are almost entirely filled out with bone. The dotted line indicates the level of pristine bone

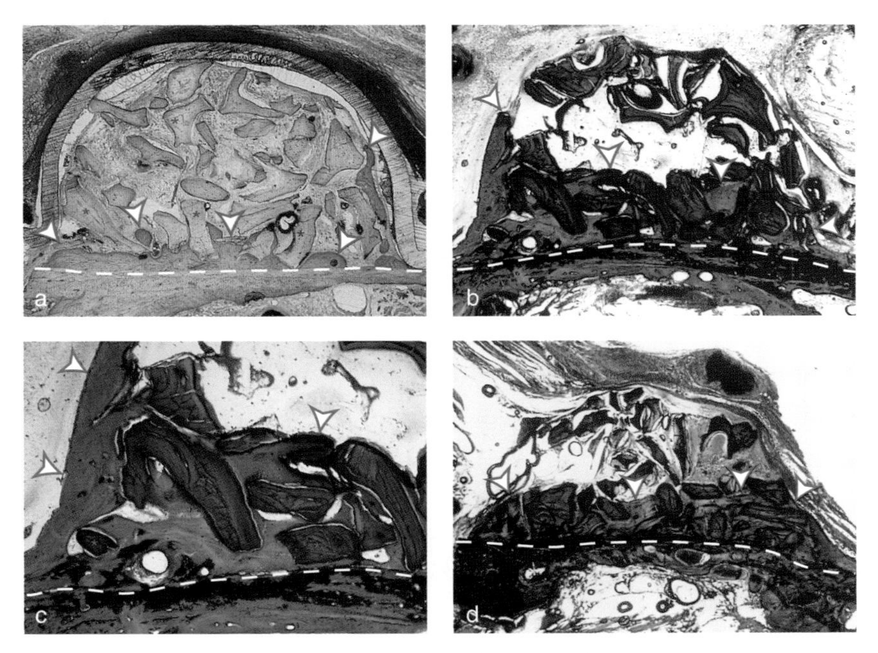

Fig. 7.6 Limited amounts of bone (arrowheads) confined in the vicinity of the pristine bone (dotted line) are observed inside capsules grafted with unsintered DBB after four (a) or 12months (b) of healing. The new bone grows in continuity with the host bone and in contact with the DBB particles (stars) (c), which occupy the major portion of the capsules. The amount of new bone remains basically stable for at least six months after capsule removal (d)

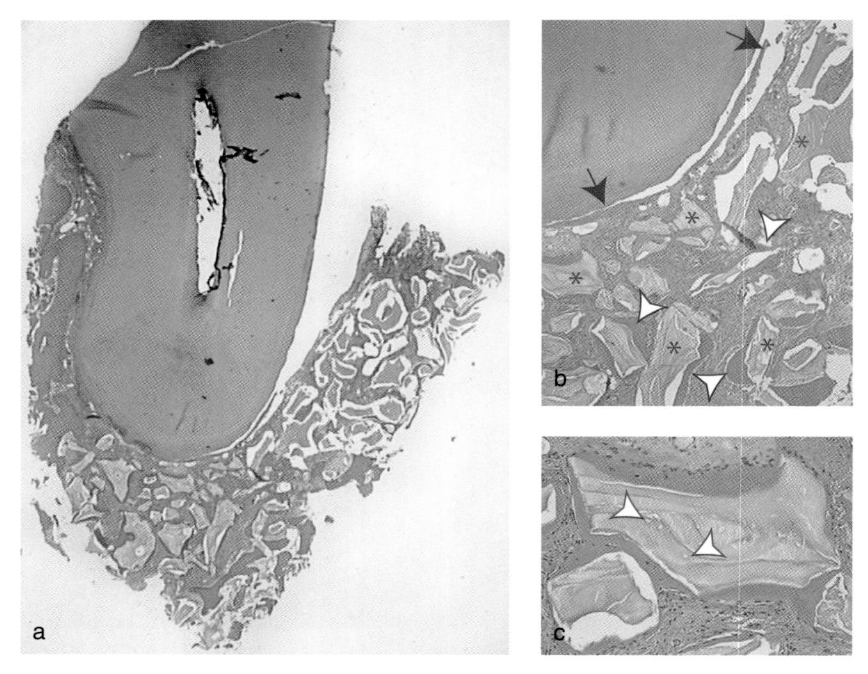

Fig. 7.7 Overview of a root with neighboring tissues removed six months after treatment with unsintered DBB+GTR (a). New cementum (arrows) with inserting collagen fibers and a new bone-like tissue (arrowheads) in direct contact with DBB particles (star) can be observed (b). A substantial portion of the defect was occupied by graft particles with empty osteocytic lacunae (arrowheads) embedded in a periodontal ligament-like connective tissue (c)

Section III

Soft Tissue Technologies

14

Meniscus Repair Techniques

F. Alan Barber[1] and Michael H. Boothby[2]

Abstract: The human meniscus is a critical element to normal knee structure and function. These crescent-shaped cartilages distribute loads, and aid in joint lubrication, stability, congruence and proprioception. An appreciation of the structure and function of the meniscus, along with its related biomechanics, proves useful in understanding its pathologic states. Various types of meniscus tears are discussed, as well as the basic science and clinical evidence of the healing potential of a tear. While most meniscus tears can be treated with simple debridement, several methods exist for meniscus repair, including suture repairs and device repairs. Accompanying the discussion of techniques, clinical evidence is used to illustrate which meniscal tears are likely to heal successfully and the biomechanical data of each type of repair. A discussion of rehabilitation protocols following meniscus repair examines the benefits and risks of early motion, weight bearing and a return to sport. The final section concerns current trends in meniscus repair, and the possible future modalities that may be employed to make meniscus repair easier and more successful.

Keywords: Meniscus repair; repair device, meniscus healing; biodegradable, arthroscopy, meniscus tear.

14.1. Introduction

The human meniscus performs many important functions in the knee. It efficiently disperses loads across the surface of the knee articular cartilage during weight bearing [1–2], contributes to the mechanics of joint lubrication, joint stability, joint congruence, proprioception [3] and articular cartilage nutrition [4–5]. An intact meniscus is even more important for anterior cruciate ligament (ACL) deficient knees to protect them from arthritic changes [6].

[1] Plano Orthopedic and Sports Medicine Center, Plano, TX
[2] Southwest Orthopedic Associates, Fort Worth, TX

From: *Orthopedic Biology and Medicine: Musculoskeletal Tissue Regeneration, Biological Materials and Methods*
Edited by W. S. Pietrzak © Humana Press, Totowa, NJ

The natural history of the meniscectomized knee raises concerns about the long-term risk of the development of degenerative arthritis. Even so, arthroscopic partial meniscectomy is still one of the most common arthroscopic procedures and very few meniscus repairs are performed [7]. Meniscal repair is desirable for selected tears possessing a good blood supply. Meniscal repair is especially appropriate for young, active individuals undergoing associated ACL reconstruction or articular cartilage-resurfacing procedures.

In general meniscal repairs can be performed four ways: open, inside-out, outside-in and all-inside. Combinations of two of these techniques are called "hybrid repairs." Open repair was initially reported by Annandale in 1885, but was not widely performed [8]. Later, King [9] documented that, with an _adequate blood supply, meniscal healing could occur in dogs. Henning pioneered arthroscopic inside-out repair in the early 1980s [10–12], with subsequent contributions by Clancy and Graf [13], Rosenberg, et al. [14] and Cannon and Morgan [15–16].

Although open techniques were initially popular [17–18], they were slowly replaced by arthroscopic inside-out approaches [10–11, 19] which minimized the risks associated with open surgery and provided access to difficult-to-reach areas of the meniscus. Later, an outside-in approach was developed [20–21] which further decreased the risk of damage to the posterior neurovascular structures. Currently, all-inside techniques for posterior horn tears of the menisci are common [22]. These avoid a posterior capsular exposure and further reduce the potential for neurovascular damage. All-inside techniques employ meniscal repair devices which offer the advantages of simplicity, decreased surgical times and reduced neurovascular risk. The purpose of this chapter is to review various meniscal repair techniques currently in use and review various meniscal repair devices.

14.2. Basic Science

14.2.1. Meniscus Form and Function

The menisci are crescent-shaped structures with a triangular cross section. This dense fibrocartilage is primarily Type 1 collagen and can be functional without severe degradation during the entire life of the patient. Peripherally, the meniscus is connected to the joint capsule via coronary attachments. The vascular supply comes from the periphery into the central meniscus (Fig. 14.1) [23]. India ink staining has shown that the peripheral third of the menisci is vascular (called the "red/red" zone), while the middle third is less vascular (the "red/white" zone) and the inner third is avascular (the "white/white" zone) [23–24]. This is significant when discussing repair techniques since a good vascular supply is the single most important factor influencing the healing potential of the torn meniscus.

The meniscus functions to deepen the articular surfaces of the tibial plateau. This, in turn, helps to increase the weight bearing surface area of the articular surface and lowers overall contact stresses. The menisci changes vertically oriented compression stresses into radial hoop stresses borne by the entire cartilage. The menisci also function as secondary stabilizers to tibial translation and rotation, especially in the face of absent, injured or incompetent stabilizing ligaments. The menisci maintain spacing between the femur and tibia, allowing for the free diffusion of joint fluid in the knee which is critical in maintaining nutrition and lubrication of articular cartilage.

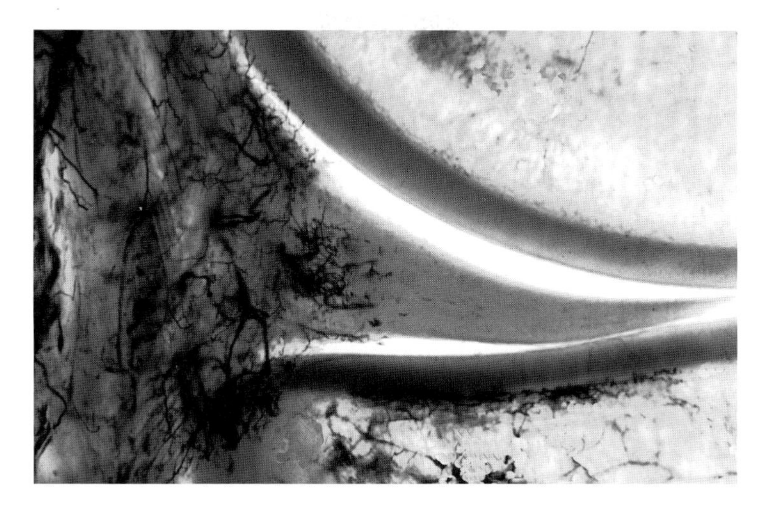

Fig. 14.1 The menisci are crescent-shaped structures with a triangular cross sectional dimension. The vascular supply comes from the periphery into the central meniscus (courtesy of Steven P. Arnoczky D.V.M.)

14.2.2. Biology of Meniscus Healing

The meniscus is a mostly avascular structure that rarely heals spontaneously when torn. A small tear may progress to a larger tear or may stabilize, but degenerate into nonfunctional tissue. When repairing the meniscus it is important to use techniques that optimize healing. Tissue preparation is very important. Rasping of the perimeniscal synovium above and below the meniscus stimulates a synovial healing response. Studies have shown that rasping some isolated, incomplete or complete, stable meniscus tears may lead to healing without fixation [25–27]. Meniscal tears which may be rasped and left to heal *in situ* include nondegenerative peripheral red-red vertical tears associated with an acute ACL injury that are less than 10 mm in length and have minimal displacement (less than 5 mm of excursion). Other examples would be posterior horn lateral meniscus tears central to the popliteus tendon, and incomplete radial or flap tears. These have been reported to have a high clinical success rate if left alone to heal after an ACL reconstruction [28].

Creating vascular access channels or trephination of the meniscus can also improve healing of meniscus tissue. Research in dogs has shown that creating vascular access channels can bring sufficient circulation into a meniscus to produce fibrovascular healing in the avascular areas of the meniscus [24]. Partial thickness trephination of the peripheral meniscus rim is also beneficial [25]. The technique can be carried out using a coring device or an 18-gauge spinal needle to puncture the meniscal tear site and adjacent tissue, thereby providing channels for capillary ingrowth from the peripheral vascular supply. The addition of a fibrin clot to the meniscal repair site has been suggested to enhance healing [29]. Henning [30] has reported that the addition of a fibrin clot decreased failures of isolated meniscal repairs from 61 percent to 8 percent.

14.2.3. Tear Patterns and Ability to Heal

It is important to understand which types of meniscal tears have the ability to heal and which do not. Meniscal tears can be classified into three basic

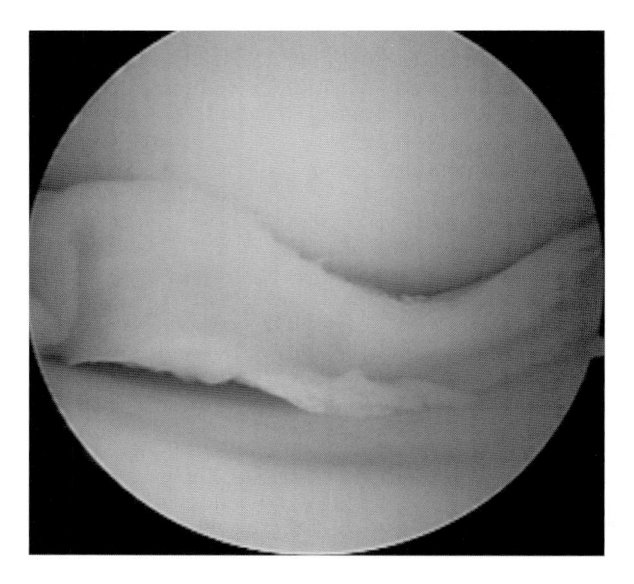

Fig. 14.2 Bucket handle meniscal tear

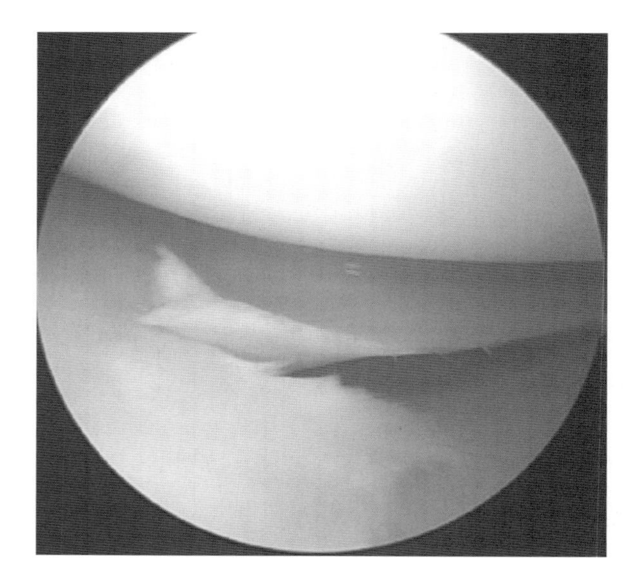

Fig. 14.3 Radial meniscal tear

types: bucket handle (Fig. 14.2), radial (Fig. 14.3), horizontal (Fig. 14.4) or complex combinations of these tears (Fig. 14.5). Each tear should be systematically evaluated intra-operatively to assess the tear pattern and its potential for healing. Initially, the surface of both menisci should be probed out to the peripheral synovial meniscal junction. Once the tear type, location and extent of the tear have been determined, the next step is to consider tissue vascularity. The literature indicates that tears within 3 mm of the meniscosynovial junction should be considered vascular. Tears 5 mm or more from the meniscosynovial junction should be considered avascular unless there is direct evidence to the contrary. Tears in the 3 to 5 mm zone have variable vascularity [23–24]. When

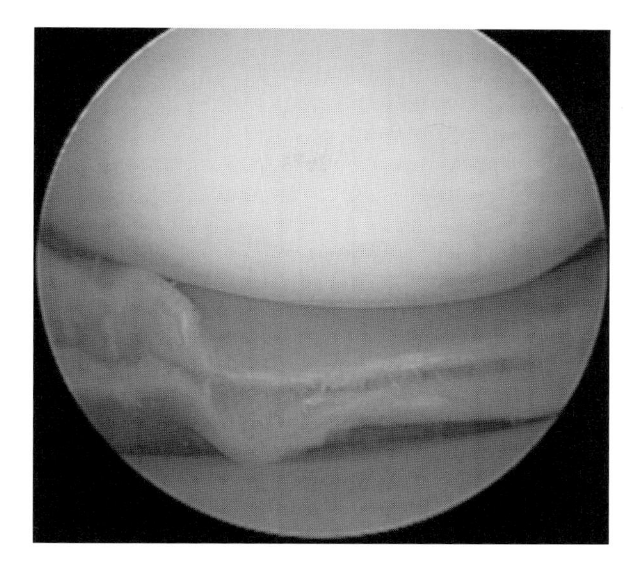

Fig. 14.4 Horizontal meniscal tear

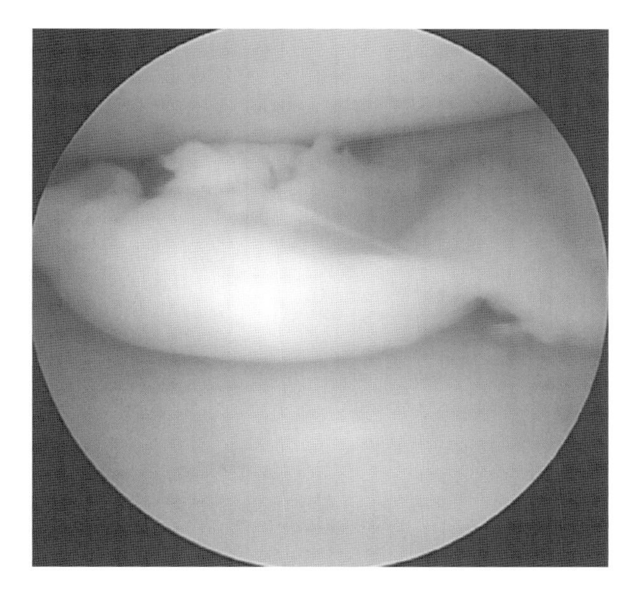

Fig. 14.5 Complex meniscal tear

evaluating vertical longitudinal tears that are oblique in one or more planes, a clinical judgment has to be made as to whether or not most of the tear is in the vascular zone are amenable to repair.

14.2.4. Scientific Study of Meniscal Healing

Several studies have examined the healing time of repaired meniscal tissue. The force required to tear repaired versus normal menisci was studied in rabbits as a function of time [31]. Simulated lesions were created in rabbit menisci and assigned to one of three treatment groups: no treatment, repair with sutures or repair with fibrin sealant. The rabbit menisci were allowed to heal for six or 12 weeks before being harvested. The energy required to tear the suture-repaired meniscal scar was 26.3 percent at six weeks and 23.3 percent at 12 weeks, when compared with the healthy meniscus. The energy required to tear the fibrin glue-repaired scar was 42.50 percent and 42.51 percent for six and 12 weeks respectively, when compared with the healthy meniscus. Therefore, even after 12 weeks of healing, the scar was still significantly weaker than a normal meniscus. Morgan, et al. [32] reported 74 arthroscopic meniscus repairs evaluated by second-look arthroscopy, noting that about four months was required for visual evidence of meniscus healing.

The amount of fixation strength needed to maintain the meniscus in a reduced position during ambulation and rehabilitation has also been studied. The forces in the knee can be as high as four times body weight during walking [32]. The menisci transmit from 55 percent [34] to 99 percent [35] of that load across the knee. The compressive loads are transmitted across the meniscus in a manner that results in only a fraction of the weight being borne by a radially directed suture or meniscal repair device. Richards, et al. [36] have shown in a porcine model that peripheral meniscus tears have a compressive, not distractive, force across them during normal unloaded motion. This suggests that a repair suture or device probably functions more to align the meniscal tissue while it heals in a compressed environment than to resist distraction forces. A human cadaver study using the same experimental model with similar results is awaiting publication.

14.3. Operative Evaluation

14.3.1. Operative Treatment of Meniscus Tears

Not all meniscus tears require surgery, but there are specific indications for operative intervention. These include pain, effusion, catching, locking, buckling and persistent focal joint line tenderness unrelieved by non-operative treatment. Following the decision to operate, the next concern is whether to repair or remove the damaged meniscal cartilage.

14.3.2. To Repair or Remove

The operative management of meniscus tears is based on numerous factors. These include tear pattern, geometry, site, vascularity, size, stability, tissue viability or quality, associated pathology, age, degenerative changes, fragmentation of material and the overall benefit versus risk for the patient.

A degenerative meniscus fragment is unlikely to heal. The quality and consistency of the meniscus tissue should be carefully evaluated at the time of surgery. If the mobile meniscus fragment is substantially damaged, has radial tears in addition to a longitudinal one, has multiple longitudinal tears, or "rolls" when probed it is probably a degenerative change and should not be repaired.

In the short-term meniscal resection offers a quicker recovery than meniscus repair. However, given well-recognized development of arthritic changes after meniscectomy and the important functions performed by the meniscus, meniscal repair is anticipated to be associated with an improved prognosis. Given this information one might conclude that trying to repair all meniscal tears is prudent. This is not the case. Patient goals, recovery time, retear risks, and technical repair issues including the surgical learning curve must be considered. Trying to repair an "un-repairable" tear will lead to further morbidity including articular cartilage damage, extension of the existing meniscal tear, the development of loose bodies and re-operation. Removing part of a meniscus provides a much better long-term outcome than a total meniscectomy [37–38] due to the support provided by the peripheral circumferential meniscal collagen bands.

Consequently an important aspect of post-meniscectomy morbidity is whether the meniscal resection violates or removes the peripheral meniscal circumferential band. Interruption of this circumferential band leads to a significant disruption of meniscal biomechanics with alteration in the normal load distribution and the ability of the remaining meniscus to disperse compressive loads and hoop stresses. If segmental resection does not penetrate the circumferential band, then much of the meniscal biomechanics is maintained. Another consideration is the axial alignment of the leg. If the mechanical alignment of the lower extremity falls within the same compartment as the meniscus being removed, the outcome is worse at long-term follow-up [39–40].

14.3.3. Associated Pathology

Patients with a meniscal tear and secondary pathology, such as chondral lesions or ligament deficiency, offer further operative dilemmas. In one study 119 patients with partial meniscectomies were evaluated 12 years after the procedure and found to show a 95 percent success rate in cases in which no adjacent chondral lesions were noted at the index surgery [38]. In contrast, only 62 percent of patients with associated chondral lesions were considered successes. ACL stability plays a significant role. In a study of 167 patients with meniscal injury followed 20 years after partial meniscectomy, 92 percent with an intact ACL were found to be successful, compared to only a 74 percent success rate for those whose ACL was deficient [41].

14.4. Methods of Meniscal Repair

14.4.1. Overview

There are many methods of meniscal repair. These include both open and arthroscopic repairs, suture and device repairs, and inside-out, outside-in and all-inside repairs. A few basic principles should be followed to ensure successful meniscal healing. Once the tear to be repaired is identified, meticulous preparation of both sides of the tear (inner fragment and meniscal rim) is extremely important. This includes excision of any loose or unstable meniscal fragments or tags, and rasping on both sides of the tear site. Stimulation of the perimeniscal synovium on both the top and bottom meniscal surfaces will promote the vascular healing response. Finally, secure and correctly placed fixation is important. Vertically oriented nonabsorbable meniscal repair sutures are considered the gold standard for repair against which all other repairs are measured.

14.4.2. Suture Repair Inside-out

An arthroscopic inside-out meniscal suture repair requires the precise placement of cannulas through which flexible needles pass sutures into and through the meniscus tear. A single lumen cannula is commonly used and, in separate passes, the suture with needles on both ends is placed through the tear. These are bent, single-barreled cannulas (zone-specific) which allow access to the posterior, middle and anterior regions of the meniscus [14, 42]. Meniscal repair sutures come with long, flexible needles which fit through these cannulas. After the first end of the suture is passed through the meniscus and out the side of the knee, the other suture end is passed through the same cannula and then through the meniscus creating either a vertical or horizontal stitch.

Once both ends of suture are passed, the stitch is tied over the capsule, through the appropriate incision. Accessory incisions up to 4 to 6 cm long are made at the posterior medial and lateral joint for needle passage. Medially a small posterior incision can be made at the level of the joint line. Care should be taken to avoid the infrapatellar and descending branches of the saphenous nerve. The posterolateral incision is centered at the joint line, just posterior to the lateral collateral ligament while staying anterior to the biceps femoris tendon. With the knee flexed to 90°, the interval between the biceps muscle fascia and the posterior border of the iliotibial band is identified and incised parallel to the fibers of the iliotibial band. The peroneal nerve lies at the deep posterior border of the biceps and must be avoided.

Medial meniscal repair sutures are tied with the knee flexed at 20°. The lateral sutures are tied with the knee in 90° of flexion. If care is taken to protect and avoid the neurovascular structures, this technique is successful with few associated complications. When working on the posterior third of the meniscus, posteromedial and posterolateral incisions and a popliteal retractor are routinely used to protect and retract neurovascular structures where the needles penetrate the posterior capsule [12, 15–16].

14.4.3. Suture Outside-in Repairs

Outside-in suture repair is useful for tears in the middle and anterior thirds of the meniscus [43]. This technique uses an 18-gauge spinal needle placed from outside to inside the joint. The needle is passed through the meniscus rim and then through the meniscus body fragment. Suture material is threaded through the spinal needle reducing the risk of neurovascular injury by placing the suture passing needles well anterior to the posterior bundle with direct arthroscopic visualization. A variant of the technique developed by Johnson [44] uses a second parallel spinal needle. The suture (absorbable or nonabsorbable) is passed through one needle and is retrieved by a metal snare passed through a second needle 5 mm away from the first. The second suture end is brought out through the second needle and the knot tied outside the joint over the capsule.

An alternative outside-in technique was described by Warren [20] and Morgan [21]. As with the previous technique, a spinal needle is passed from outside to inside across the meniscus rim and fragment. An absorbable polydioxanone suture is passed through the needle and into the joint, retrieved from the front, and pulled out through an anterior portal. A "Mulberry" knot is tied on the end of the suture. Pulling on the suture end brings the knot back into the joint and snug against the meniscal surface. Traction on the suture keeps the knot against the meniscus and reduces the tear to hold the fragment in the proper position. Several sutures can be passed through the inferior or superior surfaces of the meniscus, and the adjacent sutures tied to each other over the capsule, but under the skin. Care must be taken to avoid entrapment of the neurovascular structures when tying the sutures outside the capsule. This can be used for the more anterior portions of the meniscus that cannot be reached by all-inside or by inside-out techniques.

The advantages of an outside-in repair technique include a less invasive approach, safer access to the middle and anterior horns, and the ability to use different suture patterns and materials. The disadvantages are limited access to the posterior horn and the need for accessory incisions through which to tie the sutures. It can be difficult to place sutures perpendicular to the surface of a tear that is too far posterior, and this position can result in an oblique orientation of the sutures [45]. Also, Mulberry knots used with the outside-in technique can abrade the articular surface before absorption. Of note, the outside-in technique can be used successfully as a hybrid repair to reduce and temporarily stabilize displaced bucket handle meniscus tears while they are repaired using other techniques (inside-out or all-arthroscopic).

14.4.4. All-inside Suture Repairs

Peripheral meniscus tears in the extreme posterior horn no more than 2 mm from the synovial junction can be repaired with vertically oriented all-inside sutures passed through posterior medial or posterior lateral cannulas [16, 21]. The posterior horn can be visualized with either a 30° or 70° arthroscope placed through the intercondylar notch. A large working cannula is placed into the posterior compartment from the appropriate posterolateral or posteromedial portal [21, 46]. Curved suture hooks (Conmed Corp., Largo, FL) are introduced through the cannula and passed through the capsular bed and then across the tear in the meniscus. Polydioxanone suture (#0 or #1) is fed through the suture hook and across the tear. Using arthroscopic knot tying techniques, the suture is tied inside the joint repairing the torn meniscus. Sutures are placed 3 to 4 mm apart. This technique eliminates the necessity of accessory incisions and provides safe access to the posterior horn with a minimally invasive approach. Disadvantages of this technique include the increased technical difficulty of suture management and knot tying, and its application to only a limited number of meniscus tears.

14.4.5. Device Repairs

Using an implant or device for meniscal tear reduction and fixation incorporates many of the principles of suture repair. As with suture repairs, the tear site is prepared by rasping to provide a fresh vascularized surface. The tear is reduced and measured to determine the correct device length. The device should be inserted perpendicular to the tear to maximally compress the tear site with enough meniscal tissue on both sides for a good purchase. It is critical that any portion of an implant remaining on the meniscal surface have as low a profile as possible to reduce the potential for articular cartilage abrasion [47].

Table 14.1 A comparison of meniscal repair devices

Device	Size	Material	Device Pull-out Strength *	Comment
Contour Arrow	10,13,16 mm × 1.1 mm	SR-PD(20)L(80)LA	33.6 N	Low profile head, fully barbed shaft
PolySorb Meniscal Staple	10 mm posts with 4 mm suture	82 percent PLLA 18 per-cent PGA	31.4 N	Prior posts were 7 mm, new ones 10 mm
BioStinger	10,13,16 mm × 1.25 mm	Injection molded PLLA	56.6 N	New Hornet inserter
FasT-Fix	5 mm anchors and #0 suture	PLLA or polyacetyl anchor	72 N	Two passes allows for vertical stitch
RapidLoc	5×1.5 mm anchor; 4.5× 0.25 mm TopHat; #2-0 suture	Panacryl or Ethibond Suture; PLLA or PDS TopHat & backstop	43 N	PDS TopHat has faster absorption
Mitek Meniscal Repair Device	6 mm and 8 mm	Prolene or PDS	30 N	12°, 24° & 34° curved inserters
Clearfix screw	10 × 2.0 mm	PLLA	32.5 N	Cannulated with variable pitch
Dart	10, 12, & 14 × 1.3 mm	PDLLA	72 N	Double reverse barbs
Arthrotek Staple	11 and 13 mm	82 percent PLLA 18 percent PGA	27 N	Double-pronged fixation
Trinion screw	10 and 12 mm	TMC, PLLA, & PDLLA	39 N	Threaded at both ends with central shaft

* Strength refers to the force required to disrupt a single meniscal repair device [48–49]

Meniscal repair devices can be classified as tacks, staples, screws or self-adjusting suture anchors. A comparison of some of those devices currently available is found in Table 14.1.

14.4.5.1. Tacks

Tack devices are inserted arthroscopically across a reduced meniscal tear to hold the meniscus in place so that tissue healing can occur.

The first tack device was introduced by Bionx and later purchased by Conmed Linvatec. The Meniscus Arrow (Conmed) is a bioabsorbable device initially made of self-reinforced poly-L-lactic acid (SR-PLLA) and then self-reinforced poly dextro (4 percent) levo (96 percent) lactic acid (PDLLA) [48]. The original design included a 4 mm long "T"-shaped head with a 1.1 mm diameter shaft and 10, 13 or 16 mm lengths. The reverse barbs were at right angles to the "T" head and cut by hand into the shaft. The polymer composition of the Arrow was later changed again to the current Poly dextro (20 percent) levo (80 percent) lactic acid composition. This change makes the material even more amorphous with different degradation and mechanical properties than pure PLLA. The current device has a curved, low-profile head and is named the Contour Arrow. The implant design was also changed from the 1.1 mm thick "T" head to a lower profile rounded and contoured 0.7 mm head, and barbs were added along the entire shaft.

The Meniscal Dart (Arthrex, Naples, FL) is solid (non-cannulated) poly-dextro (30 percent), levo (70 percent) lactic acid with a double reverse barb pattern and 10, 12 or 14 mm shaft lengths. The device is 1.3 mm in diameter and repairs should use a minimum of two Darts.

The BioStinger (Conmed, Largo, FL) is a cannulated device with a low profile oval head that can be seated flush to slightly dimple the meniscus tissue to reduce the possibility of articular cartilage abrasion. The BioStinger is violet-colored, 1.25 mm in diameter, made of PLLA that is injection-molded and possesses four rows of reverse barbs on all four sides of the shaft. The BioStinger is available in 10, 13 and 16 mm lengths [49–51].

14.4.5.2. Staples

Meniscal staples work similarly to tacks, but have two legs that cross the meniscal tear and a connecting piece. They are introduced arthroscopically after appropriate repair site preparation.

The Polysorb meniscal staple was originally called the SDsorb staple (Surgical Dynamics, Norwalk, CT) and is now distributed by USS Sports Medicine (United States Surgical, North Haven, CT). The staple material is an injection-molded copolymer comprised of 82 percent poly levo-lactic acid and 18 percent polyglycolic acid. The staple has two 10 mm posts connected with a 4 mm braided absorbable suture embedded in both posts. The staple is delivered by a double-barrel insertion cannula and comes in both straight and 8° curved up versions.

The Biomet meniscal staple (Biomet, Warsaw, IN) is a single rigid staple that, like the Polysorb staple, is composed of 82 percent PLLA and 18 percent polyglycolic acid. It is inserted manually or with a CO_2 powered device and is available in 11 mm or 13 mm lengths.

14.4.5.3. Self-adjusting, Suture Containing Implants

The FasT-Fix (Smith & Nephew Endoscopy, Andover, MA) consists of two 5 mm nonabsorbable polyacetyl (plastic) suture anchors connected via a preloaded, pretied, self-sliding and self-locking knot of No. 0, nonabsorbable braided polyester suture (Fig. 14.6). It is delivered with an arthroscopic 16.5-gauge insertion needle. Straight and 22° curved needles are available

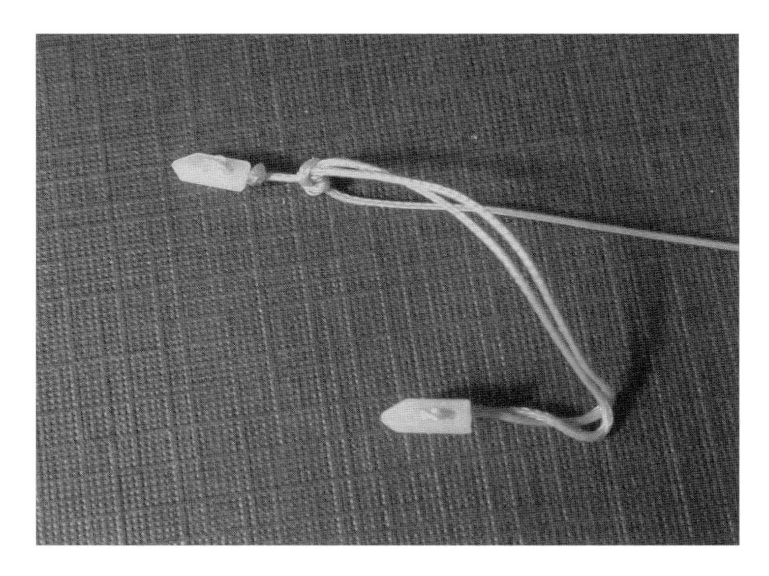

Fig. 14.6 The FasT-Fix consists of two 5 mm polyacetyl anchors connected with a preloaded, pretied, self-sliding and self-locking knot

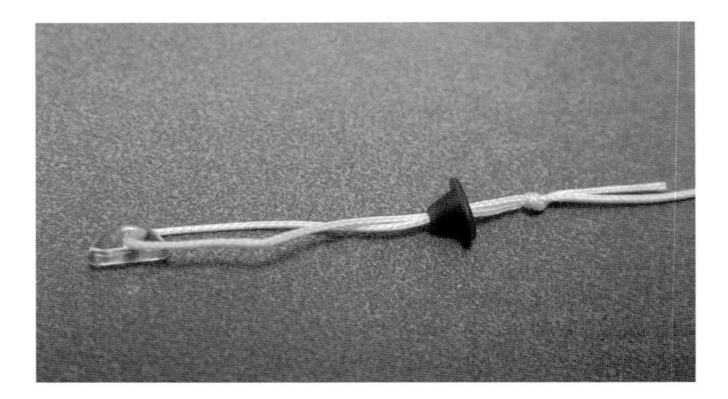

Fig. 14.7 The RapidLoc consists of a 5 mm × 1.5 mm "backstop" anchor, a connecting suture of either #2-0 absorbable Panacryl or #2-0 permanent Ethibond, and a PLLA or polydioxanone "top hat"

for implantation. The system has a split-sheath insertion cannula and separate knot pusher/suture cutter. The first of the two anchors is inserted and deployed, and then the second anchor is advanced to the end of the insertion needle and deployed as well. With both anchors solidly fixed in the meniscal tissue, the sliding, self-locking knot is pushed down the suture to tension the repair. Recent design improvements include sharper delivery needles, waxed-tip suture for easier threading and biodegradable injection molded PLLA suture anchors [4].

The Mitek RapidLoc (Mitek Products, Westwood, MA) has a 5 mm × 1.5 mm PLLA "backstop" soft tissue anchor, a connecting suture of #2-0 absorbable Panacryl or #2-0 permanent Ethibond (Ethicon, Somerville, NJ) and a PLLA or more rapidly absorbable polydioxanone "top hat" for meniscal apposition (Fig. 14.7). The soft tissue anchor "backstop" is inserted across the tear by a needle and left seated outside the capsule. The "top hat" has an overlying, pretied, self-sliding, integrated knot that can be cinched down on the suture advancing the backstop securely against the meniscus and compressing the reduced tear margins. This compresses the tear between the two suture connected anchors. The "top hat," is 4.5 mm wide and 0.25 mm thick and is seated on the femoral surface of the meniscus to provide compression across the tear site. An arthroscopic knot pusher is used to advance the top hat and seat it securely enough to dimple the meniscus material.

14.4.5.4. Miscellaneous Fixation Implants

Other types of fixation include the Clearfix Meniscal Screw (Mitek, Westwood, MA) that is a cannulated, needle-loaded, 2 × 10 mm, PLLA, variable-pitched screw that uses its threads to compress the torn meniscus [5]. The Mitek Meniscal Repair System (Mitek, Westwood, MA) is a molded polymer device available in permanent polypropylene or absorbable polydioxanone at lengths of 6 or 8 mm. This implant uses a single curved shaft connecting two perpendicular crossbars to achieve meniscal fixation. The Trinion screw (Inion Ltd, Tampere, Finland) is a cannulated, dual thread designed screw that comes in 10 mm and 12 mm lengths. It is composed of a copolymer of trimethylene carbonate (TMC), poly levo-lactic acid (PLLA) and poly dextro, levo lactic acid (PDLLA). It has threads at both ends similar of the single cannulated shaft similar to the Herbert fracture screw. Insertion is over a square needle.

14.4.5.5. Key Aspects of Device Fixation

The advantage of using an all-inside meniscal repair device is that tear fixation can be achieved quickly using an all-arthroscopic approach. The self-adjusting implants (RapidLoc and FasT-Fix) are attractive because they appear to provide a suture based meniscal repair and decreased risks of cartilage damage or implant loosening sometimes associated with rigid repair devices. A disadvantage to any implant fixation of the meniscus is the risk of retained polymer fragments, foreign body reactions, surrounding soft tissue inflammation and chondral injury [52–56]. Laboratory studies have indicated that most of these implant devices have strength profiles similar to or less than a horizontal repair suture and significantly lower than vertical mattress sutures [42, 57–60]. It is yet to be determined what level of repair strength is needed for successful meniscal healing. Perhaps simply aligning the meniscus with proper tear site preparation is all that is necessary for a successful meniscal repair. The cost of meniscal implants is substantially higher than sutures, and all of the implanted devices are associated with the potential morbidity inherent with significant learning curves [34].

14.5. Clinical Review

Repair techniques needs to be assessed to determine whether the repair will result in meniscal healing, the durability of that healing over time, and the resultant biomechanical function of the repaired meniscus. There are several reports of long-term clinical results. Eggli, et al. [61] reported a 7.5-year follow-up study of isolated repairs in ACL-stable knees with a 73 percent (38/52) meniscus healing rate. DeHaven, et al. [62] observed 30 consecutive patients (33 repaired menisci) for a minimum of 10 years after repair and reported a 79 percent meniscus repair survival rate.

Associated pathology in the injured knee can significantly diminish meniscal repair results. ACL laxity is an important factor in meniscal healing and can cause failure of the meniscal tissue to heal, or a new tear in healed tissue. The failure rate of meniscal repairs in ACL-deficient knees is nearly 46 percent, compared to 5 percent in stable or nearly stable knees [18, 62–63]. In contrast, the results have been shown to improve if ACL reconstruction is performed at the time of meniscal repair. Cannon [15] reported success in 83 percent of his 92 patients with combined cases of meniscus repair and ACL surgery, compared with his overall success rate of 75 percent.

Other factors determining repair success are tear length, the length of time after injury, associated injuries and which meniscus is injured. One study had a failure rate of 15 percent in 20 tears less than 2 cm in length, compared to a failure rate of 20 percent for 80 tears 2 to 3.9 cm, and a failure rate of 59 percent for 17 tears 4 to 5 cm [15]. Surgical timing can also be important. Cannon reported a 17 percent failure rate for 41 tears repaired less than eight weeks after injury, compared to a 28 percent failure rate for 76 tears repaired more than eight weeks after injury. Success of meniscal repair can also depend on whether the tear affects the medial or lateral meniscus. A 16 percent failure rate has been reported for 51 lateral meniscus repairs, versus a 30 percent failure rate for 66 medial meniscus repairs [15].

The choice of suture also can influence repair success. In 1997 Barrett, et al. [64] published a study examining the differences between absorbable #2-0 PDS and nonabsorbable #2-0 Ethibond in meniscal repairs using a horizontal inside-out technique. In that study 82 meniscal repairs were clinically evaluated at an average of 24.1 months. Meniscal repairs performed with permanent sutures produced better results than those done with absorbable sutures ($P = .02$).

After repair, meniscal healing can be classified as complete, partial or not healed. Direct arthroscopic visualization of the repaired tissue is the gold standard to judge this success. Magnetic resonance imaging follow-up has not been shown to be sufficiently discriminating between successful and ineffective meniscal healing to replace the necessity for repeat arthroscopic evaluation. Clinical follow-up evaluation is readily available and inexpensive, but cannot discriminate between healed or partially healed meniscus repairs and asymptomatic failures. Henning reported that two-thirds of his patients with incompletely healed or failed repairs had no accompanying symptoms of failure [12]. Morgan [65] similarly found that while all the patients in his study of second-look arthroscopies with anatomic failures were symptomatic, those patients with incompletely healed menisci were asymptomatic [65].

14.6. Clinical Results of Specific Repair Techniques

14.6.1. T-fix Suture Anchor

Barrett, et al. [66] reported the results of 21 meniscal repairs using the T-fix suture anchor with a minimum one-year follow-up. Evaluations for joint line tenderness, effusion and McMurray testing indicated that 81 percent of the repairs were successful. Avascular zone 2 repairs showed significantly lower healing rates than the peripheral zone 0 or zone 1 repairs that had a 92 percent success rate for vertical or bucket handle tears.

14.6.2. Meniscal Arrow

In 2001 Venkatachalam, et al. [67] reported on the results of 92 meniscus repairs using sutures, Arrows and T-Fix suture anchors. With an average follow-up of 21 months, the authors reported that repairs using sutures alone had higher clinical success rates (78.6 percent) than repairs using Arrows (56.5 percent) or T-fix devices (57.1 percent). The overall clinical success rate for the population was 66.1 percent. The overall complication rate of 11.3 percent included two broken Arrows as well as two Arrows that caused synovitis and articular cartilage damage. Jones, et al. [68] reported only two clinical failures requiring a second operation in 39 repaired menisci at an average follow-up time of 29.7 months. In the first 12 months, however, 31.6 percent reported transient soft tissue irritation or tenderness that generally resolved without further surgery. Petsche, et al. [69] reported two failures in 29 patients (6.8 percent) at an average follow-up time of 24 months (minimum, 12 months). Five of the patients (17.2 percent) reported local, transient skin irritation that resolved within seven months. Recently, a soft tissue complication rate of 32 percent has been reported for the Arrow [68]. Another study reported a 28 percent failure rate with significant postoperative complications, including chondral scoring, implant breakage and postoperative joint line irritation an average of 54 months after surgery [70].

14.6.3. Mitek Meniscal Repair System

The Mitek Meniscal Repair System has shown clinical promise. Laprell, et al. [71] reported 37 repaired menisci with a minimum follow-up time of 12 months. The authors found a clinical, asymptomatic success rate of 86 percent in these 37 patients.

14.7. Repair Aftercare - Rehabilitation

After successful surgical repair of a torn meniscus, controversy exists as to the postoperative rehabilitation protocol. The three main variables to consider with any rehabilitation program are when to allow motion, the weight bearing status, and when to allow pivoting sports. Clinical investigations on the effects of immobilization and restricted weight bearing provide support for more aggressive rehabilitation programs. Klein, et al. showed that immobilization and non-weight bearing in a dog model resulted in substantial atrophy of meniscus, ligament and bone [72]. In a non-weight bearing dog, atrophy was prevented by active joint motion [73]. The tensile properties of the meniscus are not significantly affected if some joint motion is allowed [74]. Prolonged immobilization after meniscal repair leads to a decrease in collagen content within the healing meniscus [75]. Taken together, this data suggests that meniscal repairs should be immediately mobilized after surgery.

Accelerated rehabilitation programs that permit early full weight bearing, unrestricted motion and no limitations on a return to pivoting sports after the postoperative effusion resolves and full motion is achieved have been described for meniscus suture repairs [63, 76–77]. The presence of an associated ACL reconstruction may make a single unified rehabilitation program for all repair techniques difficult to objectively support at this time. Some suggest identifying repairs "at risk" and protecting them postoperatively on a case-by-case basis [78]. In general, immediate full extension and flexion to 90° with protected early strengthening should be considered for most suture repairs. The newer meniscal repair devices may require a different approach. In general, rehabilitation efforts are focused on regaining full range of motion, muscle strength, flexibility and endurance. Squatting fully should not be allowed postoperatively for three months.

14.8. Current Advances and Future Possibilities

Advances in meniscal repair currently focus on the types of devices or implants used to facilitate the repair. The absorption profile of a meniscal repair device is one important biomechanical property. Materials regularly used in meniscal repair devices include poly L-lactic acid (PLLA), polyglycolic acid (PGA), polydioxanone (PDS) or derivatives of these materials (SR-PLLA, PDLLA, PLA-co-PGA). More rapidly degrading materials will hopefully decrease the risk of chondral abrasion, but joint irritation from an increased inflammatory response may be the result.

Fibrin clot techniques have been advocated to enhance meniscal healing. Recently platelet-rich fibrin matrix (PRFM) was introduced. The PRFM can deliver a more concentrated, stable fibrin matrix rich in platelets [79].

Autologous blood is centrifuged to produce platelet-rich plasma. Further centrifuging the platelet-rich plasma produces a fibrin matrix loaded with platelets that is viscous enough to be sutured. The PRFM can be inserted arthroscopically at the time of meniscal repair and held in place with the repair sutures.

The collagen meniscus implant is a biodegradable collagen matrix with possible applications in the preservation and restoration of meniscus tissue. The implant attempts to provide an environment where meniscus fibrochondrocytes and other progenitor cells can migrate into a collagen scaffold, divide and populate the scaffold. Extracellular matrix is produced which can lead to the development of new meniscus-like tissue. The collagen meniscus implant is made from bovine Achilles tendon and has a controlled resorption rate based on the degree of cross-linking. This processed collagen minimizes any immune response and the complex normal meniscus biochemical composition can be closely approximated during the production process [80–82].

Future treatments for meniscus repair may include gene therapy, stem cell therapy and tissue engineering. Goto and co-workers showed that retroviral gene transfer to a meniscal injury site is possible and that genes can be expressed locally within the injury site for several weeks [83]. This suggests that healing of the meniscus avascular areas can be improved by the transfer of genes that encode for growth factors such as PDGF, IGF-1 or hyaluronan [84–85]. Stem cells can turn into different types of tissue including bone, cartilage, muscle or tendon. Bone marrow-derived stem cells and muscle-derived stem cells persist throughout life and are accessible by biopsy. A special stem cell population derived from muscle tissue has been identified, and tissue engineering approaches are currently under development [86]. Future meniscus repair surgery may use a tissue engineered meniscus. Experimentally, meniscal cells, fibroblasts and mesenchymal stem cells have been grown on various cell matrices, including collagen-based scaffolds and biodegradable polymers [87–89].

14.9. Conclusions

The preferred approach for a symptomatic meniscal tear emphasizes meniscal tissue preservation. The surgical objective should be to remove the least amount of meniscus necessary and to repair the meniscus whenever possible. Substantial meniscus resections, whether arthroscopic or open, are to be avoided.

Failure rates are affected by initial fixation strength, cyclical stresses and associated pathology. Biomechanically, vertical sutures provide better initial fixation strength than horizontal sutures, which in turn are equivalent or superior to most of the available all-inside meniscal repair devices.

All-inside meniscal repair devices have greatly simplified the surgical technique and decreased the surgical risks of meniscal repair. They provide an attractive alternative to suture repairs. However, meniscal healing rates have not changed with the introduction of these new devices and, in fact, devices like the Meniscal Arrow have recently been reported to have success rates that are inferior to suture repairs. Surgeons should be cautious about repairing complex or degenerative meniscal tears because the healing rates are poor.

After suture meniscal repairs, the rehabilitation protocol should include unrestricted knee motion, progressive weight bearing and a rapid return to sports. However, this program has not been documented to be the best for repairs using meniscal repair devices. Aggressive programs can be implemented, but there may be an increased risk of subsequent tear or inadequate healing of the repaired meniscal tissue. The future of meniscal repair will be focused around gene therapy and tissue engineering to help develop native meniscal cells to bridge the tissue gap and stabilize meniscus tears.

References

1. Ahmed A, Burke D. In vitro measurement of static pressure distribution in synovial joints: Part I. Tibial surface of the knee. J Biomech Eng. 1983;105:216–225
2. Kurosawa H, Fukubayashi T, Nakajima H. Load-bearing mode of the knee joint: physical behavior of the knee joint with or without menisci. Clin Orthop Relat Res. 1980; 149:283–290.
3. Baratz ME, Fu FH, Mengato R. Meniscal tears: the effect of meniscectomy and of repair on intraarticular contact areas and stress in the human knee. A preliminary report. Am J Sports Med. 1986; 14:270–275.
4. Kotsovolos ES, Hantes ME, Mastrokalos DS, Lorbach O, Paessler HH. Results of all-inside meniscal repair with the FasT-Fix meniscal repair system. Arthroscopy. 2006; 22:3–9.
5. Hantes ME, Kotsovolos ES, Mastrokalos DS, Ammenwerth J, Paessler HH. Arthroscopic meniscal repair with an absorbable screw: results and surgical technique. Knee Surg Sports Traumatol Arthrosc. 2005; 13:273–279.
6. Shoemaker SC, Markolf KL. The role of the meniscus in the anterior-posterior stability of the loaded anterior cruciate-deficient knee. Effects of partial versus total excision. J Bone Joint Surg Am. 1986; 68:71–79.
7. Albrecht-Olsen P, Kristensen G, Tormala P. Meniscus bucket-handle fixation with an absorbable Biofix tack: development of a new technique. Knee Surg Sports Traumatol Arthrosc. 1993;1:104–106.
8. Annandale T. An operation for displaced semilunar cartilage. 1885. Clin Orthop Relat Res. 1990; 260:3–5.
9. King D. The healing of semilunar cartilages. 1936. Clin Orthop Relat Res. 1990; 252:4–7.
10. Henning CE. Arthroscopic repair of meniscis tears. Orthopedics. 1983;6:1130–1132.
11. Henning CE, Lynch MA, Clark JR. Vascularity for healing of meniscus repairs. Arthroscopy. 1987; 3:13–18.
12. Scott GA, Jolly BL, Henning CE. Combined posterior incision and arthroscopic intra-articular repair of the meniscus. An examination of factors affecting healing. J Bone Joint Surg Am 1986; 68: 847–861.
13. Clancy WG Jr, Graf BK. Arthroscopic meniscal repair. Orthopedics 1983; 6:1125–1129.
14. Rosenberg TD, Scott SM, Coward DB, Dunbar WH, Ewing JW, Johnson CL, Paulos LE. Arthroscopic meniscal repair evaluated with repeat arthroscopy. Arthroscopy. 1986; 2:14–20.
15. Cannon WD Jr. Arthroscopic meniscal repair, in McGinty JB, Caspari RB, Jackson RW, et al. (eds): Operative Arthroscopy. Second edition. Philadelphia, Lippincott-Raven Publishers,1996, pp 299–315
16. Cannon WD Jr, Morgan CD. Meniscal repair: arthroscopic repair techniques. Instr Course Lect. 1994; 43:77–96.
17. Cassidy RE, Shaffer AJ. Repair of peripheral meniscal tears. A preliminary report. Am J Sports Med. 1981; 9:209–214.

18. Dehaven K, Black K, Griffiths H. Open meniscus repair. technique and two to nine year results. Am J Sports Med. 1989; 17:788–795.
19. Schulte KR, Fu FH. Meniscal repair using the inside-to-outside technique. Clin Sports Med. 1996;15:455–467.
20. Warren RF. Arthroscopic meniscal repair. Arthroscopy. 1985; 1:170–172.
21. Morgan CD, Casscells SW. Arthroscopic meniscus repair: a safe approach to the posterior horns. Arthroscopy. 1986; 2:3–12.
22. Morgan CD. The "all inside" meniscus repair. Arthroscopy. 1991;7:120–125.
23. Arnoczky SP, Warren RF. Microvasculature of the human meniscus. Am J Sports Med. 1982; 10:90–95.
24. Arnoczky SP, Warren RF. The microvasculature of the meniscus and its response to injury. An experimental study in the dog. Am J Sports Med. 1983; 11:131–141.
25. Zhang Z, Arnold JA, Williams T, McCann B. Repairs by trephination and suturing of longitudinal injuries in the avascular area of the meniscus in goats. Am J Sports Med 1995; 23: 23:35–41.
26. Okuda K, Ochi M, Shu N, Uchio Y. Meniscal rasping for repair of meniscal tear in the avascular zone. Arthroscopy. 1999; 15:281–286.
27. Uchio Y, Ochi M, Adachi N, Kawasaki K, Iwasa J. Results of rasping of meniscal tears with and without anterior cruciate ligament injury as evaluated by second-look arthroscopy. Arthroscopy. 2003;19:463–469.
28. Fitzgibbons RE, Shelbourne KD. "Aggressive" nontreatment of lateral meniscal tears seen during anterior cruciate ligament reconstruction. Am J Sports Med. 1995; 23:156–159.
29. Arnoczky SP, Warren RF, Spivak JM. Meniscal repair using an exogenous fibrin clot. An experimental study in dogs. J Bone Joint Surg Am. 1988; 70:1209–1217.
30. Henning CE, Lynch MA, Yearout KM, Vequist SW, Stallbaumer RJ, Decker KA. Arthroscopic meniscal repair using an exogenous fibrin clot. Clin Orthop Relat Res. 1990; 252:64–72.
31. Roeddecker K, Muennich U, Nagelschmidt M. Meniscal healing: a biomechanical study. J Surg Res. 1994;56:20–27.
32. Morgan CD, Wojtys EM, Casscells CD, Casscells SW. Arthroscopic meniscal repair evaluated by second-look arthroscopy. Am J Sports Med. 1991;19:632–637.
33. Morrison JB. Function of the knee joint in various activities. Biomed Eng. 1969; 4:573–580.
34. Miller MD, Kline AJ, Gonzales J, Beach WR. Pitfalls associated with FasT-Fix meniscal repair. Arthroscopy. 2002;18:939–943.
35. Seedhom B, Hargreaves D. Transmission of the load in the knee joint with special reference to the role of the menisci: II. Experimental results, discussion, and conclusions. Eng in Med. 1979;8:220–228.
36. Richards DP, Barber FA, Herbert MA. Compressive loads in longitudinal lateral meniscus tears: a biomechanical study in porcine knees. Arthroscopy 2005; 21:1452–1456.
37. Hede A, Larsen E, Sandberg H. Partial versus total meniscectomy. a prospective, randomized study with long-term follow-up. J Bone Joint Surg Br. 1992; 74:118–121.
38. Schimmer RC, Brulhart KB, Duff C, Glinz W. Arthroscopic partial meniscectomy: a 12-year follow-up and two-step evaluation of the long-term course. Arthroscopy. 1998;14:136–142.
39. Fauno P, Nielsen AB. Arthroscopic partial meniscectomy: a long-term follow-up. Arthroscopy. 1992; 8:345–349.
40. Burks RT, Metcalf MH, Metcalf RW. Fifteen-year follow-up of arthroscopic partial meniscectomy. Arthroscopy. 1997; 13:673–679.
41. Neyret P, Donell ST, Dejour H. Results of partial meniscectomy related to state of the anterior cruciate ligament. review at 20 to 35 years. J Bone Joint Surg Br. 1993; 75:36–40.

42. Rimmer MG, Nawana NS, Keene GC, Pearcy MJ. Failure strengths of different meniscal suturing techniques. Arthroscopy. 1995; 11:146–150.
43. Rodeo S. Arthroscopic meniscal repair with use of the outside-to-inside technique. J Bone Joint Surg Am. 2000; 82:127–141.
44. Johnson LL. Meniscus mender II. Technical bulletin. Okemos, Michigan, Instrument Makar Inc.
45. van Trommel MF, Simonian PT, Potter HG, Wickiewicz TL. Different healing rates with the outside-in technique for meniscal repair. Am. J. Sports Med. 1998; 26: 446–452.
46. Mulhollan JS. Swedish arthroscopic approach. Orthop Clin North Am. 1982; 13:349–362.
47. Sgaglione NA, Steadman JR, Shaffer B, Miller MD, Fu FH. Current concepts in meniscus surgery: resection to replacement. Arthroscopy. 2003; 19 Suppl 1:161–188.
48. Albrecht-Olsen P, Lind T, Kristensen G, Falkenberg B. Failure strength of a new meniscus arrow repair technique: biomechanical comparison with horizontal suture. Arthroscopy. 1997; 13:183–187.
49. Barber FA, Herbert MA. Meniscal repair devices. Arthroscopy. 2000; 16:613–618.
50. Barber FA, Herbert MA, Richards DP. Load to failure testing of new meniscal repair devices. Arthroscopy. 2004; 20:45–50.
51. Barber FA, Johnson DH, Halbrecht JL. Arthroscopic meniscal repair using the BioStinger. Arthroscopy 2005; 21:744–750.
52. Whitman TL, Diduch DR. Transient posterior knee pain with the meniscal arrow. Arthroscopy. 1998; 14:762–763.
53. Menche DS, Phillips GI, Pitman MI, Steiner GC. Inflammatory foreign-body reaction to an arthroscopic bioabsorbable meniscal arrow repair. Arthroscopy. 1999;15:770–772.
54. Hechtman KS, Uribe WJ. Cystic hematoma formation following use of a biodegradable arrow for meniscal repair. Arthroscopy. 1999;15:207–210.
55. Ganko A, Engebretsen L. Subcutaneous migration of meniscal arrows after failed meniscus repair. Am J Sports Med. 2000; 28:252–253.
56. Menetrey J, Seil R, Rupp S, Fritschy D. Chondral damage after meniscal repair with the use of a bioabsorbable implant. Am J Sports Med. 2002;30:896–899.
57. Kohn D, Siebert W. Meniscus suture techniques: a comparative biomechanical cadaver study. Arthroscopy. 1989; 5:324–327.
58. Dervin GF, Downing KJ, Keene GC, McBride DG. Failure strengths of suture versus biodegradeable arrow for meniscal repair: an in-vitro study. Arthroscopy. 1997;13:296–300.
59. Post WR, Akers SR, Kish V. Load to failure of common meniscal repair techniques: effects of suture technique and suture material. Arthroscopy. 1997;13:731–736.
60. Rankin CC, Lintner DM, Noble PC, Paravic V, Greer E. A biomechanical analysis of meniscal repair. Am J Sports Med. 2002;30:492–497.
61. Eggli S, Wegmüller H, Kosina J, Huckell C, Jakob RP. Long-term results of arthroscopic meniscal repair. An analysis of isolated tears. Am J Sports Med 1995; 23:715–720.
62. DeHaven KE, Lohrer WA, Lovelock JE: Long-term results of open meniscal repair. Am J Sports Med 1995; 23:524–530.
63. Barber FA, Click SD. Meniscus repair rehabilitation with concurrent anterior cruciate reconstruction. Arthroscopy 1997; 13: 433–437.
64. Barrett GR, Richardson K, Ruff CG, Jones A. The effect of suture type on meniscus repair. A clinical analysis. Am J Knee Surg 1997;10:2–9.
65. Morgan CD, Wojtys EM, Casscells CD, Casscells SW. Arthroscopic meniscal repair evaluated by second-look arthroscopy. Am J Sports Med 1991; 19:632–637.

66. Barrett GR, Treacy SH, Ruff CG. Preliminary results of the T-fix endoscopic meniscus repair technique in an anterior cruciate ligament reconstruction population. Arthroscopy. 1997; 13:218–223.
67. Venkatachalam S, Godsiff SP, Harding ML. Review of the clinical results of arthroscopic meniscal repair. Knee. 2001; 8:129–133.
68. Jones HP, Lemos MJ, Wilk RM, Smiley PM, Gutierrez R, Schepsis AA. Two-year follow-up of meniscal repair using a bioabsorbable arrow. Arthroscopy. 2002;18:64–69.
69. Petsche TS, Selesnick H, Rochman A. Arthroscopic meniscus repair with bioabsorbable arrows. Arthroscopy. 2002;18:246–253.
70. Kurzweil PR, Tifford CD, Ignacio EM. Unsatisfactory clinical results of meniscal repair using the meniscus arrow. Arthroscopy. 2005; 21:905e1–e7.
71. Laprell H, Stein V, Petersen W. Arthroscopic all-inside meniscus repair using a new refixation device: A prospective study. Arthroscopy. 2002;18:387–393.
72. Klein L, Player JS, Heiple KG, Bahniuk E, Goldberg VM. Isotopic evidence for resorption of soft tissues and bone in immobilized dogs. J Bone Joint Surg Am. 1982; 64:225–230.
73. Klein L, Heiple KG, Torzilli PA, Goldberg VM, Burstein AH. Prevention of ligament and meniscus atrophy by active joint motion in a non-weight-bearing model. J Orthop Res. 1989;7:80–85.
74. Anderson DR, Gershuni DH, Nakhostine M, Danzig LA. The effects of non-weight-bearing and limited motion on the tensile properties of the meniscus. Arthroscopy. 1993; 9:440–445.
75. Dowdy PA, Miniaci A, Arnoczky SP, Fowler PJ, Boughner DR. The effect of cast immobilization on meniscal healing. An experimental study in the dog. Am. J. Sports Med.1995; 23: 721–728.
76. Barber FA. Accelerated rehabilitation for meniscus repairs. Arthroscopy. 1994; 10:206–210.
77. Mariani PP, Santori N, Adriani E, Mastantuono M. Accelerated rehabilitation after arthroscopic meniscal repair: a clinical and magnetic resonance imaging evaluation. Arthroscopy. 1996; 12:680–686.
78. Tenuta JJ, Arciero RA. Arthroscopic evaluation of meniscal repairs: Factors that effect healing. Am J Sports Med. 1994;22:797–802.
79. Sgaglione NA. Meniscus Repair Update: Current Concepts and New Techniques. Orthopedics 2005 28:280–286.
80. Rodkey WG, Stone KR, Steadman JR. Prosthetic meniscal replacement. In: Finerman GAM, Noyes FR, eds. Biology and biomechanics of the traumatized synovial joint: The knee as a model. Rosemont, IL: American Academy of Orthopaedic Surgeons 1992:222–231.
81. Li S-T. Biologic biomaterials: Tissue-derived biomaterials (collagen). In: Bronzino J, ed. The Biomedical Engineering Handbook. Boca Raton, FL: CRC Press 1995:627–647.
82. Stone KR, Rodkey WG, Webber RJ, McKinney LA, Steadman JR. Meniscal regeneration with copolymeric collagen scaffolds: In vitro and in vivo studies evaluated clinically, histologically, biochemically. Am J Sports Med. 1992;20:104–111.
83. Goto H, Shuler FD, Lamsam C, Moller HD, Niyibizi C, Fu FH, Robbins PD, Evans CH. Transfer of lacZ marker gene to the meniscus. J Bone Joint Surg Am. 1999; 81:918–925.
84. Bhargava MM, Attia ET, Murrell GA, Dolan MM, Warren RF, Hannafin JA. The effect of cytokines on the proliferation and migration of bovine meniscal cells. Am J Sports Med. 1999; 27:636–643.
85. Sonoda M, Harwood FL, Amiel ME, Moriya H, Amiel D. The effects of hyaluronan on the meniscus in the anterior cruciate ligament-deficient knee. J Orthop Sci. 2000;5:157–164.

86. Huard J, Acsadi G, Jani A, Massie B, Karpati G. Gene transfer into skeletal muscles by isogenic myoblasts. Hum Gene Ther. 1994; 5:949–958.
87. Cook JL, Tomlinson JL, Kreeger JM, Cook CR. Induction of meniscal regeneration in dogs using a novel biomaterial. Am J Sports Med. 1999; 27:658–665.
88. Veth RP, Jansen HW, Leenslag JW, Pennings AJ, Hartel RM, Nielsen HK. Experimental meniscal lesions reconstructed with a carbon fiber-polyurethane-poly (L-lactide) graft. Clin Orthop Relat Res. 1986; 202:286–293.
89. Ibarra C, Koski JA, Warren RF. Tissue engineering meniscus: cells and matrix. Orthop Clin North Am. 2000; 31:411–418.

15

Lessons Learned From Our First 100 Meniscus Allograft Transplants in Arthritic Knees

Kevin R. Stone[1], Ann W. Walgenbach[1], and Abhi Freyer[2]

Abstract: The meniscus performs as a knee joint stabilizer and shock absorber as the femoral condyle bears weight on the tibia, translating and rotating on the tibial plateau. A damaged meniscus is often partially removed rather than repaired. Patients without an intact meniscus have few choices: live with the pain, select joint debridement procedures, undergo meniscus allograft transplantation or undergo artificial joint replacement. Despite this, meniscus transplantation has been, until recently, a technique in its infancy. The procedure can be surgically demanding; however, recent studies suggest that meniscus transplantation is a rewarding soft tissue reconstruction that can be useful for arthritic as well as pristine knees to alleviate pain, restore function, and ultimately, delay or avoid joint arthroplasty.

Keywords: Meniscus allograft transplantation, arthritic knees.

15.1. Introduction

Meniscus allograft transplantation was first performed in humans at the turn of the century, but the cases by Milachowski in 1986 stimulated renewed interest in the field [1]. Subsequent to that time, a handful of cases were performed worldwide, but the procedure did not pick up steam until the advent of organized tissue banks in the late 1990s. Even then, meniscus transplantation lagged far behind other musculoskeletal tissue transplantations, with only a few thousand performed as late as 2004. The procedure, until recently, has been in its infancy with many lessons to be learned. This chapter will review our experience with meniscus allograft transplantation and highlight the lessons we have learned over the past few years.

[1] The Stone Clinic, San Francisco, CA
[2] Stone Research Foundation, San Francisco, CA

From: *Orthopedic Biology and Medicine: Musculoskeletal Tissue Regeneration, Biological Materials and Methods.*
Edited by W. S. Pietrzak © Humana Press, Totowa, NJ

15.2. The Meniscus: A Clinical Review

The meniscus performs as a knee joint stabilizer and shock absorber as the femoral condyle bears weight on the tibia, translating and rotating on the tibial plateau. Torn at over 1.2 million times per year in the United States, and frequently excised rather than repaired, the function of this joint cartilage becomes lost. As a result, the knee transmits force abnormally and arthritis and pain result, often years after excision. Treatment of the damaged meniscus has progressed from complete excision, which was advocated in the first three-quarters of the 20th century, to partial excision, and when possible, to repair. It was appreciated by Ahmed and Burke that the percentage and location of meniscus excision was related to the increased force concentration on the tibial plateau, with the most force concentration increase associated with excision of the posterior one-quarter of the medial meniscus [2].

Preservation of the meniscus by suture repair became slightly popular with the advent of arthroscopy and suturing devices popularized by Johnson, Lucas and Dusek, et al. [3]. However, popularity of the procedure was significantly limited due to the difficulty in performing the procedure and the belief that only the most peripheral tears could be repaired. This belief was further enforced by landmark images published by Arnoczky revealing that only the peripheral third of the meniscus had a blood supply [4]. The corollary that the inner margin tears of the avascular portion of the meniscus could not be repaired was not demonstrated; however, it became incorporated into popular belief.

Subsequent studies by Richard Webber demonstrated that the cells of the meniscus could be grown in tissue culture and could migrate [5]. Studies by Stone, et al. demonstrated that the meniscus could be regenerated when provided an appropriate regeneration template made of GAG cross-linked collagen sponges in both dogs and humans. Meniscus reconstruction using these templates is referred to as the "Collagen Meniscus Implant," or CMI, and has been approved for clinical use in Europe [6]. Efforts to regrow the entire meniscus after complete meniscectomy failed in animal models. This observation is most likely due to the biomechanical properties of the scaffold, not the regeneration potential of the meniscus. Limited regrowth options have left people without an intact meniscus with few choices: live with pain, select joint debridement procedures, undergo complete meniscus allograft transplantation, or undergo artificial joint replacement.

15.3. The Meniscus Allograft

Early efforts at meniscus allograft replacement in knees with pristine surrounding cartilage appeared to provide pain relief and durability [1, 7–12]. The few instances in which a meniscus allograft was placed in an arthritic knee were reported with relatively poor results. This became the often-repeated lore at clinical orthopaedic meetings and in the literature [8, 13–14]. However, the patients who need meniscus replacement are most commonly the 30– to 60-year-olds who have lost their meniscus, often due to sports in college, with resulting compartmental arthritic development. These patients wish to continue living an active lifestyle and want to delay artificial joint arthroplasty until they are older. To serve this need and to answer the questions, "Can meniscus replacement be performed in an arthritic knee and will it last?", we conducted a prospective outcome study and reported the results in the May 2006 issue of

Arthroscopy: The Journal of Arthroscopic and Related Surgery [15]. We will review this experience here and provide the lessons learned.

15.3.1. Patient Selection

Who is a surgical candidate for a meniscus allograft transplant? Certainly the young person who loses their lateral meniscus to an unfortunate injury or surgery is the most compelling case. Loss of the lateral meniscus always leads to significant degenerative arthritis, which must be prevented by aggressive efforts to repair or replace the meniscus at the time of injury.

Loss of the medial meniscus in a young person is slightly less significant with some whose joints degrade quickly after meniscectomy, and others whose joints degrade over the course of decades. Commonly a very large bucket- handle tear – whether due to lack of skill, confidence, or belief in the healing potential – causes a surgeon to remove rather than repair the meniscus. It is either this meniscectomy, meniscectomy a failed repair, a comminuted and degenerated meniscus, or a cystic meniscus which can often leave the patient unprotected.

Cases in the pristine cartilage setting will do well with a meniscus transplant if the surgery is performed accurately and if the rehabilitation program is protective enough to allow complete healing.

Arthritic knees present the most confusing picture; yet, arthritic patients between the ages of 30 and 60 who lost their meniscus playing high school or college sports and present with predominantly unicompartmental arthritis comprise the largest patient population asking for biologic rather than artificial joint replacement. These patients know the temporary nature of artificial materials. They know the impact sports restrictions of artificial joint replacement. They have heard the horror stories of revisions and infections. They ask the question, "Doc, is there something you can insert into my knee as a shock absorber?" They are content if surgery can be done arthroscopically and if the shock absorber can last even five years. Patients expect that the surgeon could repeat the treatment if the allograft fails or that they will eventually be "old enough" for a knee replacement.

But how arthritic is too arthritic? What are the inclusion and exclusion criteria for biologic joint replacement? Clearly, inflammatory arthritis would be too degradative an environment for cartilage transplantation of any type. Complete eburnation of a compartment with uncorrectable axis deformity prevents insertion of a new meniscus and would lead to rapid failure. However, does eburnation with a neutral or correctable axis deformity present an absolute contraindication? (Fig. 15.1) We do not believe so if the following issues can be dealt with:

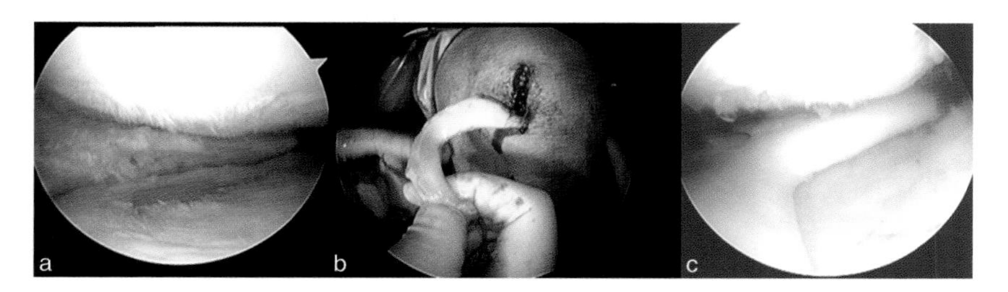

Fig. 15.1 Meniscus transplantation in the arthritic knee. (a) Loss of meniscus with exposed eburnated bone of the tibial plateau (b) Insertion of meniscal allograft into the medial arthritic compartment (c) Second-look at the meniscus allograft

Can the eburnation be treated with a cartilage grafting procedure?
We have paste grafted bipolar eburnation and performed meniscus transplants, with or without a concomitant osteotomy, in patients who absolutely refuse artificial joint replacement and understand the risks of the biologic approach [16]. One might speculate that an osteotomy alone for Grade IV arthritis might have been satisfactory, but the documented outcomes for osteotomy are short-term (five-to-seven years for good to excellent results in 80 percent of patients), and it is intuitive that if the osteotomy could be augmented by a soft tissue interpositional arthroplasty (meniscus replacement), then the outcome might be improved.

Is the majority of the pain isolated to the affected compartment?
If the patient complains of pain throughout the knee, a compartment repair is not likely to be sufficient.

Is the joint space narrowing seen on X-ray partially due to impingement of osteophytes, especially at the medial ridge?
If yes, then removal of the osteophytes can reduce the medial pain and result in a joint space appearance that is more reflective of the degree of narrowing.

Is the gait severely abnormal due to mechanical alignment reasons or due to years of favoring and compensation?
This is almost always the case because anyone living with joint pain changes their gait, loses muscle definition, wears out their shoes abnormally, and is often unaware of how much they compensate in life for these deformities. A careful physical therapy assessment and training program, concurrent with surgery and for up to a year postoperatively, can dramatically improve the outcome of the meniscus allograft transplantation procedure.

Is the other knee normal?
If no, correction of one knee without addressing the other knee leads to abnormal favoring and incomplete satisfaction. Generally, significant bilateral varus malalignment and eburnation is better treated with joint arthroplasty in middle-age and older patients. This is not only the case because of the reasons previously discussed, but also because the demands of the long-term rehabilitation program and the increased poor outcome risk of bilateral biologic joint reconstruction seems too high in our minds at this time. However, this thinking may change with improved techniques. The primary concern is the axis correction portion of the reconstruction, which still has a relatively high complication rate and uncertain outcome in middle-aged and older patients.

Is the knee unstable?
If yes, ligament reconstruction should be performed simultaneously with meniscus cartilage transplantation. The common scenarios include anterior cruciate ligament (ACL) deficiency with or without posterolateral corner laxity, and the combination of posterior cruciate ligament (PCL) laxity and medial osteoarthritis. Even in the arthritic knee, ligament reconstruction is beneficial as long as the meniscus is replaced and the arthritic cartilage surface is treated. The fear that the joint will be made "too tight" and produce more pain is unfounded. The biggest risk in all of these procedures, but especially in the combination ligament and meniscus transplantation cases, is the development of arthrofibrosis, which must be combated with an early range-of-motion (ROM) program.

Is the cartilage eburnation too far posterior?
This is a technical problem in that the arthroscopic articular cartilage grafting procedures do not reach the most posterior portions of the femoral condyles. Conversion to an open procedure may be necessary, but we have not needed to do this in our first 200 cartilage paste grafting procedures.

Is the patient contentious and non-compliant?
There is no solution for this, other than going slow and having the surgeon and rehabilitation team get to know the patient. Non-compliance remains an absolute contraindication to biologic knee reconstruction.

15.4. What is the Work-up?

15.4.1. Careful History and Physical

Careful history taking and careful physical examination are crucial initial steps.

In the history taking, the location of pain is one of the early inclusion or exclusion data points. Pain must be primarily unicompartmental. Subjective pain and functioning improvement are important considerations in determining success. A history of litigation, worker's compensation conflicts, anger at former physicians, unwillingness to take time for the rehabilitation program or unrealistic expectations of having a "normal knee" are subjective concerns which, in our hands, often lead to exclusion.

In the physical exam, observation of the patient walking and attempting to run (even in short bursts, i.e., "just to get out of the way of an oncoming truck") are usually sufficient to reveal gait abnormalities that are either correctable or potentially fatal for the biologic repair. Significant posterolateral thrust requires osteotomy. Collapsing arches with loss of motion in the ankle joints require treatment with various modalities such as heel wedges and orthotics. Loss of hip rotation and limping from causes outside of the knee joint must be addressed before the consideration of biologic joint reconstruction can proceed.

An instability examination, focusing on the presence of a pivot shift, is conducted to diagnose medial, posterior, or posterolateral instability. These can be corrected during the same surgery if the diagnosis is made in advance.

The patellofemoral exam is focused not only on the presence of the common occurrence of crepitus, but also on the presence of pain with loading. Significant anterior knee pain post-compartment correction most likely indicates poor patient selection for biologic treatments, but may be addressed with further treatment of the osteochondral defects or arthrofibrosis.

The presence of painful medial or lateral osteophytes, although easily treated, at times requires a small, open incision, as we have found the arthroscopic view deceiving. Removing impinging osteophytes leads to improvement in validated subjective questionnaire pain scores (WOMAC, IKDC, Tegner questionnaires) in our experience.

15.4.2. Careful Imaging Studies

We use current AP, 45-degree PA flexion, lateral, skyline and full-length hip-to-ankle X-ray images on all knees considered for cartilage replacement. We also use a high-field dedicated extremity 1.0 Tesla MRI (ONI Corporation) for all knees with sequences optimized for cartilage imaging.

The most important reasons for MRI in the obviously arthritic unicompartmental knee are to be sure of the status of the cartilage in the patellofemoral and lateral joints, and to assess the degree of osteonecrosis. In our opinion, neither X-ray nor MRI alone is sufficient. Additionally, for outcomes research of the cartilage transplantation procedures, preoperative and postoperative MRIs are the preferred imaging method.

15.4.3. Careful Physical Therapy Assessment

Our in-house therapy team evaluates each patient prior to surgery. The team initiates an exercise program using modalities such as heel wedges, braces, gait training, muscle strength assessment and soft tissue treatment techniques to assist patients to either avoid surgery altogether or to obtain the ideal outcome. The preoperative physical therapy sessions further serve the crucial function of identifying patients who would tend to be non-compliant with proper rehabilitation after surgical intervention.

15.4.4. Careful Nutritional Assessment

The overweight patient presents unique challenges to biologic joint reconstruction procedures and can be counseled to optimize their weight and training program. All patients are encouraged to focus on a core strengthening program with a diet supporting weight loss and strengthening. All patients are encouraged to use glucosamine as a natural anti-inflammatory and a stimulant to cartilage repair. A beverage-based supplement (Joint Juice, Inc.) may result in a higher compliance rate and enhanced bioavailability over pill-based forms.

15.5. Surgical Technique

Our surgical technique was previously published [18], and our long-term results [15] will be summarized here with a focus on surgical tips and tricks we have learned from our first 100 meniscus allograft transplants in arthritic knees.

15.5.1. Setup

Our "all-arthroscopic" meniscus transplantation technique is accomplished by having tight control of the femur because the leg often needs to be stressed in the oblique direction. This can only be accomplished with a circumferential leg holder. We prefer the Smith and Nephew Surgical Assistant Leg Holder (Smith and Nephew Inc., Memphis, Tennessee). Leg posts, human holders and open "U" designs do not permit the same angulation and easy visualization of the knee, especially for the posterior edges of the menisci. The end of the operating room table is either fully bent or removed. Instruments are placed on a Mayo stand above the patient's abdomen. No tourniquet is used; water pump infiltration provides homeostasis without the time pressure of the tourniquet.

15.5.2. Surgical Tips

15.5.2.1 Initial Preparation: Visualization

A complete arthroscopy and treatment of other issues, such as ligament instability, precedes meniscus transplantation. However, if an ACL reconstruction is to be performed, drill the holes but do not place the allograft until the end of surgery, to allow for the extra laxity necessary for visualization.

The next step to improve visualization is to trim the edges of the remaining meniscus cartilage, thereby freshening the blood supply while maintaining the rim of the meniscus to receive the allograft. Preserving the rim is the key to preventing subluxation into the medial or lateral gutter and "shrinkage" of the allograft. Avoid using any electrocautery or bipolar units on the meniscus, as blood supply determines the rate of healing. The trick to trimming the anterior one-quarter of the meniscus is to use a backbiter, both right- and left-sided. The meniscus is then needled using a smooth drill pin passed through an AO-drill guide, modified by rounding the tip of the guide to diminish the chance of scuffing the surrounding articular cartilage. The needling brings in a new blood supply and creates channels for cellular ingrowth [17]. On the medial aspect, the needle is passed repeatedly through the medial collateral ligament, creating a "Swiss cheese" effect. When valgus force is applied, opening of the joint is permitted even in the tightest of knees.

15.5.2.2. Medial Meniscus

15.5.2.2.1. Tunnel Placement: The three-tunnel technique for the medial meniscus requires that the three holes be placed optimally for meniscus insertion and fixation [18]. The posterior hole is made with a custom-modified guide that has a concave superior curvature to allow passage under the femoral condyle. The tip has a spoon to protect against unfortunate drill passage into the posterior neurovascular structures. The tip of the guide has a point, which must be placed at the bottom of the posterior medial eminence next to the PCL insertion. A drill pin is passed from the anterior tibial cortex into the spoon while watching and feeling the pin to avoid past-pointing. A 7 mm cannulated drill is then driven over the pin under direct visualization, with a curved curette positioned to catch the drill pin. If the guide pin is placed higher up or more anterior on the tibial plateau, the resulting anterior edge of the 7 mm hole will permit anterior subluxation of the meniscus, resulting in either tearing of the posterior horn or loss of flexion. This is the most common mistake in medial meniscus transplantation.

The 7 mm drill is left in place and a suture passer with a #1 nylon loop is passed up the bore and brought out through the medial portal. The drill is then removed. Prior to pulling out the nylon loop, the medial portal must be thoroughly cleared of soft tissue or else the implant will catch upon insertion. We use a large shaver, followed by an oval obturator and then followed by a large clamp spread wide in the 2 cm portal. Failure to do this leads to much frustration upon allograft insertion.

The second hole is placed one-quarter of the way around the tibia from the posterior insertion; approximately 1 cm away, but still facing the posterior aspect of the knee, not around the corner facing the medial aspect. A 4.5 mm cannulated drill is used here, since the meniscus will not be dunked into the hole. A blue PDS® suture loop is passed and brought out through the medial portal. Different size clamps are utilized to keep the sutures sorted.

The third, anterior, hole is placed by identifying the natural insertion site of the recipient, which is often over the anterior edge of the tibial plateau. A straight AO guide is placed followed by a drill pin buried only 1 cm into the bone. This is over-drilled with the 7 mm drill through the medial portal to a depth of 1 cm, thereby creating a socket to insert the anterior horn of the meniscus. A triangle drill guide is placed into the socket and a pin placed from the anterior medial tibial cortex to the tip of the guide and then over-drilled with the 4.5 mm cannulated drill. Again, a nylon suture loop is passed and exited through the medial portal.

15.5.2.2.2. Graft Preparation: Next, the meniscus allograft is prepared on the back table by separating it from the tibial plateau with a knife, retaining the periosteum at the anterior and posterior ligamentous horn insertions. A different colored, strong permanent suture is then weaved into the horns and the posterior quarter, matching the distance from the horn to the posterior hole. The bottom of the meniscus is marked with a skin marker to create "Walgenbach" lines, which assist in the differentiation between the top and bottom of the allograft should twisting occur. The horns and corner stitches are loaded into the loop stitches and pulled into the knee. A common mistake is twisting the posterior and corner stitches onto each other, which prevents seating of the allograft. This must be identified, and the meniscus must be removed and untwisted. Once seated, clamps are placed on the suture against the anterior tibia as temporary fixation.

15.5.2.2.3. Graft Fixation: We prefer an inside-out suture technique, utilizing curved, cannulated guides. We avoid making large open posterior, medial or lateral incisions and instead prefer making two or three small stab wounds, which can be stretched to retrieve the passed suture needles. We use 10-inch needles with PDS® suture, taking care to pass them both above and below the meniscus in vertical stitch orientation. It is important to note that the bottom of the allograft must be sewn to the bottom of the meniscus remnant rim; the top of the allograft to the top of the meniscus remnant. Avoid sewing directly to the synovium or the meniscus will sublux into the gutter. We sew from back to front, changing the angle for the guides as needed. When the meniscus looks balanced, the anterior, corner and posterior permanent sutures are tied while visualizing the tension on the meniscus. These sutures are tied prior to tying the knots on the middle of the meniscus to avoid pulling the horns away from the tunnel insertions. To tie the most anterior aspect of the meniscus, we use Caspari suture guides to pass two stitches and tie those to the anterior meniscus rim through the incision.

Finally, the knee is taken through a full range of motion and meniscus stability is checked with a probe.

15.5.2.3. Lateral Meniscus

The lateral meniscus insertion varies only in that a trough is made with #5.5 round burr between the anterior and posterior horns, and is checked with a curved curette. 4.5 mm drill holes are placed at either edge of the trough and sutures are passed. The meniscus allograft is trimmed with an oscillating saw and osteotomes to a 5 mm-wide block. The anterior corner and posterior sutures are placed as described above, and the meniscus is inserted with manual pressure through the slightly widened medial portal and pulled to the lateral side.

15.6. Postoperative Rehabilitation

The primary goal of the meniscus allograft rehabilitation protocol is to protect and preserve the allograft, with a secondary goal of restoring range of motion. General considerations include partial weight bearing status for four weeks postoperatively; 10 percent to 20 percent toe touch for one to two weeks; a hinged rehabilitation brace locked in full extension for four weeks postoperatively, unless otherwise indicated; regular assessment of gait to avoid compensatory patterns; regular manual mobilizations to surgical wounds and associated soft tissue to decrease the incidence of fibrosis; no resisted leg extension machines; no high-impact, cutting, or twisting activities for at least four months postoperatively; and stretching five times daily by bending the knee back as far as tolerated for 10 seconds.

The rehabilitation protocol can be described in two phases: a maximal protective phase and a moderate protective phase. The maximal protective phase is from weeks 1 to 4, and includes activities as follows:

Week 1:

- M.D. visit Day One postop to change dressing and review home program
- Icing and elevation regularly. Aim for five times per day, 15 to 20 minutes each time
- Cryotherapy machine as directed
- Soft tissue treatments to musculature for edema and pain control
- Daily manual patella glides (up/down/side-to-side) by therapist and patient
- Exercises:
  - Straight leg raise exercises (lying, seated, and standing): quadriceps/adduction/abduction/gluteal sets
  - Twice daily passive and active range-of-motion exercises
  - Theraband calf presses
  - Well-leg stationary cycling
  - Upper body training
  - Core/trunk training

Weeks 2 to 4:

- M.D. visit at eight-to-ten days postop for suture removal and check-up
- GENTLE and BRIEF pool/deep-water workouts after the first eight-to-ten days and with the use of a brace. No more than 30 minutes per workout and no more than three workouts per week
- Continue with pain control, gentle range-of-motion and soft tissue treatments M.D. visit at four weeks post-op

The moderate protective phase is from four-to-twelve weeks and includes stretching, manual treatments to restore range-of-motion, the introduction of functional exercises (i.e., partial squats, calf raises and proprioception exercises), road cycling as tolerated, slow walking on a low-impact treadmill and lateral training. Exercises increasingly focus on single-leg exercises, strength training and sport-specific training for a gradual return to activities.

Weeks 5 to 6:

- Patients progress to full weight bearing and discontinue use of rehab brace
- Increase stretching and manual treatments to improve knee range-of-motion Extension should be full and flexion should be near 100 degrees
- Incorporate functional exercises (i.e., partial squats, calf raises, mini step-ups, light leg pressing and proprioception)
- Stationary bike and progressing to road cycling as tolerated
- Slow walking on treadmill for gait training (preferably a low-impact treadmill)
- Gait training to normalize movement patterns

Weeks 7 to 8:

- Increase the intensity of functional exercises (i.e., cautiously increase depth of closed-chain exercises, shuttle/leg press). Do not overload closed- or open-chain exercises
- Continue to emphasize normal gait patterns
- Range-of-motion: Full extension and flexion to 120 degrees

Weeks 9 to 12:

- Add lateral training exercises (side step-ups, Theraband resisted side-stepping, and lateral stepping)
- Introduce more progressive single-leg exercise
- Patients should be pursuing a home program with emphasis on sport/activity-specific training
- Range of motion should be near normal

Weeks 13 to 16:

- Low-impact activities until 16 weeks
- Increase intensity of strength and functional training for gradual return to activities

15.7. Summary of Published Results

The published data of our prospective, longitudinal survival study of meniscus allograft replacement presents survival data at least two years from surgery for 45 patients with significant arthrosis (47 allografts) to determine if the meniscus can survive in an arthritic joint (Table 15.1). Data was collected for 31 men and 14 women, with mean age of 48 years (range: 14 to 69 years), with preoperative evidence of significant arthrosis and an Outerbridge classification greater than II. Failure was established by previous studies as allograft removal. No patient was lost to follow-up. The success rate was 42 of 47 allografts (89.4 percent) with a mean failure time of 4.4 years as assessed by Kaplan-Meier survival analysis. Statistical power was greater than 0.9, with $\alpha = 0.05$ and $N = 47$. There was significant mean improvement in preoperative versus postoperative self-reported measures of pain, activity, and functioning, with $p = .001$, $p = .004$ and $p = .001$, respectively, as assessed by a Wilcoxon rank-sum test with significance set as $p < .05$.

In this series, 29 allografts were cryopreserved (62 percent) and 18 were fresh-frozen allograft material (38 percent). Four of the five failures (80 percent) were of cryopreserved allograft material. A statistically significant failure rate based on allograft material was not observed, possibly because of the low number of failures.

Meniscus allografts can survive in joints with arthrosis, which challenges the contraindications of age and arthrosis severity. Figure 15.2 is representative of the level of arthrosis and long-term outcome observed in patients of this study. These results compare favorably with those in previous reports of meniscus allograft survival in patients without arthrosis [1, 7–12, 15].

15.8. Future Trends and Needs

Our experience confirms that a meniscus allograft can survive for two-to-seven years in the presence of chondromalacia in the same compartment. Whether it functions as a normal meniscus, or simply as an interpositional

Table 15.1 Summary of meniscus transplantation outcomes [15]

STUDY	Patients (Allografts)	Mean F/U Years (Range)	Mean Age Years (Range)	Allograft Material	Arthrosis Grade (n)	Failures (%)	Failure Criteria
Less Than Severe Arthrosis (OB Gr 0 - Gr III)							
Milachowski [1] (1989)	22 (22)	1.1 (0.33–2.5)	29.6 (21–45)	Deep frozen (6) Lyophilized w/ γ-irradiation (16)	Gr I (2) Gr II (10) Gr III (1) Normal (8) Unaccounted (1)	9.1	Undefined: Self assessment
Rath [10] (2001)	18 (22)	4.5 (2.0–8.1)	30 (19–41)	Deep frozen & Cryopreserved w/ bone plugs	Severe arthrosis excluded.	9.1	Allograft removal
Noyes [8] (2003)	34 (35)	3.1 (1.9–5.8)	28 (14–46)	Cryopreserved	Gr II Gr III	8.6	Allograft removal
					Total Mean Failure	**8.9% (7/79)**	
Includes Arthrosis (OB Gr IV)							
van Arkel [12] (1995)	23 (25)	3 (2–5)	41 (30–55)	Cryopreserved	Gr II (1) Gr III (23) Gr IV (1)	12	Allograft removal
Potter [9] (1996)	24 (29)	1.1 (0.25–3.4)	33.2 (24–43)	Fresh-frozen NOT γ-irradiated	Gr I–II (2) Gr III–IV (22)	3.4	Allograft removal
Cameron [7] (1997)	63 (67)	2.6 (1.0–5.5)	41 (11 pts > 50)	Fresh-frozen γ-irradiated	Gr II Gr III Gr IV	4.5	Allograft removal
Stollsteimer [11] (2000)	22 (23)	3.3 (1.1–5.8)	31 (20–42)	Cryopreserved w/ bone plugs	Gr I Gr II Gr III Gr IV	4.3	Post-Op infection & OB score
Stone (2006) [15]	45 (47)	4.5 (2–7)	48 (14–69)	Cryopreserved & fresh-frozen	Gr III (9) Gr IV (38)	10.6	Allograft removal
					Total Mean Failure	**6.8% (13/191)**	

[15] Reprinted from Arthroscopy: The Journal of Arthroscopic and Related Surgery, Vol 22. Stone KR, Walgenbach AW, Turek TJ, Freyer A, Hill M.D. Meniscus Allograft Survival in Patients with Moderate to Severe Unicompartmental Arthritis: A 2- to 7-Year Follow-up. 469–478 Copyright (2006) with permission from Arthroscopy Association of North America.

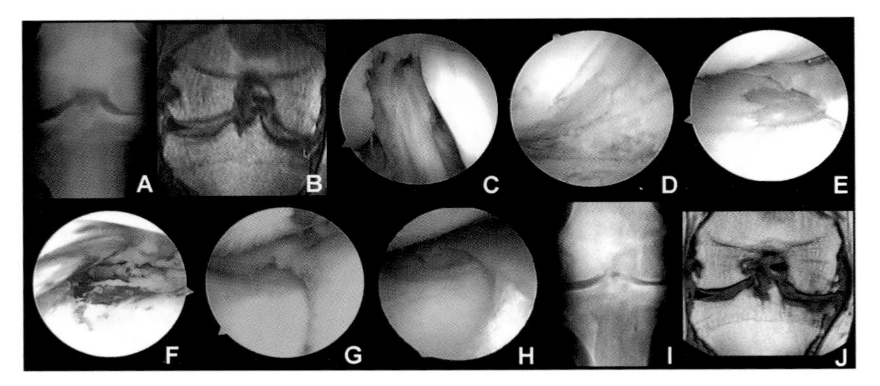

Fig. 15.2 Preoperative, operative, and postoperative images of meniscus allograft transplantation. (a) Preoperative PA flexion radiograph of a 39-year-old male one-year post-meniscectomy with noticeable joint space narrowing (b) Preoperative coronal MRI documenting lateral meniscus bucket handle tear and bipolar cartilage lesions (c) Arthroscopic view of the right knee bucket handle tear displaced into intercondylar notch (d, e) Eburnation of the femoral condyle and tibial plateau (f) Microfracture of the tibial plateau (g) Placement of the meniscus allograft (h) Arthroscopic view of the allograft 17 months postoperatively (i) AP radiograph five years postoperatively showing improved joint space (j) Five-year postoperative coronal MRI revealing the transplanted meniscus present and maturing degenerative changes

soft tissue arthroplasty, was not addressed by this study. The improvements noted in pain and functioning may be attributed to the transplant, the concomitant procedures, the rehabilitation program, or the attentive care of the medical team. The goal of the study was to determine if the graft could survive in an arthritic knee. A controlled study comparing arthroscopy with and without meniscus allograft transplantation will help clarify the implant's contribution. Compared with other outcome studies, patients in this study had successful meniscus allografts in spite of being older and having well-documented severe degenerative disease, both of which were previously believed to be contraindications for meniscal allograft transplantation. These results show that meniscal allograft transplantation can be used in higher risk patients with reasonable expectations for allograft survival. This study reveals that the previous contraindications of age and severity of arthrosis are overstated, and that these results are comparable to those of other studies whose patients were younger and without arthrosis.

15.9. Conclusions

In summary, meniscus transplantation requires attention to detail, but is a soft tissue reconstruction that can be useful for pristine as well as arthritic knees.

References

1. Milachowski KA, Weismeier CJ, Wirth CJ. Homologous meniscus transplantation: Experimental and clinical results. *Int Orthop.* 1989;13:1–11.
2. Ahmed AM, Burke DL. In-vitro measurement of static pressure distribution in synovial joints. Part I. Tibial surface of the knee. *J Biomech Eng.* 1983;105:216–25.

3. Johnson MJ, Lucas GL, Dusek JK, Henning CE. Isolated arthroscopic meniscal repair: a long-term outcome study (more than 10 years). *Am J Sports Med.* 1999 Jan-Feb;27(1):44–9.
4. Arnoczky SP, Warren RF. Microvasculature of the human meniscus. *Am J Sports Med.* 1982 Mar-Apr;10(2):90–5.
5. Webber RJ. In vitro culture of meniscal tissue. *Clin Orthop Relat Res.* 1990 Mar;(252):114–20.
6. Stone KR, Steadman JR, Rodkey WG, Li ST. Regeneration of meniscal cartilage with use of a collagen scaffold. Analysis of preliminary data. *J Bone Joint Surg Am.* 1997 Dec;79(12):1770–7.
7. Cameron JC, Saha S. Meniscal allograft transplantation for unicompartmental arthritis of the knee. *Clin Orthop Relat Res.* 1997;337:164–171.
8. Noyes FR, Barber-Westin SD. Role of meniscus allografts alone and combined with ACL reconstruction or osteochondral autograft transfer procedures. Presented at the Annual Meeting of the AOSSM, New Orleans, LA, 2003.
9. Potter HG, Rodeo SA, Wickiewicz TL, Warren RF. MR imaging of meniscal allografts: correlation with clinical and arthroscopic outcomes. *Radiology.* 1996 Feb;198(2):509–514.
10. Rath E, Richmond JC, Yassir W, Jeffreys DA, Gundogan F. Meniscal allograft transplantation two- to eight-year results. *Am J Sports Med.* 2001;29:410–414.
11. Stollsteimer GT, Shelton WR, Dukes A, Bomboy AL. Meniscal allograft transplantation: A 1-to 5-year follow-up of 22 patients. *Arthroscopy.* 2000;16:343–347.
12. van Arkel ERA, de Boer HH. Human meniscal transplantation: Preliminary results at 2 to 5-year follow-up. *J Bone Joint Surg Br.* 1995;77:589–595.
13. Fairbank TJ. Knee joint changes after meniscectomy. *J BoneJoint Surg Br.* 1976;30:664–670.
14. Zukor DJ, Cameron JC, Brooks PJ, et al. The fate of human meniscal allografts. In: Ewing W, ed. *Articular cartilage and knee joint function: Basic science and arthroscopy.* New York: Raven, 1990;147–152.
15. Stone KR, Walgenbach AW, Turek TJ, Freyer A, Hill MD. Meniscus Allograft Survival in Patients with Moderate to Severe Unicompartmental Arthritis: A 2- to 7-Year Follow-up. *Arthroscopy.* 2006; 469–478.
16. Stone KR. Articular cartilage repair—The paste graft technique. Insall JN, Scott WN, eds. *Surgery of the Knee.* Ed 3. Philadelphia: Churchill Livingstone, 2001;375–380.
17. Zhang Z, Arnold JA: Trephination and suturing of avascular meniscal tears: a clinical study of the trephination procedure. *Arthroscopy.* 1996;12(6):726–731.
18. Stone KR, Walgenbach AW. Meniscal allografting: The three tunnel technique. *Arthroscopy.* 2003;19:426–430.

16

Tissue Engineering of the Meniscus

Pieter Buma, Marloes van Meel, Tony G. van Tienen, and Rene P.H. Veth

Abstract: This chapter addresses questions related to tissue engineering of an entirely new meniscus. In particular the type and geometry of temporary scaffolds, the selection of an optimal cell type, the source of the cells and the growth factors that can be used to stimulate differentiation of cells into fibrocartilage, may all determine the final success.

Three approaches can be chosen with respect to the scaffold types used. Natural scaffolds based on tissues can be used. The disadvantage of such scaffolds is the lack of optimal mechanical properties, which are obligatory, in the highly loaded environment of the knee joint. Secondly, natural scaffolds, reconstituted from isolated naturally occurring tissue matrix components, could be an attractive alternative. An advantage is that custom-made scaffolds can be tailored for optimal tissue ingrowth, proliferation and remodelling of tissue. Thirdly, synthetic scaffolds may be fine-tuned to mechanical requirements. They have the advantage that scaffolds can be produced with optimal mechanical properties.

With respect to cells, most research so far has been focussed on autologous meniscus cells. However, their availability, particularly in clinical situations, will be limited. Therefore, research should be stimulated to investigate the suitability of other cell sources for the creation of meniscus tissue. Bone marrow stroma cells could be useful since it is well-known that they can differentiate into bone and cartilage and may possibly have paracrine effects on differentiated cell types.

With respect to growth factors, transforming growth factor-β (TGF-β) could be a suitable growth factor to stimulate cells into a fibroblastic phenotype, but unwanted effects of TGF-β introduced into a joint environment should then be prevented.

In conclusion, a meniscus seems a simple structure, but its location in a highly loaded environment makes it a challenging structure for tissue engineers.

Keywords: Growth factor, meniscus tear, cartilage degradation, osteoarthritis, repair tissue, differentiation, fibrocartilage tissue.

Department of Orthopaedics, University Medical Centre Nijmegen, Nijmegen, the Netherlands

From: *Orthopedic Biology and Medicine: Musculoskeletal Tissue Regeneration, Biological Materials and Methods*
Edited by W. S. Pietrzk © Humana Press, Totowa, NJ

16.1. Introduction

The menisci are unique wedge-shaped semi-lunar discs present in duplicate in each knee joint [1–2]. The menisci are attached to the transverse ligaments, the joint capsule, the medial collateral ligament and the meniscus-femoral ligament (laterally) [3]. Initially, the menisci were considered as functionless remains of leg muscles, but are now unquestionably thought to play a crucial role in the normal biomechanics of the knee joint, e.g., in load bearing, load distribution, shock absorption, joint lubrication and stabilization of the knee joint [4–7]. Moreover, the menisci provide stability to the injured knee when the cruciate ligaments or other primary stabilizers are deficient [5]. The ability to perform these functions is based on the anatomy in combination with intrinsic material properties, and on the presence of lubricating proteins on the surface of the meniscus. The extracellular matrix of the fibrocartilage tissue of the meniscus consists mainly of collagen Type I. In the peripheral two-thirds of the meniscus the collagen is orientated in radial and circumferential bundles [1, 8]. Particularly the circumferential Type I collagen fiber bundles give the tissue great tensile stiffness, provide resistance to radial extrusion of the meniscus and maintain the structural integrity of the meniscus during load bearing [1, 8]. Most collagen Type II is found in the inner region and is also organized in bundles [2, 9]. Proteoglycans mainly consist of large aggregating polysaccharides (glycosaminoglycans (GAGs)), with chondroitin sulphate as the dominant glycosaminoglycan and with a smaller proportion of small dermatan sulphate. Most GAGs are co-localized with the Type II collagen and are important in maintaining the viscoelastic properties, compression stiffness and tissue hydration [1, 8]. Minor extracellular matrix components are glycoproteins, elastin and small quantities of Types III and V collagen. The glycoproteins include the link proteins, the 116-k protein and a group of adhesive or potentially adhesive proteins, including Type VI collagen, fibronectin and thrombospondin [2].

The microvascular anatomy of human meniscus was investigated with the Spalteholz technique, which enables the visualization of microvascularity. Branches of the lateral, medial and middle genicular arteries supply the meniscus. A perimeniscus capillary plexus originating in the capsular and synovial tissues of the joint supplies the peripheral 10 to 25 percent of the meniscus, which is called the red zone. The transitional zone of the nonvascularized zone is the red-white zone and the inner zone is the white nonvascularized zone [10].

Meniscus lesions are among the most frequent injuries in young patients and they will inevitably lead to osteoarthritic changes of the knee articular cartilage if not treated. The avascular fibrocartilage-like tissue of the meniscus is notorious for its limited self-regenerative capacity. Various treatment options for the repair of meniscus lesions are described. In case of severe lesions the final goal will be to replace the whole meniscus by a tissue engineered construct.

Many questions remain to be answered before a tissue engineered meniscus will be available for clinical implementation. These questions are related to the selection of an optimal cell type, the source of the cells, the need to use growth factors and the type and geometry of temporary scaffolds that can be used to stimulate differentiation of cells into fibrocartilage.

16.1.1 Damage to the Meniscus

Injuries of the meniscus may be caused by a compressive force in combination with tibio-femoral rotation in the transverse plane during a movement from flexion to extension, or during rapid cutting or pivoting [11]. A number of clearly different types of lesion have been described. The circular arrangement of collagen fibrils in the central portion of the meniscus provides a functional explanation for the longitudinal orientation of the majority of tears in the meniscus [12]. One of the most prominent types is the bucket handle lesion, which is a tear in the circular direction in the white zone [13], but other more complex degenerative tears may also occur [14].

Due to the increase in popularity of arthroscopic surgery, a partial or total meniscectomy was a common surgical intervention in the 1960s and 1970s [15]. This treatment resolved the short-term pain and locking phenomena [15]. Because the osteoarthritic changes after a partial meniscectomy are not as severe as after a total meniscectomy, and since osteoarthritis develops very slowly, it took several decades before it was broadly accepted that even a partial meniscectomy inevitably generates abnormal load stresses on articular cartilage which leads to progression of osteoarthitis in the tibia and femur [15–20].

Directly after a partial meniscectomy in dogs the cut surface of the meniscus begins remodeling in most menisci. Remodeling starts with the adherence of a fibrin clot to the cut surface, which presumably is a remnant from residual haemarthroses [21]. Thereafter, re-population with fibrocytes starts and, after 12 weeks, remodeling into fibrocartilage-like tissue is found. The origin of the repair cells is unknown. They may be migrating cells from the synovium, or local proliferating meniscus fibrochondrocytes. Although partial meniscus resection is associated with less radiographic osteoarthritis over time than total meniscectomy [22], the main goal of meniscus surgery is to restore a functional meniscus and to prevent the development of degenerative osteoarthritis in the involved knee.

16.1.2. Classical Repair Techniques

In light of the progressive osteoarthritic changes a great deal of effort was put into devices that fix a loose segment or a tear on the main body of the meniscus. Two options are available. Suturing is a safe traditional procedure, but rather time-consuming [23]. More recently, suture anchors, screws, staples and a variety of other devices, which might have superior initial fixation strength, have been advocated for the rapid fixation of loose segments [23–24]. Moreover, these devices may retain their strength over time in the remodelling tissue. The main problems with all these devices are that tears in the avascular part of the meniscus may heal only slowly or not at all due to inefficient vascularization. Because of this the mechanical forces will lead to sawing of sutures or devices through the meniscus tissue in time by which mechanism the reconstruction may fail. Failure rates of such techniques of 28 percent [25] and 30 percent have been reported in literature [26].

Therefore, various procedures might be further developed for the stimulation of repair tissue in the tear gap, which might form a new stable mechanical interlock between the torn part and the main body. One of the approaches may be to use an extra fibrin clot in the tear area [27]. Fibrin could function as a scaffold that attracts cells from the existing matrix or from the synovium and, by that, stimulate repair. Another option might be to stimulate cells in the main body of the meniscus with growth factors to produce more matrix and or to migrate into the defect [28]. In this respect it is good to know that the meniscus possesses different cell populations which are characterized by different cluster of differentiation (CD) markers and pericellular matrix [29]. Also, isolated cells from the red-red, red-white and white zones of the meniscus react differently to a number of growth factors. Thus, growth factors may not have the same effect on all cells in the meniscus [30]. A different approach is to stimulate vessel ingrowth into the avascular zone. Vascular endothelial growth factor (VEGF) plays an important role in angiogenesis in fetal menisci and is downregulated in the adult meniscus [31]. Coated sutures with VEGF induced more endothelial cells in the defect site in merino sheep, but the healing of the tears was improved and immunohistochemistry showed a strong immunostaining against matrix metalloproteinase 13 (MMP-13) in the VEGF coated suture group [31]. Since MMPs might be involved in mechanically induced destruction of matrix of articular cartilage [32–34], the upregulation of MMPs by VEGF may have unwanted weakening effects on the still healthy meniscus matrix. Other techniques to locally up-regulate the activity of existing meniscus fibrocytes may be the transfer of anabolic genes into local meniscus cells. Particularly genes that up-regulate the production of matrix constituents may be interesting [35–36]. Genes that stimulate the production of extra matrix by transforming growth factor-ß (TGF-β: [37]), and genes that induce new vessel ingrowth without the unwanted effect on MMP expression (e.g., hepatocyte growth factor) may also be interesting candidates [38].

16.1.3. Repair of Tears by the Creation of an Access Channel

In light of the uncertainties concerning the stimulation of meniscus fibroblasts *in vivo* – i.e. how to stimulate their proliferation, migration into the defect and the production of enough matrix – various techniques have been advocated to stimulate healing of meniscus tears independent of the fibrocytes of the main body of the meniscus. Taking into consideration the compromised vascularization in the white zone, the concept was developed that creating an extra access channel for new vascularization from the synovium through the red zone into the tear might be helpful to stimulate repair. The channel can be left open, but then the repair appears to be limited [39]. If a scaffold material is introduced this can guide the vessel(s) and new cells into the lesion site. Scaffolds can also be used to partly replace the damaged meniscus or, in case of severe damage, to replace the whole meniscus.

16.1.4. Scaffolds for Meniscus Tissue Engineering

The ideal scaffold material should be biocompatible and biodegradable in the long term. Moreover, it should permit unrestricted cellular ingrowth, allow free diffusion of nutrients, may be used as a carrier for stimulatory and inhibitory growth factors, and it should be strong enough to withstand the load in the joint and maintain its structural integrity under these loaded conditions. Furthermore, it should have a degradation profile that allows ingrowth of new tissue and thereafter allows remodelling of these tissues under the influence of load [40]. So far, mainly two types of scaffold were used for this application:

processed or unprocessed tissues (with or without devitalization), or synthetic scaffolds based on polymers.

Tissues can be used as natural scaffold materials. Examples of tissues used for the repair of (partial) lesions are periosteal tissue, perichondral tissue, synovial flaps, small intestine submucosa and meniscus tissue itself. The success of synovial flaps was variable. In some studies repair of a tear was found, in others not. The main disadvantage of whole tissues used as scaffold material is that the initial mechanical properties and the pore geometry of the tissues cannot be varied, which may be a disadvantage. Clinical studies were performed with a fibrin clot or with infrapatellar adipose tissue. Fresh tears appear to perform better than old tears (for references see Buma, et al. [41]).

Polymers are more reliable. Generally, in the polymer implant, a fibrous tissue is formed that/which remodels into fibrocartilage. The tissue that is formed in the tear itself is mainly fibrous. The mechanical strength of the newly formed tissue, however, is still unknown [41].

16.1.5. Repair of Partial and Total Meniscus Lesions with Natural Scaffold Materials

Depending on the extent of the damage, a total or subtotal meniscectomy will need to be performed. In practice a total meniscectomy is performed if the defect of the meniscus is so large that the rim of the meniscus is interrupted, after which the remnants of the meniscus can be pushed to the periphery during load bearing. Thereby the meniscus loses its protective function in the joint. A subtotal meniscectomy is performed when the peripheral rim is still intact.

Instead of whole tissues, isolated tissue components – for instance collagens, proteoglycans or elastin molecules – can be reconstituted into tailor-made scaffolds with optimal three-dimensional architecture. The mechanical properties of such scaffolds may be a problem since, in many cases, they are too low for direct load bearing applications. The advantages of such scaffolds, however, is that they can be produced from pure tissue components with low immunogenicity, and that scaffold parameters such as porosity can be fine-tuned to the desired material properties. The most popular reconstituted scaffold for meniscus repair is based on isolated collagen molecules [42]. Based on these natural scaffold materials the group of Stone developed a meniscus implant for partial meniscus lesions [42–44]. The philosophy behind the collagen meniscus implant (CMI) is that it can act as a scaffold material to guide proliferating cells to form new meniscus tissue. The reasons to use collagen as scaffold material are the low antigenicity, the conduction of tissue regeneration in other applications, the adaptable pore size and the biological remodeling capacity of ingrown tissue [43]. The CMI is made from collagen Type I isolated from bovine tendon. Collagen fibers are coprecipitated with glycosaminoglycans (GAGs) by the addition of ammonium hydroxide and cross-linked by formaldehyde in a mold [42]. The resulting structure is sponge-like, and has an open structure of pores surrounded by collagen lamellae. The main disadvantage of the CMI implant, compared to the ideal implant, is the relatively inferior mechanical properties of the implant at implantation, which makes the initial contribution to load bearing in the partial meniscectomized knee minimal or absent.

16.1.6. Preclinical Studies with the CMI

A number of preclinical and (prospective) clinical studies tried to determine whether the CMI implant contributes to the protection of articular cartilage, and the return to daily activity and normal joint function after a meniscus trauma. For that purpose the implantations were evaluated with histology, functional scores, arthroscopy and roentgen techniques. In two preclinical studies [43–44] the ability of the scaffolds to induce cellular adherence, migration, proliferation and matrix formation *in vitro* and *in vivo* was studied. *In vitro* the depth of infiltration of seeded fibrochondrocytes into the matrix was limited, but could be improved by fibronectine [43]. *In vivo* the penetration of cells in scaffolds is generally much easier since most cells produce MMPs that may help to make the scaffolds accessible for new tissue ingrowth [45–46]. The CMI in pigs induced a mild inflammatory reaction, followed by vascular invasion and remodeling and resorption of the implant [43]. In mature canines differentiation of cells into fibrochondrocytes was found and it was concluded that the CMI induces meniscus regeneration.

Biopsies of clinical patients confirm that re-population of CMI scaffolds also occurs if they are positioned against an avascular part of the main body. An interesting point of discussion is the origin of the repair cells in the meniscus. In a partial thickness cartilage defect Hunziker already demonstrated that cells of synovial origin were able to re-populate the defect [47]. Thus, theoretically, cells that re-populate the CMI meniscus implant could originate from the main body of the meniscus, or they could originate from the synovium. Observations on clinical biopsies, which demonstrated an overgrowth of the CMI by synovial-like tissue, support a mechanism in which the CMI is re-populated by the synovium (Fig. 16.1). Also, the observation that the CMI might shrink after implantation [48] implies that synovial overgrowth of the implant is possible, since the implant is then protected from overloading by the still existing remnants of the main body of the meniscus. Shrinking of the implant would then generate a functional gap in which the synovial tissue could potentially grow freely and re-populate the collagen scaffold. A number of clinical studies were published on the CMI [42, 49–51]. The longest follow-up periods were between five and eight years [50–51]. The CMI was implantable and appeared to be safe over a three-year period. Regenerated fibrous tissue was found in defects of various sizes. After six months the original structure of the collagen network of the CMI was still present [49] and no adverse immunological reactions were reported [52]. In general most studies reported a decrease in negative clinical symptoms, an almost normal activity level of the patients, and a reduction in pain in most patients [51]. Radiographic analysis of the longer follow-up studies showed that there was no progression of osteoarthitis [50–51]. The mean age of the patients in the last study was 25 years [51].

16.1.7. Total Meniscus Replacement

Again, various options are available for the replacement of the entire meniscus including autologous tissue like tendon or synovial tissue, allograft menisci or various synthetic polymer materials. Polymers have been produced using polyglycolic acid, polylactic acid, polyurethane and combinations of these and of other copolymers, or a combination of synthetic materials with autologous tissues (see [41] for review).

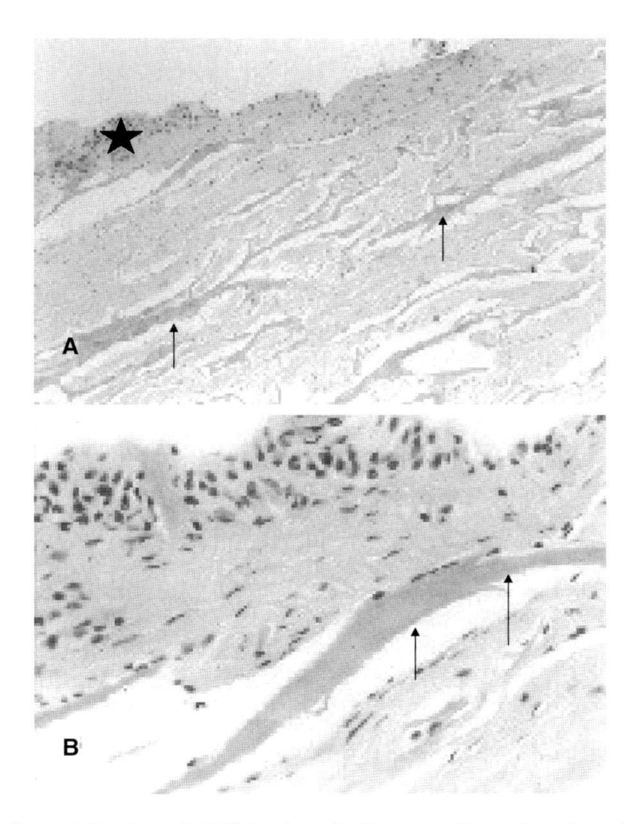

Fig. 16.1 Synovialization of CMI implant **A**. Hematoxylin and eosin stained section of surface of implanted scaffold 12 months postop. Original magnification x25 Notice collagen bundles of original implant (arrows). **B**. Magnification of **A**. On the surface of the implant a cell-rich, synovium-like tissue is present (location of asterisks in **A**). Original magnification x100. Courtesy of Dr. W.G. Rodkey (Unpublished)

With respect to the allograft meniscus, different reports mention variable results in preclinical studies. Some studies mention the prevention of osteoarthritic changes [53]; others are less positive [54]. Even though the studies of Rijk, et al. were performed in rabbits, a small animal with difficult surgery and a relatively large trauma reaction, the observation that a delayed meniscal transplantation induced even more osteoarthritic changes than a meniscectomy without transplantation is wory some [55]. From a biomechanical perspective an allograft may contribute to the restoration of the normal biomechanics of the knee joint [56].

In particular, a biodegradable porous polymer implant, which acts as a temporary scaffold to enable the regeneration of a new meniscus in time by slow degradation of the polymer and simultaneous differentiation of the ingrown fibrovascular tissue into the typical avascular meniscus fibrocartilage, may be promising. A great advantage of polymers is that the porosity, the degradation rate and the mechanical properties can be adapted to the desired specifications. In studies in our laboratory we used the porous polycaprolactone-polyurethane (PCLPU) polymer, which consists of well-defined hard segments in combination with slowly degrading polyester soft segments (Fig. 16.2) [57]. The hard

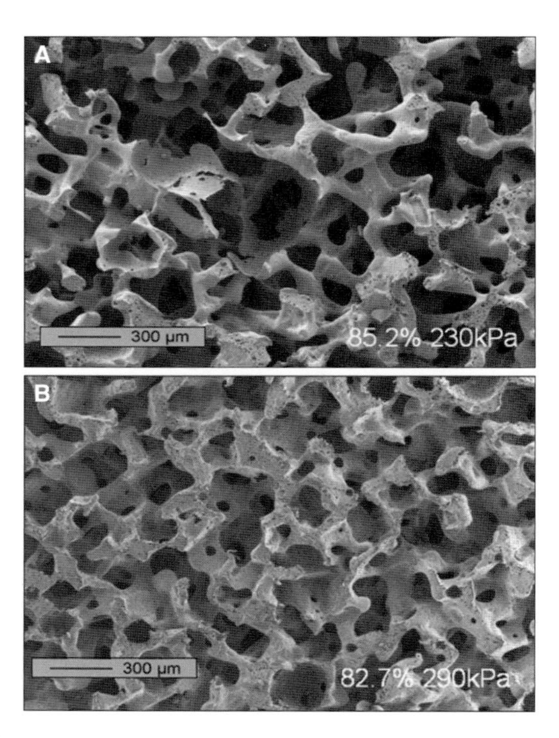

Fig. 16.2 A Scanning electron microscopic aspect of (50/50 percent epsilon-caprolacton/L-Lactide; shown in A) and estane (shown in B) porous polymers. Both polymers have micropores and larger interconnected macropores (ca 155 to 355 μm). Bars are 100 and 300 μm, respectively

segments in combination with the length of the soft segment determine the stiffness of the polymer. Both the initial mechanical properties and the pore size and geometry are important parameters for the final result. Klompmaker, et al. [58] investigated the ingrowth of new tissue into four polyurethanes with different pore sizes (50 to 90, 90 to 150, 150 to 250 and 250 to 500 μm) in wedge-shaped defects in the meniscus of rabbits. The volume percentage of macropores was 48 to 55, and total pore volume was 84 to 86 volume percent. Ingrowth into all pores was found in the scaffolds with the large pores. It was concluded that, for complete ingrowth and incorporation of partial or total meniscus prostheses, macropore sizes must be in the range of 150 to 500 μm. By varying the initial compressive modulus, the rate of ingrowth and nature of ingrown tissue could be modified. Alternatively the mechanical properties can be controlled by the degree of porosity [57, 59]. Even though polymers with a compression modulus of 40 kPa showed fast fibrous tissue ingrowth, no differentiation into fibrocartilage occurs in such scaffolds. The 100-kPa polymers, however, did show nice fibrocartilage formation [58]. Others found that the scaffolds should have an initial minimum compression modulus of 150 kPa to stimulate fibrocartilage formation [8]. Thus, for optimal ingrowth and subsequent differentiation into fibrocartilage, both pore size and initial properties are important [41].

Previously, the published results of two short-term studies (three and six month follow-up periods) used a dog model in which tissue ingrowth,

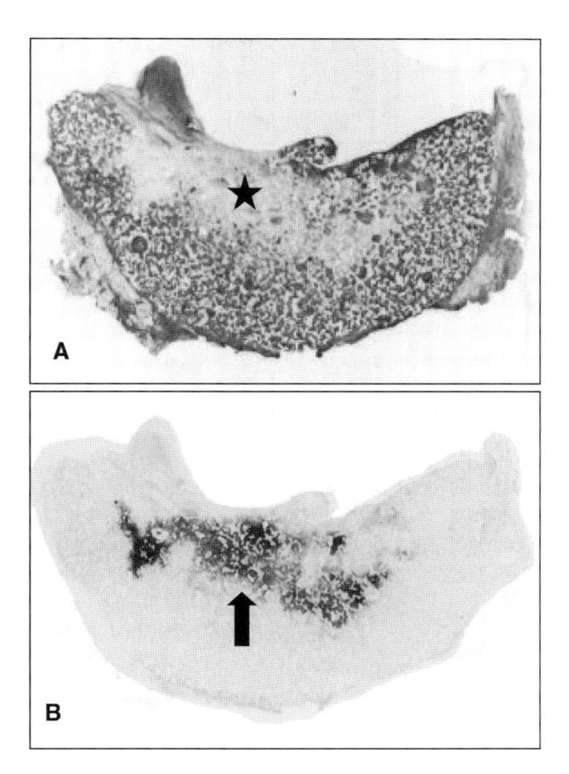

Fig. 16.3 A Overview of meniscus implant in dogs six months after the operation. The tissue is stained with an antibody to collagen Type I. Almost the entire scaffold is filled with fibrous tissue. In the central part of the scaffold the staining for collagen Type I is decreased and in this region collagen Type II staining (not shown) and toluidin blue staining was found as an indication for cartilage-like tissue formation

remodeling in the scaffold and changes in mechanical properties were analyzed [60–61]. These data were compared with results of total meniscectomy. After six months the ingrown tissue was fibrous-like in the peripheral zones of the meniscus prosthesis, but in the central areas cartilage-like tissue had developed (Fig. 16.3). The collagen bundles in the pores of the scaffold were mainly directed toward the interconnections between pores and, thus, the organization of the matrix was clearly different from the highly organized extracellular matrix of the native meniscus. The stiffness of the implant (compression modulus) after six months was intermediate between the compression modulus of the native meniscus and the porous polymer foam. Both the implant and the meniscectomy group showed a similar pattern of cartilage degeneration. The effect of polymer implants on cartilage degradation in dog models is minimal to absent [61–63]. The results of a two-year study (unpublished) with the same polymer, using an implant with a smoother surface in the same model, did not show additional chondroprotection (unpublished results).

Theoretically, scaffolds with a larger porosity might degrade slightly quicker by hydrolysis since the total surface area available for surface erosion by hydrolysis is larger. However, detailed studies are lacking so far. Furthermore, degradation should preferably lead to non-toxic products. One of the advantages of polymers is that they are highly moldable and can be manufactured into complex shapes of any size to meet the geometrical specifications set by native tissues [64–66]. Finally, the polymer may also be mixed with natural scaffold constituents like hyaluronic acid [67].

As in the collagen meniscus, extra seeded cells might enhance meniscus regeneration in polymers after transplantation. Polyglycolic acid (PGA) fiber meshes which were mechanically reinforced by bonding PGA fibers at cross points with 75:25 poly(lactic-co-glycolic) acid, were seeded with allogeneic meniscal cells. After one week of culture they were implanted into rabbits' knees and a regenerated meniscus was formed. Although the authors state that the effect on osteoarthritic changes was improved by the cell-seeding technique, no quantitative data were added to substantiate this statement [68].

16.1.8. Characterization of Meniscus Cells

The fibrochondrocytes of the meniscus appear to have considerable potential to respond to growth and other anabolic factors, which might have a function in repair or regeneration of the tissue. In this light it is relevant to know that in rabbits the level of mRNA for various matrix molecules and regulatory growth factors may differ significantly between the medial and lateral meniscus, and may be dependent on the age of the animal [69]. Webber and co-workers have developed protocols for isolation of meniscus cells [70–73]. The procedures are similar to those used for articular chondrocytes, but a few extra isolation steps are needed to free the cells from the more complex extracellular matrix. After slicing of the meniscus, the isolation starts with a short digestion in 0.05 percent hyaluronidase for five minutes and a subsequent digestion in 0.2 percent trypsin for 30 minutes, followed by the regular overnight incubation in 0.2 percent collagenase [70–73].

Isolated human meniscus cells express the collagens I, II, III and VI; the MMPs -1, -2, -3, -8 and -13; BMP-2 and -4; TGF-ß1; VEGF; insulin-like growth factor-1 (IGF-I) and IGF-II; fibroblast growth factor-2 (FGF-2); endostatin; inducible nitric oxide synthethase (iNOS); vimentin; tissue inhibitor of metallo proteinase-1 (TIMP-1), and TIMP-2; aggrecan; interleukin-1ß (IL-1ß), IL-6 and IL-18 [74]. The role of these large numbers of catabolic and anabolic factors is not known, but when using these cells in a tissue engineering approach, it should be kept in mind that part of the factors are anabolic and others are catabolic for articular cartilage.

As cells in the meniscus are diverse, it seems very likely that different cell populations are released from the matrix. Indeed, based on their morphology three different populations have been isolated from human menisci (elongated fibroblast-like cells, polygonal cells and small round chondrocyte-like cells) [75]. Moreover, cells isolated from the inner avascular part produce more GAGs in culture, compared to cells from a peripheral fibrous location [76–77]. Various studies were performed to study the effect of growth factors on meniscus fibroblasts. FGF has been shown to stimulate proliferation and matrix production of cells irrespective of their zone of origin[78]. IGF had a positive effect on the proliferation and extracellular matrix formation of all cells cultured in monolayer of all zones of the meniscus, but the effect was most prominent on fibrocytes from the avascular zone [79]. In a study in which the effects of TGF-β, IGF and bFGF on matrix production and proliferation of monolayer-cultured meniscus fibrocytes were compared, it was shown that, in contrast to the previous study, TGF had a much larger effect on matrix production than IGF, bFGF and platelet-derived growth factor (PDGF), and that TGF-β can be used to up-regulate extracellular matrix (ECM) production in monolayer cultures of meniscal fibrochondrocytes [80–81]. In a study in which meniscus fibrocytes were cultured in monolayer in chondrogenic differentiation medium with FGF, this growth factor stimulated cartilage-specific production of extracellular matrix components like GAGs, and collagen Type II [82]. Thus, TGF-β seems to be a very effective growth factor to stimulate the production of GAGs and biglycan by meniscus cells in culture [77], but the application in a joint environment may have unwanted side effects.

In light of the enormous potential of non-differentiated progenitor cells for tissue engineering of a variety of structures, mesenchymal stroma cells could be an attractive alternative cell source for meniscus tissue engineering [40]. So far, however, the types, concentration and moment/time of application of growth factors to direct the cells into a fibrocartilaginous differentiation pathway have not been elucidated yet. Possibly, the application of a particular loading pattern could prove to be essential to steer cells towards fibrocartilaginous differentiation. The main advantage of these stroma cells is, however, that they can be harvested from various locations in the body, are multipotent and are available in relatively large quantities. Mesenchymal stroma cells (MSCs) were injected into joints with an injured anterior cruciate ligament (ACL), medial meniscus and articular cartilage of the femoral condyles. At four weeks after injection of 1×10^7 MSCs into the knee, green fluorescent protein (GFP) positive cells were found in all ACLs and in six out of eight medial menisci and cartilage of femoral condyles. The transplanted cells had produced matrix that could be stained with toluidine blue, indicating matrix production by the tissue [83]. The advantage of such an approach is that it is minimally invasive, compared to conventional surgeries for these tissues [83]. An interesting effect of MSCs is that the cytokines and growth factors they produce may have both paracrine and autocrine activities [84]. Particularly the anabolic effects of these stem cells on host meniscus cells may contribute to the repair process [84].

So far, most studies have been performed with chondrocytes. The limits of scaffolds include the stress shielding of the cells by the scaffold, the effect of the scaffold on neo-tissue organization, and potential uncontrolled degradation and product toxicity. An interesting idea for meniscus repair is the concept of self-assembly of the structure in *in vitro* culture systems [85]. In a self-assembling process tissue engineered constructs are produced by seeding cells in high density in non-adhering agarose molds *in vitro* without using a scaffold [85]. With this self-assembly method, chondrocytes yielded constructs with a GAG and collagen content comparable to bovine cartilage. By 12 weeks the self-assembling process resulted in tissue engineered constructs that were hyaline-like in appearance with histological, biochemical and biomechanical properties approaching those of native articular cartilage [85]. More GAGS were present, but the collagen production was less optimal [85].

16.1.9. Combining Cells with Scaffolds

The scaffolds used so far for culture studies of meniscus cells are identical to those used for culture studies in which articular chondrocytes were used.

Popular scaffolds are fibrin [72], polyglycolic acid [86], alginate [77] and collagen Type I and II scaffolds with or without GAGs attached [87–88]. A large disadvantage of the collagen and alginate scaffolds may be the poor initial mechanical properties. Moreover, meniscus cells in these scaffolds may develop a phenotype expressing alpha-smooth muscle actin (SMA) [87–89]. This phenotype has contractile capacities, which may be very useful in wound contraction and healing but, in these relatively mechanically weak scaffolds, will lead to a considerable uncontrolled shrinkage of up to 50 percent of the construct in culture [88]. SMA is also expressed during repair of meniscus tissue [90]. SMA expression is found in the remodelling tissue at the interface of the native meniscus and a plug of meniscus tissue. However, the functional significance of SMA expression in the meniscus is not yet fully understood [90].

Also, the CMI was combined with autologous cells in a study [48] where sheep fibrochondrocytes were seeded onto the collagen scaffolds and implanted in the meniscectomized knee. Enhanced vascularization, accelerated scaffold remodelling, a higher content of newly formed extracellular matrix and lower cell numbers were noted in the pre-seeded menisci, in comparison with non-seeded controls [48]. Another important observation was that the size of the implant reduced over time. Irrespective of the scaffold type used the challenge is to find the optimal cell seeding procedure. Although the CMI is highly porous this does not mean that seeded cells can penetrate deep into the structure. In practice the pores are not orientated into one particular direction, but are distributed quite inhomogeneously, which makes penetration of seeded cells deep into the matrix quite challenging.

More mechanically firm scaffolds were used as well. Meniscal fibrochondrocytes from New Zealand white rabbits were seeded on(to) poly(glycolic acid) (PGA) scaffolds in an *in vitro* study. The results of the same cells in monolayer [80–81] were repeated [91]. TGF-beta1 stimulated both (3)H-proline and (35)S-sulfate uptake and again TGF-beta1 was more effective than IGF-I (5 ng/ml). bFGF stimulated the (3)H-proline uptake by the third week of growth factor addition. PDGF did not show notable increases in uptake [91]. Allogeneic chondrocytes of articular, auricular and costal origin of immature swine were used in combination with a vicril mesh to repair a lesion [92]. Gross mechanical testing was performed with a forceps. All tears in the lesion group(s) were repaired, but, unfortunately, no quantitative data on the mechanical strength were provided [92].

16.1.10. Mechanical Effects on Meniscus Cells

Besides scaffold materials and added growth factors, mechanical loading might have a profound effect on the differentiation and matrix production of cultured cells. In fibrochondrocytes from rat meniscus, IL-1ß induced a rapid increase in iNOS. Dynamic tensile forces could inhibit this induction of this pro-inflammatory cytokine [93]. Both (the) magnitude and frequency are important determinants of the anti-inflammatory action. Deschner, et al. [94] studied whether the receptor activator of NF-kappaB (RANK), its ligand (RANKL) or osteoprotegerin (OPG) are up- or downregulated in stretched cells. It appeared that fibrochondrocytes expressed low levels of RANKL and RANK, but high levels of OPG. When fibrochondrocytes were simultaneously subjected to cyclic tensile strain (CTS) and IL-1ß, expression of RANKL and RANK was significantly downregulated, compared to that of IL-1ß-stimulated unstretched cells. The inhibitory effect of CTS on the IL-1ß-induced upregulation of RANKL and RANK was sustained and depended on magnitude and frequency [94].

Hydrostatic pressure seems to have a profound effect during the self-assembling process of chondrocytes [95–96]. Cells cultured in scaffolds are also sensitive to mechanical stimulation [97]. Culturing meniscus cells in a rotating wall incubator, which induces a microgravity environment, in agarose and a nonwoven polymer mesh ([poly(glycolic acid) resulted in more than twice the amount of sulphated glycosaminoglycans and three times the amount of collagen, compared to static agarose constructs at week 7 [97].

16.6. Future Trends and Needs

Despite all the effort put into procedures for meniscus repair, the effects of these procedures on the prevention of articular cartilage degeneration have been disappointing so far in most studies. Although a meniscus phenotype of cells in constructs can be established [60–61], articular degeneration still occurs both in reconstructed menisci as well as in prosthetic replacement [61, 98–99]. From a series of ongoing experiments in our laboratory using a polyurethane-based reconstruction method and meniscus prosthesis we get the strong impression that the articular cartilage degradation takes place particularly during the first period after implantation [60–61].

More factors may be involved in the generation of osteoarthritic changes. They may be related to the initial bare surface of the implant, the trauma reaction in a small joint and the initial mechanical properties of the implant. With respect to the surface of the implant the bare polymer implant material initially has poor surface characteristics with respect to a smooth frictionless movement of the implant in a joint environment. Studies in which the movement of such an implant in a human knee was analyzed confirmed that it does not move frictionless in cadaver knees [100]. The resulting higher sheer stresses at the surface of the knee, in combination with the traumatized joint in which the implant is placed, may lead to initial cartilage damage. One way to avoid this initial damage by high friction of the implant could be to coat the implant materials with substances to promote a smooth, frictionless movement in the joint. Hyaluronic acid and the other constituents of GAGs – such as the highly hydrated chondroitin sulphate, keratan-sulphate and/or dermatan-sulphate – could be used for this purpose. A non-sulphated glycosaminoglycan, hyaluronic acid (HA) is present in high quantities in the synovial fluid and has a function in the lubrication of the joint. Currently, this substance is used as an injectable material to relieve complaints associated with severe osteoarthritis in patients. It also seems to have a protective effect on cartilage degeneration when used in animal models to prevent damage to the cartilage by surgical interventions [101–102]. HA can also be used as a building block for drug delivery, tissue engineering, wound repair and viscosupplementation [103]. Cell culture studies have already demonstrated HA to promote the proliferation of meniscus cells without altering the morphology of the cells or the GAG synthesis of the cells [75]. Polymers based on starch could also be tested as a coating material; they have already been considered as useful candidates for tissue engineering applications [104–105]. Finally, the coatings of biomaterials with proteins rich in RGD peptides are currently used for tissue engineering of bone [106–107], but could also be very useful for meniscus tissue engineering. A second approach to decrease the initial friction is to pre-seed the scaffolds with cells that can produce matrix before they are implanted [108].

A second issue is the operation technique. Any operation in a joint environment will induce a cascade of catabolic factors in the joint. This might lead to destruction of articular cartilage or weakening of the matrix due to depletion [109]. To avoid this trauma reaction it is essential to develop minimally invasive surgical techniques for animal studies as well, so that the induced trauma is as small as possible.

The third factor is the initial mechanical properties of the scaffolds. When mechanical properties of the scaffolds are insufficient, osteoarthritic changes can occur before the infiltrated tissue has differentiated into the typical fibrocartilage that increases the mechanical properties of the implanted scaffold. Because of the relatively poor initial mechanical properties of many scaffolds, pre-seeding the scaffold for a few days and subsequently implanting it subcutaneously in the animal to be treated for a period of time (depending on the animal model) to allow tissue ingrowth could be an option. This may allow the construct to improve its mechanical properties so that it can be used to replace the meniscus [108]. The alternative is to make implants that perfectly match both the geometry of the implant site and have the same initial mechanical properties as the native meniscus.

Finally, although not proven, the meniscus cells are probably quite firmly encapsulated in their matrix. In cartilage, migration of chondrocytes in the matrix is limited. Also, after a cartilage trauma the cells on the edge of the trauma have become necrotic or apoptotic, which might make the integration of tissue engineered constructs for meniscus repair, that were completely differentiated *in vitro*, difficult [110]. Therefore, procedures are tested to partially remove the superficial matrix to allow the still healthy chondrocytes to move to the interface with the implanted scaffold. A treatment with hyaluronidase or collagenase could be a tool to reach this goal in articular cartilage [111], although clinical implementation of such a technique might be difficult.

16.7. Conclusion

Tissue engineering of an entire new meniscus remains challenging. Scaffolds need to be able to resist the high forces in a joint environment. Scaffolds available so far are based on collagens and polymers, and scaffolds based on collagen are mechanically too weak to replace the entire meniscus; however, they may be useful for guided tissue regeneration of meniscus tissue. Scaffolds based on polymers are more suitable from a mechanical point of view, but the search is still for scaffolds that can protect the articular cartilage from further degradation and that have optimal pore geometry to guide tissue ingrowth and differentiation. Growth factors may be helpful, but their use in a joint environment may have unwanted effects on other tissues.

References

1. Ghosh P, Taylor TK. The knee joint meniscus. A fibrocartilage of some distinction. Clin Orthop 1987 Nov;224:52–63.
2. McDevitt CA, Webber RJ. The ultrastructure and biochemistry of meniscal cartilage. Clin Orthop 1990 Mar;252:8–18.
3. Sweigart MA, Athanasiou KA. Toward tissue engineering of the knee meniscus. Tissue Eng 2001 Apr;7(2):111–29.
4. Walker PS, Erkman MJ. The role of the menisci in force transmission across the knee. Clin Orthop 1975;109:184–92.
5. Fithian DC, Kelly MA, Mow VC. Material properties and structure-function relationships in the menisci. Clin Orthop 1990 Mar;252:19–31.
6. Arnoczky SP. Breakout session 4: Meniscus. Clin Orthop 1999 Oct;367:S293–S295.
7. DeHaven KE. The role of the meniscus. In: Ewing JW, editor. Articular cartilage and knee joint function: Basic science and arthroscopy.New York: Raven Press, Ltd.; 1990. p. 103–15.
8. Setton LA, Guilak F, Hsu EW, Vail TP. Biomechanical factors in tissue engineered meniscal repair. Clin Orthop 1999 Oct;367:S254–S272.
9. Kambic HE, McDevitt CA. Spatial organization of types I and II collagen in the canine meniscus. J Orthop Res 2005 Jan;23(1):142–9.
10. Arnoczky SP, Warren RF. Microvasculature of the human meniscus. Am J Sports Med 1982 Mar;10(2):90–5.
11. Brindle T, Nyland J, Johnson DL. The Meniscus: Review of Basic Principles With Application to Surgery and Rehabilitation. J Athl Train 2001 Apr;36(2):160–9.
12. Petersen W, Tillmann B. Collagenous fibril texture of the human knee joint menisci. Anat Embryol (Berl) 1998 Apr;197(4):317–24.
13. Ververidis AN, Verettas DA, Kazakos KJ, Tilkeridis CE, Chatzipapas CN. Meniscal bucket handle tears: a retrospective study of arthroscopy and the relation to MRI. Knee Surg Sports Traumatol Arthrosc 2006 Apr;14(4):343–9.
14. Christoforakis J, Pradhan R, Sanchez-Ballester J, Hunt N, Strachan RK. Is there an association between articular cartilage changes and degenerative meniscus tears? Arthroscopy 2005 Nov;21(11):1366–9.
15. Burks RT, Metcalf MH, Metcalf RW. Fifteen-year follow-up of arthroscopic partial meniscectomy. Arthroscopy 1997 Dec;13(6):673–9.
16. Allen PR, Denham RA, Swan AV. Late degenerative changes after meniscectomy. Factors affecting the knee after operation. J Bone Joint Surg Br 1984 Nov;66(5):666–71.
17. Appel H. Late results after meniscectomy in the knee joint. A clinical and roentgenologic follow-up investigation. Acta Orthop Scand Suppl 1970;133:1–111.
18. Hede A, Svalastoga E, Reimann I. Articular cartilage changes following meniscal lesions. Repair and meniscectomy studied in the rabbit knee. Acta Orthop Scand 1991 Aug;62(4):319–22.
19. Cox JS, Nye CE, Schaefer WW, Woodstein IJ. The degenerative effects of partial and total resection of the medial meniscus in dogs' knees. Clin Orthop 1975;109:178–83.
20. Maletius W, Messner K. The effect of partial meniscectomy on the long-term prognosis of knees with localized, severe chondral damage. A twelve- to fifteen-year followup. Am J Sports Med 1996 May;24(3):258–62.
21. Arnoczky SP, Warren RF, Spivak JM. Meniscal repair using an exogenous fibrin clot. An experimental study in dogs. J Bone Joint Surg Am 1988 Sep;70(8):1209–17.
22. Englund M, Lohmander LS. Risk factors for symptomatic knee osteoarthritis fifteen to twenty-two years after meniscectomy. Arthritis Rheum 2004 Sep;50(9):2811–9.
23. Farng E, Sherman O. Meniscal repair devices: a clinical and biomechanical literature review. Arthroscopy 2004 Mar;20(3):273–86.
24. Miller MD, Kline AJ, Jepsen KG. "All-inside" meniscal repair devices: an experimental study in the goat model. Am J Sports Med 2004 Jun;32(4):858–62.

25. Kurzweil PR, Friedman MJ. Meniscus: Resection, repair, and replacement. Arthroscopy 2002 Feb;18(2 Suppl 1):33–9.
26. Lee GP, Diduch DR. Deteriorating outcomes after meniscal repair using the Meniscus Arrow in knees undergoing concurrent anterior cruciate ligament reconstruction: increased failure rate with long-term follow-up. Am J Sports Med 2005 Aug;33(8):1138–41.
27. Sethi PM, Cooper A, Jokl P. Technical tips in orthopaedics: meniscal repair with use of an in situ fibrin clot. Arthroscopy 2003 May;19(5):E44.
28. Bhargava MM, Hidaka C, Hannafin JA, Doty S, Warren RF. Effects of hepatocyte growth factor and platelet-derived growth factor on the repair of meniscal defects in vitro. In Vitro Cell Dev Biol Anim 2005 Sep;41(8–9):305–10.
29. Verdonk PC, Forsyth RG, Wang J, Almqvist KF, Verdonk R, Veys EM, et al. Characterisation of human knee meniscus cell phenotype. Osteoarthritis Cartilage 2005 Jul;13(7):548–60.
30. Bhargava MM, Attia ET, Murrell GA, Dolan MM, Warren RF, Hannafin JA. The effect of cytokines on the proliferation and migration of bovine meniscal cells. Am J Sports Med 1999 Sep;27(5):636–43.
31. Petersen W, Pufe T, Starke C, Fuchs T, Kopf S, Raschke M, et al. Locally applied angiogenic factors–a new therapeutic tool for meniscal repair. Ann Anat 2005 Nov;187(5–6):509–19.
32. Kurz B, Lemke AK, Fay J, Pufe T, Grodzinsky AJ, Schunke M. Pathomechanisms of cartilage destruction by mechanical injury. Ann Anat 2005 Nov;187(5–6):473–85.
33. Stoop R, van der Kraan PM, Buma P, Hollander AP, Poole AR, van den Berg WB. Denaturation of type II collagen in articular cartilage in experimental murine arthritis. Evidence for collagen degradation in both reversible and irreversible cartilage damage. J Pathol 1999 Jul;188(3):329–37.
34. Stoop R, Buma P, van der Kraan PM, Hollander AP, Clark-Billinghurst R, Robin-Poole A, et al. Differences in type II collagen degradation between peripheral and central cartilage of rat stifle joints after cranial cruciate ligament transection. Arthritis Rheum 2000 Sep;43(9):2121–31.
35. Goto H, Shuler FD, Lamsam C, Moller HD, Niyibizi C, Fu FH, et al. Transfer of lacZ marker gene to the meniscus. J Bone Joint Surg Am 1999 Jul;81(7):918–25.
36. Martinek V, Usas A, Pelinkovic D, Robbins P, Fu FH, Huard J. Genetic engineering of meniscal allografts. Tissue Eng 2002 Feb;8(1):107–17.
37. Goto H, Shuler FD, Niyibizi C, Fu FH, Robbins PD, Evans CH. Gene therapy for meniscal injury: enhanced synthesis of proteoglycan and collagen by meniscal cells transduced with a TGFbeta(1)gene. Osteoarthritis Cartilage 2000 Jul;8(4):266–71.
38. Hidaka C, Ibarra C, Hannafin JA, Torzilli PA, Quitoriano M, Jen SS, et al. Formation of vascularized meniscal tissue by combining gene therapy with tissue engineering. Tissue Eng 2002 Feb;8(1):93–105.
39. Gao JZ. [Experimental study on healing of old tear in the avascular portion of menisci in dogs]. Zhonghua Wai Ke Za Zhi 1990 Dec;28(12):726–9, 782.
40. Arnoczky SP. Building a meniscus. Biologic considerations. Clin Orthop Relat Res 1999 Oct;(367 Suppl):S244–S253.
41. Buma P, Ramrattan NN, van Tienen TG, Veth RP. Tissue engineering of the meniscus. Biomaterials 2004 Apr;25(9):1523–32.
42. Rodkey WG, Steadman JR, Li ST. A clinical study of collagen meniscus implants to restore the injured meniscus. Clin Orthop 1999 Oct;367:S281–S292.
43. Stone KR, Rodkey WG, Webber RJ, McKinney L, Steadman JR. Future directions. Collagen-based prostheses for meniscal regeneration. Clin Orthop 1990 Mar;252:129–35.
44. Stone KR, Rodkey WG, Webber R, McKinney L, Steadman JR. Meniscal regeneration with copolymeric collagen scaffolds. In vitro and in vivo studies evaluated clinically, histologically, and biochemically. Am J Sports Med 1992 Mar;20(2):104–11.

45. van Susante JLC, Pieper J, Buma P, van Kuppevelt TH, van BH, van der Kraan PM, et al. Linkage of chondroitin-sulfate to type I collagen scaffolds stimulates the bioactivity of seeded chondrocytes in vitro. Biomaterials 2001 Sep;22(17):2359–69.
46. Buma P, Pieper JS, vanTienen T., van Susante JL, van der Kraan PM, Veerkamp JH, et al. Cross-linked type I and type II collagenous matrices for the repair of full-thickness articular cartilage defects–a study in rabbits. Biomaterials 2003 Aug;24(19):3255–63.
47. Hunziker EB, Rosenberg LC. Repair of partial-thickness defects in articular cartilage: cell recruitment from the synovial membrane. J Bone Joint Surg Am 1996 May;78(5):721–33.
48. Martinek V, Ueblacker P, Braun K, Nitschke S, Mannhardt R, Specht K, et al. Second generation of meniscus transplantation: in-vivo study with tissue engineered meniscus replacement. Arch Orthop Trauma Surg 2006 May;126(4):228–34.
49. Reguzzoni M, Manelli A, Ronga M, Raspanti M, Grassi FA. Histology and ultrastructure of a tissue-engineered collagen meniscus before and after implantation. J Biomed Mater Res B Appl Biomater 2005 Aug;74(2):808–16.
50. Steadman JR, Rodkey WG. Tissue-engineered collagen meniscus implants: 5- to 6-year feasibility study results. Arthroscopy 2005 May;21(5):515–25.
51. Zaffagnini S, Giordano G, Vascellari A, Bruni D, Neri MP, Iacono F, et al. Arthroscopic collagen meniscus implant results at 6 to 8 years follow up. Knee Surg Sports Traumatol Arthrosc 2006 Jul 15.
52. Alhalki MM, Howell SM, Hull ML. How three methods for fixing a medial meniscal autograft affect tibial contact mechanics. Am J Sports Med 1999 May;27(3):320–8.
53. Aagaard H, Jorgensen U, Bojsen MF. Reduced degenerative articular cartilage changes after meniscal allograft transplantation in sheep. Knee Surg Sports Traumatol Arthrosc 1999;7(3):184–91.
54. Rijk PC, de Rooy TP, Coerkamp EG, Bernoski FP, Van Noorden CJ. Radiographic evaluation of the knee joint after meniscal allograft transplantation. An experimental study in rabbits. Knee Surg Sports Traumatol Arthrosc 2002 Jul;10(4):241–6.
55. Rijk PC, Van Eck-Smit BL, Van Noorden CJ. Scintigraphic assessment of rabbit knee joints after meniscal allograft transplantation. Arthroscopy 2003 May;19(5):506–10.
56. Alhalki MM, Hull ML, Howell SM. Contact mechanics of the medial tibial plateau after implantation of a medial meniscal allograft. A human cadaveric study. Am J Sports Med 2000 May;28(3):370–6.
57. Heijkants RG, Calck RV, van Tienen TG, de Groot JH, Buma P, Pennings AJ, et al. Uncatalyzed synthesis, thermal and mechanical properties of polyurethanes based on poly(epsilon-caprolactone) and 1,4-butane diisocyanate with uniform hard segment. Biomaterials 2005 Jul;26(20):4219–28.
58. Klompmaker J, Jansen HWB, Veth RPH, Nielsen HKL, de Groot JH, Pennings AJ. Porous implants for knee joint meniscus reconstruction: a preliminary study on the role of pore sizes in ingrowth and differentiation of fibrocartilage. Clinical Materials 1993;14:1–11.
59. Moroni L, Poort G, Van KF, de W, Jr., van Blitterswijk CA. Dynamic mechanical properties of 3D fiber-deposited PEOT/PBT scaffolds: an experimental and numerical analysis. J Biomed Mater Res A 2006 Sep 1;78(3):605–14.
60. Tienen TG, Heijkants RG, de Groot JH, Schouten AJ, Pennings AJ, Veth RP, et al. Meniscal replacement in dogs. Tissue regeneration in two different materials with similar properties. J Biomed Mater Res B Appl Biomater 2006 Feb;76(2):389–96.
61. Tienen TG, Heijkants RG, de Groot JH, Pennings AJ, Schouten AJ, Veth RP, et al. Replacement of the knee meniscus by a porous polymer implant: a study in dogs. Am J Sports Med 2006 Jan;34(1):64–71.

62. Klompmaker J, Veth RP, Jansen HW, Nielsen HK, de Groot JH, Pennings AJ, et al. Meniscal repair by fibrocartilage in the dog: characterization of the repair tissue and the role of vascularity. Biomaterials 1996 Sep;17(17):1685–91.
63. Tienen TG, Heijkants RG, Buma P, de Groot JH, Pennings AJ, Veth RP. A porous polymer scaffold for meniscal lesion repair–a study in dogs. Biomaterials 2003 Jun;24(14):2541–8.
64. Cima LG, Vacanti JP, Vacanti C, Ingber D, Mooney D, Langer R. Tissue engineering by cell transplantation using degradable polymer substrates. J Biomech Eng 1991 May;113(2):143–51.
65. Cao Y, Vacanti JP, Paige KT, Upton J, Vacanti CA. Transplantation of chondrocytes utilizing a polymer-cell construct to produce tissue-engineered cartilage in the shape of a human ear. Plast Reconstr Surg 1997 Aug;100(2):297–302.
66. Vacanti JP, Morse MA, Saltzman WM, Domb AJ, Perez-Atayde A, Langer R. Selective cell transplantation using bioabsorbable artificial polymers as matrices. J Pediatr Surg 1988 Jan;23(1 Pt 2):3–9.
67. Chiari C, Koller U, Dorotka R, Eder C, Plasenzotti R, Lang S, et al. A tissue engineering approach to meniscus regeneration in a sheep model. Osteoarthritis Cartilage 2006 Oct;14(10):1056–65.
68. Kang SW, Son SM, Lee JS, Lee ES, Lee KY, Park SG, et al. Regeneration of whole meniscus using meniscal cells and polymer scaffolds in a rabbit total meniscectomy model. J Biomed Mater Res A 2006 Jun 15;77(4):659–71.
69. Hellio Le Graverand MP, Reno C, Hart DA. Gene expression in menisci from the knees of skeletally immature and mature female rabbits. J Orthop Res 1999 Sep;17(5):738–44.
70. Webber RJ, Zitaglio T, Hough AJ, Jr. In vitro cell proliferation and proteoglycan synthesis of rabbit meniscal fibrochondrocytes as a function of age and sex. Arthritis Rheum 1986 Aug;29(8):1010–6.
71. Webber RJ, Zitaglio T, Hough AJ, Jr. Serum-free culture of rabbit meniscal fibrochondrocytes: proliferative response. J Orthop Res 1988;6(1):13–23.
72. Webber RJ, York JL, Vanderschilden JL, Hough-AJ J. An organ culture model for assaying wound repair of the fibrocartilaginous knee joint meniscus. Am J Sports Med 1989 May;17(3):393–400.
73. Webber RJ. In vitro culture of meniscal tissue. Clin Orthop 1990 Mar;252:114–20.
74. Hoberg M, Uzunmehmetoglu G, Sabic L, Reese S, Aicher WK, Rudert M. [Characterisation of human meniscus cells]. Z Orthop Ihre Grenzgeb 2006 Mar;144(2):172–8.
75. Nakata K, Shino K, Hamada M, Mae T, Miyama T, Shinjo H, et al. Human meniscus cell: characterization of the primary culture and use for tissue engineering. Clin Orthop Relat Res 2001 Oct;(391 Suppl):S208–S218.
76. Tanaka T, Fujii K, Kumagae Y. Comparison of biochemical characteristics of cultured fibrochondrocytes isolated from the inner and outer regions of human meniscus. Knee Surg Sports Traumatol Arthrosc 1999;7(2):75–80.
77. Collier S, Ghosh P. Effects of transforming growth factor beta on proteoglycan synthesis by cell and explant cultures derived from the knee joint meniscus. Osteoarthritis Cartilage 1995 Jun;3(2):127–38.
78. Tumia NS, Johnstone AJ. Promoting the proliferative and synthetic activity of knee meniscal fibrochondrocytes using basic fibroblast growth factor in vitro. Am J Sports Med 2004 Jun;32(4):915–20.
79. Tumia NS, Johnstone AJ. Regional regenerative potential of meniscal cartilage exposed to recombinant insulin-like growth factor-I in vitro. J Bone Joint Surg Br 2004 Sep;86(7):1077–81.
80. Pangborn CA, Athanasiou KA. Effects of growth factors on meniscal fibrochondrocytes. Tissue Eng 2005 Jul;11(7–8):1141–8.

81. Pangborn CA, Athanasiou KA. Effects of growth factors on meniscal fibrochondrocytes. Tissue Eng 2005 Jul;11(7–8):1141–8.
82. Adesida AB, Grady LM, Khan WS, Hardingham TE. The matrix-forming phenotype of cultured human meniscus cells is enhanced after culture with fibroblast growth factor 2 and is further stimulated by hypoxia. Arthritis Res Ther 2006;8(3):R61.
83. Agung M, Ochi M, Yanada S, Adachi N, Izuta Y, Yamasaki T, et al. Mobilization of bone marrow-derived mesenchymal stem cells into the injured tissues after intraarticular injection and their contribution to tissue regeneration. Knee Surg Sports Traumatol Arthrosc 2006 Dec;14(12):1307–14.
84. Caplan AI, Dennis JE. Mesenchymal stem cells as trophic mediators. J Cell Biochem 2006 Apr 17.
85. Hu JC, Athanasiou KA. A self-assembling process in articular cartilage tissue engineering. Tissue Eng 2006 Apr;12(4):969–79.
86. Ibarra C, Jannetta C, Vacanti CA, Cao Y, Kim TH, Upton J, et al. Tissue engineered meniscus: a potential new alternative to allogeneic meniscus transplantation. Transplant Proc 1997 Feb;29(1–2):986–8.
87. Mueller SM, Shortkroff S, Schneider TO, Breinan HA, Yannas IV, Spector M. Meniscus cells seeded in type I and type II collagen-GAG matrices in vitro. Biomaterials 1999 Apr;20(8):701–9.
88. Mueller SM, Schneider TO, Shortkroff S, Breinan HA, Spector M. alpha-smooth muscle actin and contractile behavior of bovine meniscus cells seeded in type I and type II collagen-GAG matrices. J Biomed Mater Res 1999 Jun 5;45(3):157–66.
89. Zaleskas JM, Kinner B, Freyman TM, Yannas IV, Gibson LJ, Spector M. Growth factor regulation of smooth muscle actin expression and contraction of human articular chondrocytes and meniscal cells in a collagen-GAG matrix. Exp Cell Res 2001 Oct 15;270(1):21–31.
90. Kambic HE, Futani H, McDevitt CA. Cell, matrix changes and alpha-smooth muscle actin expression in repair of the canine meniscus. Wound Repair Regen 2000 Nov;8(6):554–61.
91. Pangborn CA, Athanasiou KA. Growth factors and fibrochondrocytes in scaffolds. J Orthop Res 2005 Sep;23(5):1184–90.
92. Weinand C, Peretti GM, Adams SB, Jr., Randolph MA, Savvidis E, Gill TJ. Healing potential of transplanted allogeneic chondrocytes of three different sources in lesions of the avascular zone of the meniscus: a pilot study. Arch Orthop Trauma Surg 2006 Nov;126(9):599–605.
93. Ferretti M, Madhavan S, Deschner J, Rath-Deschner B, Wypasek E, Agarwal S. Dynamic biophysical strain modulates proinflammatory gene induction in meniscal fibrochondrocytes. Am J Physiol Cell Physiol 2006 Jun;290(6):C1610–C1615.
94. Deschner J, Wypasek E, Ferretti M, Rath B, Anghelina M, Agarwal S. Regulation of RANKL by biomechanical loading in fibrochondrocytes of meniscus. J Biomech 2006;39(10):1796–803.
95. Hu JC, Athanasiou KA. The effects of intermittent hydrostatic pressure on self-assembled articular cartilage constructs. Tissue Eng 2006 May;12(5):1337–44.
96. Hu JC, Athanasiou KA. The Effects of Intermittent Hydrostatic Pressure on Self-Assembled Articular Cartilage Constructs. Tissue Eng 2006 May 1.
97. AufderHeide AC, Athanasiou KA. Comparison of scaffolds and culture conditions for tissue engineering of the knee meniscus. Tissue Eng 2005 Jul;11(7/8):1095–104.
98. van Tienen TG, Heijkants RG, de Groot JH, Pennings AJ, Poole AR, Veth RP, et al. Presence and mechanism of knee articular cartilage degeneration after meniscal reconstruction in dogs. Osteoarthritis Cartilage 2003 Jan;11(1):78–84.
99. Messner K, Kohn D, Verdonk R. Future research in meniscal replacement. Scand J Med Sci Sports 1999 Jun;9(3):181–3.

100. ampen A, et al. Prosthetic replacement of the medial meniscus in cadaveric knees: does the prosthesis mimic the functional behavior of the native meniscus? Am J Sports Med 2004 Jul;32(5):1182–8.
101. Kobayashi K, Amiel M, Harwood FL, Healey RM, Sonoda M, Moriya H, et al. The long-term effects of hyaluronan during development of osteoarthritis following partial meniscectomy in a rabbit model. Osteoarthritis Cartilage 2000 Sep;8(5): 359–65.
102. Han F, Ishiguro N, Ito T, Sakai T, Iwata H. Effects of sodium hyaluronate on experimental osteoarthritis in rabbit knee joints. Nagoya J Med Sci 1999 Nov;62(3–4):115–26.
103. Luo Y, Prestwich GD. Hyaluronic acid-N-hydroxysuccinimide: a useful intermediate for bioconjugation. Bioconjug Chem 2001 Nov;12(6):1085–8.
104. Marques AP, Reis RL, Hunt JA. The biocompatibility of novel starch-based polymers and composites: in vitro studies. Biomaterials 2002 Mar;23(6):1471–8.
105. Gomes ME, Reis RL, Cunha AM, Blitterswijk CA, de Bruijn JD. Cytocompatibility and response of osteoblastic-like cells to starch-based polymers: effect of several additives and processing conditions. Biomaterials 2001 Jul;22(13):1911–7.
106. Alsberg E, Anderson KW, Albeiruti A, Franceschi RT, Mooney DJ. Cell-interactive alginate hydrogels for bone tissue engineering. J Dent Res 2001 Nov;80(11):2025–9.
107. Itoh D, Yoneda S, Kuroda S, Kondo H, Umezawa A, Ohya K, et al. Enhancement of osteogenesis on hydroxyapatite surface coated with synthetic peptide (EEEEEEEPRGDT) in vitro. J Biomed Mater Res 2002 Nov;62(2):292–8.
108. Ibarra C, Koski JA, Warren RF. Tissue engineering meniscus: cells and matrix. Orthop Clin North Am 2000 Jul;31(3):411–8.
109. Stoop R, Buma P, van der Kraan PM, Hollander AP, Billinghurst RC, Meijers TH, et al. Type II collagen degradation in articular cartilage fibrillation after anterior cruciate ligament transection in rats. Osteoarthritis Cartilage 2001 May;9(4):308–15.
110. van de Breevaart BJ, In der Maur CD, Bos PK, Feenstra L, Verhaar JA, Weinans H, et al. Improved cartilage integration and interfacial strength after enzymatic treatment in a cartilage transplantation model. Arthritis Res Ther 2004;6(5): R469–R476.
111. Bos PK, DeGroot J, Budde M, Verhaar JA, van Osch GJ. Specific enzymatic treatment of bovine and human articular cartilage: implications for integrative cartilage repair. Arthritis Rheum 2002 Apr;46(4):976–85.
112. Rodkey JG, Steadman JR, Li S-T. Collagen scaffolds: A new method to preserve and restore the severely injured meniscus. Sports Medicine and Arthroscopy Review 2006;7:63–73.

17

Osteochondral Grafts

Simon Görtz, Michael B. Boyd, and William D. Bugbee

Abstract: Hyaline articular cartilage is a unique, highly specialized tissue with a distinct architecture that lacks intrinsic means to heal effectively when injured in the adult. Symptomatic osteoarticular defects continue to be a formidable challenge for the clinical and the scientific communities alike. Of the various surgical treatment options that have been proposed to this end, only osteochondral grafting techniques reliably restore appropriate hyaline tissue in acquired articular cartilage lesions, especially when these involve the subchondral bone. Both autologous and allogeneic graft sources are available to the surgeon, who must consider the unique qualities and characteristics of either approach in the treatment algorithm. Autografts and allografts alike adhere to a common methodology, relying on osseous healing of mature osteochondral constructs to transplant the adherent viable articular cartilage. The required surgical technique is straightforward and reproducible but requires precision to restore articular surface congruity, achieve reliable bony ingrowth and, ultimately, clinical success. Scientific investigation to further validate empirical clinical practice and to improve implant quality and safety is ongoing and holds great promise for the future of osteochondral grafting in general, as well as bioengineered scaffolds and allogeneic tissue as a cell source in particular.

Keywords: Osteochondral autograft, OAT, OATS, mosaicplasty, osteochondral allografts, allografting, allograft bone, cartilage transplant, allogeneic, autologous chondrocyte.

17.1. Introduction

Hyaline articular cartilage is an avascular and insensate tissue that allows low friction transmission of physiologic loads in diarthrodial joints. Ideally, the functional structure of articular cartilage is maintained in homeostasis over

Department of Orthopaedic Surgery, University of California at San Diego, La Jolla, CA

From: *Orthopedic Biology and Medicine: Musculoskeletal Tissue Regeneration, Biological Materials and Methods.*
Edited by W. S. Pietrzak © Humana Press, Totowa, NJ

the lifetime of an individual. However, mature hyaline cartilage is relatively hypocellular and incapable of mounting an effective repair response when injured in the skeletally mature adult [1–2].

Partial-thickness chondral lesions often remain occult due to the insensate nature of articular cartilage and even small, focal full-thickness lesions can remain asymptomatic. While the natural progression of degenerative changes and associated disability is multifactorial, increasing defect size contributes to the development of symptoms and, ultimately, osteoarthritis [3]. Progressive enlargement of articular defects may involve loss of containment in the articular cartilage, leading to increases in load bearing and stress concentration at the defect rim [4].

The treatment threshold for surgical intervention is not unequivocal, but patients with symptomatic lesions are generally considered as candidates for cartilage procedures. Of the many different techniques that have been proposed over time, the ones that are in common use today include marrow-stimulating techniques such as micro-fracture, autologous chondrocyte implantation in its different variations, and osteochondral grafting using autologous or allogeneic tissue [5].

Marrow-stimulating techniques are commonly considered as an initial reparative treatment option for relatively small, contained articular cartilage lesions because they are simple to perform, economical and often appropriate and effective. However, these efforts generally result in fibrocartilagenous repair with biomechanical properties and wear characteristics that are inferior to that of hyaline cartilage [6].

Autologous chondrocyte implantation (ACI) has gained popularity over the last decade as a restorative procedure. Criticisms of ACI include the high cost of culturing and expanding chondrocytes, the invasive, two-step nature of the procedure, the steep learning curve associated with the technique, and the inconsistent hyaline quality of the resultant tissue as it matures [7]. Consequent generations of ACI have tried to address some of the issues of donor site morbidity and graft hypertrophy by introducing collagen patches for coverage and by seeding the cultured chondrocytes in artificial scaffolds [8].

The use of osteochondral grafts of autologous or allogeneic origin is well supported on a basic science level and has a long successful clinical history as a means of biologic resurfacing [9–10]. While either application has unique advantages and challenges, both subscribe to a common paradigm of transplanting mature hyaline cartilage containing viable chondrocytes attached to subchondral bone to restore the architecture and characteristics of native tissue in acquired osteoarticular defects. By transplanting structurally complete osteochondral units with an intact tidemark, the fixation issue is mostly relegated to that of osseous ingrowth [11].

One obvious disadvantage of autologous graft sources is that the maximum graft surface area is self-limited by donor volume, to small and medium-sized lesions (Fig. 17.1a). This is especially true in the previously injured and/or operated knee, where suitability regarding tissue quality and overall joint topography has to be critically assessed. Also, donor site morbidity can significantly add to the disease burden during intra-articular transfer, or even introduce it if the transfer is inter-articular (e.g., knee to ankle) [10]. However, autologous grafting does hold advantages over other graft sources, such as fresh osteochondral allografting. It is relatively cheap, immediately available, nonantigenic, and osteogenetic, leading to reliable osteointegration [12].

One advantage of osteochondral allografting is that even very large and multiple lesions can be addressed with a solid orthotopic graft that reproduces the anatomy of the native joint both macroscopically and microscopically, without the risk of inducing donor site morbidity (Fig. 17.1b). No other current cartilage repair procedure can match the versatility of osteochondral allografts when addressing complex lesions in topographically challenging environments, especially if they present with an osseous deficiency. Obvious drawbacks to the methodology are the scarcity of organ donor tissue, financial and logistical issues of procurement, and residual risk of infection, albeit small [13].

The surgical techniques for either graft source are straightforward but require precision to restore articular surface congruity while maximizing the potential for bony healing [14]. The mosaicplasty technique incorporates multiple, small

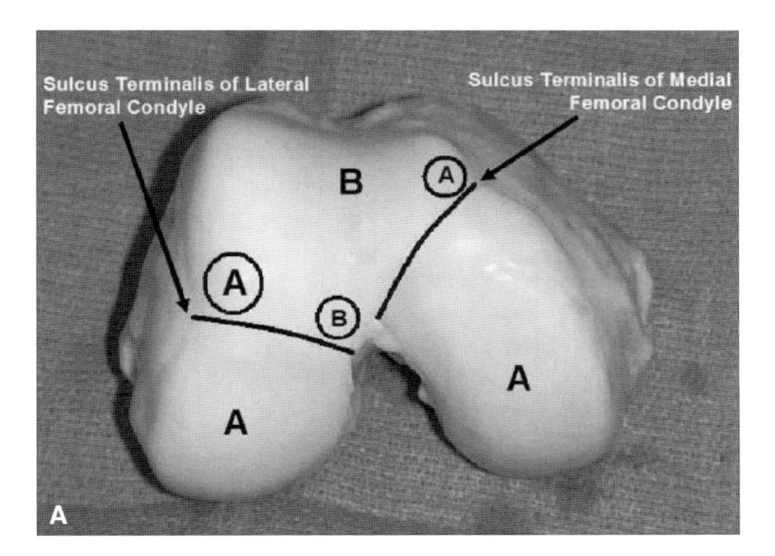

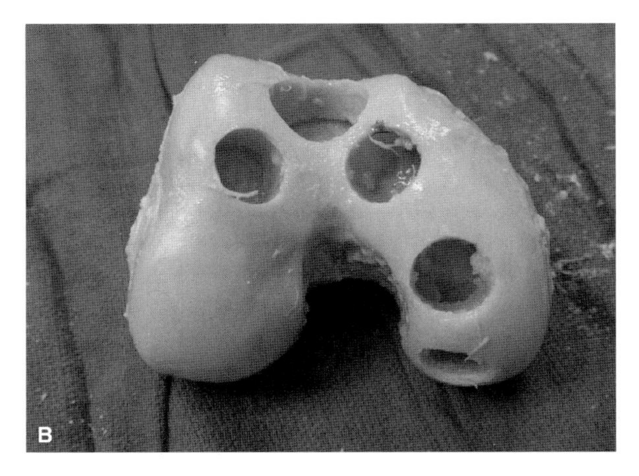

Fig. 17.1a Anatomical locations of commonly described autologous osteochondral donor sites (circled) with corresponding target areas on the articular surface of a distal femur **b** Intraoperative view of a distal femoral allograft showing actual donor sites of multiple plugs used in the resurfacing of multifocal articular cartilage defects

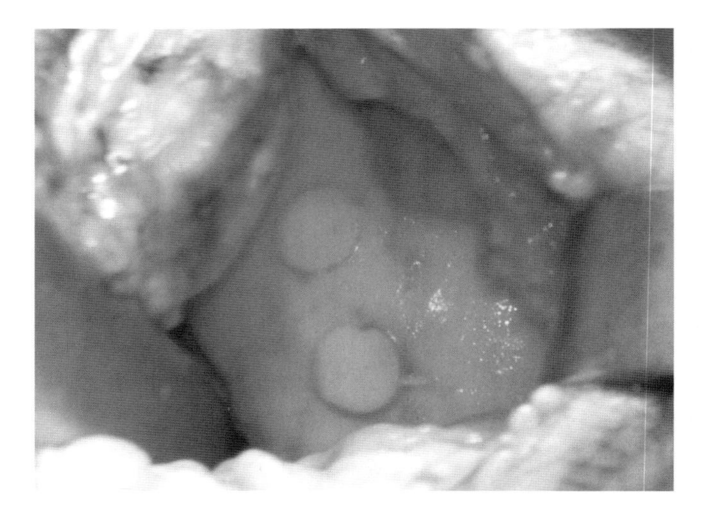

Fig. 17.2 Intraoperative view of two autologous osteochondral plugs used to stabilize a ICRS Grade II osteochondritis dissecans lesion in the typical anatomical location on the lateral margin of the medial femoral condyle

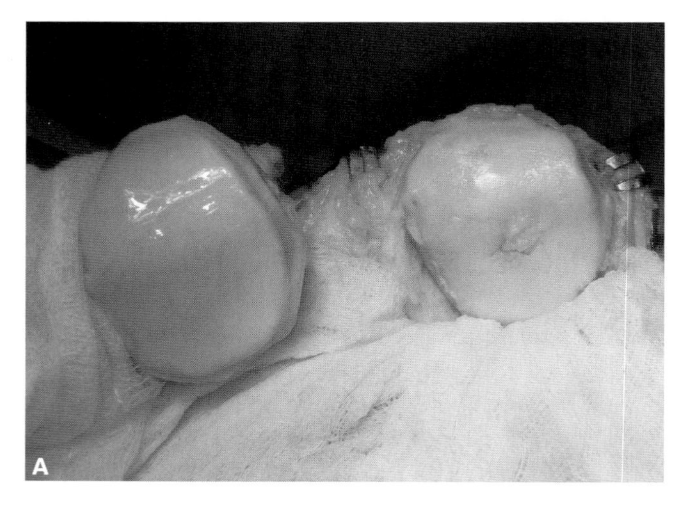

Fig. 17.3 **a** Intraoperative view of a full thickness articular cartilage lesion on a medial patellar facet with corresponding donor patella for comparison **b** Same patellar lesion cored to healthy subchondral bone Note central hole indicating position of removed guide pin **c** Dowel patellar allograft in place Note ink mark indicating adequate cephalad positioning and restoration of appropriate surface anatomy

autologous grafts, with fibrocartilage to fill in the space between osteochondral grafts, whereas the osteochondral autologous transfer system (OATS) utilizes bigger and fewer dowels [10] (Fig. 17.2). Osteochondral allografting employs orthotopic donor tissue (Fig. 17.3a) to recreate topographically appropriate articular surface anatomy (Fig. 17.3c), using either dowels that are analogous to the OATS grafts (Fig. 17.4), especially for contained small- to medium-sized condylar lesions that are accessible, while larger, more complex lesions (Fig. 17.5a) can be addressed with freehanded shell grafts [15] (Fig. 17.5b).

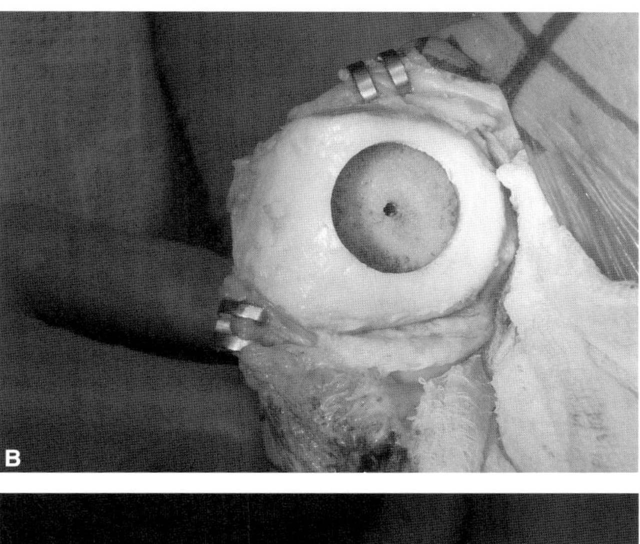

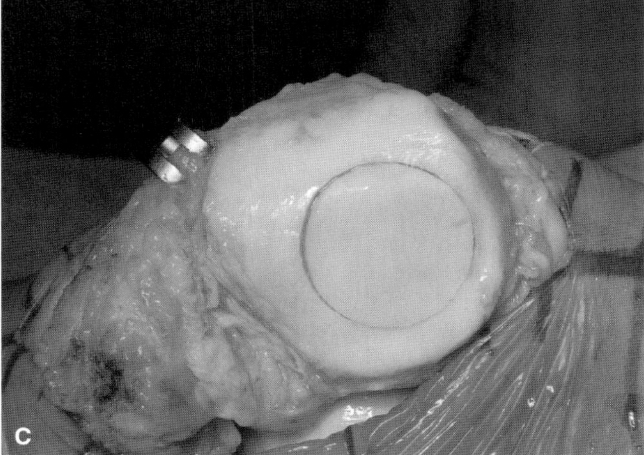

Fig. 17.3 (continued)

The use of osteochondral grafts of either origin is well established in the knee and ankle and is the subject of ongoing investigation, with indications continuously expanding in other joints.

17.2. Concepts and Basic Science

17.2.1. Properties of Hyaline Cartilage

Hyaline cartilage possesses characteristics that make it ideally suitable for transplantation. As an avascular and alymphatic tissue, its metabolic needs are met through pressurized diffusion from the synovial fluid, and it does not require innervation for function. Also, it is relatively hypocellular due to the relatively high amount of extracellular collagen matrix synthesized by the interspersed chondrocytes [5]. Thus, the common paradigm of osteochondral grafting techniques is the transplantation of articular cartilage containing viable chondrocytes, which are essential to maintain tissue homeostasis and, thus, the

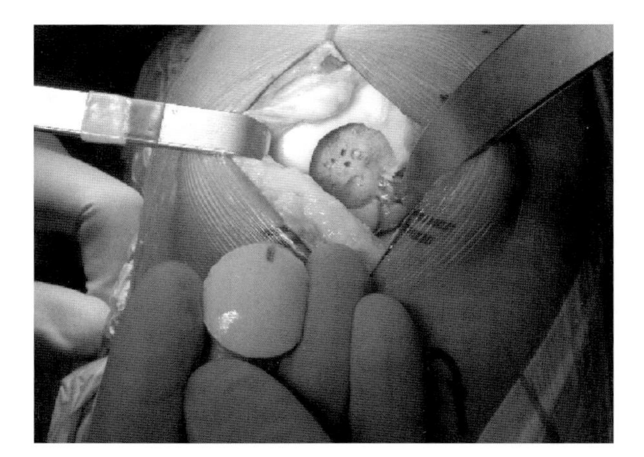

Fig. 17.4 Intraoperative view of a surgically prepared osteochondritis dissecans lesion in typical location, with corresponding osteochondral allograft dowel prior to implantation Note ink mark to ensure properly oriented implantation and proper anatomical relief of the graft

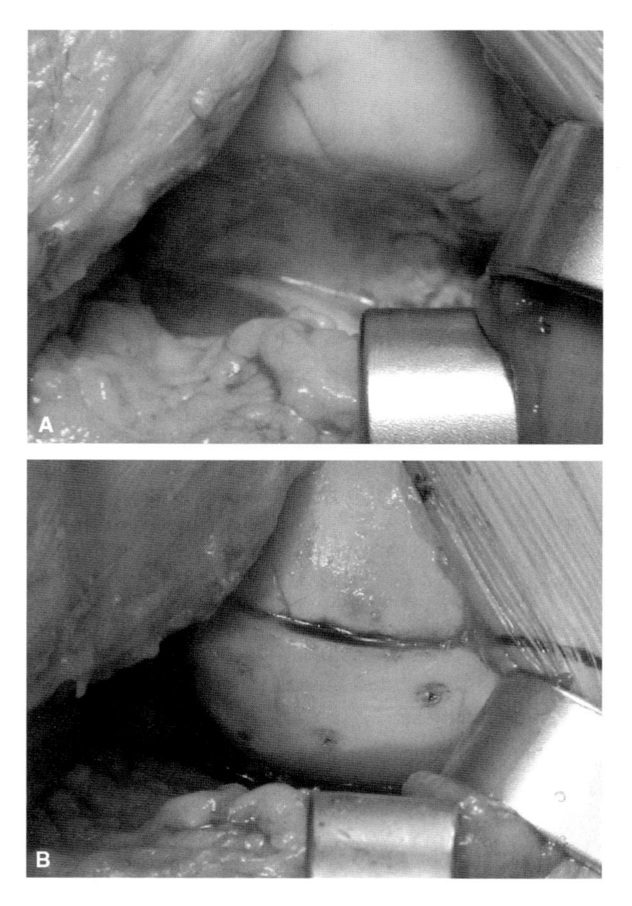

Fig. 17.5 **a** Intraoperative view of massive osteochondritis dissecans lesion of a medial femoral condyle demonstrating a substantial osseous defect **b** Same condylar lesion with orthotopic osteochondral shell allograft in place Note polydiaxone pins used for fixation

structural integrity of the surrounding collagen matrix that is responsible for the biomechanical properties of the cartilage organ.

17.2.2. Graft Storage and Chondrocyte Viability

Animal studies have shown that cell viability, as well as the structural and biochemical properties of the cartilage, are retained after autologous osteochondral grafting, while displaying donor site healing responses and host site cartilage thickness mismatches similar to those encountered in the human model [15].

Load bearing placement improved chondrocyte viability of press-fit cryopreserved osteochondral allografts in an animal model presented by Gole, et al. [16]. Likewise, retrieval studies have demonstrated that, with fresh, cold-stored osteochondral allografts, viable chondrocytes are present and mechanical properties of the matrix are maintained many years after transplantation in the human, providing proof of concept [11, 17]. This is significant, as articular cartilage undergoes deterioration when stored for prolonged periods of time, as evidenced by reduced chondrocyte viability and metabolism [18–20]. While this is not a relevant concern in single step autologous grafting, the issue has gained importance with a recent trend by tissue banks to hold allogeneic tissue for a minimum of 14 days prior to release for transplantation to allow microbiology testing to be completed, which is in contrast to empirical practice of transplanting fresh tissue within seven days of recovery. This change in clinical practice is in concordance with studies that have suggested that fresh allograft storage is reasonable beyond two weeks after graft harvest if stored under hypothermal conditions in nutritive culture medium containing amino acids, glucose, and inorganic salts [21]. This protocol constitutes the current gold standard and has been proven to preserve chondrocyte viability and structural integrity of the matrix with cell density, viability, and metabolic activity remaining essentially unchanged from baseline for as many as 14 days. While the hyaline matrix remains largely intact long beyond that, chondrocytes in stored allograft tissue deteriorate significantly after 28 days [22–23].

Fresh-frozen allografts are generally considered unsuitable for cartilage resurfacing and reserved for bulk allografting in major osseous reconstruction as it does reduce immunogenicity of the graft, especially the osseous component, at the cost of eliminating more than 95 percent of viable chondrocytes in the articular cartilage portion of osteochondral grafts. This invariably leads to deterioration of the collagen matrix over time, presumably because there are insufficient surviving cells within the matrix to maintain tissue homeostasis [24].

Cryopreservation involves the freezing of whole tissue grafts in a nutritive medium in an attempt to improve the shelf life and, thus, availability of allograft tissue. Studies employing this preservation method have shown variable, albeit generally reduced, levels of cell viability after cryoinjury to isolated chondrocytes. However, so far there has been no scientific proof for sufficient chondrocyte survival in osteochondral grafts using this technique [25].

However, even in viable cartilage, mechanical or thermal insult during harvest or implantation can lead to macroscopic injury and can induce chondrocyte necrosis and apoptosis. This particularly pertains to the cut graft margins during harvest, as well as the graft articular surface during implantation. This preferentially affects the superficial zone of articular cartilage, which is significant because chondrocytes in this zone of cartilage secrete the superficial zone protein lubricin, which contributes to the friction-lowering effect of synovial fluid [26]. On the other hand, superficial zone protein in synovial fluid is also likely to inhibit graft-to-host adhesion and ingrowth of opposing cartilage margins [27].

Marginal cell death, coupled with the inherent hypocellularity of articular cartilage, further helps to explain the lack of graft-host interface integration observed after implantation of osteochondral grafts over time [1]. This problem is obviously multiplied with the number of plugs used, as the portion of marginal cartilage in the overall surface increases. Given the fact that the interstitial bony bridges between mosaicplasty plugs heal over with fibrocartilage at best, this can have a significant impact on the overall quality of the repair tissue. Huntley, et al [28] used confocal laser scanning microscopy to demonstrate a significant marginal zone of cell death in osteochondral dowels after harvest with use of the mosaicplasty technique and concluded that up to one-third of a mosaicplasty surface is not comprised of viable hyaline cartilage. Evans, et al. [29] demonstrated the advantages of using manual punches over power trephines during plug harvest, as the latter proved technically more difficult and resulted in more gross and light microscopic damage to the osteochondral grafts, with thermal necrosis being one possible cause.

The articular surface of osteochondral grafts is prone to impaction injury during implantation if excessive compressive force is used during seating of the dowels. Borazjani, et al. [26] showed marked cell apoptosis was induced in the superficial layer of transplanted osteochondral plugs and concluded that the amplitude, more than frequency, of peak forces during implantation was responsible for triggering apoptotic cascades that lead to chondrocyte death, particularly in the superficial zone.

Optimizing cartilage health and protecting chondrocyte viability are critical to the long-term success of any cartilage restoration procedure. Care must be taken during harvest, storage, and implantation of osteochondral grafts to protect the integrity of the cartilage transplant and to maximize successful outcomes.

17.2.3. Osseous Issues

The second integral component of any osteochondral graft is the osseous portion. Conceptually, this functions as the underlying support structure for the articular cartilage and serves as a vehicle for attachment and fixation of the graft to the host.

In current practice osteochondral allografts are not HLA or blood type matched between donor and recipient. Although patients immunologically tolerate allografts from a clinical perspective, they do elicit a variable cellular-mediated immune response [30]. Because hyaline cartilage is relatively immunoprivileged [31], it is likely that this phenomenon is conveyed by the bone and associated marrow elements, as with any type of allogeneic bone graft [32–33]. Thus, immune response is generally considered clinically irrelevant [34], yet allografts tend to demonstrate slower and less extensive bone formation and neovascularization and are more prone to bone resorption [12]. Since it merely serves as an osteoconductive scaffold for healing to the host by creeping substitution, which is a rate limited process, this allogeneic potential should be minimized along with the transplanted bone wherever possible, without compromising stability of the graft as warranted by the clinical situation [24].

The osseous portion of autografts varies considerably from that of allografts, in that it is considered osteogenic and generally is incorporated rapidly and completely [12]. Postoperative hemarthrosis and, subsequently, arthrofibrosis due to bleeding from the donor site are concerns with autologous osteochondral grafting. Retrograde filling of the created defects using different artificial fillers has been investigated and proven helpful in preventing postoperative hemarthrosis and in creating a scaffold for the fibrocartilage repair process [35]. While the optimal length is debatable, bottomed plugs offer the most stable construct [36–37], their stability increasing with diameter. Since there are no immunological concerns, autologous plugs can be transplanted with more bone stock for press-fit stability if necessary [14], whereas the osseous portion of an osteochondral allograft is usually limited to depth of a few millimeters and gains press-fit stability through a wider base radius. However, depending on the clinical situation, the allograft may contain more copious amounts of bone, as required to restore injured or absent subchondral tissue [38].

17.3. Review of Preclinical Studies

17.3.1. Contact Pressures and Surface Topography

Historically, the intercondylar notch and lateral trochlea were presumed to be non-load bearing and were the recommended donor sites for autologous osteochondral grafting (Fig. 17.1a). Recent reports have demonstrated that these areas do bear significant weight, which can theoretically contribute to increased donor-site morbidity. In a cadaveric study utilizing stereophotogrammetry, Ahmad, et al. [39] studied the contact pressures and surface curvature in osteochondral autografting. They reported that the lateral trochlea was the most involved in loading, followed by the intercondylar notch. The distal medial trochlea was the least involved in loading.

Garretson, et al. [40] further analyzed the contact pressures in the patellofemoral joint. They concluded that the loading on the medial trochlea is less than on the lateral trochlea. They further suggested that because the lateral trochlea is wider than the medial side, the medial trochlea might best be suited for smaller donor plugs (<5 mm). Larger plugs could be taken from the lateral trochlea, starting proximal to the sulcus terminalis (where the lowest contact pressures of the lateral trochlea were measured).

Utilizing customized software and fresh cadaveric femurs, Bartz, et al. [41] also studied the topography of the femoral condyles. They found that grafts taken from the far medial and lateral margins of the femoral trochlea, just proximal to the sulcus terminalis, provided the most accurate reconstruction of the surface anatomy of central lesions in the weight bearing portion of either femoral condyle. Smaller grafts (4 or 6 mm) from the lateral intercondylar notch can also provide precise matches to similar lesions; however, significant inaccuracies are noted when the lateral intercondylar notch grafts are increased in size (8 mm). In addition, they concluded that the concave central intercondylar notch grafts do not match the topography of the convex femoral condyles. Ahmad et, al. [39] described similar findings. They found that the intercondylar notch donor best matched the topography of the central trochlea. Also, the curvatures of the medial and lateral trochlea better matched the recipient sites at the femoral condyles.

A biomechanical study by Koh, et al. [42] on cadaveric pig knees looked at the effect of angled osteochondral grafting on contact pressures. They found that slightly countersunk grafts and angled grafts with the highest edge placed flush to neighboring cartilage demonstrated fairly normal contact pressures. On the other hand, elevated angled grafts increased contact pressures by as much as 40 percent, making them biomechanically disadvantageous. They concluded that it is more favorable to leave a graft slightly countersunk than elevated with respect to the neighboring cartilage.

17.4. Clinical Review

17.4.1. Operative Techniques

17.4.1.1. Osteochondral Autografting Technique – Knee

The technique can be performed through standard arthrotomy, mini-arthrotomy and/or arthroscopically. Nevertheless, the surgeon should always prepare for conversion to standard arthrotomy as certain locations, i.e., the posterior femoral condyle, may be difficult to access with less invasive approaches. The patient is positioned in a supine fashion to allow for full flexion of the knee. Preoperative antibiotics are administered. A tourniquet is recommended to assist with intraoperative visualization.

The lesion is accessed and measured after cartilage and subchondral bone have been debrided to healthy margins. At this point the surgeon makes a determination on the osteochondral autografting technique to be implemented (OATS versus mosaicplasty). In current practice available donor plug sizes vary from 2.7 to 10 mm, depending on the technique utilized and the size of the chondral lesion. The surgeon should consider the articular topography when deciding between OATS and mosaicplasty. In general, matching articular geometry becomes more difficult with larger donor plugs. In addition, the potential for donor-site morbidity increases with larger dowels.

Under direct visualization the appropriately sized tubular T-handled recipient harvester is tapped perpendicular to the defect to a minimum depth of 10 mm for standard cartilage lesions (Fig. 17.6). The depth can be increased to as much as 25 mm for significant osteochondral conditions, i.e., osteochondritis dissecans. The harvester chisel is then removed by rotating the driver 90° clockwise, then 90° counterclockwise.

Utilizing the same technique with a slightly larger T-handled harvester, the donor graft is taken from the far medial or lateral margin of the trochlea, just proximal to the sulcus terminalis. Alternatively, a smaller graft can be taken from the lateral intercondylar notch. After verifying the donor graft's depth measurement, it is then transplanted into the recipient site utilizing the donor tube harvester, which dilates the cartilage layer with its beveled edge creating a tight press-fit. The last 1 mm of impaction should be performed by lightly tapping an oversized bone tamp over the cartilaginous cap. If necessary, the osseous portion of the graft can be shortened to allow the cartilage cap to lie flush with the surrounding articular surface. If required, the process is repeated until the lesion is covered with healthy hyaline cartilage. A 1 to 2 mm bone bridge between recipient sites is recommended to help achieve a tight press fit. These bridges fill with fibrocartilage. In addition, careful spacing of the plugs is essential. To avoid premature amputation of the graft, the osseous

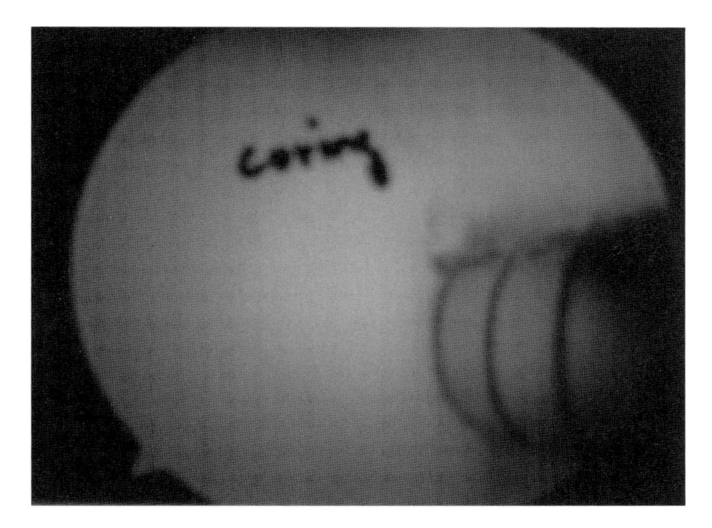

Fig. 17.6 Arthroscopic view of a recipient harvester tapped into a femoral osteochondral lesion. Note depth gauge indicating adequate resection level. (Photo courtesy of Bert Mandelbaum, MD)

portions should not intersect with one another. This can be most problematic with longer grafts (25 mm) obtained in areas of the knee where there is high curvature, i.e., the posterior femoral condyle. Finally, to prevent recipient tunnel wall fracture, each plug transfer should be completed prior to proceeding with additional recipient sockets.

The surgeon may choose to retrofill the created defects to minimize donor site morbidity. Osteobiologic plugs that correspond to the diameters of commercial coring devices are available for this purpose (Fig. 17.7). Following the graft process, surface congruity is confirmed, and the joint is put through a range of motion to ensure graft stability and lack of impingement. The knee is closed in a standard fashion over a drain after irrigation of the joint and inspection for loose bodies.

17.4.1.2. Osteochondral Allografting Technique – Knee

The technique of fresh osteochondral allografting generally relies on an open procedure, including an arthrotomy of variable size (depending on the position and dimension of the lesion). Usually the patients have had previous surgery or are at least fully imaged; otherwise, a diagnostic arthroscopy can be performed prior to the allografting procedure to confirm adequacy of the available graft. It is the responsibility of the surgeon to inspect the graft and to confirm the adequacy of the size match and quality of the tissue prior to surgery.

The patient is positioned supine with a proximal thigh tourniquet, as above. A leg or foot holder can help to position and maintain the leg in between 70° and 100° of flexion. For most femoral condyle lesions, eversion of the patella is not necessary.

A standard midline incision is made and elevated subcutaneously, depending on the location of the lesion (either medial or lateral), and the joint is entered by incising the fat pad without disrupting the anterior horn of the meniscus or damaging the articular surface. In some cases where the lesion is posterior or very large, the meniscus must be detached and reflected; generally, this can be

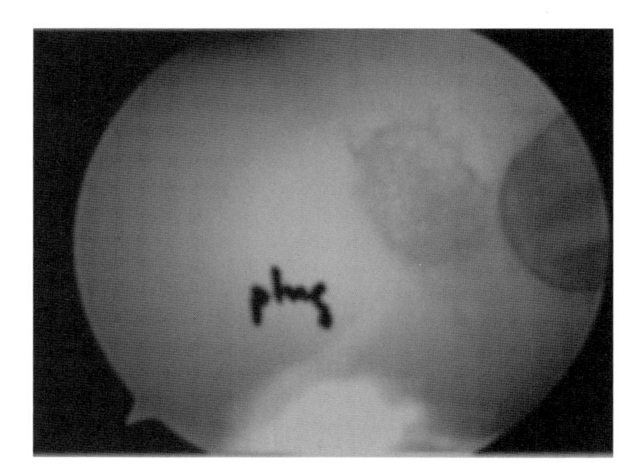

Fig. 17.7 Arthroscopic view of an implanted osteobiologic plug tamped flush with the surrounding articular cartilage. (Photo courtesy of Bert Mandelbaum, MD)

done safely, leaving a small cuff of tissue adjacent to the anterior attachment of the meniscus. Once the joint capsule and synovium have been incised and retractors have been carefully placed, the knee is brought to a degree of flexion that presents the lesion into the arthrotomy site. The lesion then is inspected and palpated with a probe to determine the extent, margins, and maximum size.

The two commonly used techniques for the preparation and implantation of osteochondral allografts include the press-fit plug technique (Fig. 17.4) and the shell graft technique (Fig. 17.5b). Each technique has advantages and disadvantages. The press-fit plug technique is similar, in principle, to autologous osteochondral transfer systems described above. This technique is optimal for contained condylar lesions between 15 and 35 mm in diameter. Fixation is generally not required, due to the stability achieved with the press fit. Disadvantages include the fact that very posterior femoral and trochlear lesions are not conducive to the use of a circular coring system and may be more amenable to shell allografts. Additionally, the more ovoid a lesion in shape, the more normal cartilage which needs to be sacrificed at the recipient site in order to accommodate the circular donor plug. Shell grafts are technically more difficult to perform and typically require fixation. However, depending on the technique employed, less normal cartilage may need to be sacrificed.

17.4.1.2.1. Surgical Technique – Dowel Allograft: As with autologous dowels, there are several proprietary instrumentation systems that are currently available for the preparation and implantation of press-fit dowel allografts up to 35 mm in diameter, and surgical techniques are similar.

After a size determination is made, a guide wire is driven into the center of the lesion, perpendicular to the curvature of the articular surface. The size of the graft is then determined utilizing sizing dowels, remembering that overlapping dowels (in a "snowman" or "mastercard" configuration) can possibly deliver the best area fit. The remaining articular cartilage is scored to subchondral bone, and a core reamer is used to remove the articular cartilage remnants and at least 3 to 4 mm of subchondral bone (Fig. 17.3b). In deeper lesions fibrous and sclerotic bone is removed to a healthy, bleeding osseous base, not to exceed 10 mm in depth. Lesions below this depth should be curetted manually, and packed morselized autologous bone graft should be utilized to fill any deeper or more extensive osseous defects. Circumferential depth measurements of the prepared recipient site are made after the guide pin has been removed.

The graft is then placed into a graft holder or held manually with bone holding forceps. The correspondent anatomic location is identified on the graft and, after a circular saw guide has been placed in the position – again perpendicular to the articular surface – an appropriate sized tube saw is used to core out the graft. Prior to removing the graft from the condyle, identifying marks are made to ensure proper orientation. Once the dowel is removed, the recipient's depth measurements are transferred to the graft. This graft is then cut with an oscillating saw and trimmed with a rasp to the precise thickness in all four quadrants. The deep edges of the bone plug can be further chamfered with a rongeur and bone rasp to ease insertion.

The graft is then irrigated copiously with a high pressure lavage to remove all marrow elements possible, and the recipient site can be dilated using a slightly oversized tamp. This may ease the insertion of the graft to prevent excessive impact loading of the articular surface when the graft is inserted, while compacting the subchondral bone to prevent subsidence of the graft. At this time any remaining osseous defects are bone grafted to a level base. The allograft is then inserted by hand in the appropriate rotation and is gently tamped into place until it is flush, again minimizing mechanical insult to the articular surface of both the graft and surrounding native tissue.

After the graft is seated, additional fixation with absorbable polydioxanone pins can be added if necessary, particularly if the graft is large or has an exposed edge within the notch. The knee is then brought through a complete range of motion to confirm that the graft is stable and there is no catching or soft-tissue obstruction. The wound is then copiously irrigated, and routine closure is performed.

17.4.1.2.2. Surgical Technique – Shell Allograft: The defect is identified through the previously described arthrotomy and the dimensions of the lesion are marked with a surgical pen. Minimizing the sacrifice of normal cartilage, a geometric shape is created that is amenable to handcrafting a shell graft. A #15 scalpel blade is used to demarcate the lesion, and sharp ring curettes are used to remove all tissue inside this mark. Using both motorized burrs and sharp curettes, the lesion is debrided down to a depth of 4 to 5 mm. The shape is transferred to the graft, which is molded in a freehand fashion, initially slightly oversizing the graft and carefully removing excess bone and cartilage from the template as necessary through multiple trial fittings. If there is deeper bone loss in the defect, more bone can be left on the graft and the defect can be grafted with cancellous bone prior to graft insertion. The graft and host bed are then copiously irrigated and the graft placed flush with the articular surface. The need for fixation is based on the degree of inherent stability. Bioabsorbable pins, as previously described, are typically used when fixation is required (Fig. 17.5b), but countersunk compression screws may be used as an alternative, optimally avoiding the weight bearing portion. After cycling the knee through a full range of motion and irrigating the joint, standard closure is performed.

17.4.2. Postoperative Protocol

Patients are kept on a touchdown weight bearing restriction for four to eight weeks after autologous grafting and slightly longer for allografts, depending on the size and position of the graft(s) and radiographic evidence of bony healing. Quadriceps strengthening and early range of motion are encouraged. Closed-chained exercises are introduced at four weeks. The return to weight bearing is gradual. Patients return to full daily activities by three to four months. Typically, braces are not utilized, unless the grafting involves the patellofemoral joint, where flexion is limited to <45° for the first four to six weeks, or in cases where bipolar tibial femoral grafts are used, an unloader or range of motion brace is used to prevent excessive stress on the grafted surfaces.

17.4.3. Clinical Results

17.4.3.1. Selected Studies about Osteochondral Autografting in the Knee [Table 17.1]

Hangody, et al. [43] reported on their 10-year clinical experience with autologous osteochondral mosaicplasty. They performed 831 mosaicplasties, involving 597 femoral condyles, 118 patellofemoral (patella and/or trochlea) joints, 76 talar domes, 25 tibial condyles, six capitulum humeri, six femoral heads and three humeral heads. Concomitant surgery (ACL reconstruction, realignment procedures and meniscal surgeries) was performed on 85 percent of the patients. They demonstrated good-to-excellent results in 92 percent of the patients in the femoral condyle group, 87 percent of those who had tibial grafts, 79 percent of those who underwent patellofemoral joint mosaicplasties, and 94 percent of those who had talar resurfacings. Long-term donor site morbidity was found in 3 percent of the patients.

Marcacci, et al. [44] reported on 37 athletes younger than 50 years of age with at least a two-year follow-up. In this study 23 of 37 (62 percent) patients underwent an associated procedure with arthroscopic mosaicplasty of the femoral condyle. These patients demonstrated 78 percent good-to-excellent results. Five patients were unable to return to sports. Twenty-seven patients returned to sports at the same level, and five patients returned at a lower level. Medial

Table 17.1 Selected outcomes of osteochondral autografting in the knee

Study	Site of Lesion	No. of Knees	Average Follow-up	Outcome
Hangody, et al.	Femur	597	1–10 y	92 % G/E
Hangody, et al.	PFJ	118	1–10 y	79 % G/E
Hangody, et al.	Tibia	25	1–10 y	87 % G/E
Marcacci, et al.	Femur	37	2.0 y	78 G/E
Jakob, et al.	Femur	52	3.1 y	92 I
Chow, et al.	Femur	30	3.8 y	83 % G/E
Outerbridge, et al.	Femur	18	7.6 y	81 % H
Karataglis, et al.	Femur & PFJ	37	3.1	87 % H

Abbreviatons:
PFJ = patellofemoral joint
G/E = good/excellent; I = improved knee function; H = high functional level

femoral condyle lesions statistically did not fare as well as lateral condyle lesions. Donor site morbidity was not an identifiable problem in this case series.

In a study by Jakob, et al. [45], 92 percent (48 of 52) of patients demonstrated improved knee function at the latest follow-up (average 37 months) from open knee mosaicplasty. In 30 of 52 patients (58 percent), a concomitant procedure was performed. Four patients required re-operation because of graft failure.

With a mean follow-up of 45.1 months, Chow, et al. [46] reported on 30 patients who had undergone arthroscopic autologous osteochondral transplantation to the femoral condyle. Good-to-excellent results were seen in 83 percent (25 of 30) patients. Lysholm scores increased from an average of 43.6 preoperatively to a mean of 87.5 postoperatively. Two (7 percent) patients had poor results and later underwent total knee arthroplasty.

Outerbridge, et al. [47] followed 18 knees for an average of 7.6 years after osteochondral autografting of the femoral condyle utilizing the ipsilateral lateral patellar facet as the donor graft. They reported an increase in Cincinnati knee scores from an average preoperative level of 37 to an average final follow-up level of 85. Eighty-one percent (13 of 16) of the patients returned to a high functional level. Twelve percent (2 of 16) of the patients experienced moderate patellofemoral joint symptoms. Nevertheless, all patients were satisfied with the procedure results and, given the choice, would have the same surgery done for an identical lesion on the contralateral knee.

Most recently Karataglis, et al. [48] reported on their mid- and long-term functional outcomes of 36 patients (37 knees) who underwent the OATS technique with average follow-up of 36.9 months. The lesions were located on the femoral condyle in 26 cases, on the trochlea in seven cases, and on the patella in four cases. Thirty-two out of 37 patients (86.5 percent) reported significant improvement of their preoperative symptoms. All but five patients had returned to previous daily activities and work. Eighteen patients returned to playing sports. Nine patients required second look arthroscopies because of swelling, pain, or clicking. In two of those cases the grafts were found to be loose and required revision. Symptoms improved significantly in four out of those nine patients after repeat arthroscopy. Donor-site morbidity was not seen.

17.4.3.1.1. Other Body Sites – Autografting: Osteochondral autografting is performed on various other joints, including the ankle (talus), the hip (femoral head), the shoulder (humeral head), and the elbow (humeral capitellum). The donor grafts are obtained from the knee, usually via a mini-arthrotomy. Unfortunately, this potentially introduces donor-site morbidity to a previously uninvolved joint. The technique can be challenging as it may be difficult to re-establish articular surface topography in these joints, and plug-host cartilage thickness mismatch is a concern. It may be appropriate to harvest the graft with a certain degree of obliquity to better match the radius of curvature of these unique bones.

Utilizing coronal MRI of the talus and distal femur of five matched cadavers, Marymont, et al. [49] performed computer reconstructions to assess the mismatch issues of the femoral condyle and talus. They found that the donor site with the least amount of step-off and closest surface contour of the medial talus is the superolateral femoral condyle. Unfortunately, long-term studies involving the above-mentioned joints with sufficient patient numbers are lacking.

17.4.3.2. Selected Clinical Studies about Osteochondral Allografting in the Knee [Table 17.2]

Garrett [50] reported on the experience with fresh osteochondral allografts used as both a press-fit plug and large shell graft in the treatment of 17 patients with osteochondritis dissecans, all of whom had undergone previous surgery. Sixteen of 17 (94 percent) reported relief of symptoms at two- to nine-year follow-up.

Emmerson, et al. [51] presented the results of 68 knees in 65 patients with OCD of the femoral condyle (Fig. 17-5a), treated with fresh osteochondral allografts implanted within five days of recovery. Patients were pre- and post-operatively evaluated using an 18-point modified D'Aubigne and Postel scale, which measures function, range of motions and absence of pain, allotting one to six points each, for a maximum of 18 points. There were 48 males and 17 females, with a mean age of 27 years (range 15 to 54). All lesions were grade III to IV OCD; 39 involved the medial femoral condyle and 29 the lateral femoral condyle. All had undergone an average of 1.7 previous surgeries. Average allograft size was 7.4 cm^2. Mean follow-up was 5.8 years (range 2 to 19); one patient was lost to follow-up. Overall, 47 of 68 (69 percent) knees were rated good or excellent, scoring 15 or above on the 18-point scale. The average clinical score improved from 13.0 preoperatively to 16.7 postoperatively ($p < 0.05$). Eight patients had re-operations on the allograft, with a mean time to re-operation of 56 months. Subjective knee function improved from a mean of 3.5 to 8.2 on a 10-point scale for the 51 patients who completed questionnaires.

Between 1997 and 2004, 43 patients with isolated cartilage lesions of the femoral condyle were treated with fresh osteochondral allografting at our institution [52]. The study population included 23 males and 20 females and had a mean age of 35 years. Twenty-nine lesions involved the medial femoral condyle, 13 the lateral femoral condyle, and one was bilateral. All patients had undergone prior surgery. Mean allograft area was 5.88 cm^2. Thirty-eight of 43 (88 percent) were considered successful (score 15 or greater on the 18-point modified D'Aubigne and Postel scale) at mean 4.5 years of follow-up.

Park, et al. [53] reported on our experience with osteochondral allografting in 37 patients who carried a clinically established and radiographically confirmed

Table 17.2 Selected outcomes of osteochondral allografting in the knee

Author	Site of Lesion	Diagnosis/ Indication	Number of Patients	Mean Follow–up	Successful Outcome
Chu	Knee	Multiple	55	6.2 Years	84 % G/E
McDermott	Knee	Trauma	50	3.8 Years	76 % SCS
Ghazavi	Knee	Trauma	126	7.5 Years	f85 % SVS
Beaver	Knee	Trauma	92	14.0 Years	63 % SVS
Aubin	Femur	Trauma	60	10.0 Years	85 % SVS
Görtz	Femur	Trauma	43	4.5 Years	88 % G/E
Garrett	Femur	OCD	17	2-9 Years	94 % G/E
Emmerson	Femur	OCD	68	5.8 Years	69 % G/E
Bugbee	Knee	Osteonecrosis	21	5.3 Years	88 % G/E
Park	Knee	Osteoarthrosis	37	3.0 Years	76 % G/E

Abbreviations:
SCS = Successful; SVS = Survivorship; G/E = Good/Excellent

diagnosis of advanced knee arthrosis. Nineteen grafts were unipolar, 10 bipolar, five included multiple surfaces and mean graft area was $10.5\,cm^2$. With a mean follow-up of three years, 28 of 34 patients who followed up were considered successes of fresh osteochondral allografting with objectively and subjectively statistically significant improvement ($p < 0.01$).

In a study reporting on the use of allografts in the salvage of 21 knees (17 patients) with established severe osteonecrosis of the knee [54], 15 were satisfied with their treatment and 14 felt that the overall condition of their knee was improved. This challenging salvage situation dealt with a relatively young patient population (average age, 30 years; range 16 to 68) and, after a mean follow-up of 5.3 years, none of the knees required conversion to total knee arthroplasty.

Chu [55] reported on 55 consecutive knees undergoing osteochondral allografting on diagnoses such as traumatic chondral injury, avascular necrosis, osteochondritis dissecans, and patellofemoral disease. The mean age of this group was 35.6 years, with follow-up averaging 75 months (range 11 to 147 months). Of the 55 knees, 43 were unipolar replacements and 12 were bipolar resurfacing replacements. On an 18-point scale, 45 of 55 (76 percent) of these knees were rated good to excellent, and 3 of 55 were fair. Of note, 36 of the 43 knees (84 percent) that underwent unipolar femoral grafts, but only six of the 12 knees (50 percent) with bipolar grafts, were rated good to excellent.

McDermott, et al. [56] reported on 100 patients treated with fresh osteochondral grafts implanted within 24 hours of recovery. Fifty patients had a unifocal traumatic defect of the tibial plateau or femoral condyle, 38 of which (76 percent) were considered successful at an average follow-up of 3.8 years. Patients with osteoarthritis and osteonecrosis did worse.

Ghazavi [57] reported on 126 knees in 123 patients with an average follow-up of 7.5 years. One-hundred-five of 123 (85 percent) patients were rated as successful, while the remaining 18 had failed. Advanced age (>50 years old), bipolar defects, malalignment and workers' compensation cases were considered main factors related to failure.

Beaver, et al. [58] performed a survivorship study on 92 knees allografted for posttraumatic cartilage lesions with failure defined as the need for a revision operation or the persistence of symptoms. There was a 75 percent success rate at five years, 64 percent at 10 years, and 63 percent at 14 years. Advanced age (>60) and bipolar defects were again identified as factors for failure.

Aubin, et al. [59] later followed up on 60 patients, 41 of whom (68 percent) had undergone simultaneous realignment osteotomy and 10 (15 percent) concomitant meniscal transplantation. Kaplan-Meier survivorship analysis showed 51 grafts (85 percent) surviving at 10 years, and 44 (74 percent) at 15 years.

17.4.3.2.1. Other Body Sites – Allografting: The use of fresh allografts for bipolar resurfacing of the tibiotalar joint is unique, as this has not been proven reliably successful in other joints; this also reflects the limited options for the younger individual with end-stage arthrosis of the tibiotalar joint. Osteochondral (uni- or bipolar) allografting of the tibiotalar joint with posttraumatic arthrosis, as well as partial talar grafts for osteonecrosis or osteochondritis dissecans lesions not amenable to OATS or other restorative procedures, has shown acceptable long-term success and the ability for future revision or conversion if necessary, making osteochondral allografting a promising alternative management strategy in the treatment algorithm for ankle arthropathy [60].

Use of osteochondral allografts in femoral and humeral heads has also been described, mostly for traumatic osteochondral lesions and osteonecrosis. Other indications in the hip, shoulder, and conceivably other joints are evolving, although little published data on such applications is currently available.

17.5. Future Trends and Needs

While osteochondral grafting has proven invaluable in the treatment of osteoarticular lesions of varying degrees and etiologies, additional research is needed to further validate and expand clinical application.

Chondrocyte necrosis and apoptosis due to mechanical insult during both harvest and implantation are effects, which are only now beginning to be quantified, and which continue to present a challenge in regards to tissue quality for allograft and autograft tissue alike. As these concerns become better understood, efforts can be focused on preserving chondrocyte viability by minimizing these deleterious effects on graft tissue. One obvious approach to a mechanical problem is a mechanical solution through advances in instrumentation, from better blade geometry [28] to impaction devices and techniques that reduce trauma to the articular organ during implantation [26].

Enzymatic pretreatment of graft tissue [61] or the use of growth factors [62] as an interventional strategy to improve integration with host tissue and to increase interfacial strength at the repair site has been investigated with promising results. Another investigational approach is the use of caspase inhibitors to block these key trigger enzymes in the apoptotic pathway and to make the graft construct more resilient against superphysiologic loads during impaction [63]. Allograft tissue, in particular, lends itself to these supplemental approaches. The respective agents can simply be added to the storage media and remain there long enough for slow diffusion into the graft tissue to occur. Immunomodulation of allograft tissue to make it perform akin to host tissue is poised to take on a bigger role as immune system interactions and the intricacies of the antigenic behavior of graft tissue continue to be conceptualized.

Bioengineered biphasic scaffolds are now being used for retrograde filling of autologous osteochondral donor sites and have evolved to the point where many surgeons are advocating their use as a primary implant to reduce overall surgical trauma and disease burden on the joint. While this currently constitutes an off-label use of the devices and no long-term results on this practice exist at this time, it is not unlikely that biphasic scaffolds are going to make OATS autografting obsolete, while utilizing the same technique for implantation.

Advances in the field of tissue engineering promise the development of novel constructs, consisting of a matrix that can be seeded with chondrocytes of either autologous or allogeneic sources over an osteoinductive base optimized for fixation. Allogeneic chondrocytes are an appealing cell source for tissue engineering applications because they can obviate the need for autologous harvest surgery and dramatically shorten the time course of treatment by being made available "off the shelf." Gene typing allows for the identification, isolation, and expansion of young cell lines with great chondrogenic potential, which could then be used to make the supply of suitable transplant tissue temporally independent through cell expansion and storage. This symbiosis allows not only for functionally superior cartilage restoration alternatives but also effectively addresses two inherent limitations of fresh osteochondral allografting, namely donor tissue availability and timely patient-donor allocation.

17.6. Conclusions

Osteochondral grafting is a scientifically validated and intuitively reasonable approach to the treatment of osteoarticular defects, as it is the only restorative method that re-introduces structurally mature and appropriate hyaline and subchondral tissue into acquired articular surface defects. While both graft sources represent a common cartilage organ transplantation paradigm and are complementary, each of the graft sources has its unique, reciprocal challenges with regard to tissue availability and safety. The discerning surgeon is responsible for communicating these considerations to the patient, appropriately weighing them in the treatment algorithm and managing them accordingly.

Autograft is immediately, yet not abundantly, available and, thus, limited in its application, while allograft tissue must be allocated and processed, but allows solid, orthotopic reconstruction of even very large and topographically complex defects. Autologous tissue is theoretically safer to use and is not antigenic, but its use carries the tangible risk of donor-site morbidity.

The surgical technique for either method is uncomplicated and reproducible, but requires precision to attain predictable and reliable results. Clinical applications continue to evolve in regard to other joints and optimizing implant quality, both through adjustments in the methods of harvest and delivery, as well as modulation of the graft environment, especially during the storage interval. Technical advances in tissue engineering hold promise for allogeneic chondrocytes as a cell source and improving scaffold design to further optimize retro- and, especially, anterograde defect coverage.

References

1. Mankin HJ. The response of articular cartilage to mechanical injury. J Bone Joint Surg Am 1982;64(3):460–6.
2. Buckwalter JA. Articular cartilage. Instr Course Lect 1983;32:349–70.
3. Hjelle K, Solheim E, Strand T, Muri R, Brittberg M. Articular cartilage defects in 1,000 knee arthroscopies. Arthroscopy 2002;18(7):730–4.
4. Guettler JH, Demetropoulos CK, Yang KH, Jurist KA. Osteochondral defects in the human knee: influence of defect size on cartilage rim stress and load redistribution to surrounding cartilage. Am J Sports Med 2004;32(6):1451–8.
5. Alford JW, Cole BJ. Cartilage restoration, part 1: basic science, historical perspective, patient evaluation, and treatment options. Am J Sports Med 2005;33(2):295–306.
6. Mithoefer K, Williams RJ, 3rd, Warren RF, Wickiewicz TL, Marx RG. High-Impact Athletics After Knee Articular Cartilage Repair: A Prospective Evaluation of the Microfracture Technique. Am J Sports Med 2006.
7. Knutsen G, Engebretsen L, Ludvigsen TC, et al. Autologous chondrocyte implantation compared with microfracture in the knee. A randomized trial. J Bone Joint Surg Am 2004;86-A(3):455–64.
8. Bartlett W, Skinner JA, Gooding CR, et al. Autologous chondrocyte implantation versus matrix-induced autologous chondrocyte implantation for osteochondral defects of the knee: a prospective, randomised study. J Bone Joint Surg Br 2005;87(5):640–5.
9. Czitrom AA, Langer F, McKee N, Gross AE. Bone and cartilage allotransplantation. A review of 14 years of research and clinical studies. Clin Orthop Relat Res 1986(208):141–5.

10. Bobic V. [Autologous osteo-chondral grafts in the management of articular cartilage lesions]. Orthopade 1999;28(1):19–25.
11. Kandel RA, Gross AE, Ganel A, McDermott AG, Langer F, Pritzker KP. Histopathology of failed osteoarticular shell allografts. Clin Orthop Relat Res 1985(197):103–10.
12. Burchardt H. The biology of bone graft repair. Clin Orthop Relat Res 1983(174):28–42.
13. Görtz S, Bugbee WD. Fresh osteochondral allografts: graft processing and clinical applications. J Knee Surg 2006;19(3):231–40.
14. Duchow J, Hess T, Kohn D. Primary stability of press-fit-implanted osteochondral grafts. Influence of graft size, repeated insertion, and harvesting technique. Am J Sports Med 2000;28(1):24–7.
15. Lane JG, Massie JB, Ball ST, et al. Follow-up of osteochondral plug transfers in a goat model: a 6-month study. Am J Sports Med 2004;32(6):1440–50.
16. Gole MD, Poulsen D, Marzo JM, Ko SH, Ziv I. Chondrocyte viability in press-fit cryopreserved osteochondral allografts. J Orthop Res 2004;22(4):781–7.
17. Czitrom AA, Keating S, Gross AE. The viability of articular cartilage in fresh osteochondral allografts after clinical transplantation. J Bone Joint Surg Am 1990;72(4):574–81.
18. Williams RJ, 3rd, Dreese JC, Chen CT. Chondrocyte survival and material properties of hypothermically stored cartilage: an evaluation of tissue used for osteochondral allograft transplantation. Am J Sports Med 2004;32(1):132–9.
19. Pearsall AWt, Tucker JA, Hester RB, Heitman RJ. Chondrocyte viability in refrigerated osteochondral allografts used for transplantation within the knee. Am J Sports Med 2004;32(1):125–31.
20. Robertson CM, Allen RT, Pennock AT, Bugbee WD, Amiel D. Upregulation of apoptotic and matrix-related gene expression during fresh osteochondral allograft storage. Clin Orthop Relat Res 2006;442:260–6.
21. Ball ST, Amiel D, Williams SK, et al. The effects of storage on fresh human osteochondral allografts. Clin Orthop Relat Res 2004(418):246–52.
22. Williams SK, Amiel D, Ball ST, et al. Prolonged storage effects on the articular cartilage of fresh human osteochondral allografts. J Bone Joint Surg Am 2003; 85-A(11):2111–20.
23. Allen RT, Robertson CM, Pennock AT, et al. Analysis of stored osteochondral allografts at the time of surgical implantation. Am J Sports Med 2005;33(10):1479–84.
24. Enneking WF, Campanacci DA. Retrieved human allografts: a clinicopathological study. J Bone Joint Surg Am 2001;83-A(7):971–86.
25. Pegg DE, Wusteman MC, Wang L. Cryopreservation of articular cartilage 1: Conventional cryopreservation methods. Cryobiology 2006.
26. Borazjani BH, Chen AC, Bae WC, et al. Effect of impact on chondrocyte viability during insertion of human osteochondral grafts. J Bone Joint Surg Am 2006;88(9):1934–43.
27. Englert C, McGowan KB, Klein TJ, Giurea A, Schumacher BL, Sah RL. Inhibition of integrative cartilage repair by proteoglycan 4 in synovial fluid. Arthritis Rheum 2005;52(4):1091–9.
28. Huntley JS, Bush PG, McBirnie JM, Simpson AH, Hall AC. Chondrocyte death associated with human femoral osteochondral harvest as performed for mosaicplasty. J Bone Joint Surg Am 2005;87(2):351–60.
29. Evans PJ, Miniaci A, Hurtig MB. Manual punch versus power harvesting of osteochondral grafts. Arthroscopy 2004;20(3):306–10.
30. Phipatanakul WP, VandeVord PJ, Teitge RA, Wooley PH. Immune response in patients receiving fresh osteochondral allografts. Am J Orthop 2004;33(7):345–8.
31. O'Sullivan N, Ibusuki S, Yaremchuk Y, Randolph M. Antigenicity of Isolated Allogeneic Human Chondrocytes for Cartilage Tissue Engineering. 6th Symposium of the International Cartilage Repair Society 2006(Podium Presentation 10b-2):42.

32. Friedlaender GE, Horowitz MC. Immune responses to osteochondral allografts: nature and significance. Orthopedics 1992;15(10):1171–5.
33. Strong DM, Friedlaender GE, Tomford WW, et al. Immunologic responses in human recipients of osseous and osteochondral allografts. Clin Orthop Relat Res 1996(326):107–14.
34. Arnoczky SP. The biology of allograft incorporation. J Knee Surg 2006;19(3):207–14.
35. Feczko P, Hangody L, Varga J, et al. Experimental results of donor site filling for autologous osteochondral mosaicplasty. Arthroscopy 2003;19(7):755–61.
36. Kock NB, Van Susante JL, Buma P, Van Kampen A, Verdonschot N. Press-fit stability of an osteochondral autograft: Influence of different plug length and perfect depth alignment. Acta Orthop 2006;77(3):422–8.
37. Kordas G, Szabo JS, Hangody L. Primary stability of osteochondral grafts used in mosaicplasty. Arthroscopy 2006;22(4):414–21.
38. Görtz S, Bugbee WD. Allografts in articular cartilage repair. J Bone Joint Surg Am 2006;88(6):1374–84.
39. Ahmad CS, Cohen ZA, Levine WN, Ateshian GA, Mow VC. Biomechanical and topographic considerations for autologous osteochondral grafting in the knee. Am J Sports Med 2001;29(2):201–6.
40. Garretson RB, 3rd, Katolik LI, Verma N, Beck PR, Bach BR, Cole BJ. Contact pressure at osteochondral donor sites in the patellofemoral joint. Am J Sports Med 2004;32(4):967–74.
41. Bartz RL, Kamaric E, Noble PC, Lintner D, Bocell J. Topographic matching of selected donor and recipient sites for osteochondral autografting of the articular surface of the femoral condyles. Am J Sports Med 2001;29(2):207–12.
42. Koh JL, Kowalski A, Lautenschlager E. The effect of angled osteochondral grafting on contact pressure: a biomechanical study. Am J Sports Med 2006;34(1):116–9.
43. Hangody L, Fules P. Autologous osteochondral mosaicplasty for the treatment of full-thickness defects of weight-bearing joints: ten years of experimental and clinical experience. J Bone Joint Surg Am 2003;85-A Suppl 2:25–32.
44. Marcacci M, Kon E, Zaffagnini S, et al. Multiple osteochondral arthroscopic grafting (mosaicplasty) for cartilage defects of the knee: prospective study results at 2-year follow-up. Arthroscopy 2005;21(4):462–70.
45. Jakob RP, Franz T, Gautier E, Mainil-Varlet P. Autologous osteochondral grafting in the knee: indication, results, and reflections. Clin Orthop Relat Res 2002(401):170–84.
46. Chow JC, Hantes ME, Houle JB, Zalavras CG. Arthroscopic autogenous osteochondral transplantation for treating knee cartilage defects: a 2- to 5-year follow-up study. Arthroscopy 2004;20(7):681–90.
47. Outerbridge HK, Outerbridge RE, Smith DE. Osteochondral defects in the knee. A treatment using lateral patella autografts. Clin Orthop Relat Res 2000(377):145–51.
48. Karataglis D, Green MA, Learmonth DJ. Autologous osteochondral transplantation for the treatment of chondral defects of the knee. Knee 2006;13(1):32–5.
49. Marymont JV, Shute G, Zhu H, et al. Computerized matching of autologous femoral grafts for the treatment of medial talar osteochondral defects. Foot Ankle Int 2005;26(9):708–12.
50. Garrett JC. Fresh osteochondral allografts for treatment of articular defects in osteochondritis dissecans of the lateral femoral condyle in adults. Clin Orthop Relat Res 1994(303):33–7.
51. Emmerson BC, Görtz S, Jamali AA, Chung CB, Amiel D, Bugbee WD. Fresh Osteochondral Allografting in the Treatment of Osteochondritis Dissecans of the Femoral Condyle. Read at the 2006 Symposium of the International Cartilage Repair Society 2006, San Diego, CA, January 9–11, 2006; Paper 10c-8.
52. Görtz S, Ho A, Bugbee W. Fresh Osteochondral Allograft Transplantation for Cartilage Lesions in the Knee. Read at the American Academy of Orthopaedic Surgeons 73rd Annual Meeting 2006, Chicago, IL, March 22–26, 2006; Paper #151.

53. Park DY, Chung CB, Bugbee WD. Fresh Osteochondral Allografts for Younger, Active Individuals with Osteoarthrosis of the Knee. Read at the American Academy of Orthopaedic Surgeons 73rd Annual Meeting 2006, Chicago, IL, March 22–26, 2006; Paper #152.
54. Bugbee WD, Khadivi B. Fresh Osteochondral Allografting in the Treatment of Osteonecrosis of the Knee. Read at the 71st Annual Meeting of the American Academy of Orthopaedic Surgeons 2004, San Francisco, CA, March 10–14, 2004; Paper #108.
55. Chu CR, Convery FR, Akeson WH, Meyers M, Amiel D. Articular cartilage transplantation. Clinical results in the knee. Clin Orthop Relat Res 1999(360):159–68.
56. McDermott AG, Langer F, Pritzker KP, Gross AE. Fresh small-fragment osteochondral allografts. Long-term follow-up study on first 100 cases. Clin Orthop Relat Res 1985(197):96–102.
57. Ghazavi MT, Pritzker KP, Davis AM, Gross AE. Fresh osteochondral allografts for post-traumatic osteochondral defects of the knee. J Bone Joint Surg Br 1997;79(6):1008–13.
58. Beaver RJ, Mahomed M, Backstein D, Davis A, Zukor DJ, Gross AE. Fresh osteochondral allografts for post-traumatic defects in the knee. A survivorship analysis. J Bone Joint Surg Br 1992;74(1):105–10.
59. Aubin PP, Cheah HK, Davis AM, Gross AE. Long-term followup of fresh femoral osteochondral allografts for posttraumatic knee defects. Clin Orthop Relat Res 2001(391 Suppl):S318–27.
60. Görtz S, Bugbee WD. Fresh Osteochondral Allograft Resurfacing of the Ankle. Oper Tech Orthop 2006;16(4):244–49.
61. van de Breevaart Bravenboer J, In der Maur CD, Bos PK, et al. Improved cartilage integration and interfacial strength after enzymatic treatment in a cartilage transplantation model. Arthritis Res Ther 2004;6(5):R469–76.
62. Siebert CH, Schneider U, Sopka S, Wahner T, Miltner O, Niedhart C. Ingrowth of osteochondral grafts under the influence of growth factors: 6-month results of an animal study. Arch Orthop Trauma Surg 2006;126(4):247–52.
63. D'Lima D, Hermida J, Hashimoto S, Colwell C, Lotz M. Caspase inhibitors reduce severity of cartilage lesions in experimental osteoarthritis. Arthritis Rheum 2006;54(6):1814–21.

18

Autologous Chondrocyte Cartilage Repair

Stefan Marlovits

Abstract: Articular cartilage injuries are one of the most common types of injuries seen in orthopaedic practice. The treatment of articular cartilage damage remains a challenge because cartilage has a limited capacity for spontaneous repair after traumatic insult or degenerative joint disease. As a result, several therapeutic strategies have been developed to restore articular cartilage and produce a durable repair. Surgical therapeutic efforts to treat cartilage defects have focused on delivering new cells capable of chondrogenesis into the lesions. Autologous chondrocyte transplantation (ACT) is an advanced, cell-based, orthobiologic technology used for the treatment of chondral defects of the knee, which has been in clinical use since 1987. With ACT, good to excellent clinical results are seen in isolated posttraumatic lesions of the knee joint in the younger patient, with the formation of hyaline or hyaline-like repair tissue. In the classic ACT technique, chondrocytes are isolated from small slices of cartilage harvested arthroscopically from a minor weight bearing area of the injured knee. The cells are expanded in vitro in cell culture and re-implanted beneath a periosteal patch covering the cartilage defect. ACT provides significant and long-term benefits for patients, with diminished pain and improved function in most cases. Most complications are directly related to the periosteal graft with periosteal hypertrophy, delamination of the transplant, arthrofibrosis and transplant failure. The need for a periosteal flap, and the complications associated with the periosteal flap, have led to the development of biomaterials as carriers for chondrocytes. Thus, efforts are now focused toward a tissue engineering approach, which combines laboratory-grown cells with appropriate three-dimensional biocompatible scaffolds, as in matrix-associated autologous chondrocyte transplantation (MACT). These biomaterials secure the cells in the defect area and enhance their proliferation and differentiation.

Department of Traumatology, Medical University of Vienna, Vienna, Austria

From: *Orthopedic Biology and Medicine: Musculoskeletal Tissue Regeneration, Biological Materials and Methods*
Edited by W. S. Pietrzak © Humana Press, Totowa, NJ

Keywords: Autologous chondrocyte transplantation (ACT), matrix-associated autologous chondrocyte transplantation (MACT), cartilage defect, surgical cartilage repair, tissue engineering.

18.1. Introduction

Articular cartilage injury and degeneration present challenging problems for orthopaedic surgeons. Every year in the United States over 500,000 arthroplastic procedures are performed; these include 125,000 total hip and 150,000 total knee arthroplasties, and 41,000 open and arthroscopic procedures to repair cartilaginous defects of the knee [1]. Symptomatic full-thickness chondral lesions in the knee pose a difficult management issue for orthopaedists and patients. The prevalence of chondral injuries in an orthopaedist's practice was noted in a retrospective review of 31,516 knee arthroscopies [2]. There were 41 percent Outerbridge Grade III chondral injuries and 19.2 percent Outerbridge Grade IV chondral injuries.

Articular cartilage can tolerate a tremendous amount of intensive and repetitive physical stress. However, it manifests a striking inability to heal after even the most minor injury. Cartilage's response to injury differs from that of other tissues because of its avascularity, the immobility of chondrocytes and the limited ability of mature chondrocytes to proliferate and alter their synthetic patterns. Both the remarkable functional characteristics and the healing limitations reflect the intricacies of its structure and biology. Cartilage is composed of chondrocytes embedded within an extracellular matrix of collagens, proteoglycans and noncollagenous proteins. Together, these substances maintain the proper amount of water within the matrix, which confers its unique mechanical properties. The stringent structural and biological requirements imply that any tissue capable of successful repair or replacement of damaged articular cartilage should be similarly constituted [3].

Symptomatic relief may be temporarily improved by arthroscopic lavage and debridement [4]. Marrow stimulation techniques aim to provide repair tissue of fibrocartilage, which has inferior mechanical properties to hyaline cartilage. Osteochondral autografts or allografts require converting a chondral lesion to an osteochondral injury to effect articular repair [5]. Further therapeutic efforts have focused on bringing in new cells capable of chondrogenesis [3]. An advanced, cell-based, orthobiologic technology, used for the treatment of chondral defects was introduced into clinical practice in the mid-1990s. With autologous chondrocyte transplantation (ACT), good to excellent clinical results have been seen in isolated posttraumatic lesions of the knee joint in the younger patient, with the formation of hyaline or hyaline-like repair tissue [6–7]. Further improvements in tissue engineering have contributed to the next generation of ACT techniques, where cells are combined with resorbable biomaterials in matrix-associated autologous chondrocyte transplantation (MACT) [8].

18.2. Basic Science of Cartilage

18.2.1. Cartilage Biology

The complex structures of synovial joints, developed and progressively refined over hundreds of millions of years, are formed by an arrangement of multiple distinct tissues, including the joint capsule, ligaments, the meniscus, the subchondral bone, the synovial tissue and the hyaline articular cartilage [9]. These tissues are self-renewing, respond to alterations in use and provide stable movement with a level of friction less than that achieved by any prosthetic joint. The tissue that contributes the most to these extraordinary functional capacities is the hyaline articular cartilage. It varies in thickness, cell density, matrix composition and mechanical properties within the same joint, among joints and among species; however, in all synovial joints, it consists of the same components, has the same general structure and performs the same functions [10].

Grossly and histologically, adult articular cartilage appears to be a simple inert tissue. When examined from inside a synovial joint, normal articular cartilage appears as a slick, firm surface that resists deformation. Light microscopy shows that it consists primarily of extracellular matrix, with only one type of cell – the chondrocyte – and that it lacks blood vessels, lymphatic vessels and nerves [9]. Articular cartilage is composed of a hydrated gel matrix that contains Type II collagen fibers and sulfated mucopolysaccharies. The matrix macromolecules are synthesized by chondrocytes. Collagen fibrils, principally Type II and cross-linked with Type IX, provide the framework that lends cartilage its tensile strength and structure. The specific deep, crescent arcades of collagen and superficial tangential arrangement are the key to the mechanical integrity and function of normal articular cartilage. Articular cartilage specifically lacks Types I and X collagen, which are often a precursor to endochondral ossification and are normally found in the hypertrophic chondrocytes of the growth plate in skeletally immature bones.

Typically, articular cartilage is divided into four zones: superficial; middle (or transitional); deep (or radial), and the zone of calcified cartilage [11]. Chondrocytes from the different zones differ in size, shape and metabolic activity [12–13]. The relative size and appearance of these zones vary among species and among joints within the same species; although each zone has different morphological features, the boundaries between the zones cannot be sharply defined. Nonetheless, recent biological and mechanical studies have shown that the zonal organization has functional importance. Variations in the matrix within zones allow the distinction of three compartments, or regions: a pericellular region; a territorial region, and an interterritorial region. The pericellular and territorial regions appear to serve the needs of chondrocytes, binding the cell membranes to the matrix macromolecules and protecting the cells from damage during loading and deformation of the tissue. They may also help to transmit mechanical signals to the chondrocytes when the matrix deforms during joint-loading. The primary function of the interterritorial matrix is to provide the mechanical properties of the tissue [9].

Within normal articular cartilage there is only one type of cell: the highly specialized chondrocyte [9]. Chondrocytes from different cartilage zones differ in size, shape and probably metabolic activity [14–16], but all of these cells contain the organelles necessary for matrix synthesis, including endoplasmic reticulum and Golgi membranes. They also frequently contain intracytoplasmic filaments, lipid, glycogen and secretory vesicles, and at least some chondrocytes have short cilia extending from the cell into the matrix [9]. The rate of metabolic activity and the ability of chondrocytes to respond to various challenges is related to the age of the organism [17]. In young animals chondrocytes proliferate, dividing rapidly, and exhibit high rates of matrix synthesis. Once skeletal maturity is reached, their cellular processes slow down, their cell numbers decrease and they rarely divide under normal conditions [18–20]. This fact is important, not only for the interpretation of results of various experimental animal studies on cartilage repair, but also because of its influence on the relative abilities of patients to heal joint surface defects [3].

The matrix of the articular cartilage consists of two major components: the tissue fluid and the framework of structural macromolecules that give the tissues form and stability [9]. Water contributes as much as 80 percent of the wet weight of articular cartilage, and the interaction of the water with the matrix macromolecules substantially influences the mechanical properties of the tissue [9, 21–22]. The structural macromolecules of cartilage, i.e., collagens, proteoglycans and noncollagenous proteins contribute 20 to 40 percent of the wet weight of the tissue [9]. At least 90 percent to 95 percent of the collagen present in articular cartilage is Type II and forms the primary component of the cross-banded fibrils [23–27]. Articular cartilage contains two major classes of proteoglycans: large aggregating proteglycan monomers or aggrecans, and small proteoglycans including decorin, biglycan and fibromodulin [27–30]. The proteoglycan monomers consist of a central protein core with multiple sulfated glycosaminoglycans bound to it. The glycosaminoglycan sidechains, because of the high concentration of anionic charge, bind cations and are hydrophilic [3]. Aggrecans have large numbers of chondroitin-sulfate and keratan-sulfate chains attached to a protein core filament. The small non-aggregating proteoglycans have shorter protein cores than aggrecan molecules; unlike aggrecans, they do not fill a large volume of the tissue or contribute directly to the mechanical behavior of the tissue. Instead, they bind to other macromolecules and probably influence cell function. Decorin and fibromodulin bind with Type II collagen meshwork [27, 31–33]. Biglycan is concentrated in the pericellular matrix and may interact with Type VI collagen [27]. These molecules appear to help organize and maintain the macromolecular structure of the matrix.

The model of a partially hydrated, compressed matrix also helps explain the mechanical and nutritional aspects of hyaline cartilage [34–36]. The close spacing between highly concentrated negatively charged groups contributes to substantial osmotic pressure and charge-to-charge repulsion, responsible for a good deal of the compressive stiffness of hyaline cartilage [35, 37–38]. Under compression interstitial fluid flows out of the permeable collagen-proteoglycan matrix and, when the load is removed, fluid flows back into the tissue. The low permeability of articular cartilage prevents fluid from being quickly squeezed out of the matrix [35]. This allows the fluid phase to "protect" the solid phase of articular cartilage from the shock of high-impact/rapid-loading situations [35]. During the first few seconds of hydrostatic loading, as much as 75 percent of the compressive stress is borne by the fluid phase. After a prolonged period of continuous loading, mechanical equilibrium is reached after the fluid phase has been expressed from cartilage. In this situation all of the load is supported by the solid phase [3]. The interaction between the solid and fluid phases is also responsible for carrying nutrients into the matrix, and conveying metabolites away. This could be a major reason why repair tissue so often appears healthy early on, and then degenerates over time. Nutrition of the chondrocytes occurs by diffusion, which depends on the viscoelastic properties of articular cartilage. It is possible that, if repair tissue differs mechanically from normal articular cartilage, this will lead to alteration in chondrocyte metabolism, with eventual lack of support of the matrix [3].

18.2.2. Cartilage Healing

The body reacts in a uniform fashion when responding to injury. Although there are certain characteristics specific to individual tissues and organs, the general pattern requires two essential ingredients. The presence of specific cells is essential, not only to clean up necrotic material, but also to synthesize new tissue. These cells are either derived from the replication of cells *in situ*, or from cells that have migrated from the wound margin or enter the area by blood vessels. The second requirement is a vascular supply. The vascular system supplies many of the cells mentioned and is also a source of many bioactive molecules, such as growth factors, chemotactic, mitogenic and cytotactic factors, and others that are needed to create the proper biochemical environment for healing. With these basic ingredients, the response to injury is usually described as consisting of three phases: the phase of necrosis; the inflammatory phase, and the remodeling phase [3, 20].

The response of cartilage to injury differs from the classic response because of two important features of the structure of cartilage, of which the most important is its avascular status [20]. The second and third phases of healing are largely mediated by the vascular system and, thus, all the inflammatory and reparative aspects that the vascular system provides are not available to cartilage [20]. The second difference is that the chondrocytes are literally imprisoned in a mesh of collagen and proteoglycan, unable to migrate to the injury site from adjacent healthy cartilage [3]. These conditions will be different if the cartilage injury penetrates through the subchondral plate, providing a pathway to the highly vascular bone [20].

18.2.3. Cartilage Injury

Injury to articular cartilage can be classified into three categories:

1) microdamage or repetitive trauma to the matrix and cells
2) partial-thickness injuries or chondral fractures, representing injury to and macro-disruption of the articular surface, without violation of the subchondral plate
3) osteochondral or full-thickness penetrating injuries, representing injury to the articular surface with extension through the tidemark and into the underlying subchondral bone

The specific response to each type of injury differs in both timing and overall quality of repair [1]. Microdamage to the cells and matrix of articular cartilage, without gross disruption of the articular surface, can be sustained by a single severe impact or by repetitive blunt trauma. Numerous investigators have found repetitive loading of cartilage to result in increased hydration, cellular degeneration and/or death, disruption of collagen ultrastructure with loss of proteoglycans, thickening of subchondral bone, and fissuring, ulceration and softening of the articular surface, with loss of its compressive and tensile stiffness [1, 39–40].

Partial-thickness defects lie entirely within the confines of cartilage tissue itself and do not penetrate beyond the calcified cartilage into subchondral bone; thus, they cannot be accessed by blood-borne cells, nor by macrophages or mesenchymal stem cells located within the bone marrow space. The lesion does not heal and its appearance several months after injury is similar to that observed at the onset [41–46]. As the cartilaginous matrix deterioration progresses, the inability of the surviving chondrocytes to repair the damaged tissue and prevent further damage may result in further degradation of the surrounding articular surface [20].

Full-thickness defects span the entire depth of articular cartilage and also penetrate the subchondral bone marrow; they are, therefore, readily accessible to blood cells, macrophages and mesenchymal cells which reside within this space. When a full-thickness defect is artificially created, blood from the marrow wells up into the lesion, and a space-filling fibrin clot containing inflammatory cells is formed; mesenchymal cells subsequently appear, and these differentiate into chondrocytes [41–42, 47–49]. Although full-thickness defects become filled with repair tissue that bears a superficial resemblance to hyaline cartilage, this does not persist. Indeed, the repair tissue usually undergoes degeneration within six to 12 months [48–49].

18.2.4. Clinical Classification of Articular Defects

Before repair is attempted, the extent of injury must be assessed. Two major systems have been used to classify and report the severity of articular injuries based on arthroscopic appearance [50].

The Outerbridge classification system was developed to assess chondromalacia of the patella and is often used to classify cartilage injuries of the other articular surfaces of the knee. It documents the progression of cartilaginous defects, primarily according to their depth. Grade 0 represents normal articular cartilage. With grade I defects there is softening and swelling of the cartilage. A grade II defect is a partial-thickness defect; it demonstrates early fissuring on the surface, but it does not reach the subchondral bone, nor does its size exceed 0.5 inch. With grade III defects there is fissuring to the level of the subchondral bone in an area with a diameter > 0.5 inch. Bone is not visibly exposed. In grade IV injuries the subchondral bone is exposed. Clinically, this classification is widely employed, with defect size specified separately [51].

In an alternative system Bauer and Jackson classify lesions of the articular surface according to cartilage fracture patterns [52]. The Bauer and Jackson classification is useful in a descriptive sense as to the initial chondral lesion and its potential cause. For instance, grades I through IV are usually associated with recent trauma; grades V and VI are usually older injuries that may have progressed from an earlier grade, or may represent early degenerative joint disease.

18.2.5. Current Treatment Options

If cartilage repair is to occur, the environment has to be therapeutically manipulated so that the deficiencies inherent in articular cartilage are overcome. Most efforts have focused on correcting the two main shortcomings of articular cartilage: introducing new cells capable of chondrogenesis and facilitating access to the vascular system. Many methods have been used, with varying success in animal studies and clinical trials. These include shaving or debridement of damaged articular cartilage, perforation of the subchondral plate by multiple drill holes or abrasion, osteotomies, and transplantation of osteochondral shell grafts, perichondrium, periosteum, chondrocytes and mesenchymal stem cells [53]. Synthetic gels and implants, such as carbon fiber pads, biodegradable matrices and collagen gels have been used by themselves or as carriers for chondrocytes or growth-stimulating factors. Biological adhesives have been developed as a means to facilitate bonding between native tissue and implanted materials. Allograft tissue and cells have been studied, along with the effect of cryopreservation on subsequent chondrogenesis [3].

18.4. Autologous Chondrocyte Transplantation

There has been a fairly long history of interest in the transplantation of isolated chondrocytes to achieve the healing of cartilage lesions. Smith isolated articular cartilage chondrocytes in 1965 [54]. Chesterman and Smith performed experiments on the transplantation of isolated chondrocytes into cartilage defects in rabbit humeri, and also into the cancellous bone of the iliac crest [17]. In 1971 Bentley and Greer transplanted chondrocytes isolated from young rabbits into the articular surfaces of adult rabbit knees [55]. They concluded that these cells survived, produced matrix, and were incorporated into the articular defects. They also observed that chondrocytes of epiphyseal origin were superior to those of articular origin. Green reported on the use of rabbit chondrocytes grown in culture and subsequently implanted as allografts [56]. Aston and Bentley, in 1982, cultured articular and epiphyseal chondrocytes for up to six weeks [57]. They produced 30 times the number of original cells and found that these cells produced a matrix similar to hyaline cartilage that was positive for Type II collagen.

18.4.1. Review of Preclinical Studies

The basic concept and principle of ACT is a three-step procedure: from a small biopsy of hyaline cartilage, chondrocytes are isolated and expanded in an *in vitro* process (Fig. 18.1). The primary goal of the initial chondrocyte cell culture is to increase the number of cells to provide a sufficient number to fill

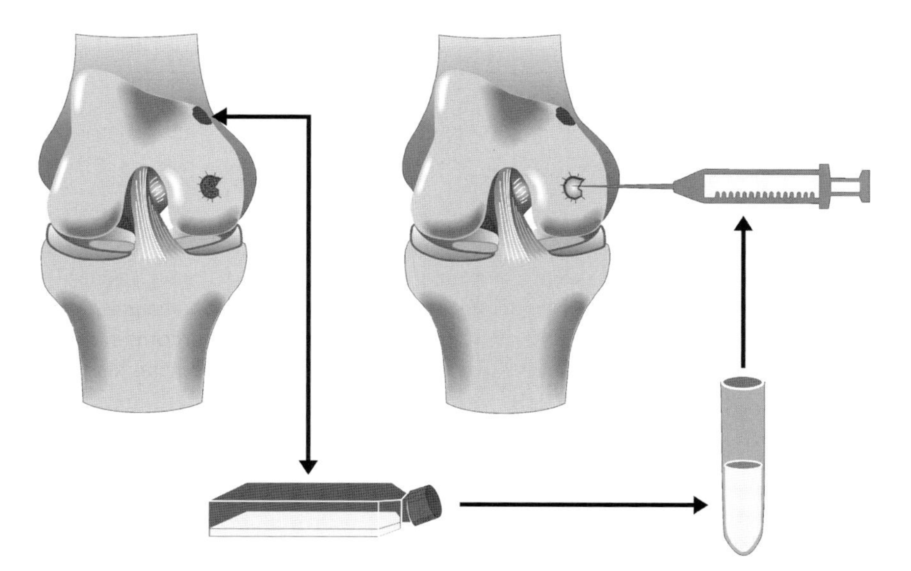

Fig. 18.1 Basic concept of ACT (autologous chondrocyte transplantation) with cell harvesting, expansion in monolayer cell-culture and implantation

a focal defect of articular cartilage. Once a sufficient number of cells has been obtained, the chondrocytes are implanted into the cartilage defect beneath a sealed periosteal flap. After implantation, the cells begin the production of a cartilage matrix that gradually fills out the cartilage defect in the defect area.

In this protocol the periosteal flap is sutured to the surrounding cartilage tissue with its cambium layer facing the defect void, and the cavity below the periosteal flap is filled with autologous chondrocytes, which had been expanded *in vitro* [58–59]. The periosteal flap is inserted in this reversed position to prevent the loss of transplanted cells from the defect void. But, apart from serving the function of a lid, the reversed periosteal flap establishes an unusual and interesting microtopographic situation, in that the repair response can be activated from the cambial layer downward, toward the floor of the defect. There are three hypotheses regarding the physiologic nature of the repair process. One is that the implanted chondrocytes re-populate the area of the defect and produce new cartilage matrix. The periosteal patch functions solely as a watertight seal, which isolates the chondrocytes and permits them to incubate, differentiate and fill the cartilage defect. The second possible explanation is that growth factors in the periosteum are able to stimulate the cultured chondrocytes to divide. The third is that the implant and periosteal patch stimulate chondrocytes in adjacent cartilage, in the subchondral bone or in the periosteum, to enter the defect and repair it. In addition, the periosteal patch may act as a protective semipermeable membrane that allows nutrients from the synovial fluid to nourish the implanted chondrocytes [50, 58].

The technique of ACT was originally developed in experiments involving rabbits by Grande, et al., [60–61] and, more recently, by Brittberg, et al. [62]. In originally studying this possibility, Grande, et al. found that 82 percent of cartilage was reconstituted in rabbits that had received transplants of autologous chondrocytes grown *in vitro*. This compared with a defect fill of only 18 percent in ungrafted controls. Chondrocytes labeled with tritiated thymidine before transplantation accounted for 8 percent of the total number of cells in the healing tissue that filled the defects [61]. Hence, the implanted cells were partly or fully responsible for the repair tissue. Using polarized light microscopy, these investigators showed that the matrix was composed predominantly of Type II collagen. The material properties of the repair tissue were not examined.

Brittberg, et al. studied rabbit patellar lesions that extended through the full thickness of the articular cartilage, but did not invade the subchondral plate [62]. There were four experimental groups: periosteal cover alone; carbon fiber scaffolds with a periosteal cover; autologous chondrocytes with a periosteal cover, and carbon fiber scaffolds seeded with autologous chondrocytes and covered with periosteum. Both groups that included chondrocyte implants demonstrated significantly more repair tissue and a better histological score than their respective controls. In comparing the two groups that received autologous chondrocytes (with and without carbon fiber scaffolds), the 12-week results were similar, but, by 52 weeks, there were more signs of deterioration in the carbon fiber group than in the group with chondrocytes alone. The repair tissue appeared predominantly hyaline-like and most cells were in a cluster formation [62].

This technique also was investigated with the use of a chondral defect model in dogs, without penetration of the subchondral bone, by Breinan, et al. [63].

Twelve to 18 months after the operation those authors were unable to confirm that articular cartilage had been regenerated in the defects that had been treated with transplantation of chondrocytes under a periosteal flap, those that had been treated with a periosteal flap alone, or those that had been left untreated. Furthermore, they could detect no significant differences with regard to any of the parameters that had been used to assess the quality of healing. Damage to adjacent cartilage was attributed to suturing of the periosteal flap to the cartilage [63–65]. In this study postoperative animal care was not controlled, and no measures were taken to ensure that the sutured periosteal flaps were maintained in position by partial or complete immobilization of the joints. Furthermore, the authors made no attempts to ascertain whether the sutured flaps had, indeed, remained in place after one or several months.

The sequence of events that occur after chondrocyte transplantation has been summarized by Itay, et al. [66]. Their observations are based on their model of homologous embryonal chicken chondrocytes embedded in a biological resorbable immobilization vehicle and transplanted into full-thickness osteochondral defects in rooster tibiotarsal joints. The *proliferative* stage takes place during the first four weeks, and is characterized by a rapid increase in the number of chondrocytes and small amounts of extracellular glycosaminoglycan production. Between four and eight weeks the *maturation* stage takes over, and cartilage is formed. The cells differentiate, presumably based on their location within the defect and as a response to local nutritional and mechanical factors. As rates of cellular proliferation decrease, rates of matrix synthesis correspondingly increase. The final stage occurs between two and six months after transplantation and is termed the *transformation* stage. In the subchondral region vascular elements proliferate and penetrate the subchondral portion of the implant. Chondrocytes in this region undergo degenerative changes and are replaced by primary osteons, and the subchondral bone plate is reconstituted. Although the exact nature of the events may vary, depending on certain factors (such as depth of defect, use of synthetic or biological carrier systems and addition of growth factors), this sequence is consistent with the general understanding of chondrogenesis and with observations on other experimental studies of chondrocyte transplantation [3].

18.4.2. Clinical Review

18.4.2.1. Indications

The recommended indications for ACT include patients with focal, full-thickness chondral defects of the femoral condyles, trochlea and osteochondritis dissecans. Relative indications include patellar, tibial or multiple defects, and are evaluated by surgeons based on the available treatment options for each clinical situation. In addition to the knee joint, ACT is performed in the ankle and hip.

The prerequisites for this technique in the knee require appropriate biomechanical alignment, ligamentous stability and range of motion. Patients with abnormal biomechanical alignment, such as a varus knee, may require corrective high tibial osteotomy to alleviate the abnormal force concentration within the involved knee compartment [67]. Patients with patellar tracking abnormalities would require realignment of the extensor mechanism prior to, or in conjunction with, ACT for a patellar or trochlea defect. Anterior cruciate ligament-deficient patients, likewise, require ligament reconstruction in conjunction with ACT for femoral condyle defects. It should be noted, however, that patients with long-standing ligamentous deficiency or biomechanical abnormalities are more likely to have greater degrees of co-existing degenerative changes and, therefore, may not be suitable candidates for this reason. The same is true of patients who have long-standing changes following a distant total menisectomy. For patients with inflammatory arthritis and moderate and severe degenerative joint disease, ACT is not recommended [68]. Hence, preoperative weight bearing radiographic evidence of joint space narrowing, osteophyte formation, subchondral bony sclerosis or cyst formation is a useful screening tool in eliminating patients with osteoarthritis from treatment with ACT [69]. Magnetic resonance (MR) imaging is also helpful in determining the extent of a chondral injury or subtle chondromalacic changes [70]. The gold standard for determining whether a symptomatic patient is a candidate for ACT is a normal radiograph, accompanied by an arthroscopic assessment [5].

18.4.2.2. Surgical Procedure

Arthroscopic assessment of the joint and possible biopsy for articular cartilage culturing requires a careful and systematic evaluation of the articular surfaces with an arthroscopic probe to demonstrate and determine the extent of the symptomatic lesion. The opposing tibial articular surface must be probed throughout to ensure that the mensicus is intact, the articular surface is healthy and, with chondromalacia, that no greater than superficial fissuring is present. The femoral condyle lesion should be assessed from its anterior to posterior length to determine whether it is a contained or an uncontained lesion. The quality and thickness of the surrounding articular cartilage should also be assessed [5].

If a lesion is considered appropriate for ACT, a biopsy of healthy cartilage is taken for enzymatic digestion and for cell culturing. The most common sites for biopsy are the superior medial edge of the trochlea and the intercondylar notch. Biopsy instruments may include ring curettes or sharp gouges. A cartilage piece of approximately 5 mm width by 1 cm in length, with a weight of 200 mg to 300 mg, contains approximately 200,000 to 300,000 cells that can be enzymatically digested and expanded *in vitro* to approximately 12 million cells per 0.4 cc culture media per implantation vial [5].

After four to six weeks of cultivation time the steps in open chondrocyte implantation include arthrotomy, defect preparation, periosteum procurement, periosteum fixation, periosteum watertight integrity testing, autologous fibrin glue sealant, chondrocyte implantation, wound closure and rehabilitation (Fig. 18.2). Adequate exposure of the cartilage defect is crucial for good suturing technique of the periosteum. For a unicondylar injury, a medial or lateral parapatellar arthrotomy is used. This is usually done through a midline incision or a longitudinal parapatellar incision. For multiple lesions, a traditional medial parapatellar arthrotomy is often required with subluxation or dislocation of the patella with hyperflexion. Cartilage defect preparation is critical and radical debridement of all fissured and undermined articular cartilage surrounding the full-thickness chondral injury to healthy contained cartilage is desirable. Small ring or closed curettes are used to debride the degenerating articular cartilage back to healthy host cartilage. Maintaining an intact subchondral bone plate without subchondral bone bleeding is important. It is essential not to perforate the subchondral bone plate, such that a mixed stem cell population does not

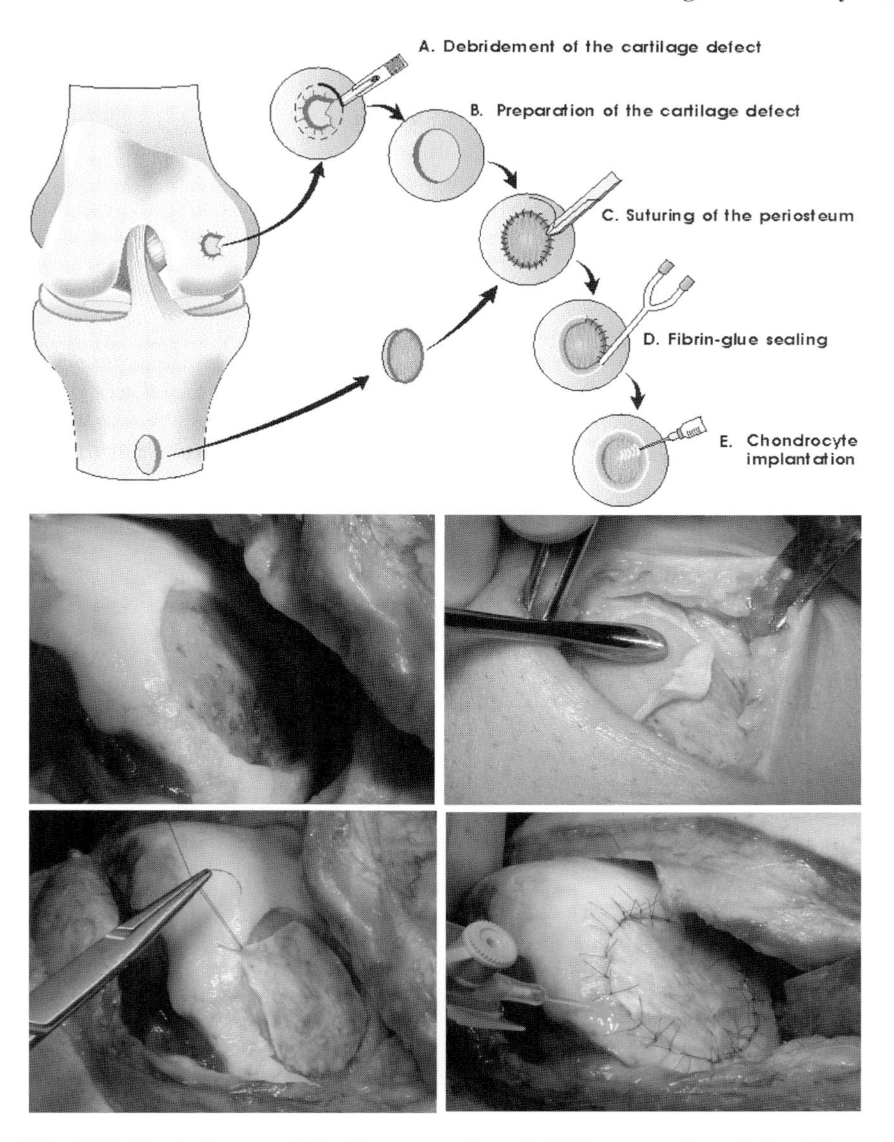

Fig. 18.2 Surgical steps of the first generation of ACT: preparation of the defect, periosteal harvest, suturing the periosteum over the defect, watertightness testing, application of fibrin glue sealant and chondrocyte implantation. The clinical pictures show the preparation of the cartilage defect on the medial femoral condyle down to the subchondral bone, the harvesting of the periosteum, the suturing of the periosteum over the cartilage defect and the application of the cell through a syringe (clinical picture from Lars Peterson, Sweden)

populate the chondral defect in addition to the *in vitro*-grown chondrocytes. A mixed cell population will favor the formation of fibrocartilage, whereas chondrocytes alone can contribute to the formation of hyaline cartilage. If there is any bleeding of the bony bed, this can usually be stopped by using a combination of thrombin and epinephrine soaked in a surgical swab that is applied to the defect and gently pressed for several minutes. Upon removal, if there continues to be some bleeding, a small drop of fibrin glue will usually suffice to make the defect dry. Once a healthy defect bed is prepared, it is templated with sterile tracing paper. A sterile marker can be used to template the defect and it can be cut out to fit the defect perfectly.

The easiest and most suitable location for periosteum procurement is from the proximal medial tibia, distal to the pes anserinus insertion on the subcutaneous border. At this site, there is subcutaneous fat, a very thin fascial layer, and the periosteum is easily accessed. Once defect size has been assessed and templated, a second incision is made approximately a fingerbreadth distal to the pes anserinus insertion, in the center of the medial subcutaneous border of the tibia. Subcutaneous fat is incised initially and then scissor dissection will reveal the shiny white proximal tibial periosteum. The template is then placed on the periosteum or, alternatively, it is marked with a ruler and a sterile marking pen. A small sharp periosteal elevator is then useful in very gently advancing the periosteum from its bony bed and preventing it from under rolling so that it does not rip. It is important to handle the periosteum delicately so that it is not perforated, and so that it is kept moist and does not undergo shrinkage or cambium cell death. Its orientation is always maintained such that the cambium layer is facing toward the subchondral bone plate.

There are three goals of periosteum fixation: provide a watertight membrane that acts as a mechanical seal; establish a semipermeable membrane for intra-articular synovial nutrition to chondrocytes, and maintain a viable periosteal cambium layer of cells so that interactive growth factors between chondrocytes and periosteum may enhance chondrocyte growth. Sutures are placed through the periosteum and then the articular surface, the knots being tied in the side of the periosteum such that they remain below the level of the adjacent cartilage. Periosteum watertight integrity testing is assessed by using a plastic angiocath with a syringe filled with saline. The angiocath is placed deep to the periosteum into the defect and, by gently filling the defect with saline, a meniscus should rise to the opening if the defect is watertight. The saline is then aspirated from the defect and, if water integrity cannot be obtained simply by a suture technique, then a fibrin sealant is used. After sealing the defect, water integrity is tested once more. The saline is then aspirated from the defect bed and the autologous chondrocyte suspension is delivered through the superior opening of the periosteal defect margin down to the base of the defect. As the angiocath is withdrawn, cells are injected until a meniscus comes to the surface. When the defect is filled with cells, final sutures are used to close the injection site, which is then sealed with fibrin glue as well. The procedure is now completed, and drains are not used within the joint, so as not to damage the periosteal patch or suck out the cells from the defect. When drains are needed, it should be without suction. The wound is then closed in layers, and a soft dressing is applied to the knee. Prophylactic intravenous cephalosporin antibiotics are used for 24 to 48 hours after surgery [5].

18.4.2.3. Postoperative Rehabilitation

There are three main goals in the postoperative period: to enhance chondrocyte regeneration and decrease the likelihood of intra-articular adhesions with aggressive range of motion exercises; to protect weight bearing for six to 12 weeks after surgery to prevent the likelihood of periosteal overload and central degeneration or delamination of the graft, and isometric muscle exercises to regain muscle tone and prevent atrophy. The concept of a time course of healing of ACT follows clinical observations of a composite of improving patient symptomatology, as well as arthroscopic second looks accompanied by an animal model that assessed the histologic appearance of healing transplants.

The stages of proliferation (zero to six weeks), transition or maturation (seven to 26 weeks), and remodeling or transformation (27 weeks onward) have been described. Proliferation denotes the rapid response of defect filling with primitive repair tissue by six weeks, which is soft. The transitional phase demonstrates macromolecular matrix production histologically, and clinically, the graft starts to "firm up," taking on the texture of a gelatin. The remodeling stage demonstrates further cellular activity, with matrix production accompanied by further mechanical hardening. The grafts are vulnerable to injury during these stages of healing when, mechanically, the grafts are not as firm as the adjacent articular surfaces.

Continuous passive motion (CPM) is instituted as soon as possible after the operation, or starting the next day. With weight bearing femoral condyles, CPM is increased to regain a full range-of-motion, to patient tolerance, with a very slow cycle setting of approximately two minutes. CPM is used for approximately six to eight hours daily for up to six weeks postoperatively. This is based on experimental work that has demonstrated an enhancement of the quality of repair tissue via this modality, as well as a clinical work, which has demonstrated an increased repair tissue fill with the use of CPM six to eight hours per day for six to eight weeks postoperatively [71–72]. Weight bearing for the femoral condyles is protected at touch weight bearing status for six weeks postoperatively on crutches. Thereafter, weight bearing is increased to full body weight by 12 weeks postoperatively. Each patient's progress is individualized and is guided by symptoms. If weight bearing discomfort, catching, locking or swelling of the knee occur, then the weight bearing status and activity level are decreased as tolerated by the patient. These signs may indicate that the graft is undergoing overload, with stimulation of the subchondral bone and resulting in pain for the patient. On average, it is four to 4.5 months before patients have discarded their canes and are walking relatively comfortably with a small effusion [73].

18.4.2.4. Clinical Outcome

A variety of outcome measures are in clinical use, but studies commonly apply a combination of the following: arthroscopy, MRI, clinical assessment and histology. Arthroscopic visual evaluation and probing are still the best source of information on the state of the repaired and surrounding area, but this invasive method inevitably involves surgery and anesthesia. The use of arthroscopic indenters adds comparative biomechanical measurements (cartilage stiffness testing) to visual arthroscopic evaluation. MR imaging is becoming an increasingly effective, noninvasive method of assessing articular cartilage defects and repairs [74–76]. Advanced MR imaging has been developed using additional articular cartilage and subchondral protocols [77–79].

The clinical outcome instruments used for the assessment of articular cartilage repair are different, validated knee-specific and life quality scores (the International Knee Documentation Committee [IKDC] form, the Tegner activity scale, the Cincinnati knee scale, the Hospital for Special Surgery knee scale, the Western Ontario and McMaster Universities Osteoarthritis Index

[WOMAC], the Knee Society knee scale, the Knee injury and Osteoarthritis Outcome Score [KOOS] and the Lysholm knee scale). A morphological catalogue for assessing cartilage repair is provided by the International Cartilage Repair Society (ICRS), which could also be used for the validation of other techniques, such as MRI, mechanical testing and biomarkers [80].

Based on the successful results obtained in animal studies, Brittberg, et al. [81], in Sweden decided to attempt the same technique in patients with cartilage defects of the knee. The initial 23 patients ranged in age from 14 to 48 years. All had symptomatic cartilage defects, ranging in size from 1.6 to 6.5 cm^2. Thirteen patients had femoral condylar defects due to trauma, and three had localized osteochondral lesions due to osteochondritis dissecans. Seven patients suffered debilitating defects of the patella: six had chondromalacia and one had a trauma-related defect. Two years postoperatively, 14 patients with femoral condylar transplants had good to excellent results. Two patients followed for the longest period maintained excellent results at 55 and 59 months postoperatively. The two patients with poor results suffered severe central wear in their grafts, with locking and pain 11 and 14 months after the procedure. Among patients who had received patellar grafts, two of seven had results graded excellent or good, while three patients had fair results, and two had poor results. The two patients with poor results had severe chondromalacia and underwent a second operation for debridement and resection of the failed graft and subchondral bone. Pain and crepitus were considerably reduced following the surgery, and knee-locking or catching ceased completely during the 16- to 66-month follow-up (mean, 39 months). At the second arthroscopy, biopsy specimens extending to the subchondral bone were taken from the central part of the transplant. Biopsy specimens were obtained from 15 of the 16 patients with femoral transplants. Eleven of these 15 biopsy specimens revealed an intact articular surface with a hyaline appearance; chondrocytes were present in lacunae, and metachromatic staining was comparable to that of the surrounding cartilage. Immunohistochemical staining for Type II collagen was positive for five of the femoral transplant biopsy specimens tested. These findings indicate that near normal hyaline cartilage had regenerated in the defect. In most of the biopsy specimens, remnants of the periosteal tissue were seen close to the articular surface. Specimens from four patients contained areas of irregular fibrous tissue surrounded by more hyaline-like tissue. Of the seven patients with patellar transplants only one biopsy specimen revealed an intact articular surface and a hyaline appearance. The other six biopsy specimens revealed central areas of fibrous tissue surrounded by more hyaline tissue. In summary, this initial series of 23 patients yielded highly promising results. Further follow-up confirmed the results of femoral condyle grafts as stated. The authors of the study hypothesize that the poorer results obtained in patients with patellar defects could be attributed to patellar mistracking and could be further improved by correcting these abnormalities concurrently with the implantation.

Gillogly reported his experience in 41 knees undergoing ACT [82]. The average size of the defects was 5.74 cm^2, indicating very large lesions. The average age was 36.2 years and ranged from 14 to 52 years of age. The medial femoral condyle was the most frequent defect site with 27 defects, followed by the lateral femoral condyle (12), trochlea (seven) and patella (six), and one in the lateral tibial plateau. Six patients had osteochondritis dissecans of a femoral condyle, four in the medial condyle and two in the lateral condyle. Nineteen patients underwent concomitant procedures at the time of the implantation for anterior cruciate ligament reconstruction (seven), anteromedialization of the tibial tubercle (12), high tibial osteotomy (one) and meniscal transplant (one). 22 (88 percent) of 25 patients with over a one-year follow-up (range = 12–36 months), patients showed significant improvement and were rated as good, very good or excellent using the Knee Society and Modified Cincinnati rating scales. One patient underwent debridement of hypertrophy of the repair cartilage at six months, and two patients undergoing concomitant procedures required arthroscopic lysis of adhesions for decreased motion at five and six months postoperatively [68].

Minas reported about a group of 44 patients with a follow-up after 12 and 24 months [83]. After one year 72 percent of treated patients improved, whereas 14 percent had no change and 14 percent reported deterioration of the symptoms. Significant initial improvement in quality of life, and in several knee scores, was also consistent after 24 months [83].

In 2000 Peterson reported about 101 patients two to nine years after ACT [7]. Good to excellent clinical results were found in 93 percent of the patients with isolated defects on the femoral condyle, in 67 percent with multiple lesions (defined as multiple femoral lesions in combination with lesions on the trochlea or patella), 89 percent with ostechondritis dissecans, 65 percent with lesions of the patella and 75 percent with lesions of the femoral condyle associated with rupture of the anterior cruciate ligament. Of those 101 patients, seven had transplant failures. In 37 patients a biopsy of the repair tissue was performed during a control arthroscopy. In 17 of these patients (45.9 percent), a homogenous matrix with low cell density, was found and characterized as hyaline-like. Peterson also demonstrated the close correlation between regeneration of hyaline-like cartilage and good clinical results. It was pointed out that initially good clinical results of ACT also correlate with good clinical results in the long-term [7].

In an international multicenter study with over 1,051 patients most cartilage defects were localized on the medial femur condyle, with an average size of 4.6 cm^2, and were described as almost exclusively grade III and IV. Evaluation of 34 patients at 36 months by the surgeon resulted in improvement in 25 patients (73.6 percent), deterioration in three (8.8 percent) and unchanged symptoms in six (17.6 percent). Evaluation by the patients resulted in improvement in 27 patients (77.2 percent), deterioration in four (11.4 percent) and no change in four (11.4 percent) [84].

In 2001 Minas reported about implantation of autologous chondrocytes in patients with simple (isolated unipolar) and complex (multifocal) defects [85]. He also reported about a salvage group of patients with focal defects in joints with radiological signs of early osteoarthritis. In 22 of 169 patients (13 percent) a failure of the implantation was observed, which usually occurred early after implantation (<12 months). In the reported cases the reasons for transplant failure were missing integration or delamination of transplant (13 out of 22), insufficient rehabilitation (two of 22), traumatic occurrence after implantation (four of 22) and progressive degeneration (three of 22). Improvement was achieved in over 80 percent of the patients [85].

In a prospective study, Horas compared ACT with osteochondral transplantation in 40 patients [86]. In the ACT group the mean defect size was

3.86cm^2, compared to the control group with 3.63cm^2. Clinical outcome was similar in both groups two years postoperatively, although the ACT group had a prolonged rehabilitation period. The most significant difference was seen morphologically in control biopsies, with the expected appearance of hyaline cartilage in the osteochondral transplanted group, and fibrous cartilage in the ACT group [86].

In a further prospective study Bentley, et al. studied 100 patients (mean age, 31.3 years; range, 16 to 49 years) with symptomatic chondral and osteochondral lesions of the knee [87]. The patients were randomized to undergo either ACT or mosaicplasty. Most lesions were posttraumatic, and the mean size of the defects was 4.66cm^2. The mean duration of symptoms was 7.2 years, and the mean number of previous operations, excluding arthroscopy, was 1.5. The mean duration of follow-up was 19 months. The clinical outcome of both groups one year postoperatively revealed no statistically significant difference. An excellent or good result was achieved in the ACT group in 88 percent, and in the mosaicplasty group in 69 percent. Arthroscopy at one year demonstrated an excellent or good repair in 82 percent of the ACT procedures, and in 34 percent of the mosaicplasties. All five patellar mosaicplasties failed [87].

Knutsen, et al. studied 80 patients who had symptomatic focal cartilage lesions of the femoral condyles measuring 2 to 10cm^2 [88]. The patients were randomized into two groups: those treated with ACT and those treated with micro-fracture. At two years both groups had significant clinical improvement and there were small differences between the two treatment groups. According to the SF-36 physical component score at two years postoperatively, the improvement in the micro-fracture group was significantly better than that in the autologous chondrocyte implantation group. Younger and more active patients did better in both groups. There were two failures in the ACT group and one in the micro-fracture group. No serious complications were reported. Two years postoperatively, arthroscopy with biopsy for histological evaluation was carried out and obtained in 84 percent of the patients. The histological evaluation of repair tissues showed no significant differences between the two groups. The authors concluded that both methods had acceptable short-term clinical results and there was no significant difference in macroscopic or histological results between the two treatment groups, and no association between the histological findings and clinical outcome at the two-year time-point [88].

18.4.2.5. Complications

The incidence of treatment failure for ACT is low, with the most widely reported causes due to either post-implantation trauma, noncompliance with rehabilitation, returning too early to high impact sports, progressive osteoarthritis or graft delamination. Age, duration of symptoms and the number of prior surgical procedures are the most significant adverse prognostic factors. The most common problems after ACT include early incomplete periosteal graft incorporation into host cartilage and late hypertrophic periosteal response [89]. Periosteal delamination may present with painful catching or complete locking of the knee, depending on whether it is just marginal, partial or complete. It is best managed by sharp excision arthroscopically. The remaining defect may be left alone if it is marginal, and micro-fractured if it is small; a repeat ACT is indicated if it is larger. Periosteal hypertrophy usually occurs 10 percent to 15 percent of the time, at seven to nine months after the cell transplantation. Patients may present with new onset catching from a previously smooth-tracking knee, with symptoms of pain and effusion. If this should occur, the activity level should be decreased and arthroscopic evaluation is recommended. The hypertrophy is normally controlled by trimming the graft to the level of the surrounding cartilage with a motorized shaver. Intra-articular adhesions are uncommon except in the case of large grafts using the femoral periosteum from an intra-articular location. This may enhance intra-articular fibrosis and possibly heterotopic ossification in the quadriceps muscle. If this occurs, adhesions are best released with arthroscopic electrocautery, or gentle shaving and a gentle manipulation after the intra-articular adhesions are released and the grafts are visualized.

18.5. Future Trends and Needs

Despite the promising clinical results obtained, the use of ACT carries a number of limitations essentially related to the complexity of the surgical procedure and the biological response of the periosteum [53, 90]. Thus, efforts are now focused on a tissue engineered approach which combines laboratory-grown cells with appropriate three-dimensional biocompatible scaffolds for the purpose of generating new tissues or tissue equivalents. Tissue engineering has emerged as a potentially new therapy and there would be numerous advantages inherent in such an approach as applied to articular cartilage repair [91–92]. The need for donor tissue would be decreased through *in vitro* amplification of autogenous or allogenic chondrocytes. The scaffolds, by providing an initial framework, could temporarily stabilize the chondrocytes in the defect and direct their spatial distribution within the repair tissue, before the synthesis of collagen and proteoglycan. Given a material of suitable mechanical properties, arthroscopic implantation may be feasible [91]. Such materials can be used as carriers for various growth factors and other bioactive molecules to enhance the environment for cartilage healing. The repair of larger surface defects or, in theory, the entire condyle could be addressed by the fabrication of chondrocyte-polymer composites with specific three-dimensional shapes. The initial mechanical properties, as well as the rate of biodegradation, could be manipulated to support the healing process.

The choice of the scaffold used for the implantation of cells, and which serves as a matrix for their expansion within the defect void, is critical. The matrix should be composed of a material that is biocompatible, mechanically stable and amenable to rapid remodeling; it should also possess properties that ensure its adequate adhesion to the defect surfaces and facilitate the integration of repair- and native-tissue matrices. Bioincompatibility of the matrix may elicit a foreign body, giant-cell reaction or an immunological response, which could delay the formation of cartilage and bone [59]. Investigators have reported that implants formed from a variety of biologic and nonbiologic materials, including treated cartilage and bone matrices, collagens alone, collagens with hyaluronan, fibrin, carbon fiber, hydroxylapatite, porous polylactic acid, polytetrafluoroethylene, polyester and other synthetic polymers, facilitate restoration of an articular surface [93–99]. These efforts have modified the technique of classical ACT and lead to the formation of new generations of cell-based cartilage repair procedures.

The second generation of ACT includes the use of a bilayer collagen membrane, rather than the periosteal flap. These purpose-designed biomaterials are sutured over the prepared cartilage defect and the cell suspension is injected underneath. The use of collagen membrane simplifies the surgical procedure and reduces the length and number of the incisions, thus reducing the overall surgical morbidity. Furthermore, the complication rates of periosteal hypertrophy could be reduced. For example, the use of Chondro-Gide® membrane, a bilayer Type I/Type III collagen scaffold (Geistlich Biomaterials, Pharma AG, Wolhausen, Switzerland), as a chondrocyte cover, results in satisfactory repair and does not appear to show evidence of hypertrophy at one-year arthroscopy, compared to periosteum [100].

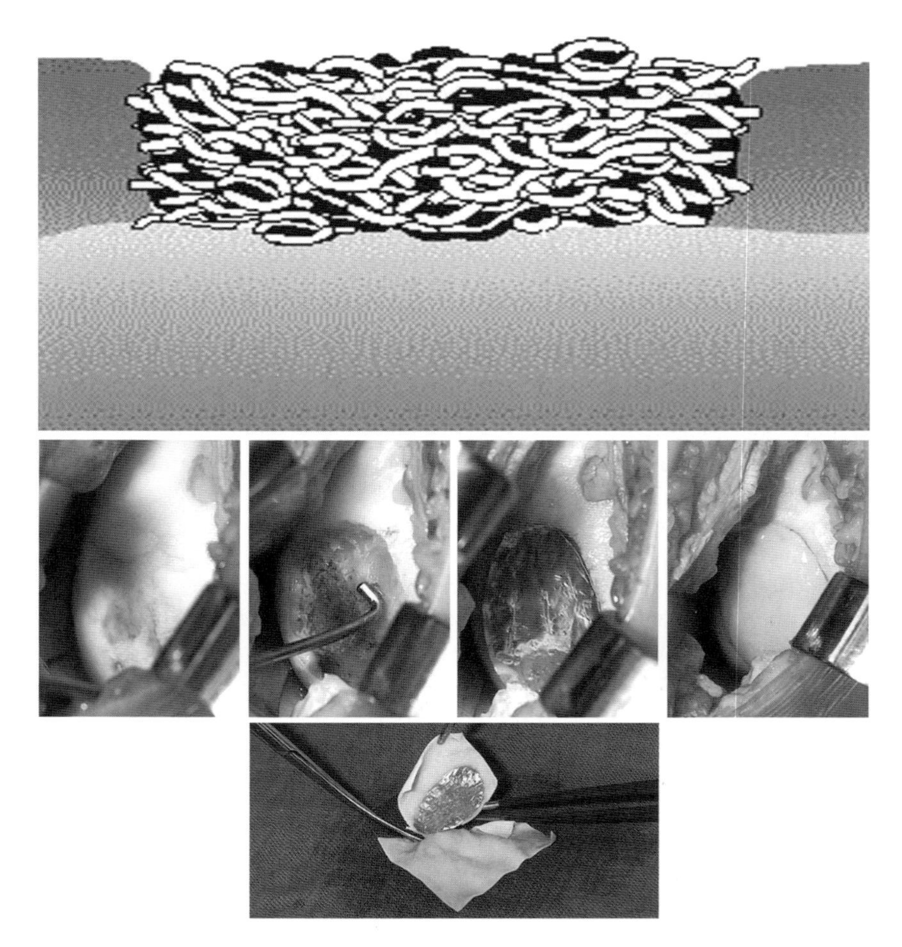

Fig. 18.3 Next generation of ACT: biomaterials seeded with chondrocytes are trimmed to exactly match the defect size and implanted without the use of a periosteal cover or fixing stitches Matrix-associated autologous chondrocyte transplantation (MACI®) using a collagen membrane. The clinical pictures show the cartilage defect on the medial femoral condyle, the preparation of the defect down to the subchondral bone, the use of a template for the graft preparation and the fixation of the graft with fibrin glue in the cartilage defect

Further technological advances have led to the third generation of ACT with the use of biomaterials seeded with chondrocytes as carriers and scaffolds for cell growth. This composite "all-in-one" tissue engineered approach combines cultured chondrocytes with three-dimensional biocompatible scaffolds. After debridement of the defect, the biomaterials with seeded cells are trimmed to exactly match the defect size and implanted without the use of a periosteal cover or fixing stitches (Fig. 18.3). In most techniques only fibrin glue is used for the fixation of the graft. Because there is no requirement for periosteal harvesting and stitching the cover over the recipient site, a mini-arthrotomy technique can be used. Resorbable collagen membranes, mainly shaped in a bilayer of Type I/Type III collagen scaffold, such as Chondro-Gide® (Geistlich Biomaterials, Pharma AG, Wolhausen, Switzerland) or Maix® collagen membrane (Matricel, Herzoenrath, Germany), have been used as cell carriers for the MACI® technique (MACI®: Matrix-induced Autologous Chondrocyte Implantation, Verigen, Leverkusen, Germany and Genzyme, Boston, MA, USA). Another biomaterial in routine clinical use is the hyaluronan-based biodegradable polymer scaffold, Hyaff®-11 (Fida Advanced Biopolymers, Abano Terme, Italy), in combination with autologous chondrocytes, Hyalograft® C [101–103]. Other biomaterials that are in experimental and clinical use are polymers of polylactide and polyglycolide (Ethicon, Norderstedt, Germany), which may offer new possibilities for cartilage repair, and are used for cartilage repair as Bioseed®-C (Freiburg, Germany) [104]. A biphasic membrane combines a collagen network with a chondoritin matrix and this has been tested in clinical studies (Novocart® 3D, Tetec Aesculap Braun, Tuttlingen, Germany). Another new technology uses a three-dimensional collagen gel consisting of Type I collagen as a three-dimensional carrier for the cells (CaReS®, Arthro Kinetics, Esslingen Germany). In contrast to the other techniques, the isolated chondrocytes are immediately cultivated in the collagen gel with no expansion in monolayer culture.

The lack of studies that directly compare different types of artificial matrices makes it difficult to evaluate their relative merits, but the available reports have shown that this approach can contribute to restoration of an articular surface [97–98, 105–106]. Clinical data for the matrix-associated cartilage cell transplantation have been mostly collected in observational studies. In a clinical pilot study the attachment rate of the MACI® technique was determined. The chondrocyte-scaffold construct was implanted and fixed in full-thickness, weight bearing cartilage defects of the femoral condyle with fibrin glue only and with no further surgical fixation. Sixteen patients were followed prospectively, and the early postoperative attachment rate at 34.7 (range, 22 to 47) days after the scaffold implantation, was determined with the use of high resolution MRI. In 14 of 16 patients (87.5 percent) a completely attached graft was observed and, in two patients, a partial attachment and complete detachment, respectively. In conclusion, the implantation and fixation of a cell-scaffold construct in a deep cartilage defect of the femoral condyle with fibrin glue only and with no further surgical fixation leads to a high attachment rate [107]. Cherubino used the MACI® technique in 13 patients with an average age of 35 years and a mean defect size of $3.5cm^2$. Improvement in clinical outcome could be found 6.5 (range, two to 15) months after the surgery in all patients [108]. In a cohort study with 67 patients, a fleece composed of autologous chondrocytes grown on a scaffold entirely made of Hyaff 11, an esterified derivative of hyaluronic acid, was used to treat cartilage defects of the knee (Hyalograft® C). After 17.5 months a subjective improvement was reported by 97 percent of the group. Objective evaluation of knees showed improvement in 87 percent, with an increase in quality-of-life in 94 percent. In the majority of analyzed control biopsies, hyaline-like regenerative tissue could be found [101]. The results of an ongoing multicenter clinical study with the use of Hyalograft® C for the treatment of cartilage defects of the knee, and the clinical results were presented on a cohort of 141 patients, with follow-up assessments ranging from two to five years (average follow-up time: 38 months). At follow-up 91.5 percent of patients improved according to the IKDC subjective evaluation; 76 percent and 88 percent of patients had no pain or mobility problems. Furthermore, 95.7 percent of the patients had their treated knee rated as normal or nearly normal, as assessed by the surgeon. The arthroscopic evaluation of the cartilage repair side was graded as normal or nearly normal in 96.4 percent of the scored knees. In addition, the majority of the second-look biopsies of the grafted site were assessed histologically as hyaline-like [102].

18.6. Conclusion

On the basis of published results, ACT can be considered an efficient and safe therapeutic option for the treatment of large and profound cartilage defects of the knee. The best results have been reported for posttraumatic lesions and osteochondritis dissecans.

In the planning and restoration of an articular defect, any significant comorbidity must be diagnosed and corrected, i.e., a meniscal deficiency, ligament laxity or mechanical malalignment of the tibiofemoral or patellofemoral joint. Uncorrected meniscal deficiency and ligament laxity are a contraindication for cartilage restoration procedures. Most patella and trochlear cartilage restoration procedures should be combined with patella realignment procedures. A high tibial osteotomy is required to correct the varus angulation of the lower limb mechanical axis when performing a cartilage restoration procedure in the medial compartment of a varus knee. For valgus angulation of a knee joint, a distal femoral osteotomy is required to restore the mechanical axis to neutral. It is important to carefully plan a sequence of surgical and rehabilitation options, and to consider staging procedures if necessary.

Patient selection and surgical technical expertise are factors that directly contribute to the success of ACT surgery. In addition, patient-related factors, as well as the biological characteristics and potency of the expanded chondrocytes and their quality assurance, are of increasing significance. The loss of specific morphological, biochemical and physiological characteristics of cultured chondrocytes can be altered by modification of cell culture conditions. This leads to the conclusion that there are biologically defined boundaries for cartilage-specific qualities *in vitro*. Further relevant factors include the harvesting technique of the periosteal patch, the amount of transplanted cells and the biology of the subchondral bone. Rehabilitation is also a critical factor in the outcome of ACT and should be carefully planned.

The next generations of ACT, with a combination of biomaterials and cultivated cells, already demonstrates biological and surgical advantages.

References

1. Chen FS, Frenkel SR, Di Cesare PE. Repair of articular cartilage defects: part I. Basic Science of cartilage healing. Am J Orthop 1999;28:31–3.
2. Curl WW, Krome J, Gordon ES, Rushing J, Smith BP, Poehling GG. Cartilage injuries: a review of 31,516 knee arthroscopies. Arthroscopy 1997;13:456–60.
3. Newman AP. Articular cartilage repair. Am J Sports Med 1998;26:309–24.
4. Hubbard MJ. Articular debridement versus washout for degeneration of the medial femoral condyle. A five-year study. J Bone Joint Surg Br 1996;78:217–9.
5. Minas T, Peterson L. Advanced techniques in autologous chondrocyte transplantation. Clin Sports Med 1999;18:13–44.
6. Peterson L, Brittberg M, Kiviranta I, Akerlund EL, Lindahl A. Autologous chondrocyte transplantation. Biomechanics and long-term durability. Am J Sports Med 2002;30:2–12.
7. Peterson L, Minas T, Brittberg M, Nilsson A, Sjogren-Jansson E, Lindahl A. Two- to 9-year outcome after autologous chondrocyte transplantation of the knee. Clin Orthop 2000:212–34.
8. Marlovits S, Zeller P, Singer P, Resinger C, Vecsei V. Cartilage repair: generations of autologous chondrocyte transplantation. Eur J Radiol 2006;57:24–31.
9. Buckwalter JA, Mankin HJ. Articular cartilage: tissue design and chondrocyte-matrix interactions. Instr Course Lect 1998;47:477–86.
10. Mow VC, Ratcliffe A, Rosenwasser MP, Buckwalter JA. Experimental studies on repair of large osteochondral defects at a high weight bearing area of the knee joint: a tissue engineering study. J Biomech Eng 1991;113:198–207.
11. Poole AR, Pidoux I, Reiner A, Rosenberg L. An immunoelectron microscope study of the organization of proteoglycan monomer, link protein, and collagen in the matrix of articular cartilage. J Cell Biol 1982;93:921–37.
12. Aydelotte MB, Greenhill RR, Kuettner KE. Differences between sub-populations of cultured bovine articular chondrocytes. II. Proteoglycan metabolism. Connect Tissue Res 1988;18:223–34.
13. Aydelotte MB, Kuettner KE. Differences between sub-populations of cultured bovine articular chondrocytes. I. Morphology and cartilage matrix production. Connect Tissue Res 1988;18:205–22.
14. Flannery CR, Hughes CE, Schumacher BL, Tudor D, Aydelotte MB, Kuettner KE, Caterson B. Articular cartilage superficial zone protein (SZP) is homologous to megakaryocyte stimulating factor precursor and Is a multifunctional proteoglycan with potential growth-promoting, cytoprotective, and lubricating properties in cartilage metabolism. Biochem Biophys Res Commun 1999;254:535–41.
15. Schumacher BL, Hughes CE, Kuettner KE, Caterson B, Aydelotte MB. Immunodetection and partial cDNA sequence of the proteoglycan, superficial zone protein, synthesized by cells lining synovial joints. J Orthop Res 1999;17:110–20.
16. Hauselmann HJ, Flechtenmacher J, Michal L, Thonar EJ, Shinmei M, Kuettner KE, Aydelotte MB. The superficial layer of human articular cartilage is more susceptible to interleukin-1-induced damage than the deeper layers. Arthritis Rheum 1996;39:478–88.
17. Chesterman PJ, Smith AU. Homotransplantation of articular cartilage and isolated chondrocytes. An experimental study in rabbits. J Bone Joint Surg [Br] 1968;50:184–97.
18. Stockwell RA. The cell density of human articular and costal cartilage. J Anat 1967;101:753–63.
19. Mankin HJ. The effect of aging on articular cartilage. Bull N Y Acad Med 1968;44:545–52.
20. Mankin HJ. The response of articular cartilage to mechanical injury. J Bone Joint Surg [Am] 1982;64:460–6.

21. Lai WM, Mow VC, Roth V. Effects of nonlinear strain-dependent permeability and rate of compression on the stress behavior of articular cartilage. J Biomech Eng 1981;103:61–6.
22. Maroudas A, Schneiderman R. "Free" and "exchangeable" or "trapped" and "non-exchangeable" water in cartilage. J Orthop Res 1987;5:133–8.
23. Bruckner P, Mendler M, Steinmann B, Huber S, Winterhalter KH. The structure of human collagen type IX and its organization in fetal and infant cartilage fibrils. J Biol Chem 1988;263:16911–7.
24. Diab M. The role of type IX collagen in osteoarthritis and rheumatoid arthritis. Orthop Rev 1993;22:165–70.
25. Diab M, Wu JJ, Shapiro F, Eyre D. Abnormality of type IX collagen in a patient with diastrophic dysplasia. Am J Med Genet 1994;49:402–9.
26. Diab M, Wu JJ, Eyre DR. Collagen type IX from human cartilage: a structural profile of intermolecular cross-linking sites. Biochem J 1996;314:327–32.
27. Roughley PJ, Lee ER. Cartilage proteoglycans: structure and potential functions. Microsc Res Tech 1994;28:385–97.
28. Hardingham T, Bayliss M. Proteoglycans of articular cartilage: changes in aging and in joint disease. Semin Arthritis Rheum 1990;20:12–33.
29. Poole AR, Rosenberg LC, Reiner A, Ionescu M, Bogoch E, Roughley PJ. Contents and distributions of the proteoglycans decorin and biglycan in normal and osteoarthritic human articular cartilage. J Orthop Res 1996;14:681–9.
30. Rosenberg L, Choi HU, Tang LH, Pal S, Johnson T, Lyons DA, Laue TM. Proteoglycans of bovine articular cartilage. The effects of divalent cations on the biochemical properties of link protein. J Biol Chem 1991;266:7016–24.
31. Hedbom E, Heinegard D. Interaction of a 59-kDa connective tissue matrix protein with collagen I and collagen II. J Biol Chem 1989;264:6898–905.
32. Hedbom E, Heinegard D. Binding of fibromodulin and decorin to separate sites on fibrillar collagens. J Biol Chem 1993;268:27307–12.
33. Hedlund H, Mengarelli-Widholm S, Heinegard D, Reinholt FP, Svensson O. Fibromodulin distribution and association with collagen. Matrix Biol 1994;14:227–32.
34. Kwan MK, Lai WM, Mow VC. Fundamentals of fluid transport through cartilage in compression. Ann Biomed Eng 1984;12:537–58.
35. Mow VC, Holmes MH, Lai WM. Fluid transport and mechanical properties of articular cartilage: a review. J Biomech 1984;17:377–94.
36. Hardingham TE, Muir H, Kwan MK, Lai WM, Mow VC. Viscoelastic properties of proteoglycan solutions with varying proportions present as aggregates. J Orthop Res 1987;5:36–46.
37. Mow VC, Ratcliffe A, Poole AR. Cartilage and diarthrodial joints as paradigms for hierarchical materials and structures. Biomaterials 1992;13:67–97.
38. Mow VC, Ateshian GA, Spilker RL. Biomechanics of diarthrodial joints: a review of twenty years of progress. J Biomech Eng 1993;115:460–7.
39. Radin EL, Ehrlich MG, Chernack R, Abernethy P, Paul IL, Rose RM. Effect of repetitive impulsive loading on the knee joints of rabbits. Clin Orthop 1978;131:288–93.
40. Dekel S, Weissman SL. Joint changes after overuse and peak overloading of rabbit knees in vivo. Acta Orthop Scand 1978;49:519–28.
41. Mankin HJ. The reaction of articular cartilage to injury and osteoarthritis (second of two parts). N Engl J Med 1974;291:1335–40.
42. Mankin HJ. The reaction of articular cartilage to injury and osteoarthritis (first of two parts). N Engl J Med 1974;291:1285–92.
43. Kim HK, Moran ME, Salter RB. The potential for regeneration of articular cartilage in defects created by chondral shaving and subchondral abrasion. An experimental investigation in rabbits. J Bone Joint Surg [Am] 1991;73:1301–15.
44. Hunziker EB, Rosenberg LC. Repair of partial-thickness defects in articular cartilage: cell recruitment from the synovial membrane. J Bone Joint Surg Am 1996;78:721–33.

45. Wei X, Gao J, Messner K. Maturation-dependent repair of untreated osteochondral defects in the rabbit knee joint. J Biomed Mater Res 1997;34:63–72.
46. Namba RS, Meuli M, Sullivan KM, Le AX, Adzick NS. Spontaneous repair of superficial defects in articular cartilage in a fetal lamb model. J Bone Joint Surg [Am] 1998;80:4–10.
47. Mitchell N, Shepard N. The resurfacing of adult rabbit articular cartilage by multiple perforations through the subchondral bone. J Bone Joint Surg [Am] 1976;58:230–3.
48. Altman RD, Kates J, Chun LE, Dean DD, Eyre D. Preliminary observations of chondral abrasion in a canine model. Ann Rheum Dis 1992;51:1056–62.
49. Shapiro F, Koide S, Glimcher MJ. Cell origin and differentiation in the repair of full-thickness defects of articular cartilage. J Bone Joint Surg Am 1993;75:532–53.
50. Minas T, Nehrer S. Current concepts in the treatment of articular cartilage defects. Orthopedics 1997;20:525–38.
51. Outerbridge RE. The etiology of chondromalacia patellae. J Bone Joint Surg [Br] 1961;43:752–67.
52. Bauer M, Jackson RW. Chondral lesions of the femoral condyles: a system of arthroscopic classification. Arthroscopy 1988;4:97–102.
53. Hunziker EB. Articular cartilage repair: basic science and clinical progress. A review of the current status and prospects. Osteoarthritis Cartilage 2002;10:432–63.
54. Smith AU. Survival of frozen chondrocytes isolated from cartilage of adult mammals. Nature 1965;205:782–4.
55. Bentley G, Greer RB 3rd. Homotransplantation of isolated epiphyseal and articular cartilage chondrocytes into joint surfaces of rabbits. Nature 1971;230:385–8.
56. Green WT, Jr. Articular cartilage repair. Behavior of rabbit chondrocytes during tissue culture and subsequent allografting. Clin Orthop 1977;124:237–50.
57. Aston JE, Bentley G. Repair of articular surfaces by allografts of articular and growth- plate cartilage. J Bone Joint Surg [Br] 1986;68:29–35.
58. Brittberg M, Lindahl A, Nilsson A, Ohlsson C, Isaksson O, Peterson L. Treatment of deep cartilage defects in the knee with autologous chondrocyte transplantation. N Engl J Med 1994;331:889–95.
59. Hunziker EB. Articular cartilage repair: are the intrinsic biological constraints undermining this process insuperable? Osteoarthritis Cartilage 1999;7:15–28.
60. Grande DA, Singh IJ, Pugh J. Healing of experimentally produced lesions in articular cartilage following chondrocyte transplantation. Anat Rec 1987;218:142–8.
61. Grande DA, Pitman MI, Peterson L, Menche D, Klein M. The repair of experimentally produced defects in rabbit articular cartilage by autologous chondrocyte transplantation. J Orthop Res 1989;7:208–18.
62. Brittberg M, Nilsson A, Lindahl A, Ohlsson C, Peterson L. Rabbit articular cartilage defects treated with autologous cultured chondrocytes. Clin Orthop 1996;326:270–83.
63. Breinan HA, Minas T, Hsu HP, Nehrer S, Sledge CB, Spector M. Effect of cultured autologous chondrocytes on repair of chondral defects in a canine model. J Bone Joint Surg Am 1997;79:1439–51.
64. Hunziker EB, Kapfinger E. Removal of proteoglycans from the surface of defects in articular cartilage transiently enhances coverage by repair cells. J Bone Joint Surg Br 1998;80:144–50.
65. O'Driscoll SW. The healing and regeneration of articular cartilage. J Bone Joint Surg Am 1998;80:1795–812.
66. Itay S, Abramovici A, Nevo Z. Use of cultured embryonal chick epiphyseal chondrocytes as grafts for defects in chick articular cartilage. Clin Orthop 1987;220:284–303.
67. Coventry MB, Ilstrup DM, Wallrichs SL. Proximal tibial osteotomy. A critical long-term study of eighty-seven cases. J Bone Joint Surg Am 1993;75:196–201.

68. Gillogly SD, Voight M, Blackburn T. Treatment of articular cartilage defects of the knee with autologous chondrocyte implantation. J Orthop Sports Phys Ther 1998;28:241–51.
69. Rosenberg TD, Paulos LE, Parker RD, Coward DB, Scott SM. The forty-five-degree posteroanterior flexion weight-bearing radiograph of the knee. J Bone Joint Surg [Am] 1988;70:1479–83.
70. Marlovits S, Singer P, Zeller P, Mandl I, Haller J, Trattnig S. Magnetic resonance observation of cartilage repair tissue (MOCART) for the evaluation of autologous chondrocyte transplantation: determination of interobserver variability and correlation to clinical outcome after 2 years. Eur J Radiol 2006;57:16–23.
71. Salter RB. The biologic concept of continuous passive motion of synovial joints. The first 18 years of basic research and its clinical application. Clin Orthop 1989;242:12–25.
72. O'Driscoll SW, Salter RB. The induction of neochondrogenesis in free intra-articular periosteal autografts under the influence of continuous passive motion. An experimental investigation in the rabbit. J Bone Joint Surg [Am] 1984;66:1248–57.
73. Hambly K, Bobic V, Wondrasch B, Van Assche D, Marlovits S. Autologous chondrocyte implantation postoperative care and rehabilitation: science and practice. Am J Sports Med 2006;34:1020–38.
74. Peterfy CG, Linares R, Steinbach LS. Recent advances in magnetic resonance imaging of the musculoskeletal system. Radiol Clin North Am 1994;32:291–311.
75. Recht M, Bobic V, Burstein D, Disler D, Gold G, Gray M, Kramer J, Lang P, McCauley T, Winalski C. Magnetic resonance imaging of articular cartilage. Clin Orthop 2001;391 Suppl:S379–96.
76. Trattnig S. Overuse of hyaline cartilage and imaging. Eur J Radiol 1997;25:188–98.
77. Imhof H, Nobauer-Huhmann IM, Krestan C, Gahleitner A, Sulzbacher I, Marlovits S, Trattnig S. MRI of the cartilage. Eur Radiol 2002;12:2781–93.
78. Marlovits S, Striessnig G, Resinger CT, Aldrian SM, Vecsei V, Imhof H, Trattnig S. Definition of pertinent parameters for the evaluation of articular cartilage repair tissue with high-resolution magnetic resonance imaging. Eur J Radiol 2004;52:310–9.
79. Recht M, White LM, Winalski CS, Miniaci A, Minas T, Parker RD. MR imaging of cartilage repair procedures. Skeletal Radiol 2003;32:185–200.
80. Mainil-Varlet P, Aigner T, Brittberg M, Bullough P, Hollander A, Hunziker E, Kandel R, Nehrer S, Pritzker K, Roberts S, Stauffer E. Histological assessment of cartilage repair: a report by the Histology Endpoint Committee of the International Cartilage Repair Society (ICRS). J Bone Joint Surg Am 2003;85-A Suppl 2:45–57.
81. Brittberg M, Lindahl A, Nilsson A, Ohlsson C, Isaksson O, Peterson L. Treatment of deep cartilage defects in the knee with autologous chondrocyte transplantation. N Engl J Med 1994;331:889–95.
82. Gillogly SD, Voight M, Blackburn T. Treatment of articular cartilage defects of the knee with autologous chondrocyte implantation. J Orthop Sports Phys Ther 1998;28:241–51.
83. Minas T. Chondrocyte implantation in the repair of chondral lesions of the knee: economics and quality of life. Am J Orthop 1998;27:739–44.
84. Erggelet C, Browne JE, Fu F, Mandelbaum BR, Micheli LJ, Mosely JB. Autologous chondrocyte transplantation for treatment of cartilage defects of the knee joint. Clinical results. Zentralbl Chir 2000;125:516–22.
85. Minas T. Autologous chondrocyte implantation for focal chondral defects of the knee. Clin Orthop 2001:291 Suppl:S349–61.
86. Horas U, Pelinkovic D, Herr G, Aigner T, Schnettler R. Autologous chondrocyte implantation and osteochondral cylinder transplantation in cartilage repair of the knee joint. A prospective, comparative trial. J Bone Joint Surg Am 2003;85-A:185–92.
87. Bentley G, Biant LC, Carrington RW, Akmal M, Goldberg A, Williams AM, Skinner JA, Pringle J. A prospective, randomised comparison of autologous chondrocyte implantation versus mosaicplasty for osteochondral defects in the knee. J Bone Joint Surg Br 2003;85:223–30.

88. Knutsen G, Engebretsen L, Ludvigsen TC, Drogset JO, Grontvedt T, Solheim E, Strand T, Roberts S, Isaksen V, Johansen O. Autologous chondrocyte implantation compared with microfracture in the knee. A randomized trial. J Bone Joint Surg Am 2004;86-A:455–64.
89. Wood JJ, Malek MA, Frassica FJ, Polder JA, Mohan AK, Bloom ET, Braun MM, Cote TR. Autologous cultured chondrocytes: adverse events reported to the United States Food and Drug Administration. J Bone Joint Surg Am 2006;88:503–7.
90. Brittberg M, Peterson L, Sjogren-Jansson E, Tallheden T, Lindahl A. Articular cartilage engineering with autologous chondrocyte transplantation. A review of recent developments. J Bone Joint Surg Am 2003;85-A Suppl 3:109–15.
91. Freed LE, Grande DA, Lingbin Z, Emmanual J, Marquis JC, Langer R. Joint resurfacing using allograft chondrocytes and synthetic biodegradable polymer scaffolds. J Biomed Mater Res 1994;28:891–9.
92. Freed LE, Vunjak-Novakovic G, Biron RJ, Eagles DB, Lesnoy DC, Barlow SK, Langer R. Biodegradable polymer scaffolds for tissue engineering. Biotechnology (N Y) 1994;12:689–93.
93. Hanff G, Sollerman C, Abrahamsson SO, Lundborg G. Repair of osteochondral defects in the rabbit knee with Gore-Tex (expanded polytetrafluoroethylene). An experimental study. Scand J Plast Reconstr Surg Hand Surg 1990;24:217–23.
94. Klompmaker J, Jansen HW, Veth RP, Nielsen HK, de Groot JH, Pennings AJ. Porous polymer implants for repair of full-thickness defects of articular cartilage: an experimental study in rabbit and dog. Biomaterials 1992;13:625–34.
95. Messner K, Gillquist J. Synthetic implants for the repair of osteochondral defects of the medial femoral condyle: a biomechanical and histological evaluation in the rabbit knee. Biomaterials 1993;14:513–21.
96. Vacanti CA, Kim W, Schloo B, Upton J, Vacanti JP. Joint resurfacing with cartilage grown in situ from cell-polymer structures. Am J Sports Med 1994;22:485–8.
97. Hendrickson DA, Nixon AJ, Grande DA, Todhunter RJ, Minor RM, Erb H, Lust G. Chondrocyte-fibrin matrix transplants for resurfacing extensive articular cartilage defects. J Orthop Res 1994;12:485–97.
98. Sams AE, Nixon AJ. Chondrocyte-laden collagen scaffolds for resurfacing extensive articular cartilage defects. Osteoarthritis Cartilage 1995;3:47–59.
99. Oka M, Chang YS, Nakamura T, Ushio K, Toguchida J, Gu HO. Synthetic osteochondral replacement of the femoral articular surface. J Bone Joint Surg Br 1997;79:1003–7.
100. Haddo O, Mahroof S, Higgs D, David L, Pringle J, Bayliss M, Cannon SR, Briggs TW. The use of chondrogide membrane in autologous chondrocyte implantation. Knee 2004;11:51–5.
101. Pavesio A, Abatangelo G, Borrione A, Brocchetta D, Hollander AP, Kon E, Torasso F, Zanasi S, Marcacci M. Hyaluronan-based scaffolds (Hyalograft C) in the treatment of knee cartilage defects: preliminary clinical findings. Novartis Found Symp 2003;249:203–17; discussion 29–33, 34–8, 39–41.
102. Marcacci M, Berruto M, Brocchetta D, Delcogliano A, Ghinelli D, Gobbi A, Kon E, Pederzini L, Rosa D, Sacchetti GL, Stefani G, Zanasi S. Articular cartilage engineering with Hyalograft C: 3-year clinical results. Clin Orthop 2005;435:96–105.
103. Marcacci M, Kon E, Zaffagnini S, Vascellari A, Neri MP, Iacono F. New cell-based technologies in bone and cartilage tissue engineering. II. Cartilage regeneration. Chir Organi Mov 2003;88:42–7.
104. Erggelet C, Sittinger M, Lahm A. The arthroscopic implantation of autologous chondrocytes for the treatment of full-thickness cartilage defects of the knee joint. Arthroscopy 2003;19:108–10.
105. Muckle DS, Minns RJ. Biological response to woven carbon fibre pads in the knee. A clinical and experimental study. J Bone Joint Surg [Br] 1990;72:60–2.
106. Brittberg M, Faxen E, Peterson L. Carbon fiber scaffolds in the treatment of early knee osteoarthritis. A prospective 4-year followup of 37 patients. Clin Orthop 1994;435:155–64.

107. Marlovits S, Striessnig G, Kutscha-Lissberg F, Resinger C, Aldrian SM, Vecsei V, Trattnig S. Early postoperative adherence of matrix-induced autologous chondrocyte implantation for the treatment of full-thickness cartilage defects of the femoral condyle. Knee Surg Sports Traumatol Arthrosc 2005;13:451–7.
108. Cherubino P, Grassi FA, Bulgheroni P, Ronga M. Autologous chondrocyte implantation using a bilayer collagen membrane: a preliminary report. J Orthop Surg (Hong Kong) 2003;11:10–5.

19

Autograft and Allograft ACL Reconstruction: Construct Rationale

Keith W. Lawhorn[1] and Stephen M. Howell[2]

19.1. Introduction

Anterior cruciate ligament (ACL) surgery continues to evolve despite the high rates of success with current techniques. Graft sources, fixation devices, tunnel techniques and instrumentation have all increased in an effort to improve successful ACL surgery while minimizing complications. Technology and basic science research continue to fuel these changes, leading to improved fixation, more rapid healing and lower complication rates.

For many years and still today, many surgeons considered the autologous bone-patella tendon-bone graft (BPTB) to be the "gold-standard" grafts for ACL reconstruction. However, with the advent of newer fixation devices designed specifically for soft tissue graft fixation, hamstring grafts and tibialis allografts have provided clinical outcomes similar to BPTB ACL reconstruction while avoiding the significant morbidity of BPTB graft harvest [1–5]. These newer devices provide not only better fixation properties of soft tissue grafts, but also take advantage of the superior properties of soft tissue grafts making these grafts advantageous to BPTB grafts in many ways. With increased graft sources and reconstruction constructs, ACL surgeons now possess greater techniques and options when managing the ACL deficient knee.

Not only has the development of newer implants for ACL fixation in many ways revolutionized how surgeons approach ACL reconstruction, but so too has newer tunnel placement instrumentation and tunnel techniques. Surgeons today now have the ability to position tibial tunnels using either intra-articular soft tissue or bony landmarks with the goal of anatomically positioning graft tunnels and minimizing the complications of impingement [6–13]. Anatomically positioning an impingement-free ACL graft with

---

[1]Advanced Orthopaedics and Sports Medicine Institute, Fairfax, VA
[2]Department of Mechanical and Aeronautical Engineering, University of California at Davis, Davis, CA

From: *Orthopedic Biology and Medicine: Musculoskeletal Tissue Regeneration, Biological Materials and Methods*
Edited by W. S. Pietrzak © Humana Press, Totowa, NJ

tensile behavior similar to the native ACL is imperative to the success of the reconstruction, regardless of graft source and the fixation.

Lastly, technology and basic science research continues to move forward in an attempt to improve the rate of healing of soft tissue grafts to bone, and to develop a true engineered ACL graft substitute. Improving the reliability and speed of healing would lessen the risks for fixation failure and increase the safety of aggressive rehabilitation. Engineering a tissue substitute would obviate the need for graft harvest and the risks associated with allograft use. Thus, this chapter will focus on the rationale of the recent technological and innovative advancements in fixation, soft tissue graft utilization, tunnel positioning techniques and future biologic augmentation devices that will continue to shape how surgeons approach ACL reconstruction.

19.2. Basic Science

19.2.1. Graft Source

19.2.1.1. Autografts

The use of soft tissue grafts for ACL reconstruction have increased in popularity over the years, due to the documented success of ACL reconstruction with these grafts and the low morbidity of medial hamstring harvest [1–2, 5, 14]. The gracilis and semitendinosis tendons are the most commonly used soft tissue autografts and have several advantages over bone plug autografts, such as the BPTB and quadriceps tendon bone grafts. Soft tissue autografts avoid the problems associated with harvesting graft tissue from the knee extensor mechanism. Chronic anterior knee pain, kneeling pain, quadricep weakness, patella tendon rupture, infrapatellar contracture syndrome, patella fracture, patella-femoral arthritis and late flexion contractures of the knee can occur as a result graft harvest from the extensor mechanism [3, 15]. These problems are largely avoided with the use of a hamstring graft, thereby minimizing the morbidity of graft harvest. Additionally, the complete return of flexion strength and the regeneration of these tendons following harvest has been documented in a large percentage of patients [14, 16–18].

The ability to double loop the semitendinosis and gracilis tendons (DLSTG) results in an autogenous graft source with greatest strength (4,304 to 4,590 N) and stiffness (861–954 N/mm) of any autogenous graft source available for ACL reconstruction [19–20]. In fact, the DLSTG is approximately twice as strong and twice as stiff as a 10 mm BPTB graft. However, maximum hamstring graft properties require equal graft tensioning of all of the graft bundles. Therefore, fixation devices need to afford the surgeon the ability to equally tension all four bundles of a DLSTG at the time of fixation, otherwise overall graft properties may not be at a maximum. Additionally, a "double bundle graft" secured in a single bone tunnel in the femur using a rigid cross-pin better duplicates the reciprocal behavior of the native two-bundle ACL, which does not occur with a single bundle bone plug graft such as a BPTB graft [21].

Graft healing and remodeling of a DLSTG differs from that of a bone plug graft as well. Bone plug grafts such as the BPTB graft experience a more rapid rate of mechanical fixation, most likely secondary to the mechanical fit of the bone plug in the tunnel [22–23]. Healing of the bone tunnel around the bone plug occurs fairly rapidly (six weeks) and the graft tissue itself becomes the weak link [24–25]. After six weeks patella tendon graft failure tends to occur within the graft substance and not at the fixation sites. The intra-articular tendinous portion of the graft undergoes central necrosis during the healing and remodeling process [24–25]. It is believed this necrosis occurs because the grafts are avascular, the native tendinous cells do not survive the transfer and the relatively large cross sectional area associated with single bundle bone plug grafts cannot be nourished via passive diffusion of nutrients from the joint fluid alone. As the remodeling process progresses, eventually the necrotic areas remodel once the tendinous graft has been re-populated by cells of synovial origin [26]. For a DLSTG the intra-articular biologic healing and remodeling of the tendinous portions of the graft occur more rapidly than for BPTB since the graft does not experience necrosis [27]. The absence of necrosis during remodeling of the DLSTG may be because the cross sectional areas of each bundle are less than the tendinous portion of single bundle bone plug grafts and the tissue can be nourished via passive synovial diffusion without the need for a vascular supply. However, the incorporation and biologic healing of a soft tissue graft to bone may take longer, based on the mechanical properties of the biologic interface. Studies have demonstrated the mechanical strength of the biologic interface of a soft tissue graft is less than a bone plug graft early after implantation, most likely because of the lack of mechanical interference fit of a soft tissue graft in the bone tunnel and possibly due to more rapid healing of the bone plug to the tunnel wall [22–23].

19.2.1.2. Allografts

Like soft tissue autografts, soft tissue allograft use has also increased over the years. There are multiple reasons for the increase in soft tissue allograft use. The ability to loop and fixate soft tissue grafts using newer fixation devices result in excellent graft fixation construct properties exceeding that of bone plug allograft sources [28–29]. Additionally, soft tissue allografts are more readily available than bone plug grafts and simply increase the overall availability of allograft tissue for ACL reconstruction. Each cadaver provides two DLSTG, two anterior tibialis and two posterior tibialis grafts, compared to just two BPTB grafts and two Achilles tendon grafts. Soft tissue allografts used for primary ACL reconstruction avoid any morbidity of graft harvest, decrease operative times and minimize surgical scars. Allograft tissue can be ideal in ACL revision surgery and multi-ligament knee reconstruction procedures where autograft tissue is limited. Strength and stiffness of single loop tibialis tendons are greater, compared to bone plug allografts (BPTB, Achilles, Quad tendon bone) [19]. Furthermore, the biomechanical properties of soft tissue allografts are less affected by aging than has been demonstrated with BTPB grafts [29–30].

However, as with all graft sources, there are disadvantages associated with allograft use. Infectious disease transmission, the rate and consistency of biologic incorporation as well as costs associated with allografts raise concerns that detract from allograft tissue being an ideal graft source in all patients. Allograft use carries with it the inherent possibility of transferring an infectious disease from donor to recipient [31]. Although the risk is low, bacteria, hepatitis, HIV and syphilis can be transmitted from donor to recipient. There is also the theoretical possibility of transmitting slow viruses (prions) with allograft use [32]. Irradiation of the soft tissue allografts with high dose (>3Mrad) radiation can sterilize allograft tissue, destroying bacteria and viruses including HIV and hepatitis [31]. Bone plug allografts may still be capable of transmitting hepatitis despite treatment with 3 Mrad irradiation [31]. Although, allograft irradiation will reduce the risk of disease transmission, it does so at the expense of diminishing the biomechanical properties of the tissue. Newer screening tests such as polymerase chain reaction (PCR) and nucleic acid testing (NAT) improve the detection of viral and bacterial DNA and RNA, and may increase the accuracy of identifying infected donor tissue and minimizing false-negatives. By improving the sensitivity and specificity of infected donor tissue identification, the risk of bacterial and viral disease transmission should be less, thereby increasing the safety of allograft use. These newer techniques could potentially decrease the need for graft irradiation and other sterilization techniques that may affect allograft properties. Unfortunately, many tissue banks do not currently perform these tests on allograft tissue routinely. In the meantime, surgeons can minimize complications associated with infected allograft tissue by only using tissue processed from a tissue bank accredited by the American Association of Tissue Banks (AATB). All tissue banks are regulated by the FDA, however tissue banks may voluntarily become accredited by the AATB. The AATB provides guidance and standards that compliment those of the FDA to further ensure tissue banks meet the safety standards for donor screening, tissue procurement, processing and storage, all in an effort to prevent disease transmission and to optimize clinical outcomes. Therefore, it is imperative that surgeons know the source of their allograft tissue as well as the testing and treatments performed on the allograft tissue, particularly if they rely on the hospital or a surgery center to obtain the allograft tissue for their patients.

Biologic incorporation and costs associated with allografts are additional considerations associated with the use of allograft tissue. Biologic incorporation of allografts may take longer than autogenous graft sources used for ACL reconstruction. Regardless of the preservation technique – fresh-frozen or cryopreservation – any viable donor cells at the time of transplantation do not survive the transplantation process. Allograft healing and incorporation depend solely on recipient cellular re-population of the graft [26]. This re-population of the graft must occur in parallel or prior to the healing and incorporation of the graft tissue. Late failure rates of allograft ACL reconstruction may be higher when compared to autograft reconstruction. Costs of allografts can be expensive, however; the costs may be offset by shorter operative times.

19.2.2. Fixation

19.2.2.1. Fixation Principles

The principles of securing a soft tissue graft include the use of fixation devices that have high strength, high stiffness, resist slippage under submaximal cyclic load conditions, promote biologic incorporation and safely allow for aggressive rehabilitation. In addition to these important principles, surgeons must also understand how to interpret the biomechanical studies providing this data. Surgeons who understand how the biomechanical data was determined for different fixation devices can better determine the best fixation for their patients.

Much of the data presented in the literature with regard to fixation devices is time of implantation data. However, time of implantation data may not accurately reflect the properties of an ACL construct weeks to months after reconstruction. An *in vivo* study evaluating the properties of two different types of tibial fixation devices showed the properties of the devices were different four weeks after implantation [33]. Surgeons must consider the testing conditions used in biomechanical studies, such as rate of loading, test loads and the testing model. Because testing conditions and models can vary between studies, it becomes difficult to directly compare the results between studies. Rather, surgeons must rely on the data obtained for given devices tested similarly in the same study. The testing model is important because fixation studies performed in animal bone (bovine, porcine, calf) overestimate the fixation strength and stiffness while underestimating the slippage as demonstrated with cancellous devices such as the interference screw, intrafix and centraloc devices [34–35]. Lastly, many studies report strength as ultimate tensile failure rather than yield load. Yield load represents the failure of a device fixation before catastrophic failure, such as graft rupture or pullout, and device breakage (ultimate tensile failure). Yield loads may represent plastic deformation of the graft tissue or the slippage of the graft tissue from the fixation. Yield loads are more clinically relevant than ultimate tensile failure loads. Lastly, submaximal cyclical load to failure data is most important in terms of device performance clinically. Cyclical testing best mimics the rehabilitation of ACL reconstructed knees since patients are cyclically loading their grafts with tensile loads less than failure loads. Devices and graft fixation constructs that perform poorly under cyclical conditions demonstrate greater amounts of graft slippage during testing and may fail to survive the designated cyclical loading protocol. Devices that perform poorly under these conditions experimentally may also perform poorly clinically, especially in the setting of an aggressive rehabilitation protocol. Recent cyclical load studies of soft tissue graft ACL constructs *in vitro* demonstrate changes in laxity are due to slippage of the graft from the fixation devices, rather than intrinsic changes in graft length such as graft elongation and stretch-out [36–38]. Surgeons, therefore, must not rely solely on one parameter to determine the best fixation of a soft tissue graft since some implants may exhibit good fixation strength, but poor stiffness or slippage data, while others may exhibit good stiffness, but poor strength and slippage data. Surgeons should consider all biomechanical parameters, how the data was collected and the model the testing was performed on to objectively choose the best fixation devices based on sound scientific evidence.

19.2.2.2. Femoral Fixation

A myriad of femoral fixation devices exist for soft tissue ACL graft fixation. Cross-pin devices such as the EZLoc, Bone Mulch Screw (BMS), RigidFix and Transfix devices afford the best tensile failure load data than other forms of femoral fixation, such as interference screw fixation and suture posts. Surgeons choose to use the various devices for a number of reasons. For femoral fixation, we prefer the EZLoc or Bone Mulch Screw devices (Fig. 19.1). The BMS is used primarily in revision cases where patients have had a two-incision approach for tunnel placement using a bone plug graft and interference screw fixation for their primary ACL reconstruction. The EZLoc and Bone Mulch Screw both provide high strength and stiffness fixation with minimal slippage under cyclical loading conditions [35, 39]. When tested in young human femurs the strength of the BMS is 1,126N and it has a stiffness of 225N/mm.

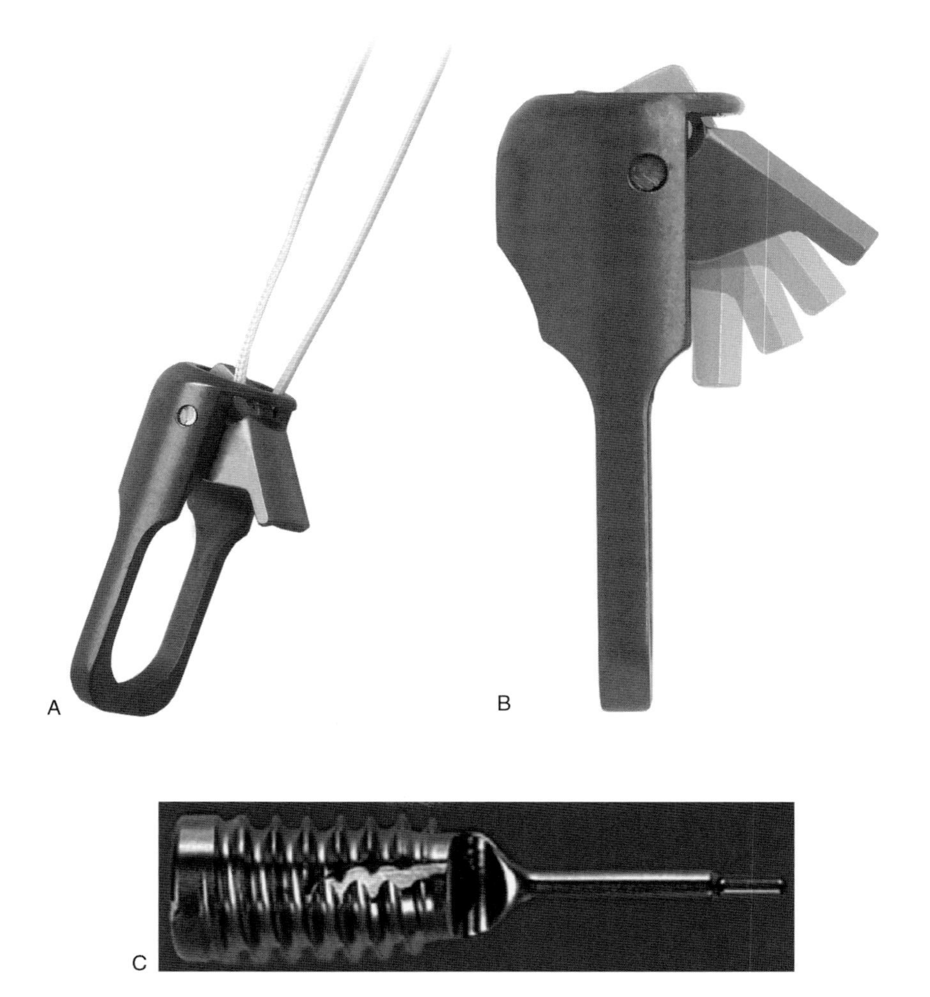

Fig. 19.1 (A) EZLoc device (B) EZLoc showing deployable lever (C) bone mulch screw

The strength of the EZLoc is greater than 1,400N tested on the bench-top. The stiffness of the EZLoc implant fixed in human bone is infinite since the device is seated directly against cortical bone. The slippage of the implant and graft, therefore, should be negligible since the graft is looped directly over the cross-pin of the device, avoiding any linkage material. Avoiding linkage material improves the stiffness of fixation while minimizing graft motion in the bone tunnel during biologic healing to the tunnel wall. The superior biomechanical and performance properties of these implants are achieved because both devices are secured on cortical, rather than in cancellous, bone. The properties of these fixation devices allow for the safe use of an aggressive rehabilitation protocol. In fact, the BMS has been shown to safely support an aggressive rehabilitation protocol without a loss of stability between four months and two years postoperatively [40]. Recent studies demonstrate device migration with the Rigidfix device and *in vivo* deformation and cross-pin fracture of the Bio-Transfix device [41]. The EZLoc and Bone Mulch screw afford the surgeon the ability to confirm 100 percent graft capture by the fixation device. For the EZLoc, the graft is passed through the cross-pin loop outside of the patient prior to graft passage. For the BMS, the graft is pulled over the cross-pin under arthroscopic visualization confirming complete graft capture (Fig. 19.2). With the other cross-pin devices, "blind" graft passage and fixation must be performed with no guarantee of complete graft capture, and the possibility of graft laceration and damage exists with "blind" cross-pin fixation [42]. Without complete graft capture or with graft damage, the functional cross sectional area of the graft tissue is diminished, resulting in a weaker graft fixation construct. The EZLoc and BMS devices afford the surgeon the ability to equally tension all four bundles of a soft tissue graft. Because the grafts are individually pulled over the cross-pin with each of these devices, all graft bundles can be equally tensioned maximizing the properties of the graft tissue. Lastly, both of these devices can help promote the biologic healing of a soft tissue graft to the bone tunnel by allowing a snug fit in the bony tunnel. With the BMS bone graft can be packed through the central housing of the screw increasing the snugness of fit and eliminating any voids between the graft and tunnel wall. The EZLoc allows for the sizing of the graft and femoral tunnel such that the snugness of fit can be optimized at the time of graft sizing.

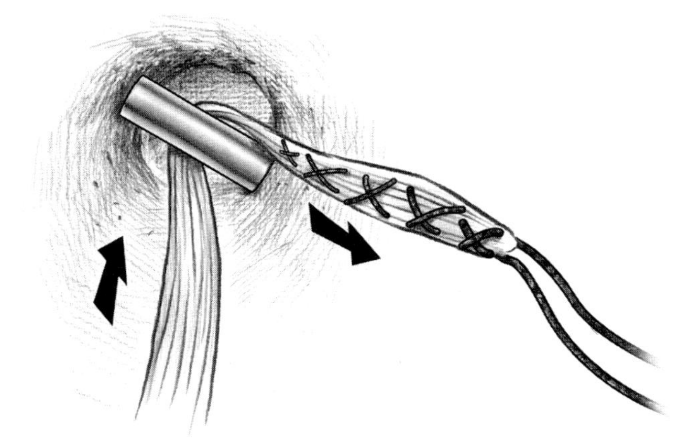

Fig. 19.2 Passage of graft over BMS cross-pin is performed under direct visualization

19.2.2.3. Tibial Fixation

The weakest link biomechanically of any ACL reconstruction is tibial fixation. As for femoral fixation, there are numerous implants designed for soft tissue graft fixation. The WasherLoc, interference screws, intrafix, centraloc, bone staples and suture posts have all been used for tibial soft tissue graft fixation. We prefer to use the WasherLoc device exclusively for tibial fixation. The WasherLoc is a screw and washer device designed to achieve distal intra-tunnel fixation using lag screw fixation to cortical bone (Fig. 19.3). As with our preference for femoral cross-pin devices, the WasherLoc graft construct has high strength (905 N) and stiffness (248 N/mm), and resistance to graft slippage under cyclical load conditions when tested in human cadaveric bone [28]. The WasherLoc fixing a double-looped hamstsring graft is the only tibial fixation device that approximates the biomechanical properties of the native

ACL when tested in human bone [43]. In addition, when tested *in vivo* in an animal model, WasherLoc fixation of a soft tissue graft has been shown to maintain its biomechanical properties over time and to promote biologic healing of the graft bone tunnel interface, a stark contrast from interference screw fixation of a soft tissue graft [33]. Another advantage of the WasherLoc is that the device allows for bone grafting of the tibial tunnel to eliminate voids, improve biomechanical properties and enhance tendon bone tunnel healing. Lastly, the biomechanical properties of the WasherLoc and its performance *in vivo* ensure safe use of aggressive rehabilitation and an early return to sports at four months with high clinical success [40].

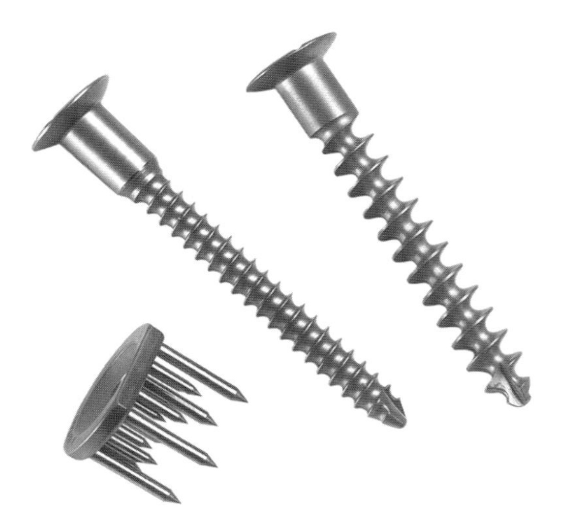

Fig. 19.3 WasherLoc tibial fixation device

19.2.3. Tunnel Placement

19.2.3.1. Principles of Correct Tunnel Placement

Correct tunnel placement is imperative to the success of any ACL reconstruction. Improper tunnel placement cannot be overcome by graft source, fixation or rehab methods. In fact, improper tunnel placement, and not graft choice, is the most common cause for complications and reconstruction failure [44]. Characteristics of proper tunnel placement include the absence of roof impingement, the absence of posterior cruciate ligament (PCL) impingement and the establishment of a tensile graft behavior similar to the native ACL. Surgeons must be cognizant of these basic requirements for tunnel placement to maximize their success rate, regardless of the tunnel techniques they utilize to position their tibial and femoral tunnels.

Roof impingement occurs when the ACL graft prematurely contacts the intercondylar roof before the knee reaches terminal extension. Roof impingement, therefore, is an error in sagittal plane positioning of the tibial tunnel. Patients experience flexion contractures and complain of difficulty achieving terminal extension [7, 12–13]. Additionally, clinical studies demonstrate increased knee laxity when roof impingement is present [6]. Roof impingement is identified postoperatively when any portion of the tibial tunnel exists anterior to Blummensat's line on a lateral radiograph with the knee in full extension [12] (Fig. 19.4). ACL grafts experiencing roof impingement demonstrate characteristic signal increase in the distal two-thirds of the graft by MRI [12, 45]. This signal increase is associated with diminished biomechanical properties of the tissue [46]. The best treatment for roof impingement is prevention. Surgeons need to account for the variability in terminal extension and the slope of the intercondylar roof (roof angle) that exist between patients when positioning the tibial tunnel. Surgeons must also know that the correlation between roof angle and knee extension is weak [7]. Therefore, surgeons must independently account for the differences in roof angle and knee extension that exist between patients when positioning the tibial tunnel for ACL reconstruction.

Posterior cruciate ligament impingement exists when the ACL graft makes contact with the PCL as the knee flexes. It occurs when the femoral tunnel is too vertical and placed at the high noon position. When using the transtibial tunnel technique, PCL impingement occurs as a result of an error in coronal plane positioning of the tibial tunnel and, therefore, also the femoral tunnel since tibial tunnel position in the coronal plane determines femoral tunnel coronal plane position. Anterior cruciate liga ment grafts experiencing PCL impingement will result in greater knee laxity and a loss of flexion because the ACL graft makes contact with the PCL as the knee flexes. This contact between the ACL graft and the native PCL results in a precipitous rise in tensile load in the ACL graft as the knee flexes. The increase in graft tension with flexion will increase the difficulty for the patient to achieve flexion and increase the risk of fixation failure and graft slippage during postoperative rehabilitation. The best treatment for PCL impingement is prevention. When using the transtibial tunnel technique, a vertical tibial tunnel in the coronal plane will lead to PCL impingement since the femoral tunnel would also be vertical. In addition, when using the transtibial tunnel technique the tibial tunnel needs to be positioned centrally or slightly lateral in the native

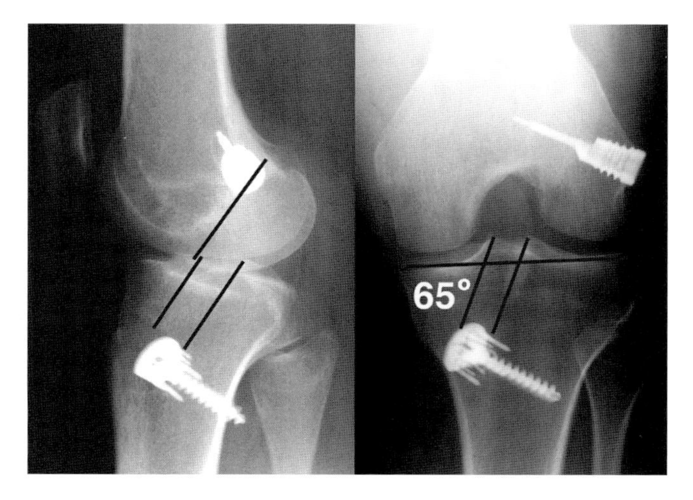

Fig. 19.4 Lateral and AP radiographs demonstrating satisfactory femoral and tibial tunnel position The single line adjacent to the femur represent Blummensat's line while the double lines adjacent to the tibia represent the anterior and posterior walls of the tibial tunnel

ACL tibial footprint between the tibial spines. Too medial placement of the tibial tunnel can also lead to PCL impingement with the transtibial technique. Therefore, accurate tunnel positioning in both the sagittal plane and coronal plane positions is imperative to avoid the complications of impingement and maximize success.

Lastly, establishment of tensile graft behavior similar to the native ACL is critical for a successful reconstruction. Provided tunnel placement is accurate and impingement free, graft behavior should be similar to the native ACL. The femoral tunnel position largely determines tensile graft behavior of an ACL reconstruction. Using the transtibial tunnel technique, femoral tunnel placement should be automatic when using femoral aimers through a tibial tunnel. Nonetheless, regardless of the technique used by the surgeon, the femoral tunnel must be positioned posteriorly and down the sidewall of the femur at the 10:00 and 2:00 positions in the right and left knees, respectively, with the superior apex of the notch representing the 12:00 position.

19.2.3.2. Tibial Tunnel Techniques

Numerous guide systems exist for placement of the tibial tunnel. The point-and-shoot guide, the PCL-referencing guide and the one step intercondylar roof-referencing guide (roof-referencing guide) are tibial guides used by surgeons to position the tibial tunnel. The point-and-shoot guide and the PCL-referencing guide both reference soft tissue landmarks on the tibia, including the native ACL footprint, the PCL and the anterior horn attachment of the lateral meniscus, to determine proper tibial tunnel positioning. The roof-referencing guide references the bony anatomy of the intercondylar notch and roof. The senior author has demonstrated a higher incidence of roof impingement with a point-and-shoot guide. PCL-referencing guides have proven to prevent roof impingement, but do so by positioning the tibial tunnel too posterior [8]. These soft tissue guides do not take into account the differences in roof angle and knee extension that exist between patients. We prefer to use the roof-referencing guide because it references bone with the knee in full extension and not mutable soft tissues with the knee in flexion. Referencing the bony intercondylar notch with the knee in full extension allows the surgeon to simultaneously account for the variability in roof angle and knee extension that exist between patients. The roof-referencing guide prevents roof impingement, obviates the need for a roofplasty and customizes the sagittal plane position of the tibial tunnel based on the patient's intercondylar roof anatomy (roof angle) and knee extension [6]. Avoiding a roofplasty is advantageous because bone removal from the intercondylar notch requires increased graft pretensioning to restore anteroposterior (AP) laxity of the knee, and this increased tensile load is deleterious to graft remodeling and increases the risk of graft slippage from the fixation devices [47–49]. In addition, the roof-referencing guide utilizes a coronal alignment guide to increase the accuracy of tibial tunnel placement in the coronal plane. Surgeons using a coronal alignment guide increase the accuracy of coronal plane position of the tibial tunnel when compared to surgeons who did not use a coronal alignment device [49]. Therefore, unlike all other tibial guide instrumentation systems, use of the roof-referencing guide allows surgeons to customize tibial tunnel sagittal plane position for all patients, eliminate the need for a roofplasty and accurately establish coronal plane position of the tibial tunnel, avoiding PCL impingement while accurately establishing femoral tunnel sagittal and coronal plane position when using a transtibial tunnel technique.

19.2.3.3. Femoral Tunnel Techniques

Numerous femoral tunnel techniques and guide systems exist for the creation of femoral tunnels for ACL reconstruction. Transtibial, transportal and two-incision techniques are all used with successful results. Transportal and two-incision tunnel techniques position the femoral tunnel independent of the tibial tunnel, whereas the transtibial technique utilizes instrumentation through the tibial tunnel to position the femoral tunnel. The transportal femoral tunnel technique utilizes an over-the-top femoral aimer through the medial arthroscopy portal to position the femoral tunnel, whereas the two-incision technique utilizes a lateral incision just proximal to the lateral femoral condyle, along with a "rear entry" guide to position the tunnel using arthroscopic assistance. We prefer the transtibial tunnel technique where the femoral tunnel is positioned using a femoral aimer through the tibial tunnel. With the transtibial tunnel technique, the position of the femoral tunnel should be automatic. Position of the femoral tunnel in both the sagittal and coronal planes requires precision since femoral tunnel position largely determines the tension behavior of an ACL graft. In the sagittal plane, the femoral tunnel must be placed posteriorly with only a 1 to 2 mm thick posterior wall. In the coronal plane the femoral tunnel must be between 60 and 65 degrees and placed down the sidewall of the notch to avoid PCL impingement when using the transtibial tunnel technique. Positioning the femoral tunnel precisely in the sagittal and coronal planes is imperative to establish a tension behavior in the graft similar to the native ACL. With the transtibial tunnel technique, the tibial tunnel position in the coronal plane determines the coronal plane position of the femoral tunnel because, with the use of a femoral aimer through the tibial tunnel, the surgeon can only change the coronal plane position by three to four degrees. The offset of the femoral aimers used in conjunction with sized-specific reamers will consistently position the femoral tunnel posteriorly in the sagittal plane. Therefore, with the use of a femoral aimer through the tibial tunnel (transtibial tunnel technique), femoral tunnel positioning will be automatic once the tibial tunnel is established. Therefore, surgeons have to focus on meticulously positioning just one tunnel (tibial tunnel), rather than on two independently placed tunnels, when using the transtibial tunnel technique for femoral tunnel positioning.

19.2.4. Biologic Healing and Surgical Technique

19.2.4.1. Biologic Healing of ACL Grafts

Bone plug grafts achieve initial fixation of the bone plug in the bone tunnel by mechanical fit and by healing of the tunnel around the bone plug [24–25]. Eventually, the bone plug becomes incorporated in the bone tunnel. Soft tissue grafts need to form an attachment to the bone tunnel and do not have any mechanical fixation inherent to the graft, as do bone plug grafts. Typically, this attachment of soft tissue grafts occurs through Sharpey-like fibers, particularly when distal fixation devices are used [27]. Interference screw fixation and other compressive intra-tunnel devices result in direct healing of the graft to the tunnel wall without Sharpey-like fibers and/or a fibrous interzone [50].

The rate of healing for the different interfaces (direct versus indirect) may also be different. In an animal study determining the properties of the biologic interface of a soft tissue graft in a bone tunnel, distal fixation resulted in better biomechanical properties of the biologic interface four weeks after implantation, compared to fixation of the soft tissue graft with an interference screw [33]. Therefore, indirect healing of a soft tissue graft with the development of a fibrous interzone appears to be advantageous to direct healing. Additionally, the tensile strength of the biologic bond is proportional to the surface area of the soft tissue graft and bone tunnel interface [51]. The use of non-biologic intra-tunnel fixation such as metal and bioresorbable interference screws significantly limits the surface area of the graft to bond to bone since a large percentage of the tunnel wall is "unavailable" for graft bone tunnel healing because of the space occupied by the fixation device. Therefore, we advocate the use of biologically active intra-tunnel fixation (bone graft), particularly on the tibial side of the reconstruction. We prefer to use a cancellous bone plug graft obtained from the tibial tunnel at the time of tunnel preparation. Impacting the bone graft into the tibial tunnel eliminates any voids between the graft and bone, decreases tunnel expansion and increases the stiffness of fixation by 58N/mm when a hamstring graft is secured using the WasherLoc device in the tibia [52].

19.2.4.2. Authors' Preferred Surgical Technique

19.2.4.2.1. Set-Up / Graft Harvest and Preparation: Position the patient supine on the operating table. Stabilize the leg using a lateral post or leg holder. Place a pneumatic tourniquet around the proximal thigh. Perform an exam under anesthesia prior to prepping the leg. Prep and drape the lower extremity to ensure ample space between the leg holder and the knee joint to allow for ease of passage of the EZLoc guidepin. Exsanguinate the leg and inflate the tourniquet. Make a 2 to 3 cm incision over the anteromedial tibia three fingerbreadths below the medial joint line. Expose the sartorius fascia and harvest the gracilis and semitendinosis tendons. Remove any muscle on the tendons and place a suture in each end of the tendon. Loop the graft over a suture or sizing post and pass through sizing sleeves to determine graft diameter (Fig. 19.5). Remove the tendons from their tibial insertion.

19.2.4.2.2. Tunnel Placement: Establish arthroscopy portals adjacent to the medial and lateral borders of the patella tendon. Remove the remnant torn ACL and expose the superior edge of the posterior cruciate ligament. Insert the roof-referencing tibial guide into the intercondylar notch. The dilated tip of the guide should pass between the PCL and the lateral wall without deforming the PCL. If the guide deforms the PCL, perform a lateral wallplasty until the guide freely passes into the notch (Fig. 19.6). Do not perform a roofplasty. With the tibial guide seated in the notch, position the knee in terminal extension (Fig. 19.7). Place the heel on the Mayo stand, maintaining the knee in full extension. Place the coronal alignment rod in the tibial guide and swivel the guide until this rod is parallel to the joint line (Fig. 19.7). Drill the tibial guide pin proximally until it strikes the guide tip in the notch. Remove the guide, flex the knee and tap the guide pin into the notch under direct arthroscopic visualization. The guide pin should angle away from the PCL and be located 4 to 5 mm posterior and parallel to the intercondylar roof. With the tibial guide

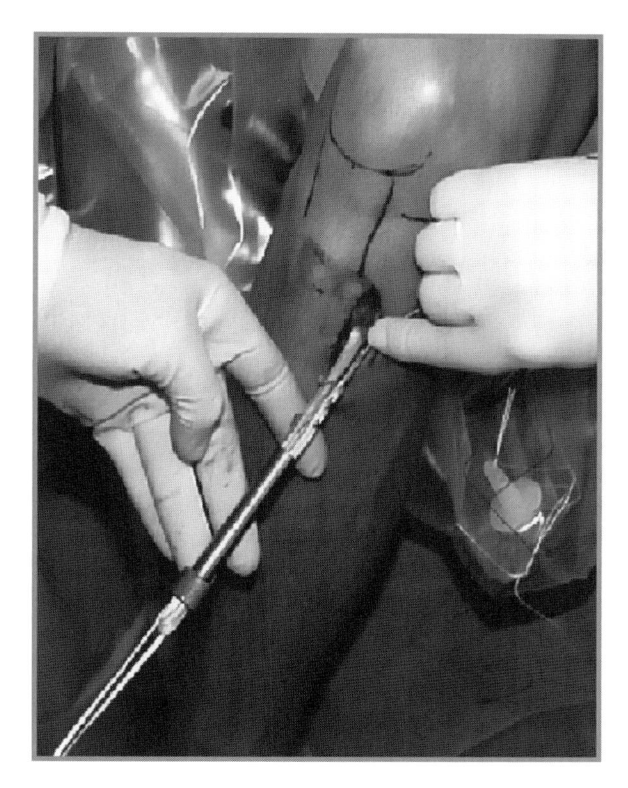

Fig. 19.5 Hamstring graft determined by double looping graft and passing through sizing sleeves before graft removal

pin in satisfactory position, ream the outer cortex of the tibia using a reamer corresponding to the graft diameter previously determined by graft sizing. Advance a 7 or 8 mm diameter coring reamer proximally using a mallet until the coring reamer strikes the subchondral bone. Remove the coring reamer with a cancellous core of compacted bone. Complete the tunnel using the appropriate diameter reamer determined by graft sizing. Pass the same sized diameter impingement rod into the tibial tunnel and advance into the notch. Extend the knee fully to ensure no evidence of roof impingement.

With the tibia tunnel properly positioned, advance a femoral aimer through the tibial tunnel and seat in the over-the-top position with the knee in flexion. Drill the long drill pin into the femur until it exits the lateral cortex. Ream the femoral tunnel over the drill pin using one-inch-long reamer tips the same diameter as the graft until the reamer exits the lateral cortex of the femur. Measure femoral tunnel length using the depth guage through the tibial tunnel. The EZLoc device comes in three lengths (short, standard and long) and four diameters (5, 6, 7/8, 9/10 mm). Use the standard length for femoral tunnels 35 to 50 mm.in length; otherwise use the short and long devices accordingly for tunnel lengths outside of the 35 to 50 mm tunnel length.

With the femoral tunnel completed, prepare the tibia for the WasherLoc fixation device. Remove a thumbnail sized area of soft tissue surrounding the tibial tunnel. Position the counterbore aimer in the tunnel aligned toward the

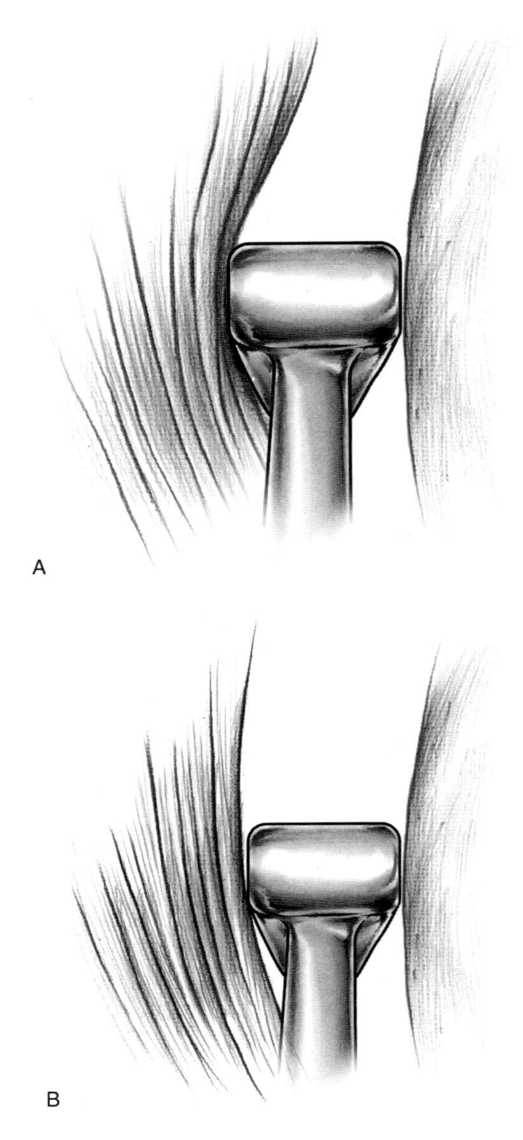

Fig. 19.6 (A) Tip of tibial guide deforms PCL when notch is too small for the graft (B) No deformation of PCL with passage of tibial guide tip in notch demonstrates adequate space for graft in notch

fibula head. Advance the counterbore awl into the distal tibial tunnel to create a pilot hole. Ream the same path with the counterbore reamer seated in the pilot hole until the reamer is flush with the posterior aspect of the distal tunnel (Fig. 19.8). Save the reamings.

19.2.4.2.3. Graft Passage and Fixation: With the tunnels completed, prepare the graft and EZLoc for passage. Pass the graft through the opening on the appropriate sized EZLoc device. Even all of the graft ends, tie the sutures together and mark the graft using a marking pen at the distance corresponding to femoral tunnel length from the tip of the deployable lever arm. With the

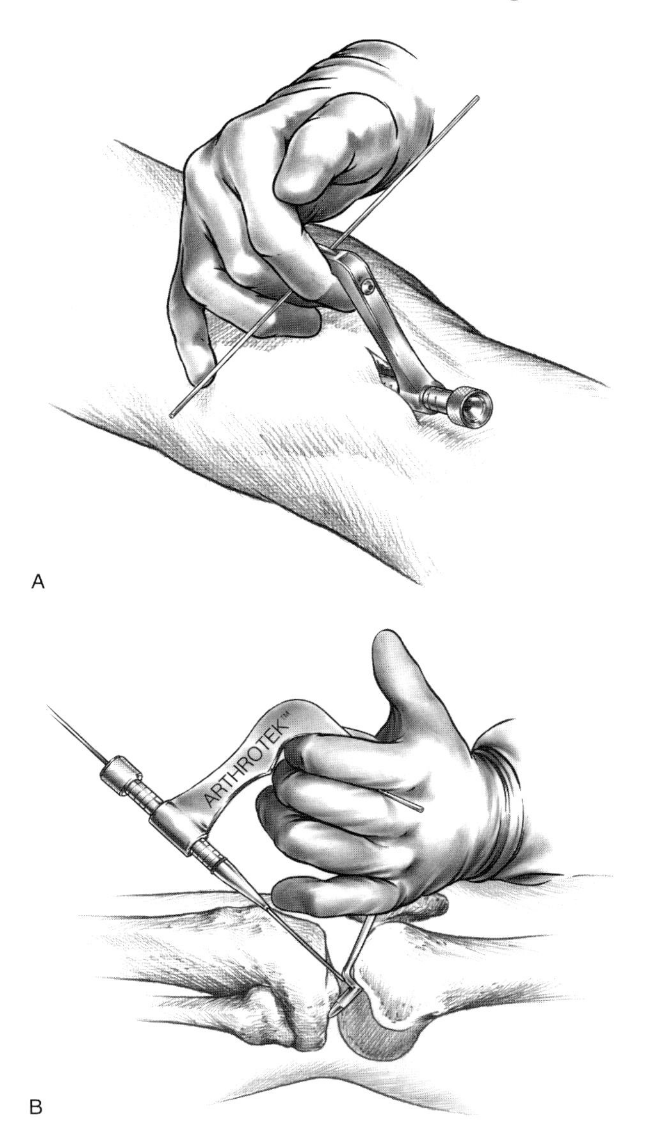

Fig. 19.7 (A) Anterior view of the tibial guide (B) Lateral view of tibial guide

EZLoc attached to the pre-packaged 16-inch passing pin and MaxBraid suture (Arthrotek, Warsaw, IN), pass the graft through the tibial tunnel and out of the femoral tunnel and lateral skin. Slowly pull the passing pin and MaxBraid suture while minimizing any bending of the passing pin to prevent premature removal of the passing pin. Engage the EZLoc in the femoral tunnel with the lever arm adjacent to the lateral wall of the tunnel (Fig. 19.9). Cut the MaxBraid suture from the passing pin and remove the passing pin, leaving the suture attached to the EZLoc device once the graft markings have entered the femoral tunnel. This should indicate the EZLoc lever arm has now been advanced proximal to the lateral cortex of the femoral tunnel (Fig. 19.10). Removing the passing pin and pulling on the MaxBraid suture deploys the

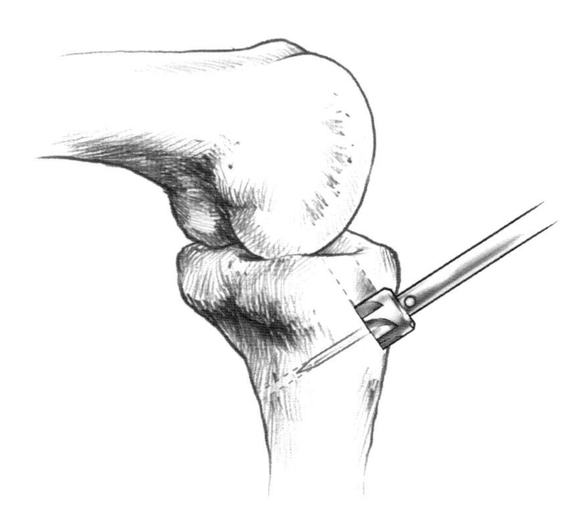

Fig. 19.8 Preparation of tibial tunnel for WasherLoc

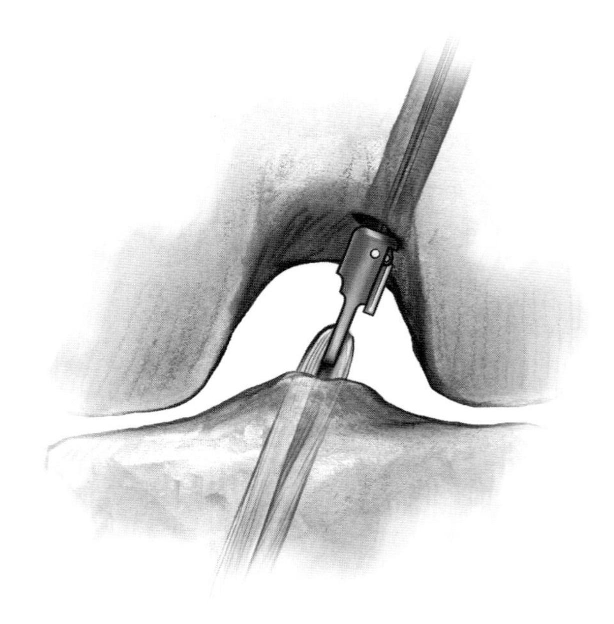

Fig. 19.9 Pull EZLoc into femoral tunnel with lever facing lateral wall of tunnel

lever arm (Fig. 19.11). With equal tension on the MaxBraid sutures exiting the femoral tunnel and the graft sutures exiting the tibial tunnel, pull the graft and EZLoc back and forth, proximal and distal, until the EZLoc is firmly seated on cortical bone (Fig. 19.12). With the EZLoc seated on the lateral cortex of the femur, pull tension on the graft sutures and cycle the knee 20 to 30 times (Fig. 19.12).

Position the knee in full extension. Pass an impingement rod through the graft sutures and have an assistant pull on the rod to tension all bundles

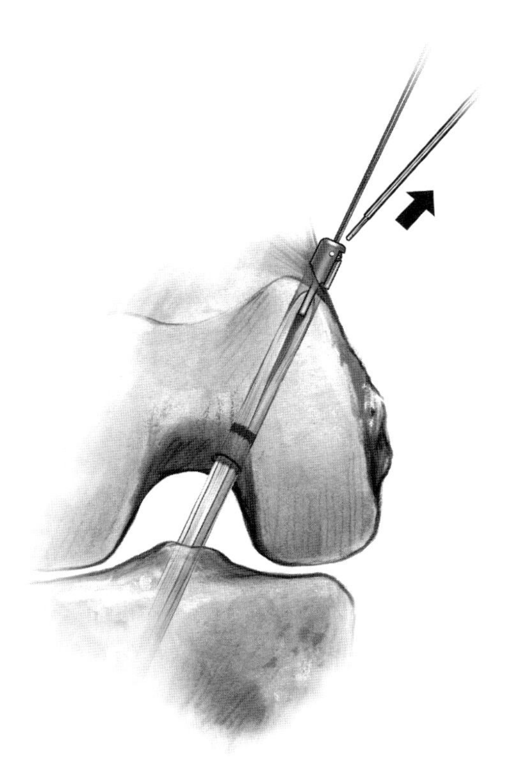

Fig. 19.10 EZLoc pulled through femoral tunnel until it exits lateral cortex The passing pin is removed

equally. Impact the WasherLoc washer aiming toward the fibular head. Drill the far cortex in the same direction using a 3.2 mm drill bit. Use a depth gauge to measure the screw length and place the appropriate length 6.0 mm cancellous screw. Dilate the tibial tunnel anterior to the graft and WasherLoc using the conical dilator by hand or gently using a mallet. Once dilated, impact the harvested core of cancellous graft by striking the inner plunger within the coring reamer. Remove excess graft and perform a Lachman's test for stability (Fig. 19.13). Remove the MaxBraid suture from the EZLoc device. Close the wound in layers and deflate the tourniquet.

Postoperatively, the patient can weight bear as tolerated brace-free. Patients who participate in an aggressive rehabilitation protocol speed recovery and improve outcomes. Typically, patients can safely return to unrestricted activity at four months, provided muscle strength of the operative lower extremity is 85 percent the normal contralateral leg.

19.3. Future Trends

The use of autogenous bone grafting of the tibial tunnel is a cost-effective method to enhance the rate of biologic healing. Other methods have also demonstrated improved rates of biologic healing, including the use of periosteal grafts and various growth factors. Platelet-derived growth factor (PDGF),

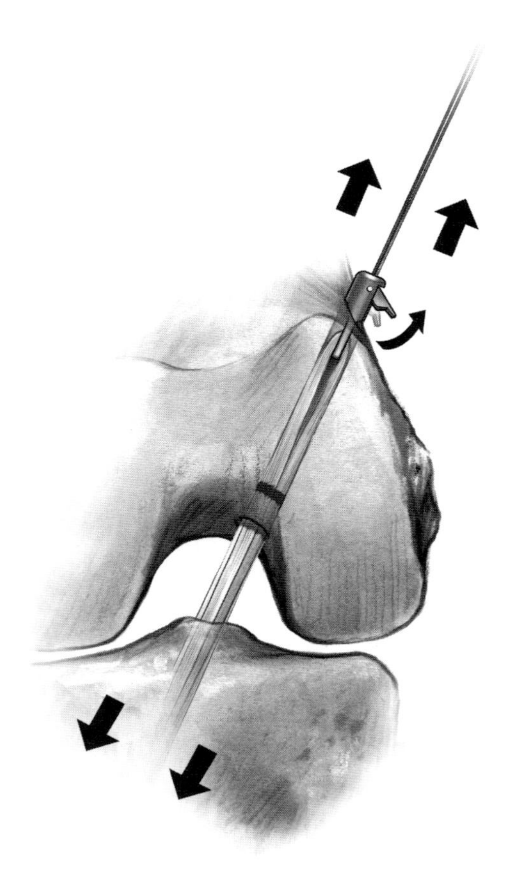

Fig. 19.11 Tension is pulled alternately on the graft sutures and the EZLoc until the EZLoc is firmly seated against the lateral cortical bone of the femur

transforming growth factor-beta (TGF-beta), insulin-like growth factor (IGF), fibroblast growth factor (FGF) and epidermal growth factor (EDF) all have the potential to improve ligament healing [53]. The use of mesenchymal stem cells (MSCs) has also been shown to improve the biomechanical properties of a tendon graft in an animal model. Additionally, MSCs demonstrated increased presence of cartilage cells at the tendon bone tunnel interface, better duplicating the chondral transition that exists with the normal ACL insertion [54]. Currently, the use of these growth factors and MSCs has been solely for research purposes and not clinical application.

In an effort to eliminate the morbidity of autogenous graft harvest and the risks of disease transmission with allograft use, tissue engineering along with the use of growth factors and gene therapy may allow scientists and surgeons to develop an ACL graft substitute in the laboratory [53]. The use of tissue scaffolds, both natural and synthetic, must allow for cell adhesion, growth and matrix production. Extrinsic cell stimulation via growth factors and mechanical conditions may modulate cellular response, improving matrix production. However, to date, no engineered construct with the appropriate biologic makeup and mechanical properties has been developed for use in the *in vivo*

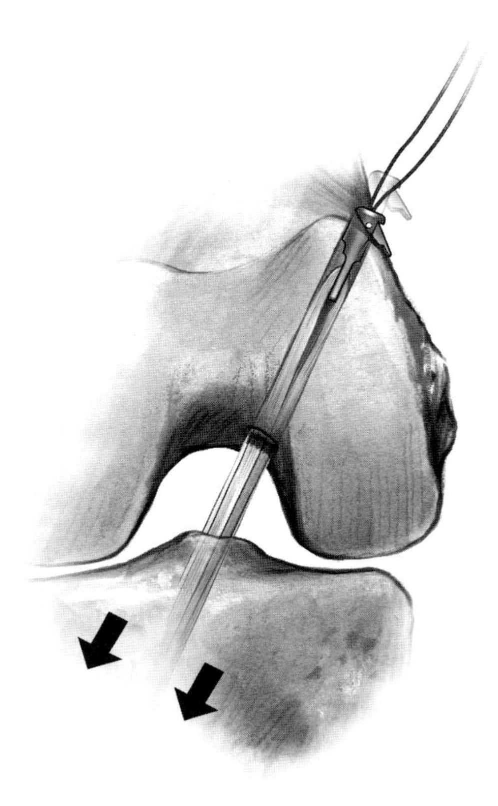

Fig. 19.12 With the EZLoc seated against the femoral cortex, tension is pulled on the graft sutures while the knee is cycled 20 to 30 times

setting. Additional research is ongoing to develop a tissue engineered scaffold that will mimic the mechanical properties and function of the native ACL with long-term durability.

19.4. Conclusions

Anterior cruciate ligament surgery continues to evolve, despite the high rates of clinical success. Technological advancements in fixation have increased the reconstructive constructs available to surgeons. Technological advancements in instrumentation for tunnel placement have improved consistency in tunnel placement while avoiding the complications of graft impingement. Together these advancements allow surgeons to better utilize soft tissue grafts with excellent biomechanical properties for successful ACL reconstruction. Further research continues in an effort to speed biologic healing, graft incorporation and remodeling. Tissue engineering may someday provide a graft source for reconstruction without the morbidity and risks currently associated with autologous and allograft tissues.

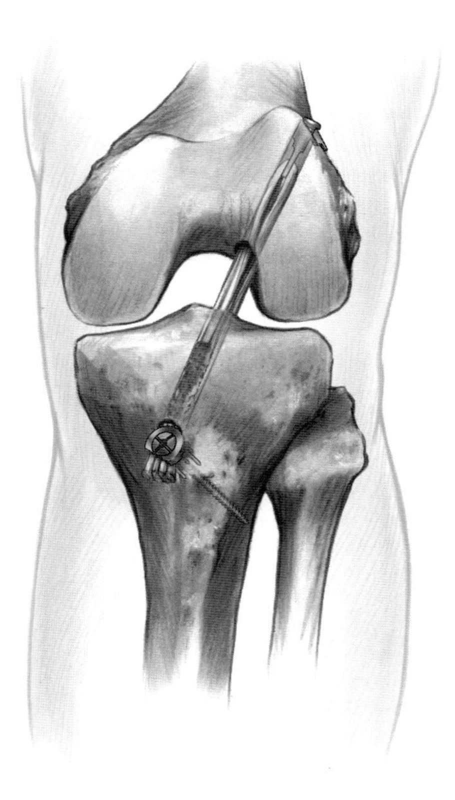

Fig. 19.13 Completed ACL reconstruction with tibial tunnel bone grafting

References

1. Boonriong T, Kietsiriroje N. Arthroscopically assisted anterior cruciate ligament reconstruction: comparison of bone-patellar tendon-bone versus hamstring tendon autograft. J Med Assoc Thai 2004; 87:1100–7.
2. Gobbi A, Mahajan S, Zanazzo M, Tuy B. Patellar tendon versus quadrupled bone-semitendinosus anterior cruciate ligament reconstruction: a prospective clinical investigation in athletes. Arthroscopy 2003; 19:592–601.
3. Miller SL, Gladstone JN. Graft selection in anterior cruciate ligament reconstruction. Orthop Clin North Am 2002; 33:675–83.
4. Tow BP, Chang PC, Mitra AK, Tay BK, Wong MC. Comparing 2-year outcomes of anterior cruciate ligament reconstruction using either patella-tendon or semi-tendinosus-tendon autografts: a non-randomised prospective study. J Orthop Surg (Hong Kong) 2005; 13:139–46.
5. Wilcox JF, Gross JA, Sibel R, Backs RA, Kaeding CC. Anterior cruciate ligament reconstruction with hamstring tendons and cross-pin femoral fixation compared with patellar tendon autografts. Arthroscopy 2005; 21:1186–92.
6. Howell SM. Principles for placing the tibial tunnel and avoiding roof impingement during reconstruction of a torn anterior cruciate ligament. Knee Surg Sports Traumatol Arthrosc 1998; 6 Suppl 1:S49–55.

7. Howell SM, Barad SJ. Knee extension and its relationship to the slope of the intercondylar roof. Implications for positioning the tibial tunnel in anterior cruciate ligament reconstructions. Am J Sports Med 1995; 23:288–94.
8. Miller MD, Olszewski AD. Posterior tibial tunnel placement to avoid anterior cruciate ligament graft impingement by the intercondylar roof. An in vitro and in vivo study. Am J Sports Med 1997; 25:818–22.
9. Morgan CD, Kalman VR, Grawl DM. Definitive landmarks for reproducible tibial tunnel placement in anterior cruciate ligament reconstruction. Arthroscopy 1995; 11:275–88.
10. Simmons R, Howell SM, Hull ML. Effect of the angle of the femoral and tibial tunnels in the coronal plane and incremental excision of the posterior cruciate ligament on tension of an anterior cruciate ligament graft: an in vitro study. J Bone Joint Surg Am 2003; 85-A:1018–29.
11. Staubli HU, Rauschning W. Tibial attachment area of the anterior cruciate ligament in the extended knee position. Anatomy and cryosections in vitro complemented by magnetic resonance arthrography in vivo. Knee Surg Sports Traumatol Arthrosc 1994; 2:138–46.
12. Howell SM, Clark JA, Farley TE. A rationale for predicting anterior cruciate graft impingement by the intercondylar roof. A magnetic resonance imaging study. Am J Sports Med 1991; 19:276–82.
13. Howell SM, Clark JA. Tibial tunnel placement in anterior cruciate ligament reconstructions and graft impingement. Clin Orthop 1992:187–95.
14. Yasuda K, Tsujino J, Ohkoshi Y, Tanabe Y, Kaneda K. Graft site morbidity with autogenous semitendinosus and gracilis tendons. Am J Sports Med 1995; 23:706–14.
15. Paulos LE, Wnorowski DC, Greenwald AE. Infrapatellar contracture syndrome. Diagnosis, treatment, and long-term followup. Am J Sports Med 1994; 22:440–9.
16. Gill SS, Turner MA, Battaglia TC, Leis HT, Balian G, Miller MD. Semitendinosus regrowth: biochemical, ultrastructural, and physiological characterization of the regenerate tendon. Am J Sports Med 2004; 32:1173–81.
17. Leis HT, Sanders TG, Larsen KM, Lancaster-Weiss KJ, Miller MD. Hamstring regrowth following harvesting for ACL reconstruction: The lizard tail phenomenon. J Knee Surg 2003; 16:159–64.
18. Rispoli DM, Sanders TG, Miller MD, Morrison WB. Magnetic resonance imaging at different time periods following hamstring harvest for anterior cruciate ligament reconstruction. Arthroscopy 2001; 17:2–8.
19. Noyes F. Biomechanical analysis of human ligament grafts used in knee-ligament repairs and reconstructions. J Bone Joint Surg Am 1984; 66a:334–52.
20. Hamner DL, Brown CH, Jr., Steiner ME, Hecker AT, Hayes WC. Hamstring tendon grafts for reconstruction of the anterior cruciate ligament: biomechanical evaluation of the use of multiple strands and tensioning techniques. J Bone Joint Surg Am 1999; 81:549–57.
21. Wallace MP, Howell SM, Hull ML. In vivo tensile behavior of a four-bundle hamstring graft as a replacement for the anterior cruciate ligament. J Orthop Res 1997; 15:539–45.
22. Papageorgiou CD, Ma CB, Abramowitch SD, Clineff TD, Woo SL. A multidisciplinary study of the healing of an intra-articular anterior cruciate ligament graft in a goat model. Am J Sports Med 2001; 29:620–6.
23. Tomita F, Yasuda K, Mikami S, Sakai T, Yamazaki S, Tohyama H. Comparisons of intraosseous graft healing between the doubled flexor tendon graft and the bone-patellar tendon-bone graft in anterior cruciate ligament reconstruction. Arthroscopy 2001; 17:461–76.
24. Arnoczky SP. Biology of ACL reconstructions: what happens to the graft? Instr Course Lect 1996; 45:229–33.

25. Arnoczky SP, Warren RF, Ashlock MA. Replacement of the anterior cruciate ligament using a patellar tendon allograft. An experimental study. J Bone Joint Surg Am 1986; 68:376–85.
26. Min BH, Han MS, Woo JI, Park HJ, Park SR. The origin of cells that repopulate patellar tendons used for reconstructing anterior cruciate ligaments in man. J Bone Joint Surg Br 2003; 85:753–7.
27. Goradia VK, Rochat MC, Grana WA, Rohrer MD, Prasad HS. Tendon-to-bone healing of a semitendinosus tendon autograft used for ACL reconstruction in a sheep model. Am J Knee Surg 2000; 13:143–51.
28. Magen HE, Howell SM, Hull ML. Structural properties of six tibial fixation methods for anterior cruciate ligament soft tissue grafts. Am J Sports Med 1999; 27:35–43.
29. Haut Donahue TL, Howell SM, Hull ML, Gregersen C. A biomechanical evaluation of anterior and posterior tibialis tendons as suitable single-loop anterior cruciate ligament grafts. Arthroscopy 2002; 18:589–97.
30. Pearsall AWt, Hollis JM, Russell GV, Jr., Scheer Z. A biomechanical comparison of three lower extremity tendons for ligamentous reconstruction about the knee. Arthroscopy 2003; 19:1091–6.
31. CDC. Hepatitis C Transmission from and Antibody-Negative Organ and Tissue Donor - United States 2000–2002. MMWR 2003; 52:273–276.
32. Barbour SA, King W. The safe and effective use of allograft tissue–an update. Am J Sports Med 2003; 31:791–7.
33. Singhatat W, Lawhorn KW, Howell SM, Hull ML. How four weeks of implantation affect the strength and stiffness of a tendon graft in a bone tunnel: a study of two fixation devices in an extra-articular model in ovine. Am J Sports Med 2002; 30:506–13.
34. Kousa P, Jarvinen TL, Vihavainen M, Kannus P, Jarvinen M. The fixation strength of six hamstring tendon graft fixation devices in anterior cruciate ligament reconstruction. Part II: tibial site. Am J Sports Med 2003; 31:182–8.
35. Kousa P, Jarvinen TL, Vihavainen M, Kannus P, Jarvinen M. The fixation strength of six hamstring tendon graft fixation devices in anterior cruciate ligament reconstruction. Part I: femoral site. Am J Sports Med 2003; 31:174–81.
36. Smith CK, Hull ML, Howell SM. Migration of radio-opaque markers injected into tendon grafts: a study using roentgen stereophotogrammetric analysis (RSA). J Biomech Eng 2005; 127:887–90.
37. Smith CK, Hull ML, Howell SM. Lengthening of a single-loop tibialis tendon graft construct after cyclic loading: a study using Roentgen stereophotogrammetric analysis. J Biomech Eng 2006; 128:437–42.
38. Roos PJ, Hull ML, Howell SM. Lengthening of double-looped tendon graft constructs in three regions after cyclic loading: a study using Roentgen stereophotogrammetric analysis. J Orthop Res 2004; 22:839–46.
39. To JT, Howell SM, Hull ML. Contributions of femoral fixation methods to the stiffness of anterior cruciate ligament replacements at implantation. Arthroscopy 1999; 15:379–87.
40. Howell SM, Hull ML. Aggressive rehabilitation using hamstring tendons: graft construct, tibial tunnel placement, fixation properties, and clinical outcome. Am J Knee Surg 1998; 11:120–7.
41. Cossey AJ, Kalairajah Y, Morcom R, Spriggins AJ. Magnetic resonance imaging evaluation of biodegradable transfemoral fixation used in anterior cruciate ligament reconstruction. Arthroscopy 2006; 22:199–204.
42. Chandratreya AP, Aldridge MJ. Top tips for RIGIDfix femoral fixation. Arthroscopy 2004; 20:e59–61.
43. Brand J, Jr., Weiler A, Caborn DN, Brown CH, Jr., Johnson DL. Graft fixation in cruciate ligament reconstruction. Am J Sports Med 2000; 28:761–74.

44. Carson EW, Anisko EM, Restrepo C, Panariello RA, O'Brien SJ, Warren RF. Revision anterior cruciate ligament reconstruction: etiology of failures and clinical results. J Knee Surg 2004; 17:127–32.
45. Howell SM, Berns GS, Farley TE. Unimpinged and impinged anterior cruciate ligament grafts: MR signal intensity measurements. Radiology 1991; 179:639–43.
46. Weiler A, Peters G, Maurer J, Unterhauser FN, Sudkamp NP. Biomechanical properties and vascularity of an anterior cruciate ligament graft can be predicted by contrast-enhanced magnetic resonance imaging. A two-year study in sheep. Am J Sports Med 2001; 29:751–61.
47. Hame SL, Markolf KL, Hunter DM, Oakes DA, Zoric B. Effects of notchplasty and femoral tunnel position on excursion patterns of an anterior cruciate ligament graft. Arthroscopy 2003; 19:340–5.
48. Karchin A, Hull ML, Howell SM. Initial tension and anterior load-displacement behavior of high-stiffness anterior cruciate ligament graft constructs. J Bone Joint Surg Am 2004; 86-A:1675–83.
49. Howell SM, Gittins ME, Gottlieb JE, Traina SM, Zoellner TM. The relationship between the angle of the tibial tunnel in the coronal plane and loss of flexion and anterior laxity after anterior cruciate ligament reconstruction. Am J Sports Med 2001; 29:567–74.
50. Weiler A, Hoffmann RF, Bail HJ, Rehm O, Sudkamp NP. Tendon healing in a bone tunnel. Part II: Histologic analysis after biodegradable interference fit fixation in a model of anterior cruciate ligament reconstruction in sheep. Arthroscopy 2002; 18:124–35.
51. Greis PE, Burks RT, Bachus K, Luker MG. The influence of tendon length and fit on the strength of a tendon-bone tunnel complex. A biomechanical and histologic study in the dog. Am J Sports Med 2001; 29:493–7.
52. Howell SM, Roos P, Hull ML. Compaction of a bone dowel in the tibial tunnel improves the fixation stiffness of a soft tissue anterior cruciate ligament graft: an in vitro study in calf tibia. Am J Sports Med 2005; 33:719–25.
53. Petrigliano FA, McAllister DR, Wu BM. Tissue engineering for anterior cruciate ligament reconstruction: a review of current strategies. Arthroscopy 2006; 22: 441–51.
54. Lim JK, Hui J, Li L, Thambyah A, Goh J, Lee EH. Enhancement of tendon graft osteointegration using mesenchymal stem cells in a rabbit model of anterior cruciate ligament reconstruction. Arthroscopy 2004; 20:899–910.

20

Tissue Engineered Anterior Cruciate Ligament Graft

Timothy M. Simon and Douglas W. Jackson

Abstract: The anterior cruciate ligament (ACL) is the most frequently ruptured ligament in the knee that is associated with functional disability. Because it lacks successful healing capabilities, it is often reconstructed. The current methods utilizing autograft and allograft tissue to reconstruct the ACL have been quite successful. However, surgeons and patients would prefer grafts without the potential for donor site morbidity (autografts) and the potential for disease transmission and unavailability (allografts). In addition, there is time necessary to shape and prepare the graft material before implantation. Tissue engineering has the potential to address some of these issues and give a more ideal graft. Trying to create a functional tissue engineered ACL graft that is available and a cost-effective, value-added alternative presents the problems and challenges of the regeneration of any tissue. The ACL presents some unique challenges ahead in developing a biological engineered tissue replacement. These unique challenges are related to its complex microanatomy, its time zero and incorporated mechanical and structural properties and its intra-articular space and intrasynovial environment. Trying to duplicate the ACL's structural and mechanical characteristics is dependent on developing, placing and properly tensioning fibers of different lengths. Its intricate macro- and microanatomy have not been duplicated to date with engineered tissue or biomaterials. The native ACL has no adjacent soft tissue, as many ligaments in the body do, that can enhance the healing process.

While biologic substitutes (naturally occurring engineered tissue) have played a major role in ACL reconstruction and serve as a source of a great deal of scientific work and precedence to build upon, regeneration of a biologic ligament outside of the human has not been clinically perfected.

Keywords: Tissue engineering, anterior cruciate ligament (ACL), ACL grafts, ACL reconstruction, ACL substitutes, biomaterials.

Orthopaedic Research Institute at the Southern California Center for Sports Medicine and Long Beach Memorial Medical Center, Long Beach, CA

From: *Orthopedic Biology and Medicine: Musculoskeletal Tissue Regeneration, Biological Materials and Methods*
Edited by W. S. Pietrzak © Humana Press, Totowa, NJ

20.1. Introduction

Few structures of its size have received as much attention from the orthopaedic scientific community as the anterior cruciate ligament (ACL). In part, this is because the ACL is one of the most commonly ruptured ligaments in the human knee. It is an injury that receives almost daily coverage on sports pages all over the world. Many high profile athletes, as well as recreational athletes, rupture their ACLs. While many of these individuals return to their chosen sports and activity level after a surgical reconstruction of the ACL, there is room for improvement as clinical challenges continue.

It has been estimated that there are more than 300,000 ACL injuries annually in the United States and, in recent years, the number of injuries appear to be [1]. Many active individuals that sustain this injury have difficulty with their knee giving way and swelling with simple daily tasks that involve changing direction and abruptly stopping when walking and running. Orthopaedic surgeons often recommend ACL reconstructive surgery for symptomatic instability and to reduce the potential for further meniscal damage.

Currently most ACL reconstructions performed in these patients use an autograft of either bone-patellar tendon-bone or hamstring tendons. These autografts have provided reasonable clinical results in long-term objective and subjective evaluations [2–3]. These tendon grafts have showed some ability to be remodeled as they are incorporated [4]. Concerns associated with the use of autograft tissues include donor site morbidity, including anterior knee pain, residual muscle weakness, and reduced range-of-motion [5–6].

Many authors have proposed the use of allografts to reconstruct both acute and chronic ACL deficiencies. They feel these donated tissues obtained from cadavers eliminate the potential for donor site morbidity and require less invasive surgical techniques. The allografts being used include patellar tendon, hamstring tendon, Achilles tendon, anterior tibial tendons, fascia lata and quadriceps tendon [7–9]. There have been problems in the past and ongoing concerns associated with allograft usage. These include the risk of disease transmission, inflammatory (acute and chronic) and immunogenic reactions [10–11], and their additional costs. In addition, they have been reported to have decreased tensile properties after certain sterilization and preservation methodologies [1] and delayed incorporation in comparison to autografts [12]. The significant histocompatibility problems in orthopaedic surgery have been a factor with larger allografts [13]. A potential problem that would develop with widespread usage of allografts for ACL reconstructions would be their availability. There are a limited number of suitable donors each year.

The desire by surgeons to have an off-the-shelf ACL substitute available without the concerns for disease transmission and reducing the time for harvesting and/or preparing the grafts, has prompted the search and ongoing interest in the biotechnology to develop biomaterials for an ideal graft. The most successful experience to date with ACL substitutes has been with the basic biological material seen throughout the animal kingdom – collagen. This collagen is obtained and transplanted as tendinous autografts and allografts. In addition to this natural occurring biologic polymer, artificial materials such as polyester, polypropylene, polyethylene, expanded polytetrafluoroethylene (Teflon) and polylactide have demonstrated suboptimal results to date [14–15].

The high degree of homology and widespread presence of collagen in native tissues in the animal kingdom make xenografts appealing if techniques can be developed to reduce many of the biocompatibility problems that exist between species. This may be achieved, in part, by genetic manipulations of the animal sources and new methods of purifying and processing the collagen from xenografts. In addition, when using collagen for grafts there is the potential to improve and or hasten their remodeling and functional incorporation. Tissue engineering in the future for an ACL ligament will involve the careful orchestration and interaction of extracellular matrices, living cells and regulatory factors to create a synergy of conductive and inductive healing strategies.

The time zero matrix at implantation, which may be biologic or synthetic, serves in a conductive manner and/or as the scaffolding for cells to adhere to and grow upon. Regulatory factors can be used in an inductive manner causing cells to proliferate, differentiate and produce new matrix. The new matrix components ideally will replace the implanted matrix scaffold, which is remodeled, replaced and/or is resorbed. The challenge remains to develop a histologically, biomechanically and functionally homologous regenerated ACL ligament.

20.2. Anterior Cruciate Ligament - Form, Function and Properties

The ACL develops in concert, and is adjacent to, the posterior cruciate ligament within the intracondylar notch of the knee. The primary role of the anterior cruciate ligament is in contributing to and providing stability in the knee. It is a "check rein" or restraint against abnormal anterior tibial translation and plays a role in controlling abnormal rotation and hyperextension of the knee joint. In addition, the ACL appears to have a limited proprioceptive sensory role providing feedback to the muscular functions about the knee. Attributable to its four bar linkage, the cruciate ligaments have a role embryologically in forming the shape of the joint during development and contribute to the final range of motion during flexion and extension.

While the ACL has an important stabilizing role in the knee joint, it does not function as an isolated structure [16–21]. The anatomy of the ACL is closely related to its functions as a constraint of knee motion [22–33]. The characterization and our understanding of the mechanical and structural properties of the ACL have increased over the past two decades. Three key factors have emerged among the clinicians doing ACL reconstructions:

Factor 1 - Different parts of the ACL carry some load at different points in the range of motion [34–35]. The ACL is important in keeping the tibia from translating anteriorly relative to the femur [36], and from rotating in the flexed knee [16, 37]. Accordingly, the ACL has different ultimate force to failure values and failure mechanisms for different loads at different knee positions [38]. The injury mode begins in that portion of the ACL that is carrying load. Therefore, when testing for the injury, the three-dimensional position of the knee should be considered when performing diagnostic testing (drawer, KT-1,000, stress roentgenograms) and surgical reconstruction.

Factor 2 - From human and animal studies, it appears that the ACL carries only a small load during normal daily activity [39–41]. Normal daily activity loads are generally only 20 percent of the ACL tensile limit [40, 42]. The ultimate force to failure value in young individuals is approximately 2,400 newtons [38, 43]. Therefore, the ACL must function with repetitive low load cycles, but must provide occasional high strength performance for transitory high loading episodes.

Factor 3 - The highest loads on the ACL are achieved by excessive internal rotation, hyperextension of the knee, excessive valgus/varus stress on the tibia with a collateral deficient knee and, especially, quadriceps extension of the knee from about 40 degrees to full extension [20, 39, 41].

Like other tendons and ligaments, the ACL is a viscoelastic structure [44]. Accordingly, when load is applied, the ACL is able to adjust its length and, thus, redistribute load and the stresses on the constituent collagen fibers. This is a potentially important consideration for graft materials used to reconstruct the ACL, especially if they are significantly different from the native material [45]. A difference in viscoelastic properties may contribute to the stretch out or creep that occurs with some graft materials, resulting in a loose but not ruptured repair.

The normal ACL is composed of collagen, elastin, proteoglycans, water and cells [46–47]. The structural base of the ACL is formed from a hierarchical arrangement of mostly Type I collagen molecules. The collagen forms fibrils that are grouped into fibers, large numbers of which form subfascicular units that are separated by columns of cells in fibrous capsules. The subfascicular units and cells are bound together into fascicles [34] that ultimately form the functional bands of the ligament [22]. The fibers in the bands are selectively recruited into tension at different joint positions and loads. The recruitment of these fibers is related to where the various fibers insert into bone. As long as the fibers reside within the area of the ACL "footprint" (Fig. 20.1) they are relatively isometric, that is, the fibers may slightly elongate, but not rupture during normal range of motion [22]. This suggests that, for restoration of

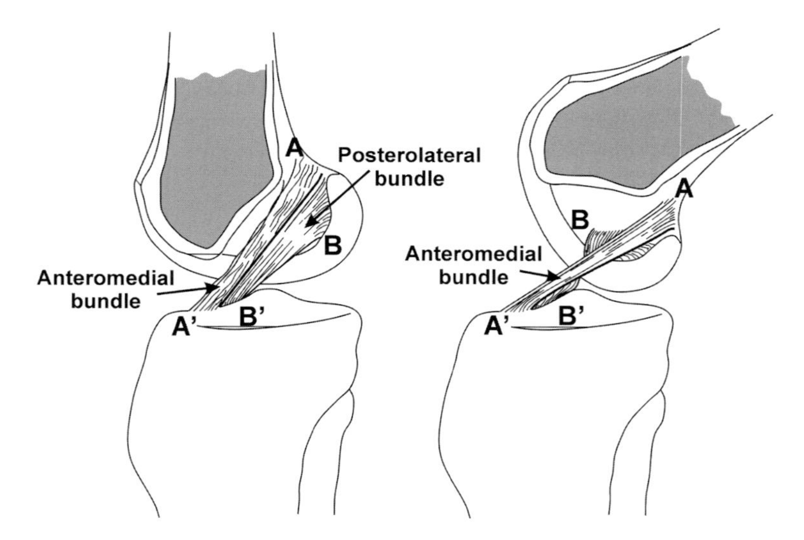

Fig. 20.1 The traditional two band description of the ACL is based on the tensioning action of the posterolateral and anteromedial fiber bundles The posterolateral bundle is taut in extension and the anteromedial bundle is taut at 60 degrees of flexion

normal ACL function, consideration should be given to duplicating the ACL placement and shape of the ACL insertion as closely as possible [22, 48].

The ACL courses anteriorly, medially and distally as it passes from femur to tibia, and twists approximately 90 degrees externally. The complex ACL structure can be simplified for surgical purposes as two ligament collagen bundles, an anteromedial and a posterolateral bundle, each of which contributes to anterior and rotational knee joint stability. The posterolateral bundle is taut in extension and the anteromedial bundle is taut at 60 degrees of flexion. This tensioning action of the posterolateral and anteromedial fiber bundles forms the basis for the traditional two-band description of the ACL. The functional interaction of the ACL components, i.e., collagen, proteoglycans, fibroblasts, blood vessels and nerves, and the effect of loading tension are still unclear. The complex microanatomy and ultrastructure of the normal human ACL are based on the interaction, orientation and spatial relationship of the matrix macromolecules and cells that compose it. To date, the mechanical and structural properties and physical characteristics of the ACL have not been duplicated successfully using autografts, allografts or synthetic substitutes. The traditional method to reconstruct the ACL utilizes a single bundle repair approach i.e., a graft with uniformly parallel fiber orientation that functions more as a "check rein" to limit the abnormal anterior tibial translation. It has been proposed that a potential improvement in reconstructed ACL outcomes may be achieved using an anatomic distinct two bundle approach [49–50]. Other techniques involve single socket femoral-two tibial tunnels, two femoral sockets-single tibial tunnel and a triple bundle approach with two femoral sockets-three tibial tunnels [51–52]. The double bundle ACL reconstruction and variants are being evaluated to see if any offer improved rotational stability and potentially longer term advantages (reducing potential development of osteoarthritis (OA)). However, long-term studies will be needed to demonstrate a better clinical outcome.

20.2.1. Microarchitecture of the Human ACL

The challenges in tissue engineering for an ACL include the native ligament having four classes of matrix macromolecules that form the molecular framework of the ACL: 1) collagen, 2) elastin, 3) proteoglycans and 4) glycoproteins. The interactions between these molecules result in the three dimensional and unique characteristics of the ACL.

Collagen structure The major matrix constituent of the ACL is collagen (about 75 percent dry weight). Approximately 90 percent is Type I collagen and most of the remaining collagen is Type III in the adult. Type III collagen is much more prevalent in fetal ACL and is sometimes referred to as embryonic or fetal collagen. Another collagen found in the ACL is Type VI (an adhesive glycoprotein) and is associated with cell attachment and enhanced cross-linking of collagen.

The diameter of the collagen fibrils varies within the ligament. Several studies have shown that the adult human ACL has a bimodal profile of collagen fibrils [53]. Most fibrils are in the 30 to 100 nm diameter range and a moderate number are greater than 100 nm. These patterns appear to vary during the aging process. At birth fibril diameters are predominantly small. With maturity more of the larger diameter fibrils are seen, but with aging the smaller fibrils again predominate [53].

Elastin Elastin comprises only about 5 percent of the molecular framework of the ACL, but its functional contribution is important. It forms networks interdigitated among collagen fascicles. Under tension the molecule is ordered and elongated. As the tension is released, the molecule takes on a coiled configuration. This behavior probably contributes to the tensile resistance and elastic recoverability of ligament tissue. It may also help restore the crimp pattern of the collagen fibril after deformation. The crimp pattern is a morphologic characteristic of ligaments such as the ACL, and manifests as a waviness of the orientated collagen at the level between collagen fiber and fascicles. The waviness period is approximately 20.6 ± 6.7 nm in the human ACL [44].

Proteoglycans and Glycoproteins Proteoglycans consist of a small protein bound to negatively charged polysaccharide chains and are associated with maintaining the molecular water balance between collagen fibrils. The glycoproteins have an important role in the complicated interactions of ligament cells and their matrix environment; however, how these functions are accomplished is poorly understood. It has been reported that the ACL has the highest proportion of glycosaminoglycans (GAG) that is two to four times the concentration present in tendons [46, 54]. These proteoglycans are also evident at the insertion sites of the collagen fibers into bone [48]. These studies suggest that the increased water associated with the GAGs in the ACL alters the viscoelastic properties and may provide additional "shock-absorbing" and load handling characteristics that are more important in ligaments than in tendons.

Cellular component Normal maintenance of the ACL is accomplished via the interaction of the cells with the matrix. The cells must synthesize new macromolecules to balance the losses due to normal degradation or microtrauma. The ACL is populated with different types of intrinsic cells. The outermost layer of the ACL is known as the epiligament and is populated with small fibrocytes and adipocytes. The epiligament continues into the substance of the ACL as the endoligament. The endoligament supports the neurovascular structures and divides the ligament into "bundles" or "fascicles" of collagen fibers [48].

Cells within the ligament substance are located between the longitudinal collagen fibers and have a variety of shapes ranging from ovoid to fusiform. It is unclear whether these cells represent a single or multiple cell population. The ovoid cells are typically arranged in columns between collagen fibers and lack extensive cytoplasmic processes. Fusiform fibrocytes are more elongated and closely approximate the dense collagen bundles. The cells are mechanically linked to the matrix through surface proteins called integrins. The integrin molecules mechanically link the matrix macromolecules to the internal cytoskeleton. Integrins participate in cell adherence, migration, proliferation and regulation of cell synthesis of new matrix macromolecules [55, 47].

20.2.2. Ligament Healing – Natural History

Following injury in extra-articular ligaments, a hematoma forms within the tissue around the ligament and functions as a chemotactic scaffold [56–57]. Inflammatory cells capable of secreting cytokines and growth factors then infiltrate the area. In the final stage of healing and maturation, fibroblasts re-populate the new tissue and synthesize collagen, which forms a vascular scar repair that is capable of further remodeling and maturing into a more organized structure. For an intra-articular ligament such as the ACL the healing response is not exactly the same. The synovial sheath blood supply is disrupted with the injury, but without formation of the functional focal hematoma. Without this hematoma scaffold, the subsequent healing events of localized chemotaxis, cytokine and growth factors are impaired [58].

Current tendon mechanical and structural properties of ACL autografts and allografts start out reasonably strong at time zero, but change during remodeling. The eventual reconstructed and remodeled ACL typically has areas of less organized structure, reduced endogenous cells owing to cell death (autografts), numerous blood vessels and inflammatory foci with exogenous cells infiltrating the graft and remodeling it with smaller diameter collagen microfibrils (Fig. 20.2). The end ACL graft is far from being like the native ACL (true regeneration). During incorporation the substance of the graft is partially broken down and replaced with a scar-like tissue [53]. This new scar collagen forms rapidly and replaces the graft's time zero collagen, and turns over with time. Initially, the replacement collagen organizes with the loading stresses. Gradual substitution results in a structure grossly resembling a ligament [4, 59, 60], but not necessarily similar at the ultrastructural level [53, 61–62]. Further, the mechanical properties of the reconstructed ligament are similar to organized scar and do not duplicate the desired ACL properties [61, 63–65]. The cells that re-populate the graft do not maintain or synthesize the tissue specific ACL structural and material properties. The results of these reconstructed ACL responses is a tissue that is weaker, and creeps (elongates) more than the native ACL [4, 66–67]. In our study the intact ACL in adult goats was subjected to a freeze-thaw technique that killed native ACL cells and destroyed the blood supply, leaving only the collagen in its original position and tension [68]. We demonstrated an increase in small diameter collagen fibrils within six months in the native ACL as the graft was re-populated with cells and vascularized. These changes in a damaged, yet otherwise intact ACL were comparable to those autogenous grafts and allograft reconstruction of the ACL in the goat model at six months [12]. This illustrated some of the intrinsic difficulties of ACL reconstruction that must be overcome to duplicate the native ACL structure.

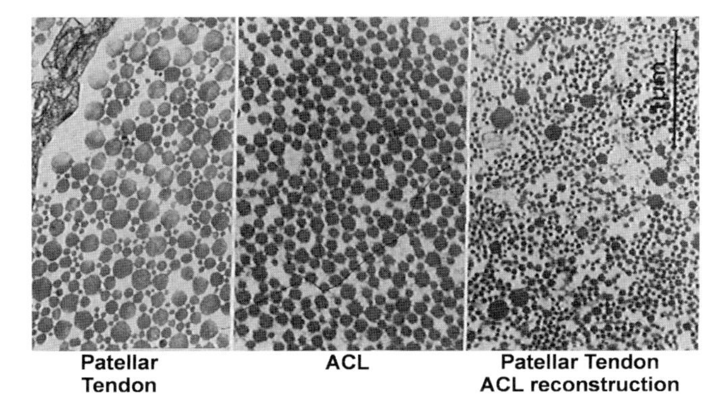

Fig. 20.2 Transmission electron micrographs showing the relative size of the collagen fibril diameters of the patellar tendon, anterior cruciate ligament and remodeled patellar tendon autograft six months after ACL reconstruction, and showing increased numbers of small diameter fibrils and residual original larger patellar tendon fibrils. Original magnification (all) x34,000

20.3. Ligament Tissue Engineerng Principles

Tissue engineering principles have been applied for years by orthopaedic surgeons performing ACL reconstructions. They have harvested a tendon (a natural occurring bioengineered collagen matrix by the body), with or without bone, and transplanted it as a scaffold providing mechanical and structural support. These matrices have living tendon cells and may have useful embedded intrinsic extracellular factors present at the time of implantation. Moreover, the graft site is prepared to encourage and induce the local environment to promote the desired remodeling (i.e., drilling the osseous tunnels and stimulating bleeding from the marrow space).

What is making us want to expand this current application of tissue engineering? Now, there are higher aspirations to produce a more organized tissue repair (i.e., closer to regeneration). To date, bone is the only musculoskeletal tissue to completely regenerate itself. The other musculoskeletal tissues (such as cartilage, ligament and tendon) repair themselves with organized scar tissue. The challenge for the clinician is to apply new technology and understanding to try and convert or alter the usual tissue repair to the regeneration of normal tissue.

20.3.1. Design Issues Relative to Cell Distribution

A very consistent and specific design is shared in nature relative to cells within the ligament. This is illustrated in the microstructure of ligament insertion into bone. It is common throughout the animal kingdom [48]. There is a transition of cells in a distinctive organization and is seen where the ACL inserts into bone. It allows a graduated change in stiffness and prevents stress concentration at the insertion site. This transition zone is important in the load transfer between the ligament and the more rigid bone, and is divided into four distinctive regions or zones. Zone 1 is ligamentous tissue that transitions into zone 2 that is fibrocartilage; zone 3 forms a transition from fibrocartilage to mineralized fibrocartilage, the outer limits of which are clearly demarcated by a "tidemark" or basophilic line that stains blue with hematoxylin. Zone 3 ultimately transitions into zone 4, which is bone. If a biologic graft biomaterial is to function as the living ACL, then an area of focus for the ACL substitute should include the graft/bone interface and how this will change and mature in the graft over time.

There are other cells within a functioning ACL. They are living, physiologically active, matrix producing cells that are capable of dynamically remodeling and repairing, within some limits, intrinsic damage within the ligament. Without living cells (i.e., ACL fibroblasts and other intrinsic cells), the ligamentous extracellular matrix and scaffold will degenerate over time. Mature ACL fibroblasts and other cells have been investigated with the hope that, after treatment with regulatory signals, the biologic clocks of these cells can be turned back, increasing their regenerative potential. Mature cell sources include fully differentiated fibrocytes or synovial cells that may be biopsied and cultured. Immature cells have also been the focus of study since, in their undifferentiated state, they have a broader potential for regeneration. Immature cell sources include autologous, pluripotential, bone marrow-derived mesenchymal stem cells or fetal cells that can be cultured into larger quantities. These cultured cells are then used to seed an engineered scaffold. The engineered scaffold, acting as a cell delivery system, is then implanted into the host target site to be reconstructed.

Initial cell studies involved culturing of two dimensional monolayers, which allow the study of cellular proliferation and processes. Studies progressed to involve three dimensional culturing techniques with sophisticated loading mechanisms to apply stresses to the growing cells, which allow further investigation of cellular differentiation. Current efforts involve three dimensional investigations of cell, matrix and regulatory factor interaction in a loading environment.

20.3.2. Viable Mature ACL

Existing literature suggested that transplanting mature living cells was important in the long-term survival of heart valve transplants [69–72]. To test this hypothesis in ACL surgery, we performed intra-articular transplantation of viable anterior cruciate ligament cells within a fresh anterior cruciate ligament allograft [73–74]. This potential for maintaining the matrix with the appropriate distribution of mature anterior cruciate ligament cells seemed ideal if the cells survived. Using a deoxyribonucleic acid (DNA) probe technique that clearly distinguished donor cells from host cells, it was shown that these viable mature anterior cruciate ligament allograft fibroblasts did not survive after transplantation in the goat model. They were replaced with host cells within a few weeks and we documented a similar remodeling process and cellular re-population in those anterior cruciate ligament allografts that did not have transplanted living cells.

A challenge involves attracting or altering specific cells that re-populate the grafts. A possible approach to this is the use of grafts containing extracellular and matrix factors. We have studied this concept by using demineralized bone. It is a repository of extracellular matrix factors. We felt this matrix might attract specific cells or modify their expression during the remodeling process. In an attempt to attract specific cells or to modify the expression of the cells that re-populate a graft, demineralized bone collagen matrix grafts were used for anterior cruciate ligament reconstruction [75–76]. In a goat model three specific and different zones of remodeling in the homogenous demineralized collagen graft were documented. These zones included bone formation within the osseous tunnels, establishment of the ligament transition zone to bone and intra-articular ligamentous remodeling devoid of the time zero cannicular structure of the collagen. The preliminary results using demineralized bone matrix, with its inherent residual extracellular and matrix factors, showed some site specific remodeling (Fig. 20.3) [75–76]. However, the intra-articular remodeling was slow and incomplete at the one-year follow-up.

20.3.3. Porosity

Pore size is an important feature when it is desirable to have cells seeded or infiltrating the scaffold material either *in vitro* or *in vivo*. Cell infiltration into the matrix interior is proportional to the material pore size or porosity. Large pore matrices allow for an even distribution of cells, while small pore matrices have a higher cell density at the surface and low cell density at the interior. A pore size of less than 60 microns permits poor cell infiltration and that of less

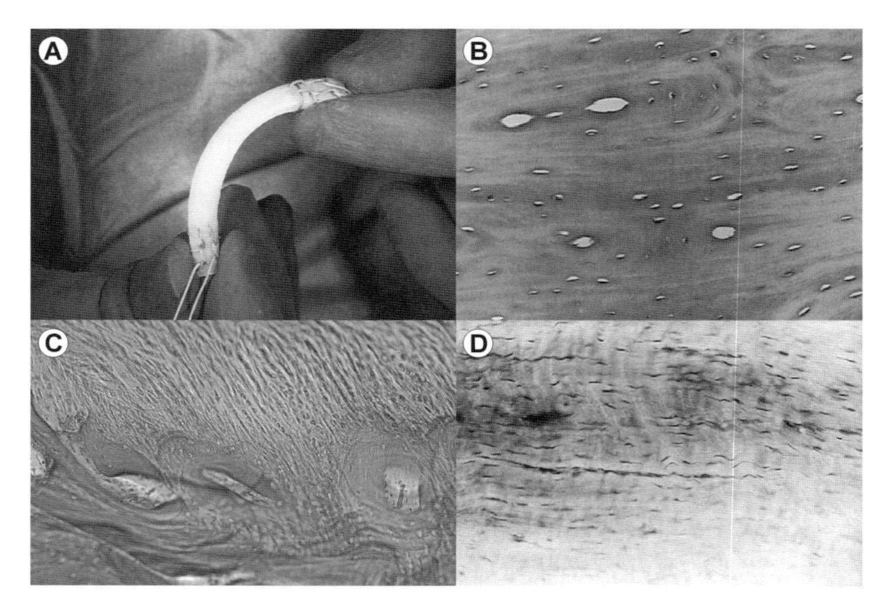

Fig. 20.3 Demineralized bone matrix (DBM) graft ACL reconstruction (A) Appearance of the graft at the time of implantation surgery Sutures were used for passing, tensioning, and fixing the graft in place (B) Histologic section showing the DBM at the time of implantation The bony architecture was intact, but acellular H&E stain, original magnification x40 (C) Histologic section showing the ligament-like collagen formed attachments to osseous tunnel walls through fibrocartilage Cells appeared organized into columns near the bone interface (lower portion of picture), one year after implantation surgery H&E stain, original magnification x40 (D) Histologic section showing the intra-articular portion of the remodeled graft with organized collagen with crimp pattern one year after surgery Toluidine blue stain, original magnification x40

than 25 microns prevents infiltration entirely. Porosity can also affect degradation rate. In contrast to what one might intuitively expect, high porosity PLA-PGA matrices show lower degradation rates than low porosity matrices. The lower porosity matrices are less able to evacuate the acidic degradation by-products that increase autocatalysis.

20.3.4. Mechanical Loading

If the stiffness of the graft is significantly greater than the ingrowing host tissue, then the graft may stress shield the tissue from mechanical loading. This can prevent it from remodeling and maturing. Cells also respond to mechanical loading stresses which can induce them to synthesize matrix and participate in remodeling [77].

Hence, the postoperative rehabilitation is as important as the operative procedure in these techniques. Motion and weight bearing are essential for healthy, transplanted or regenerated tissue nutrition and remodeling. Postoperative rehabilitation protocols have to strike a balance between the effects caused by subjecting the graft to too much load, and the stress shielding effects and degeneration that can occur when the graft sees too little motion and load.

20.3.5. Implantation Surgery Considerations

There are common ACL reconstructive techniques and issues relating to the intra-articular graft placement. These involve preparation of the intercondylar notch, tunnel placement and fixation, avoiding impingement, fixation and postoperative care. The time frame for protection and immobilization are dependent on time zero properties of the graft, the course of remodeling and ultimate strength.

20.3.6. Biomaterials for Ligaments

The ideal ACL substitute graft would duplicate all of the mechanical and physical properties of the native ACL in terms of strength, stiffness, elasticity, compliance, size and durability without producing any untoward reactions after implantation. The strength and stiffness of a variety of biomaterials used for ACL reconstruction are shown in Table 20.1. ACL graft substitutes, whether configured as matrices, scaffolds, lattices or substrates, are intended to re-establish the complex interactions and spatial relationship of the macromolecules and cells that compose the native ACL ligament. Ideally a biologic graft would develop the specific microanatomy and macroanatomy of the normal anterior cruciate ligament. Improved weaving, knitting and braiding strategies may facilitate the use of natural and synthetic polymers. Development of new polymers and surface treatment to enhance cell attachment, growth and differentiation are an area of continuing interest to the biomaterials engineer. Drug/factor delivery by cross-linked agents to the graft material is an emerging field [78]. Moreover, genetically engineered herds of animals that produce more human-friendly collagen grafts are a novel approach for the supply and manipulation of biomaterials [79–81].

A complex array of factors must be considered when constructing a scaffold for tissue engineering. Blends and combinations of polymers of polylactic acid, polyglycolic acid, polyanhydrides, polyphosphoesters, collagen, fibrin

Table 20.1 Mechanical properties of various biomaterials used for ACL reconstruction.

Material	Ultimate Tensile Load (N)	Stiffness (N/mm)
ACL (human) [89,127–128])	2,160; 1,725–2,160; 2,195	306; 242
Dacron	3,631	420
Gore-Tex prosthesis [91, 127]	5,300; 4,830	322
Hamstring graft (human) [128]	3,790–4,140	776
Knitted PLLA-PLGA scaffold [129]	29.4	
Ligament augmentation device (LAD) [127]	1,500	36
Parallel silk matrix [89]	2,214	1740
Patellar tendon graft (human) [89]		685
PLGA braid [130]	907	
Twisted silk matrix [89]	2,337	354

and cells are being investigated [82–83]. The precise combination of matrix molecules, crosslinks and three dimensional orientation will influence the matrices adhesive and cohesive properties, porosity, cell infiltration, permeability, hydrophobicity, degradation rate and regulatory factor release profile. Academic and commercial investigators are currently working to find such an optimal matrix for cartilage and connective tissue engineering.

20.3.7. Natural

20.3.7.1. Collagen

Collagen represents the major component of ligaments making up approximately 80 percent of the dry weight. It also represents a logical biomaterials choice as a potential ligament substitute. Collagen has a long history in medicine for use as suture material and for enhancing hemostasis. Collagen from bovine and ovine sources is most often used to produce extruded fibers and sheets. The collagen from these sources is processed to remove contaminating components (cells, cell fragments, etc.) that can act as foreign antigens after implantation. Generally, the intact triple helix portion of the collagen molecule is not very immunoreactive, whereas the telopeptide globular regions of the collagen can be reactive. A number of methods have been developed to process and purify collagen to address these issues [84]. In implantation studies grafts composed of parallel bovine collagen fibers, while showing fibroblast ingrowth and proliferation, failed to develop mechanical strength comparable to the native ligament [85–86]. The collagen in native ligaments has cross-links that are important for tensile strength properties, for durability and for affecting host cell response [87].

In an effort to improve the mechanical properties of collagen scaffolds, various cross-linking methods have been devised and have included chemical agents such as formaldehyde, glutaraldehyde, polyepoxy, carbodiimides, acylazide and hexmethylene diisocyanate [88]. However, toxic residues remaining in the collagen after treatment have been a problem. Physical methods have also been tried to avoid the toxic residue issues and include controlled drying, heating and exposure to gamma or ultraviolet radiation. The difficulties in controlling the cross-linking process, potential immunoreactivity and limited improvement in mechanical properties have slowed interest in collagen as a scaffold material.

20.3.7.2 Silk

Silk, like collagen, is a natural protein polymer that, when processed properly, shows some potential as a ligament scaffold material [89]. Silk is composed of a fibroin core and a sericin glue-like outer cover. It is the sericin cover that has been associated with most of the adverse and hypersensitivity issues [90]. Accordingly, sericin must be completely removed before use as a biomaterial in a living system. The fibroin core has outstanding mechanical properties and is slowly degraded by proteolytic enzymes, depending on the environment. Constructs of silk made by weaving the fibers into bundles and cords have been reported to have mechanical properties similar to the ACL [89, 91]. The silk fibers lose tensile strength by one year *in vivo* and are undetectable at two years [89]. Human bone marrow derived stem cells seeded onto silk scaffolds when subjected to rotational and translational stresses *in vitro* have been reported to produce collagen and other fibroblastic characteristics [91–92].

When the silk is properly processed it is biocompatible and has a predictable bioresorption rate and has had a long history of use as surgical sutures. There is a paucity of further *in vivo* studies reported.

20.3.8. Synthetic

Interest in the use of synthetic material to reconstruct the human ACL began in the early 20th Century, but it was not until the 1970s that several investigators began to focus on the search for an artificial substitute for the ACL. The present status of prosthetic devices suggests they have a very limited clinical indication. Initially, results were encouraging for isolated ACL injuries [14–15, 93–95]; however, problems with their use persist [96–97]. Results have been disappointing for their use in complex knee instabilities and salvage cases. It has been reported that 40 percent to 78 percent of prosthetic ligaments used for ligament reconstruction over the past 10 to 15 years have failed [98–101]. Early (within one year) and late failures of the devices were observed.

The ideal synthetic ligament should be tissue compatible and biomechanically competent. It should not incite any abnormal inflammatory response. If it induces a reaction, it should be directed to the induction of fibrous tissue ingrowth. The material should be free of any systemic side effects and should be nonmutagenic. The surgical technique for placement should be reliable and reproducible. When used, the graft should have a similar load deformation curve to the normal ACL and restore joint kinematics. Such criteria are not dissimilar for other biologic grafts.

20.3.8.1. Non-resorbable Polymers

To date the synthetic ligaments that have been used clinically consist of homogenous polymers that do not duplicate the mechanical and surface properties of the complex ACL. Some of the synthetic polymers that were recently used included the Gore-Tex® prosthetic ligament, composed of expanded polytetrafluoroethylene (Gore-Tex® is a registered trademark of W. L. Gore, Flagstaff, AZ); the ligament augmentation device (LAD® - original trademark registered to 3M Company, St. Paul, MN [trademark now cancelled]), composed of woven polypropylene, and the Stryker-Dacron® ligament prosthesis that is a composite of Dacron® tapes wrapped in a Dacron® sleeve (Dacron® is a registered trademark of Invista, Inc. Wichita, KS and licensed to Unifi Inc.) [14–15]. Attempts are being made to improve upon the currently available synthetics that have been used in the recent past. Early fragmentation of carbon fiber implants has been partially amended by the application of a resorbable coat of either a copolymer or collagen. The result was an observable reduction in intrasynovial carbon fibers. Filamentous carbon fiber implants have been used to replace the ACL in dogs [102–103] and treat tendon injuries in horses [104]. Similar to the carbon fiber treatment, Dacron® implants were coated with silicone to decrease abrasion, but 70 percent of these prototypes failed in two to four years. The compact Gore-Tex® II ligament, which has a "tighter" braid or weave design than its predecessor, lasts twice as long in abrasion testing and significantly improves the non-wear parameters (cyclic elongation, bending fatigue and ultimate tensile strength) [15].

Synthetic ligaments have been proposed for use as permanent ligaments, temporary stents or as scaffolds. Permanent ligaments such as the Gore-Tex® and the Stryker-Dacron® prostheses have high strength and increased resistance to fatigue failure. These grafts are permanent. Their time zero properties are unchanged unless they fail. They do not rely on the eventual contribution from tissue ingrowth. A stent differs as it is a temporary synthetic ligament. The polypropylene LAD is an example of a stent. It functions to augment the strength of a concurrent biologic reconstruction. Theoretically, with time, the role of the LAD decreases as the tissue strength increases. A scaffold device differs in that it allows or promotes the ingrowth of autogenous tissue. The scaffold device material becomes a composite with the biologic ingrowth.

Unlike their biologic counterparts, there are more complications associated with the failure of a synthetic ligament, which are often related to polymer wear debris in the joint [98–100, 105–108]. This has been a persistent problem with the current group of synthetic devices and has reduced their use to the point that some are no longer available. Newer material and design approaches may potentially provide a more ideal prosthetic ligament in the future.

20.3.8.2. Resorbable Polymers

Polylactic acid (PLA) is an aliphatic polyester that degrades into lactic acid. The resorption rate varies depending on molecular weight, size, shape and implantation site, and ranges from 10 to 48 months [109]. From *in vivo* studies done in sheep, the PLA reconstructed ACL had only 12.3 percent of the ultimate tensile strength after 48 weeks [110]. Attempts to use PLA in combination with collagen also failed to improve overall mechanical strength of the graft substitute because of poor integration between the PLA and collagen [82].

20.4. Bioactive Factors – Growth Factors, Gene Therapy

Molecular biologic studies led to the discovery of a new class of small protein regulatory factors. These factors, called growth factors and morphogenic proteins, regulate cell differentiation, control phenotypic expression, act as mitogens leading to cell proliferation and stimulate matrix synthesis. The most commonly investigated include: transforming growth factor – beta (TGF-beta), bone morphogenic proteins (BMPs), platelet-derived growth factor (PDGF), insulin-derived growth factor (IDGF), endothelial growth factor (EGF) and fibroblast growth factor (FGF). TGF-beta, PDGF, EGF and FGF have reported effects on ACL cell response. These include increased collagen synthesis, proteoglycan synthesis, cell proliferation and neovascularization [111–113]. Several of these growth factors have been shown to play a role in bone and cartilage formation, and may have a role in ACL reconstruction as well for osseous tunnel healing.

The transforming growth factor superfamily is a diverse group of growth factors that are ubiquitously present and influence a wide range of body tissues and biologic processes. These growth factors act in a paracrine manner and exert their influence by binding to cell surface receptors.

Recombinant human BMPS, TGF-beta and other factors are being impregnated into cell laden matrices. In the right combinations these factors may cause migration into the scaffold of primitive stem cells by chemotaxis, binding of cells to the matrix via fibronectin, integrins and other proteins, and activation, proliferation and differentiation of cells leading to new matrix production and tissue regeneration. Controlled delivery and distribution of these powerful agents at the appropriate time and concentration is an area for further study. In addition to microspheres, nanospheres and nanofibers (nanotechnology) may provide a potential delivery mechanism. The successful use of these bioactive factors will be dependent on a better understanding of how they induce healing pathways and tissue regeneration [114–116].

20.5. Assessment of ACL Graft Performance in the Animal Model

Animal models continue to be studied for their potential to provide information about how a proposed graft substitute may respond and function in the human knee. There is currently no particular animal model that does not have drawbacks. The large animal models, at best, provide an indication that a graft may work in the human knee. In addition, the animal models do provide information about the graft being tested regarding its safety and potential long-term durability. Technical considerations in the animal models are important. There are animal-specific issues related to graft placement, tensioning and early loading, methods of fixation, protected weight bearing as well as the size of the graft device being implanted.

While there are limitations in all animal models, the larger animals such as dogs, goats, sheep and pigs have been studied to obtain more insight into the ACL graft's remodeling process. The animal model permits large numbers of similar sized animals to be studied, use of standardized or traditional surgical techniques and can provide controls for comparisons. Our group has considerable experience with the goat model [117–118]. Other authors have also reported the use of the goat model [119]. Dogs have been the primary model to show the relationship between ACL deficiency and development osteoarthritis. Consequently, inhibition of OA development by efficacious ACL reconstruction with various ligament substitutes has been pursued in studies [120–121]. Many of the techniques that were initially investigated in the canine model are now routinely used to reconstruct ACLs. Porcine models have not been widely studied for their utility in ACL reconstruction, although reports suggest the porcine ACL have some similarities with the human ACL [122]. The rabbit model has reasonably good documentation of its biochemical and mechanical properties [123], although its relatively small size makes the reproducible ACL reconstruction and fixation difficult.

A critical assessment of the incorporation and/or failure mode of various future ACL substitute grafts will require dynamic *in vivo* biological environments such as the knee in an animal model. This allows comparisons and the characterization of the structural and mechanical properties of the time zero graft after its incorporation.

20.6. Future Directions

What are the chances of the regeneration of an ACL in the future? Today we are attempting to apply tissue engineering to our medical practice, based upon about 1 percent of the knowledge base that will be discovered over the next 100 years [124]. Regenerating (tissue engineering) a site-specific normal ACL is years away. How does nature produce (embryologically) an ACL: a high concentration of pluripotent and progenitor cells, a high cell-to-extracellular-matrix ratio in comparison to most adult tissues, a highly organized and carefully orchestrated process with numerous signaling and sequential activities? The entire embryonic development and generation of a specific mature ACL takes a considerable amount of time, progressive motion and loading in utero and then eventual weight bearing.

Cells that are living, physiologically active and matrix producing within a bioengineered construct will be essential to the success of the graft. Utilization of native ACL fibroblasts that are now debrided by most surgeons may potentially be a useful cell source. Since ACL fibrocytes are capable of migration into a scaffold, it appears the scaffold itself is more an issue for ACL regeneration. If stem cells or specific pluripotential host cells prove useful in tissue engineered ACL reconstruction, then a reliable source may need to be established.

Nanotechnology The microstructure of the ACL underscores the complex interactions between forces, cells, extracellular matrix and other structural components. Nanotechnology is an emerging technology that provides new fabrication methodology at and below the microstructural level. The electrospinning process is capable of creating nanofibers from 3 nm to 1 um. Such fibers can have a variety of pore designs that provide a good environment for cell attachment and orientation [125]. When cells are seeded on longitudinally oriented nanofibers they are reported to produce more collagen matrix than random fibril patterns, suggesting a relationship between scaffold orientation and matrix synthesis [83].

Bioreactors While growing and replicating desired cells, such as ACL specific fibroblasts, outside the patient for potential use at implantation surgery is possible, this also generates logistic issues and cost factors. A ligament designed specific bioreactor in an *in vitro* controlled environment would be ideal. In addition, using autologous cells are cheaper and preferred by most patients if given a choice. Future ligament substitute grafts will be explored, grown and developed on a scaffold for subsequent ligament reconstruction in the patient. The desired cell source will be seeded onto the scaffold device. Some studies will further explore exogenous stimuli, i.e., loading stresses, to provide and upregulate collagen synthesis and extracellular matrix production [126]. The goal in this approach is to develop a graft substitute that is ready for implantation that would be functional immediately, and would ultimately remodel. incorporate and further interact with the host tissues.

Cytokine Pathways and Inflammation The knee joint can be a difficult environment in which to attempt tissue regeneration. The initial injury event leads to initiation of the cytokine pathways and inflammation. However, the proinflammatory and anti-proinflammatory cytokine pathways are quite complex with many areas of cross talking. Currently, this is making it difficult to understand the exact role(s) of these mediator molecules in ACL repair and reconstruction. The proinflammatory cytokines appear to be potential therapeutic targets for controlling the joint environment or making it more conducive for a remodeling tissue. It may be beneficial to the remodeling process if some of these cytokine pathways are controlled or inhibited for certain phases of remodeling or incorporation. In the future, these controlling factors may be incorporated into the scaffold structure for controlled release.

20.7. Conclusions

Even though the current ACL replacements are structurally and mechanically inferior, patients undergoing replacement and reconstruction procedures experience reduced disability and restored function. Tissue engineering of an ACL substitute may give the orthopaedist an alternative in the future treatment for the ruptured ACL. While significant advances have been made and are being made in the area of tissue engineering and biomaterials, additional hurdles must be overcome before such techniques can be applied clinically to the ACL. Further studies are required on the optimal combination of growth factors, the behavior of cells in a scaffold and the ideal scaffold composition. Given the complex nature of engineered tissues and the unique risks posed by them, proper testing protocols must be developed. Biocompatibility *in vitro* may not be predictive of biocompatibility *in vivo*. The effects of scaffold degradation products, particularly those of synthetic scaffolds, need to be carefully examined. For example, Poly-L-Lactate breakdown products have been shown to interfere with bone regeneration. Neoplastic potential caused by degradation products or extracorporeal culture of cells must also be evaluated. Because of the species-specific tissues and the significant expense of recombinant and other technologies involved in tissue engineering, animal studies in this field may be difficult to perform. The standard for the foreseeable future will continue to be the currently used autograft and allograft (natural occurring human collagen scaffold) tendon implant. New improvements will need to justify their additional cost and demonstrate they are value-added replacements that show superior clinical and long-term outcomes.

References

1. Fu FH, Bennett CH, Lattermann C, Ma CB. Current trends in anterior cruciate ligament reconstruction. Part 1: Biology and biomechanics of reconstruction. Am J Sports Med 1999;27:821–830.
2. West RV, Harner CD. Graft selection in anterior cruciate ligament reconstruction. J Am Acad Orthop Surg 2005;13:197–207.
3. Freedman KB, D'Amato MJ, Nedeff DD, Kaz A, Bach Jr BB. Arthroscopic anterior cruciate ligament reconstruction: a metaanalysis comparing patellar tendon and hamstring tendon autografts. Am J Sports Med 2003;31:2–11.
4. Amiel D, Kleiner JB, Roux RD, Harwood FL, Akeson WH. The phenomenon of "ligamentization": anterior cruciate ligament reconstruction with autogenous patellar tendon. J Orthop Res 1986;4:162–172
5. Bach BR Jr, Levy ME, Bojchuk J, Tradonsky S, Bush-Joseph CA, Khan NH. Single-incision endoscopic anterior cruciate ligament reconstruction using patellar tendon autograft. Minimum two-year follow-up evaluation. Am J Sports Med 1998;26:30–40.
6. Bach BR Jr, Tradonsky S, Bojchuk J, Levy ME, Bush-Joseph CA, Khan NH. Arthroscopically assisted anterior cruciate ligament reconstruction using patellar tendon autograft. Five- to nine-year follow-up evaluation. Am J Sports Med 1998;26:20–29.
7. West RV, Harner CD. Graft selections in anterior cruciate ligament reconstruction. J Am Acad Orthop Surg 2005;13:197–207.
8. Schrock KB, Jackson DW. Allograft reconstruction of the anterior cruciate ligament: Basic Science. Operative Techniques in Sports Medicine 1995;3:139–147.

9. Fu FH, Jackson DW, Jamison J, Lemos MJ, Simon TM. Allograft reconstruction of the anterior cruciate ligament. In: The Anterior Cruciate Ligament: Current and Future Concepts. Editor: Douglas W. Jackson. Raven Press, Publisher, New York, NY, 1993, pp 325–338.
10. Crawford C, Kainer M, Jernigan D, Banerjee S, Friedman C, Ahmed F, Archibald LK. Investigation of postoperative allograft-associated infections in patients who underwent musculoskeletal allograft implantation. Clin Infect Dis 2005;41:195–200.
11. Harner CD, Fu FH. The immune response to allograft ACL reconstruction. Am J Knee Surg 1993;6:45–46.
12. Jackson DW, Grood ES, Goldstein JD, Rosen MA, Kurzweil PR, Cummings JF, Simon TM. A comparison of patellar tendon autograft and allograft used for anterior cruciate ligament reconstruction in the goat model. Am J Sports Med 1993;21:176–185.
13. Rodrigo JJ, Jackson DW, Simon TM, Muto KN. The immune response to freeze-dried bone-tendon-bone ACL allografts in humans. Am J Knee Surg 1993;6(2):47–53.
14. Fowler PJ. Synthetic augmentation. In The Anterior Cruciate Ligament. Current and Future Concepts 1993 Jackson DW, Arnoczky SP, Frank CB, Woo SL-Y, Simon TM (Eds) Raven Press New York 339–342.
15. McCarthy DM, Tolin BS, Schwendeman L, Friedman MC, Woo SL-Y. Prosthetic replacement of the anterior cruciate ligament. In The Anterior Cruciate Ligament. Current and Future Concepts 1993 Jackson DW, Arnoczky SP, Frank CB, Woo SL-Y, Simon TM (Eds) Raven Press New York 343–356.
16. Ahmed AM, Burke DL, Duncan NA, Chan KH. Ligament tension pattern in the flexed knee in combined passive anterior translation and axial rotation. J Orthop Res 1992;10:854–867.
17. Haimes JL, Wroble RR, Grood ES, Noyes FR. Role of the medial structures in the intact and anterior cruciate ligament-deficient knee. Limits of motion in the human knee. Am J Sports Med 1994;22:402–409.
18. Markolf KL, Wascher DC, Finerman GA. Direct in vitro measurement of forces in the cruciate ligaments. Part II: The effect of section of the posterolateral structures. J Bone Joint Surg 1993;75A:387–394.
19. Shapiro MS, Markolf KL, Finerman GA, Mitchell PW. The effect of section of the medial collateral ligament on force generated in the anterior cruciate ligament. J Bone Joint Surg 1991;73A:248–256.
20. Shoemaker SC, Adams D, Daniel DM, Woo SL. Quadriceps/anterior cruciate graft interaction. An in vitro study of joint kinematics and anterior cruciate ligament graft tension. Clin Orthop 1993;294:379–390.
21. Wascher DC, Markolf KL, Shapiro MS, Finerman GA. Direct in vitro measurement of forces in the cruciate ligaments. Part I: The effect of multiplane loading in the intact knee. J Bone Joint Surg 1993;75A:377–386.
22. Amis AA, Dawkins GP. Functional anatomy of the anterior cruciate ligament. Fibre bundle actions related to ligament replacements and injuries. J Bone Joint Surg 1991;73B:260–267.
23. Arnoczky SP, Warren RF. Anatomy of the cruciate ligaments. In Feagin JA Jr, (Ed) The cruciate ligaments, 1988 Churchill Livingstone New York, 179–195.
24. Brantigan OC, Voshell AF. The mechanics of the ligaments and menisci of the knee joint. J Bone Joint Surg 1941;23A:44–66.
25. Furman W, Marshall JL, Girgis FG. The anterior cruciate ligament: a functional analysis based on post-mortem studies. J Bone Joint Surg 1976;58A:179–185.
26. Fuss FK. Anatomy of the cruciate ligaments and their function in extension and flexion of the human knee joint. Am J Anat 1989;184:165–176.
27. Girgis FG, Marshall JL, Monajem A. The cruciate ligaments of the knee joint. Clin Orthop 1975;106:216–231.

28. Kaplan EB. Some aspects of functional anatomy of the human knee joint. Clin Orthop 1962;23:18–29.
29. Kennedy JC, Weinberg HW, Wilson AS. The anatomy and function of the anterior cruciate ligament as determined by clinical and morphological studies. J Bone Joint Surg 1974;56A:223–235.
30. Last RJ. Some anatomical details of the knee joint. J Bone Joint Surg [Br] 1948;30B:683–688.
31. Norwood LA, Cross MJ. Anterior cruciate ligament: functional anatomy of its bundles in rotary instability. Am J Sports Med 1979;7:23–26.
32. Odensten M, Gillquist J. Functional anatomy of the anterior cruciate ligament and a rationale for reconstruction. J Bone Joint Surg 1985;67A:257–262.
33. Welsh RP. Knee joint structure and function. Clin Orthop 1980;147:7–14.
34. Dodds JA, Arnoczky SP. Anatomy of the anterior cruciate ligament: a blueprint for repair and reconstruction. Arthroscopy 1994:10;132–139.
35. Hollis JM, Woo SL-Y. The estimation of anterior cruciate ligament loads in situ: indirect methods. In The Anterior Cruciate Ligament. Current and Future Concepts 1993 Jackson DW, Arnoczky SP, Frank CB, Woo SL-Y, Simon TM (Eds) Raven Press New York 85–94.
36. O'Connor JJ, Zavatski A. Anterior cruciate ligament forces in activity. In The Anterior Cruciate Ligament. Current and Future Concepts 1993 Jackson DW, Arnoczky SP, Frank CB, Woo SL-Y, Simon TM (Eds) Raven Press New York 131–140.
37. Hefzy MS, Grood ES. Knee motions and their relations to the function of the anterior cruciate ligament. In The Anterior Cruciate Ligament. Current and Future Concepts 1993 Jackson DW, Arnoczky SP, Frank CB, Woo SL-Y, Simon TM (Eds) Raven Press New York 75–84.
38. Woo SL-Y, Blomstrom GL. The tensile properties of the anterior cruciate ligament as a function of age. In The Anterior Cruciate Ligament. Current and Future Concepts 1993 Jackson DW, Arnoczky SP, Frank CB, Woo SL-Y, Simon TM (Eds) Raven Press New York 53–62.
39. Beynnon BD, Fleming BD, Pope MH, Johnson RJ. The measurement of anterior cruciate ligament strain in vivo. In The Anterior Cruciate Ligament. Current and Future Concepts 1993 Jackson DW, Arnoczky SP, Frank CB, Woo SL-Y, Simon TM (Eds) Raven Press New York 101–12.
40. Holden JP, Grood ES, Korvick DL, Cummings JF, Butler DL, Bylski-Austrow DI. In vivo forces in the anterior cruciate ligament: direct measurements during walking and trotting in a quadruped. J Biomech 1994;27:517–526.
41. Lewis JL, Lew WD, Markolf KL. The measurement of anterior cruciate ligament loads: direct methods. In The Anterior Cruciate Ligament. Current and Future Concepts 1993 Jackson DW, Arnoczky SP, Frank CB, Woo SL-Y, Simon TM (Eds) Raven Press New York 95–100.
42. Beynnon BD, Fleming BC, Johnson RJ, Nichols CE, Renstrom PA, Pope MH. Anterior cruciate ligament strain behavior during rehabilitation exercises in vivo. Am J Sports Med 1995;23:24–34.
43. Kdolsky R, Kwasny O, Schabus R. Synthetic augmented repair of proximal ruptures of the anterior cruciate ligament. Long-term results of 66 patients. Clin Orthop 1993;295:183–189.
44. Haut RC. The mechanical and viscoelastic properties of the anterior cruciate ligament and of ACL fascicles. In The Anterior Cruciate Ligament. Current and Future Concepts 1993 Jackson DW, Arnoczky SP, Frank CB, Woo SL-Y, Simon TM (Eds) Raven Press New York 63–74.
45. King GJ, Edwards PE, Brant R, Shrive NG, Frank CB. Intraoperative graft tensioning alters viscoelastic but not failure behaviors of rabbit medial collateral ligament autografts. J Orthop Res 1995;13:915–922.

46. Amiel D, Billings E, Akeson WH. Ligament structure, chemistry and physiology. In Knee Ligaments: Structure, Function, Injury and Repair 1990 Daniel DD, Akeson WH, O'Connor JJ (Eds) Raven Press New York 77–91.
47. McDevitt CA, Marcelino J. Adhesion macromolecules of the ligament: the molecular glues in wound healing. In The Anterior Cruciate Ligament. Current and Future Concepts 1993 Jackson DW, Arnoczky SP, Frank CB, Woo SL-Y, Simon TM (Eds) Raven Press New York 179–188.
48. Arnoczky SP, Matyas JR, Buckwalter JA, Amiel D. Anatomy of the anterior cruciate ligament. In The Anterior Cruciate Ligament. Current and Future Concepts 1993 Jackson DW, Arnoczky SP, Frank CB, Woo SL-Y, Simon TM (Eds) Raven Press New York 5–22.
49. Chhabra A, Starman JS, Ferretti M, Vidal AF, Zantop T, Fu FH. Anatomic, radiographic, biomechanical, and kinematic evaluation of the ACL and its two functional bundles. J Bone Joint Surg (Am), in press 2006.
50. Zelle BA, Brucker PU, Feng MT, Fu FH.: Anatomical double-bundle anterior cruciate ligament reconstruction. Sports Med 2006;36:2:99–108.
51. Comparing graft options for ACL: Which offers the most benefits today? (www.orthosupersite.com) Orthop Today International March 2006;9:34.
52. Yasuda K, Kondo E, Ichiyama H, Tanabe Y, Tohyama H. Clinical evaluation of anatomic double-bundle anterior cruciate ligament reconstruction procedure using hamstring tendon grafts: comparisons among 3 different procedures. Arthroscopy 2006;22:240–51.
53. Oakes BW. Collagen ultrastructure in the normal ACL and in ACL graft. In The Anterior Cruciate Ligament. Current and Future Concepts 1993 Jackson DW, Arnoczky SP, Frank CB, Woo SL-Y, Simon TM (Eds) Raven Press New York 209–217.
54. Amiel D, Frank C, Harwood F, Fronek J, Akeson W. Tendons and ligaments: a morphological and biochemical comparison. J Orthop Res 1984;1:257–265.
55. Murphy PG, Frank C, Hart DA. The cell biology of ligaments and ligament healing. In The Anterior Cruciate Ligament. Current and Future Concepts 1993 Jackson DW, Arnoczky SP, Frank CB, Woo SL-Y, Simon TM (Eds) Raven Press New York 165–177.
56. Woo SL, Inoue M, McGurk-Burleson E, Gomez MA. Treatment of the medial collateral ligament injury. II: Structure and function of canine knees in response to differing treatment regimens. Am J Sports Med 1987;15:22–29.
57. Pascher A, Steinert AF, Palmer GD. Enhanced repair of the anterior cruciate ligament by in situ gene transfer evaluation in an in vitro model. Mol Ther 2004;10:327–336.
58. Hefti FL, Kress A, Fasel J, Morscher EW. Healing of the transected anterior cruciate ligament in the rabbit. J Bone Joint Surg 1991;73:373–383.
59. Amiel D, Kleiner JB, Akeson WH. The natural history of the anterior cruciate ligament autograft of patellar tendon origin. Am J Sports Med 1986;14:449–462.
60. Lane JG, Mcfadden P, Bowden K, Amiel D. The ligamentization process: a 4 year case study following ACL reconstruction with a semitendinosus graft. Arthroscopy 1993;9:149–153.
61. Ballock RT, Woo SL, Lyon RM, Hollis JM, Akeson WH. Use of patellar tendon autograft for anterior cruciate ligament reconstruction in the rabbit: a long-term histologic and biomechanical study. J Orthop Res 1989;7:474–485.
62. Shino K, Oakes BW, Horibe S, Nakata K, Nakamura N. Collagen fibril populations in human anterior cruciate ligament allografts. Electron microscopic analysis. Am J Sports Med 1995;23:203–208.
63. Jackson DW, Lemos MJ. Autograft reconstruction of the anterior cruciate ligament: bone-patellar tendon-bone. In The Anterior Cruciate Ligament. Current and Future Concepts 1993 Jackson DW, Arnoczky SP, Frank CB, Woo SL-Y, Simon TM (Eds) Raven Press New York 291–304.

64. Ng GY, Oakes BW, Deacon OW, Mclean ID, Lampard D. Biomechanics of patellar tendon autograft for reconstruction of the anterior cruciate ligament in the goat: three-year study. J Orthop Res 1995;13:602–608.
65. Beynnon BD, Johnson RJ, Fleming BC. The mechanics of anterior cruciate ligament reconstruction. In The Anterior Cruciate Ligament. Current and Future Concepts 1993 Jackson DW, Arnoczky SP, Frank CB, Woo SL-Y, Simon TM (Eds) Raven Press New York 259–272.
66. Frank CB, Jackson DW. The science of reconstruction of the anterior cruciate ligament. J Bone Joint Surg 1997;79:1556–1576.
67. Hildebrand KA, Frank CB. Scar formation and ligament healing. Can J Surg 1998;41:425–429.
68. Jackson DW, Grood ES, Cohn BT, Arnoczky SP, Simon TM. The effects of in situ freezing on the anterior cruciate ligament. An experimental study in goats. J Bone Joint Surg 1991;73A:201–213.
69. Kosek JC, Iben AB, Shumway NE, Angell WW. Morphology of fresh heart valve homografts. Surg 1969;66:269–274.
70. Mohri H, Reichenbach DD, Barnes RW, Merendino KA. A biologic study in the homologous aortic valve in dogs. J Thorac Cardiovas Surg 1967;54:622–628.
71. Mohri H, Reichenbach DD, Barnes RW, Merendino KA. Homologous aortic valve transplantation. Alterations in viable and nonviable valves. J Thorac Cardiovas Surg 1968;56:767–774.
72. O'Brien MF, Stafford G, Gardner M, Pohlner P, McGiffin D, Johnston N, Brosnan A, Duffy P. The viable cryopreserved allograft aortic valve. J Cardiac Surg 1987;2(Suppl):153–167.
73. Jackson DW, Simon TM, Kurzweil PR, Rosen MA. DNA probe analysis of fresh allograft cells after ACL reconstruction. Trans Orthop Res Soc 1991;16:184.
74. Jackson DW, Simon TM, Kurzweil PR, Rosen MA. Survival of cells after intra-articular transplantation of fresh allografts of the patellar and anterior cruciate ligament: DNA probe analysis in a goat model. J Bone Joint Surg 1992;74A:112–118.
75. Jackson DW, Simon TM, Lowery W, Gendler E. Anterior cruciate ligament reconstruction using collagen matrix derived from demineralized bone in a goat model. Trans Orthop Res Soc 1995;20:2:634.
76. Jackson DW, Simon TM, Lowery W, Gendler E. Biologic remodeling after anterior cruciate ligament reconstruction using a collagen matrix derived from demineralized bone: An experimental study in the goat model. Am J Sports Med 1996; 24:405–414.
77. Hart DA, Natsu-ume T, Sciore P, Tasevski V, Frank CB, Shrive NG, Pandalai SG. Mechanobiology: Similarities and differences between in vivo and in vitro analysis at the functional and molecular levels. Recent Res Devel Biophys Biochem. 2002;2:157–177.
78. SE Sakiyama-Elber, Hubbell JA. Functional biomaterials: Design of novel biomaterials. Ann Rev Materials Res 2001;31:183–201.
79. Ahn C, Kim JY, Lee BC, Kang SK, Lee JR, Hwang WS. The past, present, and future of xenotransplantation. Yonsei Med J 2004;45:1017–1024.
80. Cascalho M, Platt JL. The immunologic barriers to replacing damaged organs. Curr Top Microbiol Immunol 2003;278:1–21.
81. Kaiser J. Xenotransplantation: Cloned pigs may help overcome rejection. Science 2002; 295:25–27.
82. Ge Z, Yang F, Goh JC, Ramakrishna S, Lee EH. Biomaterials and scaffolds for ligament tissue engineering. J Biomed Mater Res 2006;77A:639–652.
83. Petrigliano FA, McAllister DR, Wu BM. Tissue engineering for anterior cruciate ligament reconstruction: A review of current strategies. Arthroscopy 2006;22:4:441–451.
84. Hutmacher DW, Goh C, Teoh SH. An introduction to biodegradable materials for tissue engineering applications. Ann Acad Med Singapore 2001;30:183–191.

85. Dunn MG, Liesch JB, Tiku ML, Zawadsky JP. Development of fibroblast-seeded ligament analogs for ACL reconstruction. J Biomed Mater Res 1995;29:1363–1371.
86. Bellincampi LD, Closkey RF, Prasad R, Zawadsky JP, Dunn MG. Viability of fibroblast-seeded ligament analogs after autogenous implantation. J Orthop Res 1998;16:414–420.
87. Caruso AB, Dunn MG. Changes in mechanical properties and cellularity during long-term culture of collagen fiber ACL reconstruction scaffolds. J Biomed Mater Res A 2005;73:388–397.
88. Khor E. Methods for the treatment of collagenous tissues for bioprostheses. Biomaterials 1997;18:95–105.
89. Altman GH, Horan RL, Lu HH, Moreau J, Martin I, Richmond JC, Kaplan DL. Silk matrix for tissue engineered anterior cruciate ligaments. Biomaterials 2002;23:4131–4141.
90. Chen J, Altman GH, V. Karageorgiou V, Horan R, Collette A, Volloch V, Colabro T, Kaplan DL. Human bone marrow stromal cell and ligament fibroblast responses on RGD-modified silk fibers. J Biomed Mater Res A 2003;67:559–570.
91. Vunjak-Novakovic G, Altman G, Horan R, Kaplan DL. Tissue engineering of ligaments. Ann Rev Biomed Eng 2004;6:131–156.
92. Altman GH, Horan RL, Martin I, Farhadi J, Stark PR, Volloch V, Richmond JC, Vunjak-Novakovic G, Kaplan DL. Cell differentiation by mechanical stress. FASEB J 2002;16:270–272.
93. Dahlstedt L, Dalen N, Jonsson U. Goretex prosthetic ligament vs. Kennedy ligament augmentation device in anterior cruciate ligament reconstruction. A prospective randomized 3-year follow-up of 41 cases. Acta Orthop Scand 1990;61:217–224.
94. Dahlstedt L, Dalen N, Jonsson U, Adolphson P. Cruciate ligament prosthesis vs. augmentation. A randomized, prospective 5-year follow-up of 41 cases. Acta Orthop Scand 1993;64:431–433.
95. Richmond JC, Manseau CJ, Patz R, McConville O. Anterior cruciate reconstruction using a Dacron ligament prosthesis. A long-term study. Am J Sports Med 1992;20:24–28.
96. Muren O, Dahlstedt L, Dalen N. Reconstruction of old anterior cruciate ligament injuries. No difference between the Kennedy LAD-method and traditional patellar tendon graft in a prospective randomized study of 40 patients with 4-year follow-up. Acta Orthop Scand 1995;66:118–122.
97. Noyes FR, Barber SD. The effect of a ligament-augmentation device on allograft reconstructions for chronic ruptures of the anterior cruciate ligament. J Bone Joint Surg 1992;74A:960–973.
98. Barrett GR, Line LL Jr, Shelton WR, Manning JO, Phelps R. The Dacron ligament prosthesis in anterior cruciate ligament reconstruction. A four-year review. Am J Sports Med 1993;21:367–373.
99. Dandy DJ, Gray AJ. Anterior cruciate ligament reconstruction with the Leeds-Keio prosthesis plus extra-articular tenodesis. Results after six years. J Bone Joint Surg 1994;76B:193–197.
100. Engstrom B, Wredmark T, Westblad P. Patellar tendon or Leeds-Keio graft in the surgical treatment of anterior cruciate ligament ruptures. Intermediate results. Clin Orthop 1993;295:190–197.
101. Paulos LE, Butler DL, Noyes FR, Grood ES. Intra-articular cruciate reconstruction: II. Replacement with vascularized patellar tendon. Clin Orthop Rel Res 1983;172:78–84.
102. Denny HR, Goodship AE. Replacement of the anterior cruciate ligament with carbon fibre in the dog. J Small Anim Prac 1980;21:279–286.

103. Goodship AE, Brown PN, Silver IA, Jenkins D, Kirby M. Use of carbon fibre for tendon repair. Vet Rec 1978;102:322.
104. Goodship AE, Brown PN, Yeats JJ, Jenkins DH, Silver IA. An assessment of filamentous carbon fibre for the treatment of tendon injury in the horse. Vet Rec 1980:106:217–221.
105. Demaio M, Noyes FR, Mangine RE. Principles for aggressive rehabilitation after reconstruction of the anterior cruciate ligament. Orthopedics 1992;15:385–392.
106. Kurosawa H, Yasuda K, Yamakoshi K, Kamiya A, Kaneda K. An experimental evaluation of isometric placement for extra-articular reconstructions of the anterior cruciate ligament. Am J Sports Med 1991;19:384–388.
107. Paulos LE, Rosenberg TD, Grewe SR, Tearse DS, Beck CL. The GORE-TEX anterior cruciate ligament prosthesis. A long-term follow-up. Am J Sports Med 1992;20:246–252.
108. Woods GA, Indelicato PA, Prevot TJ. The Gore-Tex anterior cruciate ligament prosthesis. Two versus three year results. Am J Sports Med 1991;19:48–55.
109. Migliaresi C, Fambri L, Cohn D. A study on the in vitro degradation of poly(lactic acid). J Biomater Sci Polym Ed 1994;5:591–606.
110. Laitinen 0, Pohjonen T, Tormala P, Saarelainen K, Vasenius J, Rokkanen P, Vainionpaa S. Mechanical properties of biodegradable poly-L-lactide ligament augmentation device in experimental anterior cruciate ligament reconstruction. Arch Orthop Trauma Surg 1993;112:270–274.
111. Meaney Murray M, Rice K, Wright RJ, Spector M. The effect of selected growth factors on human anterior cruciate ligament cell interactions with a three-dimensional collagen-GAG scaffold. J Orthop Res 2003;21:238–244.
112. Kobayashi D, Kurosaka M, Yoshiya S, Mizuno K. Effect of basic fibroblast growth factor on the healing of defects in the canine anterior cruciate ligament. Knee Surg Sports Traumatol Arthrosc 1997;5:189–194.
113. DesRosiers EA, Yahia L, Rivard CH. Proliferative and matrix synthesis response of canine anterior cruciate ligament fibroblasts submitted to combined growth factors. J Orthop Res 1996;14:200–208.
114. Moreau JE, Chen J, Bramono DS. Growth factor induced fibroblast differentiation from human bone marrow stromal cells in vitro. J Orthop Res 2005;23:164–174.
115. Hankemeier S, Keus M, Zeichen J, Jagodzinski M, Barkhausen T, Bosch U, Krettek C, Griensven MV. Modulation of proliferation and differentiation of human bone marrow stromal cells by fibroblast growth factor 2: Potential implications for tissue engineering of tendons and ligaments. Tissue Eng 2005;11:41–49.
116. Bramono DS, Richmond JC, Weitzel PP Chernoff H, Martin I, Volloch V, Jakuba CM, Diaz F, Gandhi JS, Kaplan DL, Altman GH. Characterization of transcript levels for matrix molecules and proteases in ruptured human anterior cruciate ligaments, Connect Tissue Res 2005;46:53–65.
117. Jackson DW, Simon TM. Reduced A/P translation associated with adaptive changes in the meniscus in the failed ACL reconstruction goat model. Trans Orthop Res Soc 1997;22:1:100.
118. Proctor CS, Jackson DW, Simon TM. Characterization of the replacement tissue after harvesting the central one-third of the patellar ligament: an experimental study in a goat model. J Bone Joint Surg 1997;79A:997–1006.
119. Goulet F, Rancourt D, Cloutier R. Torn ACL: a new bioengineered substitute brought from the laboratory to the knee joint. Applied Bionics Biomech. 2004;1:115–121.
120. Tashman S, Anderst W, Kolowich P, Havstad S, Arnoczky S. Kinematics of the ACL deficient canine knee during gait: serial changes over two years. J Orthop Res. 2004;22:931–941.
121. Lopez MJ, Kunz D, Vanderby R Jr, Heisey D, Bogdanske J, Markel MD. A comparison of joint stability between anterior cruciate ligament intact and deficient

knees: A new canine model of anterior cruciate ligament disruption. J Orthop Res 2003;21:224–230.

122. Xerogeanes JW, Fox RJ, Takeda Y, Kim HS, Ishibashi Y, Carlin GJ, Woo SL. A functional comparison of animal anterior cruciate ligament models to the human anterior cruciate ligament. Ann Biomed Eng 1998;26:345–352.
123. An HY, Friedman RJ. Animal selections in orthopaedic research. In: An HY, Friedman RJ, editors. Animal Models in Orthop Res. New York: CRC; 1999. 39–58.
124. Venter JC: The Medical Futures Forum: The Genome On Main Street. The Pfizer J 1998;2:13–25.
125. Lee CH, Shin HJ, Cho IH, Kang YM, Kim IA, Park KD, Shin JW. Nanofiber alignment and direction of mechanical strain affect the ECM production of human ACL fibroblast. Biomaterials 2005;26:1261–1270.
126. Altman GH, Lu HH, Horan RL, Calabro T, Ryder D, Kaplan DL, Stark P, Martin I, Richmond JC, Vunjak-Novakovic G. Advanced bioreactor with controlled application of multidimensional strain for tissue engineering. J Biomech Eng 2002;124:742–749.
127. Dunn MG. Anterior cruciate ligament prostheses. In: Pahey T, editor. Encyclopedia of Sports Med and Science. 2004. Available at http://www.sportsci.org/encyc/index.html.
128. Rittmeister M, Noble PC, Lintner DM, Alexander JW, Conditt M, Kohl HW III. The effect of strand configuration on the tensile properties of quadrupled tendon grafts. Arthroscopy 2002;18:194–200.
129. Ge Z, Goh J, Lee EH. The effects of bone marrow-derived mesenchymal stem cells and fascia wrap application to anterior cruciate ligament tissue engineering. Cell Transplant 2006;14:763–773.
130. Cooper JA, Lu HH, Ko FK, Freeman JW, Laurencin CT. Fiber based tissue-engineered scaffold for ligament replacement: Design considerations and in vitro evaluation. Biomaterials 2005;26:1523–1532.

21

Biologic Scaffold Materials for Orthopaedic Soft Tissue Reconstruction

Stephen F. Badylak

Abstract: Biologic scaffold materials composed of extracellular matrix (ECM) are being used for the repair and reconstruction of injured or weakened orthopaedic soft tissues, especially the rotator cuff. These ECM-based products differ in their tissue of origin, species of origin and the processing and sterilization procedures used to prepare such materials for human clinical use. These differences clearly alter the host tissue remodeling response, clinical course and clinical outcome. This chapter reviews the composition, preparation and mechanical and material properties of ECM scaffold materials. Preclinical and clinical studies, although relatively few in number, are also reviewed for the commercial products currently available for orthopaedic soft tissue surgical application.

Keywords: Extracellular matrix, bioscaffolds, rotator cuff, orthopaedic soft tissue, regenerative medicine, tissue engineering.

21.1. Introduction

Freshly harvested autologous tissue is commonly used as a scaffold or graft for orthopaedic soft tissue reconstruction, such as anterior cruciate ligament repair [1–5], ulnar collateral ligament repair, rotator cuff repair [6–8] and, less commonly, Achilles tendon repair. Donor tissues for these applications include the middle third of the patellar tendon [1, 9–10], semitendinosus tendon [1, 9–10], the latissimus dorsi tendon [7], the palmaris longus tendon and the fascia lata [11–13]. Synthetic biomaterials such as polytetrafluoroethylene [14–16], polyethylene terephthalate (Dacron®) and Marlex mesh are used for selected surgical procedures, more commonly in non-orthopaedic applications, when autologous tissue is either absent or otherwise unacceptable [17]. During the past five to seven years off-the-shelf biologic scaffold materials composed of extracellular matrix (ECM) have become available for the repair and

Department of Surgery, McGowan Institute for Regenerative Medicine, Department of Surgery, University of Pittsburgh, Pittsburgh, PA

From: *Orthopedic Biology and Medicine: Musculoskeletal Tissue Regeneration, Biological Materials and Methods*
Edited by W. S. Pietrzak © Humana Press, Totowa, NJ

reconstruction of injured or weakened orthopaedic soft tissues, especially the rotator cuff. The clinical products currently available include GraftJacket® (Wright Medical Technology, Inc., Arlington, TN), Restore™ (DePuy Orthopaedics®, Inc., Warsaw, IN), CuffPatch™ (Arthrotek, Warsaw, IN), TissueMend® (TEI Biosciences, Inc., Boston, MA), Zimmer® Collagen Repair Patch (Tissue Science Laboratories, Covington, GA) and OrthADAPT™ (Pegasus Biologics, Irvine, CA). These ECM- based products differ in the tissue of origin, species of origin and the processing and sterilization procedures used to prepare each material for human clinical use. These differences can clearly alter the host tissue remodeling response, clinical course and clinical outcome.

Many of the ECM scaffold materials currently available for orthopaedic applications are also used for tissue reconstruction in other body systems. The prototype of these ECMs is small intestinal submucosa (SIS). The SIS-ECM material from which the Restore™ device is manufactured is also marketed as Oasis®, Surgisis® and Durasis® for the treatment of skin wounds, general surgery applications and replacement of the dura mater, respectively. Human dermis, the material from which Graft Jacket® is constructed, is sold as Alloderm® and marketed for the treatment of skin wounds and other surgical applications. Carbodiimide cross-linked SIS-ECM, the material from which CuffPatch™ is manufactured, is available in a multilaminate form as Graft Patch™ which is sold as a general surgery soft tissue repair material. The Zimmer® Collagen Repair Patch was previously marketed as Permacol®. Permacol® is used for general surgery applications and for the treatment of skin wounds. In summary, the use of ECM scaffolds for orthopaedic soft tissue repair is certainly not unique. However, the general principles of tissue remodeling, the indications and contraindications, and the rehabilitation regimens that optimize the clinical outcomes have many common features.

Purported advantages of using ECM-derived scaffold materials, instead of purified components of the ECM such as Type I collagen or synthetic biomaterials, include their natural three-dimensional ultrastructure and their diverse composition of structural and functional proteins including collagen, elastin, growth factors and proteoglycans [18–25]. In summary, the ECM plays a generally constructive role in the processes of developmental biology and wound healing. The prospect of harnessing this constructive potential in an "off-the-shelf" product has become an interesting and popular concept. The mechanisms by which these ECM devices function as scaffold materials for orthopaedic applications have been investigated extensively for some materials and very little for other materials.

The objective of this chapter is to provide some insight into the composition, preparation, mechanical and material properties of ECM scaffold materials, and the preclinical and clinical studies that have been reported for the commercial products currently available for orthopaedic soft tissue repair and reconstruction.

21.2. Basic Science

21.2.1. Composition

Individual components of the ECM, such as collagen and hyaluronic acid, have been investigated as scaffold materials for tissue reconstruction with varying degrees of success [26–27]. The host response to an unmodified and intact ECM is different than the response to purified components of the ECM. For example, VEGF will induce angiogenesis and BMP will induce bone formation, but the amount of compound to administer, the duration of activity and appropriateness of the response is difficult to control. When ECM is used in its native state, the biologic response to the combination of components results in a more potent biologic response than would occur with individual molecules. The advantages and disadvantages of using individual components of the ECM as therapeutic interventions will not be further discussed.

The extracellular matrix represents the secreted product of resident cells within each tissue and organ, and is composed of a mixture of structural and functional proteins arranged in a unique, tissue specific three-dimensional ultrastructure. These molecules, mainly proteins, provide the mechanical strength required for proper structural support of each tissue, but perhaps more importantly serve as a conduit for information exchange (i.e., signaling) between adjacent cells and between cells and the ECM itself. The ECM is in a state of dynamic reciprocity [28] and will change in response to environmental cues such as hypoxia and mechanical loading. In the context of tissue engineering and, specifically, for rotator cuff reconstruction, use of the ECM as a scaffold provides structural support, but perhaps more importantly provides a favorable environment for constructive remodeling of the tissue.

The mechanism by which these materials function *in vivo* is related to and dependent upon the composition and the ultrastructure of the ECM, and to the methods of processing the tissues from which these ECMs are derived to obtain a commercial product.

21.2.1.1 Collagen

Collagen is the most abundant protein within mammalian ECM. Greater than 90 percent of the dry weight of the ECM from most tissues and organs is represented by collagen [29]. More than 20 distinct types of collagen have been identified, each with a unique biologic function. Type I collagen is the major structural protein present in tissues and is ubiquitous within both the animal and plant kingdoms. Type I collagen is abundant in tendinous and ligamentous structures, such as the rotator cuff, and provides the necessary strength to accommodate the uniaxial and multiaxial mechanical loading to which these tissues are commonly subjected.

Other collagen types exist in the ECM of most tissues, but typically in much lower quantities. These alternative collagen types provide distinct mechanical and physical properties to the ECM and simultaneously contribute to the population of ligands that interact with the resident cell populations. For example, Type IV collagen is present within the basement membrane of most vascular structures and within tissues that contain an epithelial cell component [30–32]. Type III collagen is found within the submucosal tissue of selected organs such as the urinary bladder; a location in which tissue flexibility and compliance are required for appropriate function as opposed to the more rigid properties required of a tendon or ligament supplied by Type I collagen [31]. Type VI collagen is a relatively small molecule that serves as a connecting unit between glycosaminoglycans and larger structural proteins such as Type I collagen, thus providing a gel-like consistency to the ECM [32]. Type VII collagen is found within the basement membrane of the epidermis and functions as an anchoring fibril to protect the overlying keratinocytes from sheer stresses [32]. Each type of collagen is the result of specific gene expression patterns as cells differentiate and tissues and organs develop and spatially organize [29, 32]. In nature collagen is intimately associated with glycosylated proteins, growth factors and other structural proteins such as elastin and laminin to provide unique tissue properties [32]. Each of these types of collagen exists within most of the ECM scaffolds that are currently marketed for rotator cuff reconstruction. It is easy to understand how the biologic response to a mixture of collagen types is different than the response to a purified form of Type I collagen.

21.2.1.2. Fibronectin

Fibronectin is second only to collagen in quantity within the ECM. Fibronectin is a dimeric molecule of 250,000 MW subunits and exists both in soluble and tissue isoforms, and possesses ligands for adhesion of many cell types [33–36]. The ECM of submucosal structures, basement membranes and interstitial tissues all contain abundant fibronectin [33, 35]. The cell friendly characteristics of this protein have made it an attractive substrate for *in vitro* cell culture and for use as a coating for synthetic scaffold materials to promote host biocompatibility. Fibronectin is found at an early stage within the ECM of developing embryos and is critical for normal biologic development, especially the development of vascular structures. Fibronectin was the first "structural" molecule identified to have a functional motif. The presence of fibronectin in a biologic scaffold material likely has a significant positive effect upon orthopaedic soft tissue remodeling.

21.2.1.3. Laminin

Laminin is a complex adhesion protein found in the ECM, especially within basement membrane ECMs [35]. This protein plays an important role in early embryonic development and is perhaps the best studied of the ECM proteins found within embryonic bodies [37]. The prominent role of laminin in the formation and maintenance of vascular structures is particularly noteworthy when considering the ECM as a scaffold for tissue reconstruction [38–39]. This protein appears to be among the first and most critical ECM factors in the process of cell and tissue differentiation. The specific role of laminin in tissue reconstruction when ECM is used as a scaffold for tissue and organ reconstruction in adults is unclear, but its importance in developmental biology suggests that this molecule is essential for self assembly of cell populations and for organized tissue development, as opposed to scar tissue formation.

21.2.1.4. Glycosaminoglycans

The ECM contains a mixture of glycosaminoglycans (GAGs) depending upon the tissue location of the ECM in the host, the age of the host and the microenvironment. The GAGs bind growth factors and cytokines, promote water retention and contribute to the gel properties of the ECM. The heparin binding properties of numerous cell surface receptors and of many growth factors (e.g., fibroblast growth factor family, vascular endothelial cell growth factor) make the heparin-rich GAGs important components of naturally occurring substrates for cell growth. The glycosaminoglycans present in ECM include chondroitin sulfates A and B, heparin, heparan sulfate and hyaluronic acid [40–41]. Hyaluronic acid has been most extensively investigated as a scaffold for tissue reconstruction and as a carrier for selected cell populations in therapeutic tissue engineering applications. The concentration of hyaluronic acid within ECM is highest in fetal and newborn tissues and tends, therefore, to be associated with desirable healing properties. The specific role, if any, of this GAG upon progenitor cell proliferation and differentiation during adult wound healing is unknown. There are currently orthopaedic products available that rely upon hyaluronic acid (e.g., Synvisc®, Genzyme Corporation, Cambridge, MA) and although its mechanism of action is not fully understood, it is generally considered to have favorable effects upon the healing of injured tissues.

21.2.1.5. Growth Factors

An important characteristic of the intact ECM that distinguishes it from other scaffolds for tissue reconstruction is its diversity of structural and functional proteins. The bioactive molecules that reside within the ECM and their unique spatial distribution provide a reservoir of biologic signals. Although cytokines and growth factors are present within ECM in very small quantities, they act as potent modulators of cell behavior. The list of growth factors found within ECM is extensive and includes vascular endothelial cell growth factor (VEGF), the fibroblast growth factor (FGF) family, stromal-derived growth factor (SDF-1), epithelial cell growth factor (EGF), transforming growth factor beta (TGF-beta), keratinocyte growth factor (KGF), hepatocyte growth factor (HGF), platelet-derived growth factor (PDGF) and bone morphogenetic protein (BMP), among others [42–44]. These factors tend to exist in multiple isoforms, each with its specific biologic activity. Purified forms of growth factors have been investigated in recent years as therapeutic methods of encouraging blood vessel formation (e.g., VEGF), stimulating deposition of granulation tissue (PDGF) and bone (BMP), and encouraging epithelialization of wounds (KGF). However, the therapeutic approach of using purified growth factors has not yielded outstanding clinical results because of the difficulty in determining optimal dose and methods of delivery, the ability to sustain and localize the growth factor release at the desired site and the inability to turn the factor "on" and "off" as needed during the course of tissue repair.

An advantage of utilizing the ECM in its native state as a substrate or scaffold for cell growth and differentiation is the presence of all the attendant growth factors (and their inhibitors) in the same relative amounts that exist in nature and, perhaps more importantly, in their native three-dimensional ultrastructure. The ECM efficiently presents these factors to resident or migrating cells, protects the growth factors from degradation and modulates their synthesis [40, 42–44]. If one considers the ECM to be a substrate for *in vitro* and *in vivo* cell growth, it is reasonable to think of the ECM as a temporary (i.e., degradable) controlled release vehicle for naturally derived growth factors. This concept is quite different than the usual consideration of an orthopaedic scaffold, which is focused upon strength and mechanical properties.

21.2.2. Structure and Biomechanical Properties

The biomechanical properties of most of the ECM scaffold materials used for rotator cuff reconstruction have not been thoroughly investigated or reported, especially as these properties change during the course of tissue remodeling [45]. There is perhaps more published regarding the mechanical and material properties of the non-chemically cross-linked SIS-ECM material than any of the other scaffold materials. The Restore™ device is composed of 10 layers

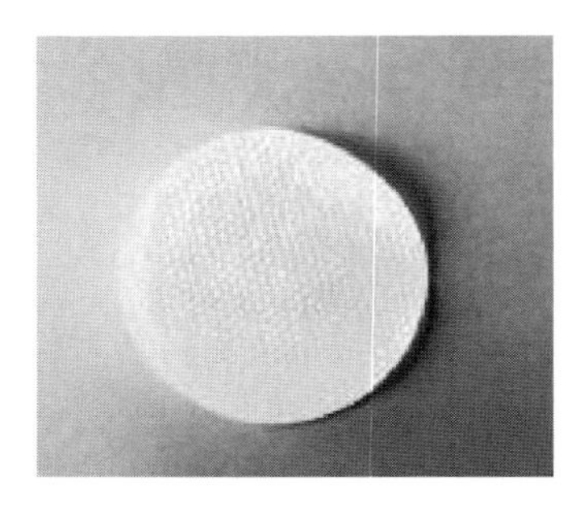

Fig. 21.1 The 10-layer SIS-ECM disc is marketed as the Restore™ device by DePuy, Inc. This multilaminate ECM biologic scaffold is used for the constructive remodeling of orthopaedic soft tissue structures

of SIS-ECM that are arranged in a specific pattern to assure isotropic mechanical properties. Figure 21.1 stated differently, the Restore™ device can be cut or sutured in any direction with resultant identical mechanical properties. The device has been engineered to have ultimate tensile strength which exceeds that of the normal human supraspinatus tendon. The suture retention properties of the Restore™ device are excellent and exceed the strength of adjacent tissues to which it is typically attached. The ball burst strength of the device (a test of multiaxial strength) typically exceeds 60 lbs, a value that exceeds that of most normal tissues. In a study that evaluated the change in strength over time following *in vivo* implantation in a dog model of abdominal wall repair, it was shown that the strength of a multilaminate SIS-ECM device decreases approximately 50 percent over the first two to three weeks following implantation, followed by an increase in strength following the remodeling process with a final value exceeding the strength of normal tissues [46]. The rate and extent of remodeling are critically dependent upon the loading following surgical implantation (rehabilitation). The optimal remodeling outcome of the Restore™ device in patients with rotator cuff repair and other soft tissue applications tends to be associated with aggressive rehabilitation protocols. The principle of "use it or lose it" applies to tissue remodeling with the use of ECM scaffolds that are degradable and replaced by host tissue. This same principle may not be true for the nondegradable scaffold materials because these materials "load protect" the adjacent remodeling soft tissue.

The imaging characteristics of scaffolds that are used for rotator cuff reconstruction and that are subjected to varying degrees of loading during rehabilitation will likely change significantly during this remodeling period. There is a significant need for studies that correlate the imaging profile of these scaffolds over time with their composition, morphology and mechanical properties.

21.2.3. Bioscaffold Degradation

Studies with radiolabeled (^{14}C) SIS-ECM in several body locations have shown a rapid rate of degradation and replacement by host tissues. Approximately 20 percent of the device is degraded by two weeks following surgical implantation, and more than 60 percent of the device is degraded by 28 days following implantation. The device is completely degraded between 60 and 90 days post-surgery and is replaced by host cells and neo-ECM that have remodeled in a site appropriate fashion [47–48]. There are no reported studies of the degradation rates of the other ECM rotator cuff repair devices and, therefore, predictions of remodeling rates are not possible. The degree of tissue remodeling, specifically rotator cuff remodeling, varies between ECM devices and between individuals and is dependent upon active rehabilitation/use. Stated differently, there is an extremely dynamic interplay between scaffold degradation and host tissue reassembly.

A recent study showed that the degradation products of ECM have the potential for biologic activity such as chemoattraction for endothelial cells, bone marrow-derived cells and other cell types [24]. Similarly, antimicrobial activity has been reported for the degradation products of ECM-derived scaffold material [25]. The above findings suggest that at least a portion of the host biologic response to ECM-derived materials is associated with and/or caused by the degradation products of the scaffold itself. Conversely, the lack of degradation of a biologic scaffold material would logically suggest that such downstream effects would not occur.

Fibrous encapsulation with implanted materials has long been associated with the inability to remove these materials from the implant site [49–50]. ECM scaffolds that are processed in such a way as to minimize degradation, for example through chemical cross-linking methodologies [51–54], are more likely to be associated with fibrous encapsulation and chronic inflammation [55–57]. There was a distinct fibrous capsule around the Permacol™ and TissueMend® devices. These devices also showed the slowest rate of scaffold degradation over the course of 112 days in a head-to-head study [58]. Although TissueMend® does not include chemical cross-linking as a processing step, the proprietary methodology of making the final product may be related to its relatively slow rate of degradation.

21.2.4. Source of Cells

Acellular ECM scaffolds marketed for rotator cuff repair at the time of implantation have, by definition, been decellularized; therefore, the cells that populate the scaffold and become part of the new tissue are of host origin. The source of these cells has not been examined or reported for any of the commercially available scaffold materials except for SIS-ECM. The source of cells that remodel SIS-ECM appears to be a combination of cells from adjacent tissue and blood-borne progenitor cells [21, 24]. Recent studies in several animal models have shown that multipotential progenitor cells of bone marrow origin are recruited to the site of the Restore™ device during its degradation phase [59]. These cells, in turn, respond to local environmental cues, such as pH, oxygen tension and, importantly, the mechanical forces (e.g., rehabilitation protocol after surgery) that direct cell differentiation and phenotype. The extent to which these marrow-derived cells participate in the remodeling process is not known with certainty, but their presence does provide a rational explanation for the site-specific differentiation of tissue, instead of the default accumulation of scar tissue that is expected in a typical adult mammalian wound healing response. The signals for recruitment of these progenitor cells appear to derive from both the intact growth factors that are part of the originally implanted scaffold, as well as newly generated bioactive molecules that result from scaffold degradation. In other words, degradation of the ECM scaffold appears to be essential to achieve the full benefit of the bioinductive properties of the scaffold. The effect of chemical cross-linking, a process that slows or eliminates scaffold degradation, upon the source of cells that participate in the remodeling process requires further investigation.

21.3. Preclinical and Clinical Studies

Each of the above-mentioned ECM-derived scaffold materials has been the subject of preclinical studies. These preclinical studies have typically focused upon an individual scaffold material or product. Very few head-to-head studies involving the commercially available products for rotator cuff repair have been conducted either *in vitro* [18, 60–62] or *in vivo* [63–70]. In addition, few of these preclinical studies have utilized a musculotendinous application as the test system [55, 63, 66, 68]. Consequently, there is relatively little clinically relevant information with which to make educated decisions regarding the selection of the most appropriate scaffold material for selected orthopaedic soft tissue applications.

The safety and mechanism of remodeling of the Restore™ device in an intra-articular environment was evaluated in a dog model in which discs of the material were placed in the stifle joint by an arthroscopic approach [71]. The findings showed no evidence for inflammation or other adverse host responses, and suggested that remodeling is critically dependent upon the microenvironment and mechanical forces. Numerous studies of the use of SIS-ECM to facilitate tissue regeneration in an intra-articular environment have been reported, all of which indicate that contact with healthy adjacent tissue is important for the remodeling process [72–77].

The effect of the SIS-ECM scaffold upon rotator cuff (infraspinatus tendon) healing has been evaluated in a dog model of full thickness tendon replacement [68] and a sheep model of tendon repair with augmentation [78]. These studies showed beneficial effects upon tendon healing and biomechanical performance of the tendons.

A study of SIS-ECM for the repair of large rotator cuff defects (supraspinatus tendon) in a rat model showed that the bioscaffold promoted neovascularization, host tissue ingrowth and increased mechanical strength that approached normal tendon tissue by 16 weeks [79]. However, the authors cautioned about the extrapolation of these results to humans with large defects, a caution that is supported by an early human clinical experience described below.

A similar study in which a full thickness replacement of the infraspinatus tendon was performed in a dog model showed that human acellular dermal matrix (the material from which Graft Jacket™ is made) caused cellular infiltration, neotendon development and excellent biomechanical properties within 12 weeks [80].

Two recent preclinical studies performed a head-to-head comparison of several commercially available ECM products for rotator cuff repair including Restore™, CuffPatch™, Graft Jacket®, TissueMend® and Permacol™. These studies compared the biomechanical properties of each device (prior to surgical implantation) [81], and the temporal histologic appearance of the remodeled devices up to 16 weeks post-surgery [58]. Results showed that CuffPatch™ and Graft Jacket® had the greatest mechanical strength prior to surgery, and that the Restore™ device showed the most rapid remodeling with organized and differentiated host tissue replacement. These studies also showed that chemical cross-linking of an ECM, such as occurs with carbodiimide treated SIS-ECM (CuffPatch™), results in significantly greater initial strength of the material, but is associated with a prolonged chronic inflammatory response. Studies in which fibrovascular ingrowth into a chemically cross-linked ECM (Permacol™) was evaluated showed very limited ability of host cells to penetrate the bioscaffold [53]. Attempts to increase fibrovascular ingrowth by laser perforation of the Permacol™ device resulted in minimal improvement [52]. These findings are consistent with those of the comparative study described above.

Because of the relatively recent introduction of ECM scaffolds into the marketplace, and the fact that human clinical studies are not required for regulatory approval, there are very few reports regarding the clinical efficacy of these ECM-based devices.

The largest number of clinical reports for a biologic scaffold device deal with the Restore™ device. The Restore™ device has been available for use longer than any of the other scaffold materials (since year 2000) and, therefore, a handful of studies have now been published. The results are mixed. A study by Metcalf, et al. showed a positive clinical outcome in 12 of 13 patients in which the Restore™ device was used for augmentation of rotator cuff repair. The study involved a one-year follow–up [82]. A study by Zalavras, et al. reported a lack of benefit in the majority patients in which the Restore™ device was used to treat massive rotator cuff defects [79]. Iannotti, et al. reported a lack of efficacy in the majority of patients treated for multi-tendon tears of the rotator cuff within which the Restore™ device was used to bridge a gap [83–84]. Both the Zalavras and Iannotti studies involved the use of the Restore™ device in an off-label application; specifically, the device was used for the repair of large defects.

A single patient report by Bhatia, et al. evaluated the use of Graft Jacket® for interpositional arthroplasty. Other than indicating "safe and reproducible" results, no additional data was provided [85].

In contrast, the use of an isocyanate cross-linked porcine dermal ECM (Permacol™) as an interpositional graft for trapeziectomy resulted in termination of a randomized study because of an adverse foreign body reaction in six of 13 patients within six months of surgery [55].

A study of 13 patients with high risk pelvic, abdominal and chest wall defects were repaired with AlloDerm (the same ECM material used in the Graft Jacket® device). These patients had severe complications including fistulous tracts and contaminated lesions. Although complications occurred in six of the 13 patients, there was no clinical evidence for infection of the ECM mesh or recurrent herniation. The authors concluded that AlloDerm can be safely used in such clinical situations [86]. It is generally accepted that naturally occurring biomaterials, such as those composed of ECM, will fare better in the presence of infection [87–89].

A similar, favorable result was reported for a 52-year-old female patient with a large ventral abdominal hernia that was repaired with the Permacol™ device. One-year follow-up showed no evidence for rejection of the device, nor evidence of recurrent hernia [90].

AlloDerm was used to cover the dorsal plating for wrist arthrodesis with favorable results. There was a decrease in adhesions, a lack of infection and generally favorable soft tissue remodeling [91]. Once again, although Alloderm is the same basic material from which Graft Jacket® is made, the study was not conducted with the commercially available product for orthopaedic surgery.

Approximately 30,000 human patients have been implanted with the Restore™ device for the treatment of musculoskeletal defects. The majority of these surgical procedures have involved repair of the rotator cuff. When the device has been used "on label" as an augmentation for the reinforcement of damaged or weakened tissue, the results have been very good. When use of the device has extended beyond label indications, such as for the replacement of large cuff defects with fatty degeneration and atrophy of the remaining cuff tissue, the results have been poor. These findings are not surprising considering the mechanism by which the device performs *in vivo* as described above. Stated differently, as with most procedures, patient selection is critical for optimal results.

Development of arthroscopic techniques for the repair of rotator cuffs with biologic scaffolds appears imminent [92]. A recent technical report documents a technique for the use of Graft Jacket® and TissueMend® in arthroscopic repair of large rotator cuff defects. Efficacy and long-term follow-up were not reported [92].

21.4. Future Trends and Needs

It seems apparent that biologic materials, such as those composed of extracellular matrix, are finding a niche in orthopaedic surgery. These materials are presently derived from a variety of species and tissue sources, and the methods for processing the different materials vary greatly. There is a strong need for studies to critically compare the effect of these differences upon safety and efficacy. Methods of tissue decellularization, variability in tissue sourcing, utilization of chemical cross-linking agents and the effects of terminal sterilization methods upon mechanical properties and the host response are all examples of factors that can markedly affect the clinical performance of a device.

Preclinical studies that directly compare commercially available devices in a clinically relevant musculotendinous application would add significantly to the information database that would benefit clinicians. Although every animal model has its limitation, head–to-head comparisons of biomaterials within the same test system provide useful information.

With continued use clinical reports will undoubtedly include information concerning long-term follow-up, the incidence of complications and the optimal indications for biologic scaffold materials in orthopaedic surgery. Prospective, randomized trials with careful patient selection will eventually provide the best guidance for use of such materials.

21.5. Conclusions

Regenerative medicine is finding its place in orthopaedic surgery through the use of biologic scaffold materials, bioactive molecules such as bone morphogenetic proteins (BMP) and cell-based therapies such as autologous chondrocyte implantation and platelet-rich plasma. There are the typical growing pains as optimal clinical indications and product processing techniques are evaluated in the clinical setting. However, it seems clear that the use of naturally occurring scaffold materials have significant potential to improve the treatment of orthopaedic soft tissue defects.

References

1. Aglietti P GF, Buzzi R, et al. Anterior cruciate ligament reconstruction: bone-patellar tendon-bone compared with double semitendinosus and gracilis tendon grafts. A prospective, randomized clinical trial. *J Bone Joint Surg Am*. 2004;86-A:2143–2155.
2. Bak K JU, Ekstrand J, et al. Results of reconstruction of acute ruptures of the anterior cruciate ligament with an iliotibial band autograft. *Knee Surg Sports* Traumatol Arthrosc. 1999;7(2):111–117.
3. Bak K SM, Hansen S, et al. Isolated partial rupture of the anterior cruciate ligament. *Knee Surg Sports Traumatol Arthrosc*. 1997;5(2):66–71.
4. Jorgensen U BK, Ekstrand J, et al. Reconstruction of the anterior cruciate ligament with the iliotibial band autograft in patients with chronic knee instability. *Knee Surg Sports Traumatol Arthrosc*. 2001;9(3):137–145.
5. Kartus J SS, Lindahl S, et al. Factors affecting donor-site morbidity after anterior cruciate ligament reconstruction using bone-patellar tendon-bone autografts. *Knee Surg Sports Traumatol Arthrosc*. 1997;5(4):222–228.
6. Cofield RH PJ, Hoffmeyer PJ, et al. Surgical repair of chronic rotator cuff tears. A prospective long-term study. *J Bone Joint Surg Am*. 2001;83-A(1):71–77.
7. Kronberg M, Wahlstrom, P., Brostrom, L.A. Shoulder function after surgical repair of rotator cuff tears. *J Shoulder Elbow Surg*. 1997;6(2):125–130.
8. Williams GR, Jr., Rockwood, C.A., Jr., Biglianim L.U., et. al. Rotator cuff tears: Why do we repair them? *J Bone Joint Surg Am*. 2004;86-A(12):2764–2776.
9. Ejerhed L KJ, Sernert N, et al. Patellar tendon or semitendinosus tendon autografts for anterior cruciate ligament reconstruction? A prospective randomized study with a two-year follow-up. *Am J Sports Med*. 2003;31(1):19–25.
10. Kartus J MT, Karlsson J. Donor-site morbidity and anterior knee problems after anterior cruciate ligament reconstruction using autografts. *Arthroscopy*. 2001;17(9):971–980.
11. Disa JJ, Goldberg, NH, Carlton, JM, et al. Restoring abdominal wall integrity in contaminated tissue-deficient wounds using autologous fascia grafts. *Plast Reconstr Surg*. 1998;101(4):979–986.
12. Haas F, Seibert, FJ, Koch, H, et al. Reconstruction of combined defects of the Achilles tendon and the overlying soft tissue with a fascia lata graft and a free fasciocutaneous lateral arm flap. *Ann Plast Surg*. 2003;51(4):376–382.
13. Williams JK, Carlson, GW, deChalain, T, et al. Role of tensor faciae latae in abdominal wall reconstruction. *Plast Reconstr Surg*. 713–718 1998;1998(101):3.
14. Aoki M, Fukushima, S, Okamura, K, et al. Mechanical strength of latissimus dorsi tendon transfer with Teflon felt augmentation. *J Shoulder Elbow Surg*. 1997;6(2):137–143.
15. Kimura A, Aoki, M, Fukushima, S, et al. Reconstruction of a defect of the rotator cuff with polytetrafluoroethylene felt graft. Recovery of tensile strength and histocompatibility in an animal model. *J Bone Joint Surg Br*. 2003;85(2):282–287.
16. Woo SL, Buckwalter, JA, et al. *Injury and repair of the musculoskeletal soft tissues: workshop*. Paper presented at: American Academy of Orthopaedic Surgeons Symposium, June 1987; Savannah, GA.
17. Ozaki J, Fujimoto, S, Masuhara, K, et al. Reconstruction of chronic massive rotator cuff tears with synthetic materials. *Clin Orthop Relat Res*. 1986;202:173–183.
18. Badylak S, Liang A, Record R, et al. Endothelial cell adherence to small intestinal submucosa: an acellular bioscaffold. *Biomaterials*. Dec 1999;20(23–24):2257–2263.
19. Badylak SF. The extracellular matrix as a scaffold for tissue reconstruction. *Seminars in Cell & Developmental Biology*. 2002;13(5):377–383.
20. Badylak SF. Xenogeneic extracellular matrix as a scaffold for tissue reconstruction. *Transpl Immunol*. Apr 2004;12(3–4):367–377.

21. Badylak SF, Park K, McCabe G, et al. Marrow-Deprived Cells Populate Scaffolds Composed of Xenogeneic Extracellular Matrix. *Experimental Hematology*. 2001;29:1310–1318.
22. Hodde J. Naturally occurring scaffolds for soft tissue repair and regeneration. *Tissue Eng*. Apr 2002;8(2):295–308.
23. Hodde JP, Record RD, Liang HA, et al. *Vascular endothelial growth factor in porcine-derived extracellular matrix. Endothelium*. 2001;8(1):11–24.
24. Li F, Li W, Johnson SA, et al. Low-Molecular-Weight Peptides Derived from Extracellular Matrix as Chemoattractants for Primary Endothelial Cells. *Endothelium*. 2004;11:199–206.
25. Sarikaya A, Record R, Wu CC, et al. Antimicrobial activity associated with extracellular matrices. *Tissue Engineering*. 2002;8(1):63–71.
26. Hahn MS, Teply, BA; Stevens, MM; Zeitels, SM; Langer, R Collagen composite hydrogels for vocal fold lamina propria restoration. *Biomaterials*. 2006;27(7):1104–1109.
27. Lisignoli GC, S; Piacentini, A; Zini, N; Noel, D; Jorgensen C; Facchini, A Chondrogenic differentiation of murine and human mesnchymal stromal cells in a hyaluronic acid scaffold: Differences in gene expression and cell morphology. *J Biomed Mater Res*. 2006;77A(3):497–506.
28. Bissell MJ, Aggeler J. Dynamic reciprocity: how do extracellular matrix and hormones direct gene expression? *Prog Clin Biol Res*. 1987;249:251–262.
29. van der Rest M, Garrone, R. The collagen family of proteins. *Faseb J*. 1992;5:2814–2823.
30. Barnard K, Gathercole LJ. Short and long range order in basement membrane type IV collagen revealed by enzymic and chemical extraction. *Int J Biol Macromol*. Dec 1991;13(6):359–365.
31. Piez KA. *Molecular and aggregate structures of the collagens*. New York: Elsevier; 1984.
32. Yurchenco P, Birk, DE, Mecham, RP *Extracellular Matrix Assembly and Structure;* 1994.
33. McPherson T, Badylak, SF Characterization of fibronectin derived from porcine small intestinal submucosa. *Tissue Eng*. 1998;4:75–83.
34. Miyamoto S, Katz BZ, Lafrenie RM, et al. Fibronectin and integrins in cell adhesion, signaling, and morphogenesis. *Ann N Y Acad Sci. Oct 23* 1998;857:119–129.
35. Schwarzbauer J. Basement membranes: Putting up the barriers. *Curr Biol*. Apr 8 1999;9(7):R242–244.
36. Schwarzbauer JE. Fibronectin: from gene to protein. *Curr Opin Cell Biol*. Oct 1991;3(5):786–791.
37. Li S, Harrison D, Carbonetto S, et al. Matrix assembly, regulation, and survival functions of laminin and its receptors in embryonic stem cell differentiation. *Journal of Cell Biology*. 2002;157(7):1279–1290.
38. Ponce ML, Nomizu M, Delgado MC, et al. Identification of endothelial cell binding sites on the laminin gamma 1 chain. *Circ Res*. Apr 2 1999;84(6):688–694.
39. Werb Z, Vu TH, Rinkenberger JL, et al. Matrix-degrading proteases and angiogenesis during development and tumor formation. *APMIS*. Jan 1999;107(1):11–18.
40. Entwistle J, Zhang S, Yang B, et al. Characterization of the murine gene encoding the hyaluronan receptor RHAMM. *Gene*. Oct 3 1995;163(2):233–238.
41. Hodde JP, Badylak SF, Brightman AO, et al. Glycosaminoglycan content of small intestinal submucosa: A bioscaffold for tissue replacement. *Tissue Eng*. 1996;2:209–217.
42. Bonewald LF. Regulation and regulatory activities of transforming growth factor beta. *Crit Rev Eukaryot Gene Expr*. 1999;9(1):33–44.
43. Kagami S, Kondo S, Loster K, et al. Collagen type I modulates the platelet-derived growth factor (PDGF) regulation of the growth and expression of beta1 integrins by rat mesangial cells. *Biochem Biophys Res Commun*. 1998;252(3):728–732.

44. Roberts R, Gallagher J, Spooncer E, et al. Heparan sulphate bound growth factors: a mechanism for stromal cell mediated haemopoiesis. *Nature*. 1988;332(6162):376–378.
45. Derwin KA, Baker, AR, Spragg, R.K, Leigh, DR, Iannotti, JP Commercial extracellular matrix scaffolds for rotator cuff tendon repair: biomechanical, biochemical, and cellular properties. *J Bone Joint Surg Am*. in press.
46. Badylak S, Kokini K, Tullius B, et al. Strength over time of a resorbable bioscaffold for body wall repair in a dog model. *J Surg Res*. Aug 2001;99(2):282–287.
47. Badylak SF, Kropp B, McPherson T, et al. Small intestional submucosa: a rapidly resorbed bioscaffold for augmentation cystoplasty in a dog model. *Tissue Eng*. Winter 1998;4(4):379–387.
48. Gilbert TW, Stewart-Akers, AM, Simmons-Byrd, A, Badylak, SF Degradation and Remodeling of Small Intestinal Submucosa in Canine Achilles Tendon Repair. *JBJS - Am*. in press.
49. Ratner BD. *Biomaterials science: an introduction to materials in medicine*. 2nd ed. Amsterdam: Boston: Elsevier Academic Press; 2004.
50. Vistnes LM, Ksander, GA, Kosek, J. Study of encapsulation of silicone rubber implants in animals. *Plast Reconstr Surg*. 1978;62(4):580–588.
51. Billiar K, Murray J, Laude D, et al. Effects of carbodiimide cross-linking conditions on the physical properties of laminated intestinal submucosa. *J Biomed Mater Res*. Jul 2001;56(1):101–108.
52. Macleod TM, Sarathchandra P, Williams G, et al. The diamond CO2 laser as a method of improving the vascularisation of a permanent collagen implant. *Burns*. Nov 2004;30(7):704–712.
53. Macleod TM, Williams G, Sanders R, et al. Histological evaluation of Permacol trade mark as a subcutaneous implant over a 20-week period in the rat model. *Br J Plast Surg*. Jun 2005;58(4):518–532.
54. MacLeod TM, Williams G, Sanders R, et al. Prefabricated skin flaps in a rat model based on a dermal replacement matrix Permacol. *Br J Plast Surg*. Dec 2003;56(8):775–783.
55. Belcher HJ, Zic R. Adverse effect of porcine collagen interposition after trapeziectomy: a comparative study. *J Hand Surg [Br]*. Apr 2001;26(2):159–164.
56. Cheung D, Brown L, Sampath R. Localized inferior orbital fibrosis associated with porcine dermal collagen xenograft orbital floor implant. *Ophthal Plast Reconstr Surg*. May 2004;20(3):257–259.
57. Saray A. Porcine dermal collagen (Permacol) for facial contour augmentation: preliminary report. *Aesthetic Plast Surg*. Sep-Oct 2003;27(5):368–375.
58. Valentin JE, Badylak, JS, McCabe, GP, Badylak, SF Extracellular Matrix bioscaffolds for Orthopaedic Applications: A Comparative Histologic Study. *J Bone Joint Surg Am*. in press.
59. Zantop T, Gilbert, TW, Yoder, MC, Badylak, SF. Extracellular Matrix Scaffolds Attract Bone Marrow Derived Cells in a Mouse Model of Achilles Tendon Reconstruction. *J Orthop Res*. 2006;24(6):1299–1309.
60. Badylak SF, Record R, Lindberg K, et al. Small intestinal submucosa: a substrate for in vitro cell growth. *J Biomater Sci Polym Ed*. 1998;9(8):863–878.
61. Jarman-Smith ML, Bodamyali T, Stevens C, et al. Porcine collagen cross-linking, degradation and its capability for fibroblast adhesion and proliferation. *J Mater Sci Mater Med*. Aug 2004;15(8):925–932.
62. Kimuli M, Eardley I, Southgate J. In vitro assessment of decellularized porcine dermis as a matrix for urinary tract reconstruction. *BJU Int*. Oct 2004;94(6):859–866.
63. Badylak S, Kokini K, Tullius B, et al. Morphologic study of small intestinal submucosa as a body wall repair device. *J Surg Res*. Apr 2002;103(2):190–202.
64. Badylak SF, Kropp B, McPherson T, et al. Small intestinal submucosa: a rapidly resorbed bioscaffold for augmentation cystoplasty in a dog model. *Tissue Eng*. Winter 1998;4(4):379–387.

65. Bano F, Barrington JW, Dyer R. Comparison between porcine dermal implant (Permacol) and silicone injection (Macroplastique) for urodynamic stress incontinence. *Int Urogynecol J Pelvic Floor Dysfunct.* Mar-Apr 2005;16(2):147–150; discussion 150.
66. Beniker D, McQuillan D, Livesey S, et al. The use of acellular dermal matrix as a scaffold for periosteum replacement. *Orthopaedics.* May 2003;26(5 Suppl): s591–596.
67. Brigido SA, Boc SF, Lopez RC. Effective management of major lower extremity wounds using an acellular regenerative tissue matrix: a pilot study. *Orthopaedics.* Jan 2004;27(1 Suppl):s145–149.
68. Dejardin LM, Arnoczky SP, Ewers BJ, et al. Tissue-engineered rotator cuff tendon using porcine small intestinal submucosa. Histologic and mechanical evaluation in dogs. *Am J Sports Med.* 2001;29(2):175–184.
69. Harper C. Permacol: clinical experience with a new biomaterial. *Hosp Med.* Feb 2001;62(2):90–95.
70. MacLeod TM, Sarathchandra P, Williams G, et al. Evaluation of a porcine origin acellular dermal matrix and small intestinal submucosa as dermal replacements in preventing secondary skin graft contraction. *Burns.* Aug 2004;30(5):431–437.
71. Fox DB, Cook, JL, Arnoszky, SP, Tomlinson, JL, Kuroki, K, Kreeger, JM, Malaviya, P Fibrochrondrogenesis of free intraarticular small intestinal submucosa scaffolds. *Tissue Eng.* 2004;10(1–2):129–137.
72. Aiken S, Badylak SF, Toombs JP, et al. Small intestinal submucosa as an intra-articular ligamentous graft material: a pilot study in dogs. *Vet Comp Orthopedics Traumatology.* 1994;7:124–128.
73. Cook JL, Fox, DB, Malaviya, P, Tomlinson, JL, Farr, J, Kuroki, K, Cook, CR Evaluation of small intestinal submucosa grafts for meniscal regeneration in a clinically relevant posterior meniscectomy model in dogs. *J Knee Surg.* 2006;19(3):159–167.
74. Cook JL, Tomlinson JL, Arnoczky SP, et al. Kinetic study of the replacement of porcine small intestinal submucosa grafts and the regeneration of meniscal-like tissue in large avascular meniscal defects in dogs. *Tissue Eng.* 2001;7(3):321–334.
75. Cook JL, Tomlinson JL, Kreeger JM, et al. Induction of meniscal regeneration in dogs using a novel biomaterial. *Am J Sports Med.* 1999;27:658–665.
76. Gastel JA, Muirhead WR, Lifrak JT, et al. Meniscal tissue regeneration using a collagenous biomaterial derived from porcine small intestine submucosa. *Arthroscopy.* Feb 2001;17(2):151–159.
77. Paulino C, Holden, D, Plouhar,P, et al. *The use of an SIS-PGA composite graft for repair of cartilage defects.* Paper presented at: 2nd SIS Symposium, December 1998; Orlando, FL.
78. Schlegel TF, Hawkins, RJ, Lewis, CW, Motta, T, Turner, AS The effects of augmentation with Swine small intestine submucosa on tendon healing under tension: histologic and mechanical evaluations in sheep. *Am J Sports Med.* 2006;34(2):275–280.
79. Zalavras C, Gardocki R, Huang E, et al. Reconstruction of large rotator cuff tendon defects with porcine small intestinal submucosa in an animal model. *J Shoulder Elbow Surgery.* 2006;15:225–231.
80. Adams JE, Zobitz, ME, Reach, JS, Jr., An, KN, Steinman, SP. Rotator cuff repair using an acellular dermal matrix graft: an in vivo study in a canine model. *Arthoscopy.* 2006;22(7):700–709.
81. Derwin K, Androjna C, Spencer E, et al. Porcine small intestine submucosa as a flexor tendon graft. *Clin Orthop.* Jun 2004(423):245–252.
82. Metcalf M, Savoie F, Kellum B. Surgical Technique for Xenograft (SIS) Augmentation of Rotator-Cuff Repairs. *Operat Tech Orthop.* 2002;12(3):204–208.
83. Iannotti JP, Codsi, MJ, Kwon, YW, Derwin, K, Ciccone, J. Porcine small intestine submucosa augmentation of surgical repair of chronic two-tendon rotator cuff tears. A randomized, controlled trial. *J Bone Joint Surg Am.* 2006;88(6):1238–1244.

84. Sclamberg SG, Tibone JE, Itamura JM, et al. Six-month magnetic resonance imaging follow-up of large and massive rotator cuff repairs reinforced with porcine small intestinal submucosa. *J Shoulder Elbow Surg*. 2004;13(5):538–541.
85. Bhatia DN, van Rooyen, KS, du Toit, DF, and de Beer, JF. Arthroscopic technique of interposisiton arthroplatsty of the glenohumeral joint. *Arthoscopy*. 2006;22(5):570 el - 575.
86. Butler CE, Prieto VG. Reduction of adhesions with composite AlloDerm/polypropylene mesh implants for abdominal wall reconstruction. *Plast Reconstr Surg*. 2004;114(2):464–473.
87. Bradham R, Cordle, F, McIver, FA. Effect of bacteria on vascular protheses. *Ann Surg*. 1961;154(suppl):187–191.
88. Bricker D, Beall, AC, DeBakey, ME. The different response to infection of autogenous vein versus Dacron arterial prosthesis. *Chest*. 1970;58:566–570.
89. Moore W, Rosson, CT, Hall, A. Effect of prophylactic antibodies in preventing bacteremic infection of vascular protheses. *Surgery*. 1971;69:825–828.
90. Liyanage S, Purohit, GS, Frye, JN, Giordano, P. Anterior abdominal wall reconstruction with a Permacol implant. 59. 2006;5(553–5).
91. Althausen P, Szabo, RM. Coverage of distal radius internal fixation and wrist fusion devices with AlloDerm. *Tech Hand Up Extrem Surg*. 2004;8(4):266–268.
92. Silberstein N. Biologic Tissue Scaffolds in Shoulder Surgery. *Orthopedic Technology Review*. Vol 7; 2005.

22

Muscle Repair after Injury and Disease

Fabrisia Ambrosio[1], Yong Li[1], Arvydas Usas[1], Michael L. Boninger[2], and Johnny Huard[1]

Abstract: Muscle injuries can greatly impair an individual's function and ability to participate in recreational and occupational activities. While differing mechanisms of muscle injury affect different aspects of skeletal muscle structure, the phases of muscle healing among the varying types of injury are remarkably preserved. The overall interrelated and overlapping phases of muscle repair involve: 1) degeneration of injured muscle fibers, 2) inflammation, 3) regeneration and, finally, 4) the development of fibrosis. In this chapter we will discuss the natural processes occurring in skeletal muscle healing, and we will provide a summary of current biological treatment techniques being investigated to restore skeletal muscle function after injury.

Keywords: Skeletal muscle, injury, regeneration, myopathy, healing.

22.1. Introduction

The function of skeletal muscle is to contract such that it exerts a force under a given set of conditions. Muscle injury, defined as "a prolonged impairment of the ability of a muscle to produce force" [1], can greatly impair an individual's function and ability to participate in recreational and occupational activities. In extreme cases the decreased ability of a muscle to produce the required output may result in death, as is often the case in Duchenne Muscular Dystrophy (DMD), where the failure of the respiratory muscles results from chronic degradation of the muscle fibers. In this chapter we will discuss the natural processes occurring in skeletal muscle healing, and we will provide a summary of current biological treatment techniques being investigated to maximize skeletal muscle function after injury and disease.

[1] Growth and Development Laboratory, Stem Cell Research Center, Department of Orthopaedic Surgery, Department of Physical Medicine and Rehabilitation, Children's Hospital of Pittsburgh, Pittsburgh, PA

[2] Department of Physical Medicine and Rehabilitation, University of Pittsburgh, Pittsburgh, PA

From: *Orthopedic Biology and Medicine: Musculoskeletal Tissue Regeneration, Biological Materials and Methods*
Edited by W. S. Pietrzak © Humana Press, Totowa, NJ

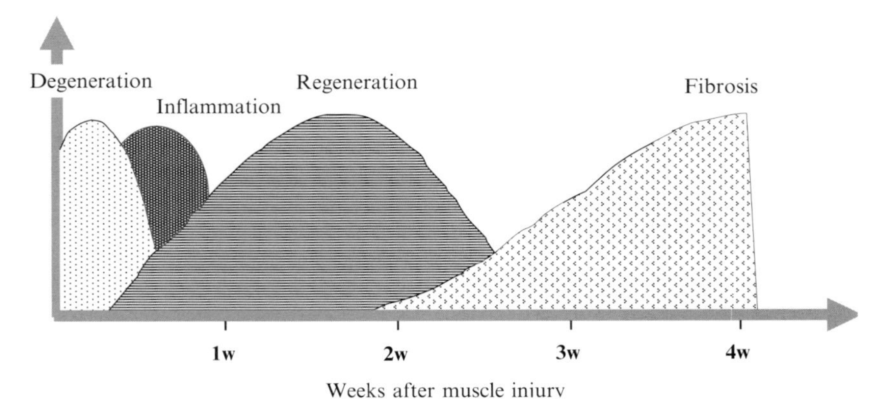

Fig. 22.1 The healing process

22.2. Cellular Processes for Muscle Repair

The overall interrelated and overlapping phases of muscle repair involve: 1) degeneration of injured muscle fibers, 2) inflammation, 3) regeneration and 4) the development of fibrosis [2] (Fig. 22.1).

22.2.1. Degeneration

Muscle damage involves a disruption in the muscle fiber and the surrounding connective tissue, including the plasma membrane and the basal lamina. Such a disruption results in the leakage of calcium into the extracellular space [3]. The influx of calcium and subsequent protease activation results in a focal necrosis of the myofibers by autodigestion, occurring within the first few days after injury, although the first signs of necrosis may be observed after only two hours from the time of injury [4]. To contain the area of autodigestion, and prevent degradation of intact myofibers, the damaged area is sealed off by the formation of "contraction zones" defined by sarcolemmal formation at the boundary of the injury [5]. These contraction zones may be observed 12 hours after injury [6].

Degeneration is promoted by local swelling and hematoma formation, in which blood vessels, activated macrophages, mononuclear cells and T-lymphocytes infiltrate the injured tissue area. Neutrophil accumulation is significant after just one hour from the time of injury [7], after which time macrophages invade the injury site. Macrophages participate primarily in phagocytosis of muscle debris and release factors, such as cytokines (interleukin-6 (IL-6), interleukin-8 (IL-8) and tumor necrosis factor-α (TNF-α)), which subsequently increase vascular permeability and stimulate inflammation. In muscle diseases such as Duchenne Muscular Dystrophy (DMD), in which myofibers lack dystrophin expression due to a mutation of the dystrophin gene, there is a subsequent deficit of membrane integrity following muscle contraction [8, 9, 10, 11,12, 13], and muscle pathology is initiated. Macrophage accumulation may hasten the decay process in the skeletal muscle. For this reason, immunosuppressive agents are often used in the treatment of DMD. The phagocytosis of the injured region by the macrophages eventually results in a "ghost-like, moth-eaten appearance" of the muscle fiber [14]. The resulting scaffolds are necessary to provide a framework for subsequent muscle fiber regeneration.

With the calcium influx that follows disruption to the myofiber's internal structure, there is a secondary increase in ultrastructural damage [3]. With the release of intracellular calcium, calpain is activated, resulting in disruption of the myofibrillar apparatus as a result of proteolysis and/or conformational changes [15]. On the other hand, calpain has also been shown to play a role in the activation of regenerative cells out of the quiescent phase [16], suggesting it also plays a role in muscle regeneration.

22.2.1.1. Intervention

Overall there has been limited research focused on finding ways to minimize muscle degradation following injury. Since degradation is initiated immediately following insult, intervention at this stage would primarily involve prophylactic medicine techniques. However, given the progressive nature of DMD as a result of chronic muscle fiber degradation, methods to minimize myofiber damage in this disease have been investigated.

It has been shown that the increased calcium levels in dystrophic muscle trigger the calpain cascade that induces the breakdown of several intracellular protein targets [17, 18]. In fact, calpains may be responsible for approximately 60 percent of skeletal muscle sarcomeric protein degradation in normal muscle [19]. Specifically, it has been shown that utrophin, a structural and functional dystrophin homolog that compensates for dystrophin deficiency in *mdx* mice [20], an animal model of DMD [21], is rapidly degraded by calpain isoforms I and II [22], suggesting a specific role for calpain in DMD pathology. Calpain inhibition has been previously investigated as a means to prevent myofiber degeneration in dystrophic muscles [23]. Spencer and Mellgren (2002) found that *mdx* mice genetically engineered to overexpress calpastatin, a specific, endogenous calpain inhibitor, demonstrated a reduction in the percentage of the total necrotic muscular cross sectional area, and a reduction in the total number of macrophage-invaded fibers, when compared to control counterparts [23]. However, it should be noted that calpain is only one mechanism by which protein degradation in dystrophic muscles is initiated, and is not the sole factor contributing to the myofibrillar death that characterizes dystrophic muscles. Whether increased calpain expression is enough to compensate for the overall degradation occurring in dystrophic muscles, or if it results in functionally significant improvements, has not yet been tested.

Clinically, β2-adregenergic agonists, such as albuterol, which increase calpastatin levels are also being investigated as pharmacological agents for the treatment of DMD [24]. Clenbuterol, another β2-adregenergic agonist, has resulted in decreased myofiber degradation [25], increased regeneration [26, 27] and even anti-atrophy effects following hindlimb unloading in rodents [28, 29, 30, 31]. In a recent pilot study nine children with either Becker or Duchenne Muscular Dystrophy participated in a crossover study in which they received two 12-week treatments (albuterol and placebo), administered orally, separated by a four-week washout period [24]. There was a significant difference in mean peak knee extensor strength between the two groups, but no significant difference in the mean peak knee flexor strength. There were no significant changes in any of the functional tests, including time to run, time to climb four stairs or time to stand from a supine position. Larger, randomized controlled clinical trials are needed to further investigate the applicability of β2-adregenergic agonists to prevent muscle degeneration in patients with DMD.

Studies have also been conducted to investigate methods for minimizing muscle fiber degeneration in *mdx* mice by blocking the pro-inflammatory cytokine, TNF-α [32–33, 34]. Grounds, et al. (2004) found that neutralizing TNF-α activity through the use of an anti-TNF-α antibody resulted in a histologically reduced breakdown of dystrophic muscle as evidenced by decreased inflammation and necrosis [32]. Authors concluded that TNF-α may trigger the degeneration-regeneration cascade by exacerbating the inflammatory response leading to an increased overall myofiber necrosis.

However, TNF-α has been shown to be very important in signaling regeneration after cardiotoxin muscle injury [35]. Chen, et al. (2005) demonstrated that TNF-α signaling is required for triggering events necessary in normal muscle regeneration, despite its role in muscle protein breakdown [35]. The absence of TNF-α resulted in morphologic and physiologic abnormalities in healing skeletal muscle after injury. In fact, TNF receptor-null mice were significantly weaker than wild type mice at approximately two weeks after freeze injury [36]. The effect of TNF-α seems to vary with the type of injury, since regeneration was not impaired in TNF-α knockout mice after crush injury [37].

22.2.2. Inflammation

Following myofiber injury, an influx of Ca^{2+} occurs within damaged cells that subsequently initiates the release of phospholipase A2. This, in turn, breaks down phospholipids within the cell wall into arachidonic acid, which is further transformed into prostaglandins via the cyclooxygenase pathway. Prostaglandins have been shown to play a role in nociception [38, 39], inflammation [40] and regeneration [41, 42]. Three isoforms of cyclooxygenase have been described [43, 44, 45, 46, 40]. Of these isoforms, Cyclooxygenase 2 (COX2) is known to play a major role in the mediation of pain and inflammation following injury [38, 39].

Of course, skeletal muscle injury results not only in the destruction of muscle fibers, but also in torn blood vessels. The resulting hematoma triggers an influx of blood-borne neutrophils, activated macrophages and T-lymphocytes within the first day from the time of exercise or injury [47, 48, 49, 50]. In fact, within 45 minutes of an exercise-induced skeletal muscle injury, a significant accumulation of intramuscular neutrophils was observed in vastus lateralis biopsies of nine healthy young men [47]. Neutrophil levels remained elevated for five days following the exercise bout [47].

Neutrophils play a role in phagocytosis and in releasing proteases that degrade damaged muscle fiber debris [51]. It is believed that neutrophils can increase muscle damage following ischemia-reperfusion injuries [52, 53, 54, 55, 56, 57, 58, 59], possibly through the generation of oxygen reactive species. It has also been reported that neutrophil-mediated damage impairs muscle contractility [59]. In a study by Walden, et al. (1990) animals treated with an intravenous injection of Vinblastine four days prior to injury demonstrated both a decreased neutrophil accumulation following ischemia-reperfusion injury, and a concomitant increase in peak isometric tension when compared to control counterparts [59]. A limitation of this study is the secondary effects of Vinblastine on blood eosinophils, blood monocytes and lymphocyte, which may also affect muscle histology and function following injury. Teixeira, et al. (2003) demonstrated that mice treated intraperitoneally with neutrophil antisera

36 hours prior to injury demonstrated an impaired regenerative capacity seven days after injury, as determined by the percentage of regenerating muscle fibers in relation to the total area of muscle damage [60]. In this model regeneration was limited by the large areas of necrotic debris that had not been removed.

Another function of neutrophils is the release of cytokines that signal monocytes. Monocytes are eventually transformed into macrophages which, in addition to their participation in phagocytosis and the removal of cellular debris, release chemoattractants to further amplify the inflammatory response. It has been suggested that macrophages release growth factors such as heparin-binding EGF-like growth factor [61], play a role in the differentiation of terminal myotubes. Heparin-binding EGF-like growth factor has also been shown to increase the likelihood for muscle cell survival under oxidative stress [62].

22.2.2.1. Intervention

Non-steroidal anti-inflammatory drugs (NSAIDs) have long been among the primary interventions used for the treatment of muscle injury. NSAIDs inhibit the cyclooxygenase pathway, thereby blocking the conversion of arachidonic acid into prostoglandins and thromboxane, inflammatory metabolites that are known to induce pain and vasodilation, among other inflammatory symptoms. It has been increasingly accepted that the use of non-selective NSAIDs both impedes muscle healing and delays long-term functional recovery following a skeletal muscle injury [63, 64]. While NSAIDs have been shown to provide an immediate improvement (increased torque production) of skeletal muscle three to seven days after exercise-induced muscle injury, subsequent deficits in muscle torque capacity have been shown with time (at 28 days) [64]. The decreased contractile function of the NSAID-treated muscles at 28 days was concomitant with a significant reduction in circulating neutrophils, when compared to untreated controls. There was, however, no significant difference in the levels of circulating monocytes between groups. Evidence suggests that the use of NSAIDs may delay soft tissue healing, since it appears that the inflammatory response contributes to cellular remodeling and eventual functional return of skeletal muscle after injury [64].

To minimize COX1-inhibiting side effects such as platelet inhibition and gastric mucosal injury, COX2-selective inhibitors have been used as a medical intervention for skeletal muscle injury. These medications provide the analgesic and anti-inflammatory effects of NSAIDS, with a decreased likelihood for undesirable side effects. However, even these selective NSAIDS may impair muscle healing. Bondensen, et al. (2004) and Shen, et al. (2005) recently demonstrated that inhibition of the COX2 pathway after muscle injury decreases the size of regenerating myofibers, increases fibrosis formation and increased coexpression of transforming growth factor- ß1 (TGF-ß1) and myostatin, two negative regulators of skeletal muscle growth [65, 66]. *In vitro*, our laboratory has demonstrated that COX2 knockout myogenic precursor cells demonstrated decreased formation of myotubes in culture, a phenomenon that was reversed with the supplementation of prostoglandins PGE_2 and $PGF_{2\alpha}$ [42]. These findings supported previous studies demonstrating a positive effect of $PGF_{2\alpha}$ on myotube formation and muscle growth [41, 67].

Along these lines we have shown that, two weeks after muscle laceration, COX2 knockout mice contained significantly fewer regenerating myofibers when compared to control counterparts with the same injury [42]. Control animals exhibited an increased functional recovery as determined by peak force production, when compared to COX2 knockout mice. Inhibition of the COX2 pathway is also associated with decreased myoblast infiltration within injured skeletal muscle [65]. It has also been suggested that COX2 inhibition impairs muscle regenerative cell activation, proliferation, differentiation and/or fusion [68]. Therefore, while reducing muscle degradation and pain by limiting inflammation may theoretically be advantageous, in fact, there appears to exist a paradoxical effect in which the application of NSAIDS, selective or non-selective, reduce the availability of important regenerative factors, and interfere with the muscle healing process, ultimately affecting functional recovery.

22.2.3. Regeneration

Mature mammalian skeletal muscle fibers are terminally differentiated and contain post-mitotic nuclei. To restore a muscle's function after injury, the damaged muscle fibers must be replaced with regenerating muscle fibers. Satellite cells, located between the basement membrane and the sarcolemma, are primarily responsible for muscle regeneration. Following injury, satellite cells are activated and proliferate [69]. Two primary populations of satellite cells have been identified [4]. The first population of committed satellite cells readily undergoes differentiation, without preceding mitosis, while the second population primarily undergoes cell division to recycle the satellite cell pool at the injured site. Recently, our laboratory described another myogenic population, muscle-derived stem cells (MDSC). MDSCs are unique in the fact that, while they follow the typical myoblast pattern of proliferation, terminal differentiation and fusion, they may also be stimulated to differentiate into a variety of other cell lineages including neural and endothelial cells [70]. This makes the use of MDSCs to improve muscle regeneration promising to address muscle fiber, neuron and vascular damage common to muscle injuries.

Regeneration occurs seven to 10 days after injury, and begins once the phagocytic cells clear necrotic tissue and quiescent satellite cells are activated by growth factors [14]. However, it has been reported that activated satellite cells and myotubes may be seen as early as three days after injury [5]. Growth factors such as basic fibroblast growth factor (bFGF), hepatocyte growth factor (HGF), nerve growth factor (NGF) and insulin-like growth factor (IGF-1) have been shown to be capable of enhancing the proliferation (self-renewal) and/or differentiation of satellite cells into myoblasts *in vitro* [71]. Kami and Senba (2002) found that leukemia inhibitory factor (LIF), a member of the IL-6 family of cytokines, may be important in mediating molecular events occurring in the early phases of regeneration [72]. It has been demonstrated that muscle loading increases IGF-1 secretion [73, 74, 75], which appears to play a role in muscle regeneration and hypertrophy. However, unlike other growth factors, IGF-1 promotes not only satellite cell proliferation, but also cell fusion [76], indicating that IGF-1 may have the capacity to stimulate regeneration through two different pathways. On the other hand myostatin, a TGF-β superfamily member, is a negative regulator of skeletal muscle regeneration [77], and seems to block quiescent satellite cells from being activated

[78, 79]. Myostatin has been observed to be present in elevated levels in cases of atrophy resulting from muscle unloading [80]. In fact, it has been shown that the absence of myostatin results in increased proliferation of satellite cells and an overall increase in the rate of the inflammatory cell response. Not surprisingly, HGF, a satellite cell activator, has been shown to be a myostatin downregulator [79].

Finally, macrophages, the largest cell population present in the injured muscle 12 hours after injury, release mediators, like chemokines, that are essential for orchestrating a satellite cell response [81, 82]. It has not only been shown that, in the absence of macrophages, muscle regeneration is absent, but also, under conditions of an enhanced macrophage response, satellite cell proliferation and differentiation is increased [81, 83]. It has also been recently reported that myogenic progenitor cells have the ability to selectively and specifically chemoattract monocytes [84]. Working within the scaffold template set up by phagocytizing macrophages, myoblasts eventually fuse to form multi-nucleated myotubes. Once the centrally-located nuclei of myotubes move to the periphery, the muscle fiber is usually considered a mature myofiber.

Studies conducted at our laboratory have shown that, in mouse models, although muscle regeneration is the body's natural repair response to skeletal muscle injury, this repair is often incomplete, and large areas of non-regenerated muscle still exist even at 35 days post-injury [85]. This results in partial functional recovery of the muscle. We are now investigating methods to maximize the regenerative response of skeletal muscle following injury.

22.2.3.1. Intervention

Growth factors, i.e. IGF-1, have been identified as being capable of stimulating and proliferating myoblasts *in vitro* [71]. Similarly, enhancing muscle regeneration through the injection of growth factors into injured skeletal muscle *in vivo* has also demonstrated an improvement in muscle healing and strength post-laceration [71]. Muscles treated with growth factors demonstrated increased twitch and tetanic tensions at 15 days post-injury [71]. However, these proteins have short biological half-lives and a rapid clearance. Therefore, large doses of these factors would likely be needed to observe a clinically significant improvement in human skeletal muscle.

The transplantation of satellite cells/myoblasts has been investigated as a means for improving regeneration in injured skeletal muscle and, in particular, dystrophic muscle. In fact, it has been shown that transplanted myoblasts can contribute to the formation of dystrophin positive myofibers within the dystrophic muscle [86–93]. However, while demonstrating the ability to restore normal histology of dystrophic muscles and to improve skeletal muscle strength, this method has shown only transient effects and remains limited by factors such as immune rejection, poor cellular survival rates and the limited distribution of transplanted cells [94–98, 2]. A main limiting step in the transplantation of myoblasts is the massive cell death occurring in the first few hours after injection, possibly a result of a triggered immune response. To make a significant contribution to the regenerating muscle, surviving cells must proliferate at high enough rates to compensate for the large number of cell deaths, rates not typically seen in transplanted cells. At this time little information exists as to the factors required for the survival, activation and proliferation ultimately affecting the engraftment of satellite cells.

Muscle derived stem cells (MDSCs) are a step closer to overcoming some of the barriers obstructing the use of myoblasts for the treatment of muscle pathologies. Muscle stem cells are defined as cells that possess the ability to produce both new muscle stem cells, as well as myoblasts, without themselves expressing markers of muscle differentiation. Neonatal MDSCs display an improved regenerative and transplantation capacity in the skeletal muscle of *mdx* mice when compared to satellite cells [99, 70]. MDSCs have the ability to proliferate *in vivo* for an extended period of time due to their high resistance to stress [100], demonstrate strong capacity for self-renewal, undergo multipotent differentiation and display immune privileged behavior [70]. The transplantation of MDSCs obtained from normal animals has the potential to create a reservoir of normal stem cells that have the capability of restoring dystrophin expression [70]. At both 30- and 90 days post-injection into young, female *mdx* muscle, MDSCs resulted in a 10-fold increase in the dystophin-positive fiber count, when compared to skeletal muscles injected with an equal number of satellite cells [70]. Further, because of the fact that MDSCs have the ability to differentiate into endothelial and neural lineages, an enhanced neural and vascular supply to the targeted skeletal muscle may enhance regeneration [70, 101].

MDSCs obtained from normal muscle have the ability to regenerate dystrophin-positive myotubes within dystrophic muscles. Contractile testing of the tibialis anterior (TA) muscles from our laboratory has shown promising, yet variable, results with the fast-twitch increase of MDSC-treated versus untreated control muscles ranging from 0.5 percent to 2.86 percent, and the percentage increase in tetanus strength ranging from 0.0 percent to 6.82 percent (unpublished data). In this study, the tibialis anteriors of four-, eight- and 10-week-old female mice were injected with 500,000 MDSCs suspended in 15 ul of saline solution. Control muscles were injected with an equal volume of saline solution. Physiological testing was performed six weeks after injection. Improvements in the physiological functioning of MDSC-treated skeletal muscle were variable, at best; therefore, presenting a significant barrier to the translation of stem cell therapy to the medical treatment of muscular dystrophy [102]. Investigations considering how to maximize functional improvements of regenerated skeletal muscle after transplantation are scarce. Clearly, a challenge in the use of MDSCs for improving dystrophic skeletal muscle healing lies in how to stimulate cell proliferation, differentiation and improvements in skeletal muscle function. Questions such as the innervation status of differentiated muscle cells following transplantation, and their ability to respond to local environmental demands may elucidate variabilities in the contractile properties of treated muscles. For example, it is possible only those MDSCs that are fusing with existing myofibers contribute to the overall force producing capacity of the muscle, whereas those MDSCs that are fusing to each other, while demonstrating histological evidence of increased regeneration, make no functional contribution because of their lack of neural stimulation.

It is well known that environmental cues resulting from muscle injury or exercise stimulate resident satellite cells to proliferate and differentiate to form multi-nucleated myotubes. Palermo, et al. (2005) suggested that a specific set of molecular cues associated with physiological stress increases the contribution of bone marrow derived stem cells (BMDCs) to skeletal muscle [103]. It has been observed that, when there is no overt injury to the skeletal muscle, there appears to be no contribution by BMDCs into skeletal muscle [104, 105]. However, when the skeletal muscle is injured, BMDCs respond to biological cues, undertake a myogenic lineage and participate in skeletal muscle regeneration [106–108]. Along these lines, when the muscle was subjected to physiological stresses such as treadmill running or mechanical overloading, there is an observed increased contribution of BMDCs to the injured muscle. In each of these investigations involving BMDCs, stem cells were administered systemically. LaBarge and Blau (2002) suggested that BMDCs respond to the skeletal muscle needs for regeneration and/or repair that result from injury or overuse [104]. Future investigations should seek to identify specific environmental or physiological factors that may lead to the high amounts of variability seen in the functional characteristics of stem cell-transplanted muscles. Coupling MDSC transplantation with an exercise protocol may prove effective in providing the transplanted cells with the environmental cues necessary to increase the physiological function of treated dystrophic muscles.

22.2.4. Fibrosis

After a muscle injury the body responds quickly by attempting to regenerate damaged muscle fibers, while also providing temporary tensile resistance through the development of scar tissue (fibrosis). Yet, even in the absence of loading, such as in instances of immobilization, fibrosis is formed [109]. Scar tissue formation usually occurs between the second and third weeks after injury. The extracellular matrix is activated and produces collagen. Types I and III collagen are the major fibrillar collagens found in muscle, and their synthesis has been shown to increase after skeletal muscle injury [110–112]. Skeletal muscle often heals with a scar in addition to the muscle fiber regeneration that occurs. In fact, it has been suggested that any factor contributing to a decreased contractile capacity of muscle, such as fibrosis, decreases the energy-absorbing capabilities of the muscle, increases the likelihood for re-injury and decreases functional capacity [113]. Further, it has been hypothesized that the persistence of scar tissue formation inhibits complete regeneration of the muscle, predisposing the muscle to recurrent injury [114]. Kaariainen, et al. (1998) investigated factors affecting risk for injury recurrence following muscle laceration [115]. They found that the site of scar tissue formation was also the site for mechanical failure during tensile strain tests until 10 days after the injury. This study was limited by the fact that it did not investigate the functional contractile properties following injury, such as strength and fatigue.

Our laboratory has identified TGF-β1 as a key factor in activating the fibrosis cascade in skeletal muscle [116]. In fact, TGF-β1 has been shown to be associated with the excessive muscle fibrosis common to the skeletal muscle of individuals with DMD [117]. TGF-β1, released by infiltrating lymphocytes, macrophages and fibroblasts, infiltrates the injury site during the inflammatory response. TGF-β1 further induces autocrine expression in local cells within the injured muscle through a positive feedback cycle [116].

22.2.4.1. Intervention

Given the fact that muscle fibrosis is a major limiting factor in the complete functional recovery of injured skeletal muscle, our laboratory has investigated several mechanisms for minimizing the fibrotic cascade after injury. Among the most promising mechanisms is through the inhibition of TGF-β1, either directly or indirectly. Gamma interferon (γINF) inhibits TGF-β1 signaling by inducing the expression of SMAD-7 [118]. SMAD-7 triggers a negative feedback loop in the TGF-β1 signal transduction pathway [118]. Our studies have shown that, not only does γINF reduce the rate of growth of muscle-derived fibroblasts *in vitro*, but it also results in a significant improvement in the contractile strength of injured skeletal muscle, when compared to saline-injected controls [119].

Ideally, however, treatment would involve not only the inhibition of fibrosis, or the enhancement of muscle regeneration, but a combination of the two. Sato and colleagues (2003) attempted to combine the regenerative abilities of IGF-1 with the antifibrotic effects of decorin, an antagonist to TGF-β1 [120]. As expected, the combination of IGF-1 and decorin was capable of improving the histological and contractile characteristics of the muscle. However, this effect was not associated with a corresponding improved physiological strength, when compared to treatment with decorin alone. It was later discovered that decorin has the ability to not only block fibrosis, but also significantly increase the number of regenerating myofibers [116]. Decorin injection after muscle laceration resulted in a near complete recovery of muscle structure and function [121]. In fact, there was no significant difference in the fast-twitch and tetanic muscle strength of the decorin-treated groups and the normal, non-injured muscle [121]. Although a major improvement in muscle healing was seen with the use of decorin, large amounts of the protein were required to observe an effect. Furthermore, the study was performed in mice and, more directly clinical investigations must be conducted to evaluate the utility of this agent in the treatment of skeletal muscle injuries in humans.

Negishi and colleagues (2005) investigated the ability of relaxin, an insulin-like growth factor, to improve muscle healing after injury [122]. Relaxin-treated skeletal muscle demonstrated enhanced muscle regeneration, decreased fibrosis and an increased strength after a laceration injury [122]. Like decorin and relaxin, suramin is an antifibrotic agent, and suramin functions by competitively binding to the TGF-β1 receptor [123–125]. Rodent model investigations have demonstrated a decrease in scar tissue formation after laceration and strain, and an increased number of regenerating myofibers and contractile characteristics that were comparable to non-injured controls [126, 127]. Suramin has the advantage of being FDA-approved, making clinical applications imminent.

22.3. Factors Affecting Muscle Healing

22.3.1. Exercise

For centuries, it has been proposed that controlled activity promotes muscle healing and return to pre-injury function levels, although this school of thought continues to be debated [128]. Without a doubt, maintenance of muscle function requires at least a minimal amount of loading. Decreased activity levels result in decreased myofiber volume, oxidative capacity and capillary density, as well as an increased connective tissue mass [129]. These effects are more severe in cases of immobilization, with subsequent myofiber degeneration and a progressively increased proportion of connective tissue composition. In cases of skeletal muscle injury literature supports the idea that exercise promotes normal growth and repair of mammalian skeletal muscle [130]. Increased muscle contraction results in an increased blood flow to the area, thereby increasing the infiltration of leukocytes and monocytes to the injured region [131]. Exercise has also been shown to increase satellite cell activation, and even increase neural recruitment [129]. The timing in which activity should be introduced after injury is still unclear. It has been suggested that premature loading of injured muscle inhibits healing by interfering with the normal inflammatory processes. However, after a brief period of immobilization, activity results in a more complete and organized muscle fiber regeneration [132], suggesting that exercise may provide benefits to muscle healing during the regenerative and remodeling stages of repair.

22.3.2. Aging and Muscle Repair

As age progresses there is not only an increased susceptibility to muscle damage [133, 134], but also an impairment of skeletal muscle regeneration in response to injury [135–137] and a prolonged recovery [138, 139]. In 1977 Snow demonstrated that, while satellite cells make up approximately 30 percent of the muscle nuclei in newborns, this percentage decreases drastically to 4.6 percent in adult and 2.4 percent in elderly mice [140]. Since then a decline in the number of satellite cells with aging has been supported [141, 142]. In humans, *in vitro* studies showed a drastic decrease in the number of satellite cells only through the first two decades, after which the population count appears to plateau [143]. Although adult human satellite cells retain their ability to proliferate through adulthood, they appear to express a reduced capacity for differentiation [137]. It has also been shown that the basal lamina thickens with age, which may impair the ability of quiescent satellite cells from being activated [140]. Finally, aging coincides with a decreased immune response after exercise-induced injury resulting from a decreased expression of pro-inflammatory genes [144].

The environment may be a key factor determining the ability for skeletal muscle regeneration after healing. In an experiment conducted by Carlson and Faulkner (1989) it was found that, when young extensor digitorum muscles (EDLs) harvested from young animals were transplanted into old hosts, the young muscles regenerated no better than the old muscles [136]. Conversely, when old EDLs were transplanted into young hosts, the transplanted muscles did not show any significant difference in regenerative capacity, when compared to young muscles that had been transplanted into young hosts [136]. Along these lines, through heterochronic parabiosis, aged muscles were exposed to circulating factors typical of young animals, and vice versa [145]. It was found that old muscles exposed to a young environment resulted in increased regenerative capacity of the cells. Authors hypothesized that systemic factors supporting regeneration in young animals control critical molecular pathways that control the regenerative capacity of satellite cells [145]. Some have observed a decreased capillary density in aged muscles when compared to young muscle counterparts, and this may help explain some of these findings [146–148].

22.3.3. Sex

Findings have demonstrated decreased skeletal muscle damage after exercise-inducing injury in female rats when compared to male counterparts [149–151]. This attenuation of post-exercise muscle damage is possibly attributed to differences in circulating levels of estrogen. Estrogen has been shown to have a protective effect on skeletal muscle in response to injury [152, 153]. Feng, et al. (2004) reported findings that the presence of estrogen not only protected skeletal muscle from strain injury, but also improved the regeneration of strain-injured muscles [154]. In a study including 16 healthy individuals, eight men and eight women, Stupka and colleagues (2000) reported gender differences in the extent of exercise-induced muscle damage [151]. This difference corresponded to a decreased inflammatory response in females. Specifically, estrogen has been shown to inhibit inflammation by limiting neutrophil infiltration [154]. Neutrophils have been implicated in exacerbating skeletal muscle damage by producing oxidizing agents. A limited neutrophil infiltration may reduce muscle damage and speed healing. However, gender-related differences in response to skeletal muscle damage have been controversial, and the physiological consequences on differing estrogen levels for muscle healing still remains unclear.

22.3.4. Muscle Fiber Type

Mammalian skeletal muscle is comprised of slow-twitch and fast-twitch myofibers, each expressing differences in mitochondrial content, vascularity, metabolic properties and function. It has been shown that the type of training affects slow-twitch and fast-twitch fiber-type expression. For example, chronic loading increases the percentage of slow-twitch fibers [155]. This is not surprising since slow fibers are characterized by an increased vascularity and number of mitochondria, allowing for an increased oxidative capacity. Similarly, it has been shown that muscle injury induces a fiber type conversion, specifically, from a fast- to slow-type [156]. The role of this fiber switching during the healing process is still unclear.

22.4. Conclusions

Muscle injury is a common occurrence and generally affects all individuals at some time; an athlete injured during a game, a soldier injured in combat, a child with congenital muscle pathology or an individual who sprains their ankle stepping off a curb. In all these types of injury, the natural healing process is remarkably similar and a loss of function resulting from delayed or incomplete healing may lead to lost time and money.

While the treatment interventions for skeletal muscle injury have remained relatively unchanged over the last few decades, ongoing research is investigating intervention methods at every level of the muscle repair process. Given that the stages of muscle healing are interrelated and overlapping, the most effective treatments are those that attend to multiple levels of the repair process. Along these lines, among the most promising interventions are those that enhance skeletal muscle regeneration while minimizing fibrosis, as these appear to be key factors in determining the extent of functional muscle healing. Exciting new research has revealed mechanisms by which fibrosis may be minimized and fiber regeneration maximized, allowing for an increased viable muscle healing and a faster, more complete return to previous activities. Although numerous biological approaches are being investigated to improve muscle healing, it is clear that exercise, sex and aging will influence the repair process.

Abbreviations: bFGF Basic fibroblast growth factor; BMDC bone marrow derived stem cell; COX-1 Cyclooxygenase-1; COX-2 Cyclooxygenase-2; DMD Duchenne Muscular Dystrophy; EDL Extensor digitorum longus; γINF Gamma interferon; HGF Hepatocyte growth factor; IGF-1 Insulin-like growth factor-1; IL-6 Interleukin-6; IL-8 Interleukin-8; LIF Leukemia inhibitory factor; MDSC Muscle-derived stem cell; NGF Nerve growth factor; NSAID Non-steroidal anti-inflammatory drug; TA Tibialis anterior; TGF-β1 Transforming growth factor-β1; TNF-α Tumor Necrosis factor-α

Acknowledgements of Grant Support: This work was supported by grants from the National Institutes of Health (NIH 1 R01 AR47973 & NIH 1 R01 AR 49684), Department of Defense, and the Beatrice Dewey Hirtzel Memorial Foundation. This work was also supported by the Henry J. Mankin Endowed Chair at the University of Pittsburgh.

References

1. Warren GL, Lowe DA, Armstrong RB. Measurement tools used in the study of eccentric contraction-induced injury. [Review] [132 refs]. Sports Medicine 27 (1):43–59, 1999.
2. Huard J, Li Y, Fu FH. Current concepts review - Muscle injuries and repair: Current trends in research. Journal of Bone and Joint Surgery-American Volume 2002; 84A: 822–832.
3. Jones DA, Jackson MJ, McPhail G, Edwards RH. Experimental mouse muscle damage: the importance of external calcium. Clinical Science 66 (3):317–22, 1984.
4. Rantanen J, Hurme T, Lukka R, Heino J, Kalimo H. Satellite cell proliferation and the expression of myogenin and desmin in regenerating skeletal muscle: evidence for two different populations of satellite cells. Laboratory Investigation 72 (3):341–7, 1995.
5. Hurme T, Kalimo H, Lehto M, Jarvinen M. Healing of skeletal muscle injury: an ultrastructural and immunohistochemical study. Medicine & Science in Sports & Exercise 23(7):801–10, 1991.
6. Papadimitriou JM, Robertson TA, Mitchell CA, Grounds MD. The process of new plasmalemma formation in focally injured skeletal muscle fibers. Journal of Structural Biology 103 (2):124–34, 1990.
7. Fielding RA, Manfredi TJ, Ding W, Fiatarone MA, Evans WJ, Cannon JG. Acute phase response in exercise. III. Neutrophil and IL-1 beta accumulation in skeletal muscle. American Journal of Physiology 265 (1 Pt 2):R166–72, 1993.
8. Menke A, Jockusch H. Decreased osmotic stability of dystrophin-less muscle cells from the mdx mouse.[see comment]. Nature 349 (6304):69–71, 1991.
9. Koenig M, Hoffman EP, Bertelson CJ, Monaco AP, Feener C, Kunkel LM. Complete cloning of the Duchenne muscular dystrophy (DMD) cDNA and preliminary genomic organization of the DMD gene in normal and affected individuals. Cell 50 (3):509–17, 1987.

10. Petrof BJ, Stedman HH, Shrager JB, Eby J, Sweeney HL, Kelly AM. Adaptations in myosin heavy chain expression and contractile function in dystrophic mouse diaphragm. American Journal of Physiology 265 (3 Pt 1):C834–41, 1993.
11. Hoffman EP, Brown RH, Jr., Kunkel LM. Dystrophin: the protein product of the Duchenne muscular dystrophy locus. Cell 51 (6):919–28, 1987.
12. Bonilla E, Samitt CE, Miranda AF, Hays AP, Salviati G, DiMauro S, Kunkel LM, Hoffman EP, Rowland LP. Duchenne muscular dystrophy: deficiency of dystrophin at the muscle cell surface. Cell 54 (4):447–52, 1988.
13. Zubrzycka-Gaarn EE, Bulman DE, Karpati G, Burghes AH, Belfall B, Klamut HJ, Talbot J, Hodges RS, Ray PN, Worton RG. The Duchenne muscular dystrophy gene product is localized in sarcolemma of human skeletal muscle. Nature 333 (6172):466–9, 1988.
14. Hill M, Wernig A, Goldspink G. Muscle satellite (stem) cell activation during local tissue injury and repair. Journal of Anatomy 203; 89-99, 2003.
15. Dedieu S, Dourdin N, Dargelos E, Poussard S, Veschambre P, Cottin P, Brustis JJ. Calpain and myogenesis: development of a convenient cell culture model. Biology of the Cell 94 (2):65–76, 2002.
16. Raynaud F, Carnac G, Marcilhac A, Benyamin Y. m-Calpain implication in cell cycle during muscle precursor cell activation. Experimental Cell Research 298 (1):48–57, 2004.
17. Alderton JM, Steinhardt RA. Calcium influx through calcium leak channels is responsible for the elevated levels of calcium-dependent proteolysis in dystrophic myotubes. Journal of Biological Chemistry 275 (13):9452–60, 2000.
18. Alderton JM, Steinhardt RA. How calcium influx through calcium leak channels is responsible for the elevated levels of calcium-dependent proteolysis in dystrophic myotubes. [Review] [41 refs]. Trends in Cardiovascular Medicine 10(6):268–72, 2000.
19. Huang J, Forsberg NE. Role of calpain in skeletal-muscle protein degradation. [erratum appears in Proc Natl Acad Sci U S A 2000 Jun 6;97(12):6920]. Proceedings of the National Academy of Sciences of the United States of America 95 (21):12100–5, 1998.
20. Blake DJ, Tinsley JM, Davies KE. Utrophin: a structural and functional comparison to dystrophin. [Review] [93 refs]. Brain Pathology 6 (1):37–47, 1996.
21. Sicinski P, Geng Y, Ryder-Cook AS, Barnard EA, Darlison MG, Barnard PJ. The molecular basis of muscular dystrophy in the mdx mouse: a point mutation. Science 244 (4912):1578–80, 1989.
22. Courdier-Fruh I, Briguet A. Utrophin is a calpain substrate in muscle cells. Muscle & Nerve 33 (6):753–9, 2006.
23. Spencer MJ, Mellgren RL. Overexpression of a calpastatin transgene in mdx muscle reduces dystrophic pathology. Human Molecular Genetics 11(21):2645–55, 2002.
24. Fowler EG, Graves MC, Wetzel GT, Spencer MJ. Pilot trial of albuterol in Duchenne and Becker muscular dystrophy. Neurology 62 (6):1006–8, 2004.
25. Navegantes LC, Machado CR, Resano NM, Migliorini RH, Kettelhut IC. Beta2-agonists and cAMP inhibit protein degradation in isolated chick (Gallus domesticus) skeletal muscle. British Poultry Science 44 (1):149–54, 2003.
26. Burniston JG, Clark WA, Tan LB, Goldspink DF. Dose-dependent separation of the hypertrophic and myotoxic effects of the beta(2)-adrenergic receptor agonist clenbuterol in rat striated muscles. Muscle & Nerve 33 (5):655–63, 2006.
27. Katoch SS, Garg A, Sharma S. Histological evidences of reparative and regenerative effects of beta-adrenoceptor agonists, clenbuterol and isoproterenol, in denervated rat skeletal muscle. Indian Journal of Experimental Biology 44 (6):448–58, 2006.
28. Yimlamai T, Dodd SL, Borst SE, Park S. Clenbuterol induces muscle-specific attenuation of atrophy through effects on the ubiquitin-proteasome pathway. Journal of Applied Physiology 99 (1):71–80, 2005.

29. Dodd SL, Koesterer TJ. Clenbuterol attenuates muscle atrophy and dysfunction in hindlimb-suspended rats. Aviation Space & Environmental Medicine 73 (7):635–9, 2002.
30. Hinkle RT, Hodge KM, Cody DB, Sheldon RJ, Kobilka BK, Isfort RJ. Skeletal muscle hypertrophy and anti-atrophy effects of clenbuterol are mediated by the beta2-adrenergic receptor. Muscle & Nerve 25 (5):729–34, 2002.
31. von Deutsch DA, Abukhalaf IK, Wineski LE, Roper RR, Aboul-Enein HY, Paulsen DF, Potter DE. Distribution and muscle-sparing effects of clenbuterol in hindlimb-suspended rats. Pharmacology 65 (1):38–48, 2002.
32. Grounds MD, Torrisi J. Anti-TNFalpha (Remicade) therapy protects dystrophic skeletal muscle from necrosis. FASEB Journal 18 (6):676–82, 2004.
33. Spencer MJ, Marino MW, Winckler WM. Altered pathological progression of diaphragm and quadriceps muscle in TNF-deficient, dystrophin-deficient mice. Neuromuscular Disorders 10(8):612–9, 2000.
34. Gosselin LE, Barkley JE, Spencer MJ, McCormick KM, Farkas GA. Ventilatory dysfunction in mdx mice: impact of tumor necrosis factor-alpha deletion. Muscle & Nerve 28 (3):336–43, 2003.
35. Chen SE, Gerken E, Zhang Y, Zhan M, Mohan RK, Li AS, Reid MB, Li YP. Role of TNF-{alpha} signaling in regeneration of cardiotoxin-injured muscle. American Journal of Physiology - Cell Physiology 289 (5):C1179–87, 2005.
36. Warren GL, Hulderman T, Jensen N, McKinstry M, Mishra M, Luster MI, Simeonova PP. Physiological role of tumor necrosis factor alpha in traumatic muscle injury. FASEB Journal 16 (12):1630–2, 2002.
37. Collins RA, Grounds MD. The role of tumor necrosis factor-alpha (TNF-alpha) in skeletal muscle regeneration. Studies in TNF-alpha(-/-) and TNF-alpha(-/-)/LT-alpha(-/-) mice. Journal of Histochemistry & Cytochemistry 49 (8):989–1001, 2001.
38. Mense S. Sensitization of group IV muscle receptors to bradykinin by 5-hydroxytryptamine and prostaglandin E2. Brain Research 225 (1):95–105, 1981.
39. Hedenberg-Magnusson B, Ernberg M, Alstergren P, Kopp S. Pain mediation by prostaglandin E2 and leukotriene B4 in the human masseter muscle. Acta Odontologica Scandinavica 59 (6):348–55, 2001.
40. Zhang Y, Shaffer A, Portanova J, Seibert K, Isakson PC. Inhibition of cyclooxygenase-2 rapidly reverses inflammatory hyperalgesia and prostaglandin E2 production. Journal of Pharmacology & Experimental Therapeutics 283 (3):1069–75, 1997.
41. Horsley V, Pavlath GK. Prostaglandin F2(alpha) stimulates growth of skeletal muscle cells via an NFATC2-dependent pathway. Journal of Cell Biology 161 (1):111–8, 2003.
42. Shen W, Prisk V, Li Y, Foster W, Huard J. Inhibited skeletal muscle healing in cyclooxygenase-2 gene-deficient mice: the role of PGE2 and PGF2alpha. Journal of Applied Physiology 101 (4):1215–21, 2006.
43. Botting RM. Mechanism of action of acetaminophen: is there a cyclooxygenase 3?. [Review] [98 refs]. Clinical Infectious Diseases 31 Suppl 5:S202–10, 2000.
44. Chandrasekharan NV, Dai H, Roos KL, Evanson NK, Tomsik J, Elton TS, Simmons DL. COX-3, a cyclooxygenase-1 variant inhibited by acetaminophen and other analgesic/antipyretic drugs: cloning, structure, and expression.[see comment]. Proceedings of the National Academy of Sciences of the United States of America 99 (21):13926–31, 2002.
45. Tilley SL, Coffman TM, Koller BH. Mixed messages: modulation of inflammation and immune responses by prostaglandins and thromboxanes. [Review] [49 refs]. Journal of Clinical Investigation 108 (1):15–23, 2001.
46. Murakami M, Naraba H, Tanioka T, Semmyo N, Nakatani Y, Kojima F, Ikeda T, Fueki M, Ueno A, Oh S, Kudo I. Regulation of prostaglandin E2 biosynthesis by inducible membrane-associated prostaglandin E2 synthase that acts in concert with cyclooxygenase-2. Journal of Biological Chemistry 275 (42):32783–92, 2000.

47. Cannon JG, Orencole SF, Fielding RA, Meydani M, Meydani SN, Fiatarone MA, Blumberg JB, Evans WJ. Acute phase response in exercise: interaction of age and vitamin E on neutrophils and muscle enzyme release. American Journal of Physiology 259 (6 Pt 2):R1214–9, 1990.
48. Tidball JG. Inflammatory cell response to acute muscle injury. [Review] [118 refs]. Medicine & Science in Sports & Exercise 27 (7):1022–32, 1995.
49. Frenette J, Cai B, Tidball JG. Complement activation promotes muscle inflammation during modified muscle use. American Journal of Pathology 156 (6):2103–10, 2000.
50. MacIntyre DL, Sorichter S, Mair J, Berg A, McKenzie DC. Markers of inflammation and myofibrillar proteins following eccentric exercise in humans. European Journal of Applied Physiology 84 (3):180–6, 2001.
51. Smedly LA, Tonnesen MG, Sandhaus RA, Haslett C, Guthrie LA, Johnston RB, Jr., Henson PM, Worthen GS. Neutrophil-mediated injury to endothelial cells. Enhancement by endotoxin and essential role of neutrophil elastase. Journal of Clinical Investigation 77 (4):1233–43, 1986.
52. Chatelain P, Latour JG, Tran D, de Lorgeril M, Dupras G, Bourassa M. Neutrophil accumulation in experimental myocardial infarcts: relation with extent of injury and effect of reperfusion. Circulation 75 (5):1083–90, 1987.
53. Engler RL, Schmid-Schonbein GW, Pavelec RS. Leukocyte capillary plugging in myocardial ischemia and reperfusion in the dog. American Journal of Pathology 111 (1):98–111, 1983.
54. Korthuis RJ, Grisham MB, Granger DN. Leukocyte depletion attenuates vascular injury in postischemic skeletal muscle. American Journal of Physiology 254 (5 Pt 2):H823–7, 1988.
55. Linas SL, Shanley PF, Whittenburg D, Berger E, Repine JE. Neutrophils accentuate ischemia-reperfusion injury in isolated perfused rat kidneys. American Journal of Physiology 255 (4 Pt 2):F728–35, 1988.
56. Mullane KM, Read N, Salmon JA, Moncada S. Role of leukocytes in acute myocardial infarction in anesthetized dogs: relationship to myocardial salvage by anti-inflammatory drugs. Journal of Pharmacology & Experimental Therapeutics 228 (2):510–22, 1984.
57. Petrone WF, English DK, Wong K, McCord JM. Free radicals and inflammation: superoxide-dependent activation of a neutrophil chemotactic factor in plasma. Proceedings of the National Academy of Sciences of the United States of America 77 (2):1159–63, 1980.
58. Romson JL, Hook BG, Kunkel SL, Abrams GD, Schork MA, Lucchesi BR. Reduction of the extent of ischemic myocardial injury by neutrophil depletion in the dog. Circulation 67 (5):1016–23, 1983.
59. Walden DL, McCutchan HJ, Enquist EG, Schwappach JR, Shanley PF, Reiss OK, Terada LS, Leff JA, Repine JE. Neutrophils accumulate and contribute to skeletal muscle dysfunction after ischemia-reperfusion. American Journal of Physiology 259 (6 Pt 2):H1809–12, 1990.
60. Teixeira CF, Zamuner SR, Zuliani JP, Fernandes CM, Cruz-Hofling MA, Fernandes I, Chaves F, Gutierrez JM. Neutrophils do not contribute to local tissue damage, but play a key role in skeletal muscle regeneration, in mice injected with Bothrops asper snake venom. Muscle & Nerve 28 (4):449–59, 2003.
61. Miyagawa J, Higashiyama S, Kawata S, Inui Y, Tamura S, Yamamoto K, Nishida M, Nakamura T, Yamashita S, Matsuzawa Y. Localization of heparin-binding EGF-like growth factor in the smooth muscle cells and macrophages of human atherosclerotic plaques. Journal of Clinical Investigation 95 (1):404–11, 1995.
62. Horikawa M, Higashiyama S, Nomura S, Kitamura Y, Ishikawa M, Taniguchi N. Upregulation of endogenous heparin-binding EGF-like growth factor and its role as a survival factor in skeletal myotubes. FEBS Letters 459 (1):100–4, 1999.

63. Almekinders LC, Gilbert JA. Healing of experimental muscle strains and the effects of nonsteroidal antiinflammatory medication. American Journal of Sports Medicine 14(4):303–8, 1986;–Aug.
64. Mishra DK, Friden J, Schmitz MC, Lieber RL. Anti-inflammatory medication after muscle injury. A treatment resulting in short-term improvement but subsequent loss of muscle function.[see comment]. Journal of Bone & Joint Surgery - American Volume 77 (10):1510–9, 1995.
65. Bondesen BA, Mills ST, Kegley KM, Pavlath GK. The COX-2 pathway is essential during early stages of skeletal muscle regeneration. American Journal of Physiology - Cell Physiology 287 (2):C475–83, 2004.
66. Shen W, Li Y, Tang Y, Cummins J, Huard J. NS-398, a cyclooxygenase-2-specific inhibitor, delays skeletal muscle healing by decreasing regeneration and promoting fibrosis. American Journal of Pathology 167 (4):1105–17, 2005.
67. Rodemann HP, Goldberg AL. Arachidonic acid, prostaglandin E2 and F2 alpha influence rates of protein turnover in skeletal and cardiac muscle. Journal of Biological Chemistry 257 (4):1632–8, 1982.
68. Bondesen BA, Mills ST, Pavlath GK. The COX-2 pathway regulates growth of atrophied muscle via multiple mechanisms. American Journal of Physiology - Cell Physiology 290 (6):C1651–9, 2006.
69. Schultz E, Jaryszak DL, Valliere CR. Response of satellite cells to focal skeletal muscle injury. Muscle & Nerve 8 (3):217–22, 1985; -Apr.
70. Qu-Petersen Z, Deasy B, Jankowski R, Ikezawa M, Cummins J, Pruchnic R, Mytinger J, Cao B, Gates C, Wernig A, Huard J. Identification of a novel population of muscle stem cells in mice: potential for muscle regeneration. Journal of Cell Biology 157 (5):851–64, 2002.
71. Menetrey J, Kasemkijwattana C, Day CS, Bosch P, Vogt M, Fu FH, Moreland MS, Huard J. Growth factors improve muscle healing in vivo. Journal of Bone and Joint Surgery-British Volume 2000; 82B: 131-137.
72. Kami K, Senba E. In vivo activation of STAT3 signaling in satellite cells and myofibers in regenerating rat skeletal muscles. Journal of Histochemistry & Cytochemistry 50 (12):1579–89, 2002.
73. DeVol DL, Rotwein P, Sadow JL, Novakofski J, Bechtel PJ. Activation of insulin-like growth factor gene expression during work-induced skeletal muscle growth. American Journal of Physiology 259 (1 Pt 1):E89–95, 1990.
74. Yan Z, Biggs RB, Booth FW. Insulin-like growth factor immunoreactivity increases in muscle after acute eccentric contractions. Journal of Applied Physiology 74 (1):410–4, 1993.
75. Yang H, Alnaqeeb M, Simpson H, Goldspink G. Changes in muscle fibre type, muscle mass and IGF-I gene expression in rabbit skeletal muscle subjected to stretch. Journal of Anatomy 190; 613-22, 1997.
76. Engert JC, Berglund EB, Rosenthal N. Proliferation precedes differentiation in IGF-I-stimulated myogenesis. Journal of Cell Biology 135 (2):431–40, 1996.
77. McPherron AC, Lawler AM, Lee SJ. Regulation of skeletal muscle mass in mice by a new TGF-beta superfamily member. Nature 387 (6628):83–90, 1997.
78. McCroskery S, Thomas M, Maxwell L, Sharma M, Kambadur R. Myostatin negatively regulates satellite cell activation and self-renewal. Journal of Cell Biology 162 (6):1135–47, 2003.
79. McCroskery S, Thomas M, Platt L, Hennebry A, Nishimura T, McLeay L, Sharma M, Kambadur R. Improved muscle healing through enhanced regeneration and reduced fibrosis in myostatin-null mice. Journal of Cell Science 118 (Pt 15):3531–41, 2005.
80. Carlson CJ, Booth FW, Gordon SE. Skeletal muscle myostatin mRNA expression is fiber-type specific and increases during hindlimb unloading. American Journal of Physiology 277 (2 Pt 2):R601–6, 1999.

81. Merly F, Lescaudron L, Rouaud T, Crossin F, Gardahaut MF. Macrophages enhance muscle satellite cell proliferation and delay their differentiation. Muscle & Nerve 22 (6):724–32, 1999.
82. Warren GL, O'Farrell L, Summan M, Hulderman T, Mishra D, Luster MI, Kuziel WA, Simeonova PP. Role of CC chemokines in skeletal muscle functional restoration after injury. American Journal of Physiology - Cell Physiology 286 (5): C1031–6, 2004.
83. Lescaudron L, Peltekian E, Fontaine-Perus J, Paulin D, Zampieri M, Garcia L, Parrish E. Blood borne macrophages are essential for the triggering of muscle regeneration following muscle transplant. Neuromuscular Disorders 9 (2):72–80, 1999.
84. Chazaud B, Sonnet C, Lafuste P, Bassez G, Rimaniol AC, Poron F, Authier FJ, Dreyfus PA, Gherardi RK. Satellite cells attract monocytes and use macrophages as a support to escape apoptosis and enhance muscle growth. Journal of Cell Biology 163 (5):1133–43, 2003.
85. Kasemkijwattana C, Menetrey J, Day CS, Bosch P, Buranapanitkit B, Moreland MS, Fu FH, Watkins SC, Huard J. Biologic intervention in muscle healing and regeneration. Sports Medicine and Arthroscopy Review 1998; 6: 95-102.
86. Karpati G, Pouliot Y, Zubrzycka-Gaarn E, Carpenter S, Ray PN, Worton RG, Holland P. Dystrophin is expressed in mdx skeletal muscle fibers after normal myoblast implantation. American Journal of Pathology 135 (1):27–32, 1989.
87. Karpati G, Holland P, Worton RG. Myoblast transfer in DMD: problems in the interpretation of efficiency. Muscle & Nerve 15 (10):1209–10, 1992.
88. Partridge TA, Morgan JE, Coulton GR, Hoffman EP, Kunkel LM. Conversion of mdx myofibres from dystrophin-negative to - positive by injection of normal myoblasts. Nature 337 (6203):176–9, 1989.
89. Huard J, Bouchard JP, Roy R, Malouin F, Dansereau G, Labrecque C, Albert N, Richards CL, Lemieux B, Tremblay JP. Human myoblast transplantation: preliminary results of 4 cases. Muscle & Nerve 15 (5):550–60, 1992.
90. Huard J, Roy R, Bouchard JP, Malouin F, Richards CL, Tremblay JP. Human myoblast transplantation between immunohistocompatible donors and recipients produces immune reactions. Transplantation Proceedings 24 (6):3049–51, 1992.
91. Tremblay JP, Malouin F, Roy R, Huard J, Bouchard JP, Satoh A, Richards CL. Results of a triple blind clinical study of myoblast transplantations without immunosuppressive treatment in young boys with Duchenne muscular dystrophy. Cell Transplantation 2(2):99–112, 1993; -Apr.
92. Vilquin JT, Wagner E, Kinoshita I, Roy R, Tremblay JP. Successful histocompatible myoblast transplantation in dystrophin-deficient mdx mouse despite the production of antibodies against dystrophin. Journal of Cell Biology 131 (4):975–88, 1995.
93. Kinoshita I, Vilquin JT, Tremblay JP. Mechanism of increasing dystrophin-positive myofibers by myoblast transplantation: study using mdx/beta-galactosidase transgenic mice. Acta Neuropathologica 91 (5):489–93, 1996.
94. Fan Y, Maley M, Beilharz M, Grounds M. Rapid death of injected myoblasts in myoblast transfer therapy. Muscle & Nerve 1919; 853-60, 1996.
95. Guerette B, Asselin I, Skuk D, Entman M, Tremblay JP. Control of inflammatory damage by anti-LFA-1: increase success of myoblast transplantation. Cell Transplantation 6 (2):101–7, 1997; -Apr.
96. Beauchamp JR, Morgan JE, Pagel CN, Partridge TA. Dynamics of myoblast transplantation reveal a discrete minority of precursors with stem cell-like properties as the myogenic source. Journal of Cell Biology 144 (6):1113–22, 1999.
97. Hodgetts SI, Beilharz MW, Scalzo AA, Grounds MD. Why do cultured transplanted myoblasts die in vivo? DNA quantification shows enhanced survival of donor male myoblasts in host mice depleted of CD4+ and CD8+ cells or Nk1.1+ cells. Cell Transplantation 9 (4):489–502, 2000; -Aug.

98. Smythe GM, Hodgetts SI, Grounds MD. Immunobiology and the future of myoblast transfer therapy. [Review] [120 refs]. Molecular Therapy : the Journal of the American Society of Gene Therapy 1(4):304–13, 2000.
99. Jankowski RJ, Deasy BM, Cao B, Gates C, Huard J. The role of CD34 expression and cellular fusion in the regeneration capacity of myogenic progenitor cells. Journal of Cell Science 115 (Pt 22):4361–74, 2002.
100. Oshima H, Payne TR, Urish KL, Sakai T, Ling Y, Gharaibeh B, Tobita K, Keller BB, Cummins JH, Huard J. Differential myocardial infarct repair with muscle stem cells compared to myoblasts. Molecular Therapy : the Journal of the American Society of Gene Therapy 12 (6):1130–41, 2005.
101. Peng H, Huard J. Muscle-derived stem cells for musculoskeletal tissue regeneration and repair. [Review] [83 refs]. Transplant Immunology 12 (3-4):311–9, 2004.
102. Mueller GM, O'Day T, Watchko JF, Ontell M. Effect of injecting primary myoblasts versus putative muscle-derived stem cells on mass and force generation in mdx mice. Human Gene Therapy 13(9):1081–90, 2002.
103. Palermo AT, Labarge MA, Doyonnas R, Pomerantz J, Blau HM. Bone marrow contribution to skeletal muscle: a physiological response to stress. Developmental Biology 279 (2):336–44, 2005.
104. Labarge MA, Blau HM. Biological progression from adult bone marrow to mononucleate muscle stem cell to multinucleate muscle fiber in response to injury. Cell 111 (4):589–601, 2002.
105. Wagers AJ, Sherwood RI, Christensen JL, Weissman IL. Little evidence for developmental plasticity of adult hematopoietic stem cells.[see comment]. Science 297 (5590):2256–9, 2002.
106. Camargo FD, Green R, Capetanaki Y, Jackson KA, Goodell MA. Single hematopoietic stem cells generate skeletal muscle through myeloid intermediates.[see comment][erratum appears in Nat Med. 2004 Jan;10(1):105 Note: Capetenaki, Yassemi [corrected to Capetanaki, Yassemi]]. Nature Medicine 9 (12):1520–7, 2003.
107. Abedi M, Greer DA, Colvin GA, Demers DA, Dooner MS, Harpel JA, Pimentel J, Menon MK, Quesenberry PJ. Tissue injury in marrow transdifferentiation. [Review] [14 refs]. Blood Cells Molecules & Diseases 32 (1):42–6, 2004; -Feb.
108. Corbel SY, Lee A, Yi L, Duenas J, Brazelton TR, Blau HM, Rossi FM. Contribution of hematopoietic stem cells to skeletal muscle.[see comment]. Nature Medicine 9 (12):1528–32, 2003.
109. Menetrey J, Kasemkijwattana C, Fu FH, Moreland MS, Huard J. Suturing versus immobilization of a muscle laceration. A morphological and functional study in a mouse model. American Journal of Sports Medicine 27 (2):222–9, 1999; -Apr.
110. Lehto M, Duance VC, Restall D. Collagen and fibronectin in a healing skeletal muscle injury. An immunohistological study of the effects of physical activity on the repair of injured gastrocnemius muscle in the rat. Journal of Bone & Joint Surgery - British Volume 67 (5):820–8, 1985.
111. Lehto M, Sims TJ, Bailey AJ. Skeletal muscle injury--molecular changes in the collagen during healing. Research in Experimental Medicine 185 (2):95–106, 1985.
112. Sasse J, von der MH, Kuhl U, Dessau W, von der MK. Origin of collagen types I, III, and V in cultures of avian skeletal muscle. Developmental Biology 83 (1):79–89, 1981.
113. Croisier JL. Factors associated with recurrent hamstring injuries. [Review] [85 refs]. Sports Medicine 34 (10):681–95, 2004.
114. Nikolaou PK, Macdonald BL, Glisson RR, Seaber AV, Garrett WE, Jr. Biomechanical and histological evaluation of muscle after controlled strain injury. American Journal of Sports Medicine 15 (1):9–14, 1987; -Feb.

115. Kaariainen M, Kaariainen J, Jarvinen TL, Sievanen H, Kalimo H, Jarvinen M. Correlation between biomechanical and structural changes during the regeneration of skeletal muscle after laceration injury. Journal of Orthopaedic Research 16 (2):197–206, 1998.
116. Li Y, Foster W, Deasy BM, Chan YS, Prisk V, Tang Y, Cummins J, Huard J. Transforming growth factor-beta 1 induces the differentiation of myogenic cells into fibrotic cells in injured skeletal muscle - A key event in muscle fibrogenesis. American Journal of Pathology 2004; 164: 1007-1019.
117. Bernasconi P, Di Blasi C, Mora M, Morandi L, Galbiati S, Confalonieri P, Cornelio F, Mantegazza R. Transforming growth factor-beta1 and fibrosis in congenital muscular dystrophies. Neuromuscular Disorders 9 (1):28–33, 1999.
118. Wen FQ, Liu X, Kobayashi T, Abe S, Fang Q, Kohyama T, Ertl R, Terasaki Y, Manouilova L, Rennard SI. Interferon-gamma inhibits transforming growth factor-beta production in human airway epithelial cells by targeting Smads. American Journal of Respiratory Cell & Molecular Biology 30 (6):816–22, 2004.
119. Foster W, Li Y, Usas A, Somogyi G, Huard J. Gamma interferon as an antifibrosis agent in skeletal muscle. Journal of Orthopaedic Research 21(5):798–804, 2003.
120. Sato K, Li Y, Foster W, Fukushima K, Badlani N, Adachi N, Usas A, Fu FH, Huard J. Improvement of muscle healing through enhancement of muscle regeneration and prevention of fibrosis. Muscle & Nerve 28 (3):365–72, 2003.
121. Fukushima K, Badlani N, Usas A, Riano F, Fu F, Huard J. The use of an antifibrosis agent to improve muscle recovery after laceration. American Journal of Sports Medicine 29 (4):394–402, 2001; -Aug.
122. Negishi S, Li Y, Usas A, Fu FH, Huard J. The effect of relaxin treatment on skeletal muscle injuries. American Journal of Sports Medicine 2005; 33: 1816-1824.
123. Schrell UM, Gauer S, Kiesewetter F, Bickel A, Hren J, Adams EF, Fahlbusch R. Inhibition of proliferation of human cerebral meningioma cells by suramin: effects on cell growth, cell cycle phases, extracellular growth factors, and PDGF-BB autocrine growth loop. Journal of Neurosurgery 82 (4):600–7, 1995.
124. Stein CA, LaRocca RV, Thomas R, McAtee N, Myers CE. Suramin: an anticancer drug with a unique mechanism of action. Journal of Clinical Oncology 7 (4):499–508, 1989.
125. Zumkeller W, Schofield PN. Growth factors, cytokines and soluble forms of receptor molecules in cancer patients. [Review] [18 refs]. Anticancer Research 15 (2):343–8, 1995; -Apr.
126. Chan YS, Li Y, Foster W, Horaguchi T, Somogyi G, Fu FH, Huard J. Antifibrotic effects of suramin in injured skeletal muscle after laceration. Journal of Applied Physiology 2003; 95: 771-780.
127. Chan YS, Li Y, Foster W, Fu FH, Huard J. The use of suramin, an antifibrotic agent, to improve muscle recovery after strain injury. American Journal of Sports Medicine 2005; 33: 43-51.
128. Buckwalter JA, Grodzinsky AJ. Loading of healing bone, fibrous tissue, and muscle: implications for orthopaedic practice. [Review] [69 refs]. Journal of the American Academy of Orthopaedic Surgeons 7 (5):291–9, 1999; -Oct.
129. Jozsa L, Kannus P, Thoring J, Reffy A, Jarvinen M, Kvist M. The effect of tenotomy and immobilisation on intramuscular connective tissue. A morphometric and microscopic study in rat calf muscles. Journal of Bone & Joint Surgery - British Volume 72 (2):293–7, 1990.
130. Markert CD, Merrick MA, Kirby TE, Devor ST. Nonthermal ultrasound and exercise in skeletal muscle regeneration. Archives of Physical Medicine & Rehabilitation 86 (7):1304–10, 2005.
131. Lieber RL, Schmitz MC, Mishra DK, Friden J. Contractile and cellular remodeling in rabbit skeletal muscle after cyclic eccentric contractions. Journal of Applied Physiology 77 (4):1926–34, 1994.

132. Jarvinen M. Healing of a crush injury in rat striated muscle. 2. a histological study of the effect of early mobilization and immobilization on the repair processes. Acta Pathologica et Microbiologica Scandinavica - Section A, Pathology 83 (3):269–82, 1975.
133. Brooks SV, Faulkner JA. Contractile properties of skeletal muscles from young, adult and aged mice. Journal of Physiology 404 :71–82, 1988.
134. Zerba E, Komorowski TE, Faulkner JA. Free radical injury to skeletal muscles of young, adult, and old mice. American Journal of Physiology 258 (3 Pt 1): C429–35, 1990.
135. Brooks SV, Faulkner JA. Contraction-induced injury: recovery of skeletal muscles in young and old mice. American Journal of Physiology 258 (3 Pt 1):C436–42, 1990.
136. Carlson BM, Faulkner JA. Muscle transplantation between young and old rats: age of host determines recovery. American Journal of Physiology 256 (6 Pt 1): C1262–6, 1989.
137. Jarvinen M, Aho AJ, Lehto M, Toivonen H. Age dependent repair of muscle rupture. A histological and microangiographical study in rats. Acta Orthopaedica Scandinavica 54 (1):64–74, 1983.
138. Dedrick ME, Clarkson PM. The effects of eccentric exercise on motor performance in young and older women. European Journal of Applied Physiology & Occupational Physiology 60 (3):183–6, 1990.
139. McBride TA, Gorin FA, Carlsen RC. Prolonged recovery and reduced adaptation in aged rat muscle following eccentric exercise. Mechanisms of Ageing & Development 83 (3):185–200, 1995.
140. Snow MH. The effects of aging on satellite cells in skeletal muscles of mice and rats. Cell & Tissue Research 185 (3):399–408, 1977.
141. Gibson MC, Schultz E. Age-related differences in absolute numbers of skeletal muscle satellite cells. Muscle & Nerve 6 (8):574–80, 1983.
142. Renault V, Thornell LE, Eriksson PO, Butler-Browne G, Mouly V. Regenerative potential of human skeletal muscle during aging.[erratum appears in Aging Cell. 2003 Feb;2(1):71 Note: Thorne Lars-Eric [corrected to Thornell Lars-Eric]]. Aging Cell 1(2):132–9, 2002.
143. Decary S, Mouly V, Hamida CB, Sautet A, Barbet JP, Butler-Browne GS. Replicative potential and telomere length in human skeletal muscle: implications for satellite cell-mediated gene therapy. Human Gene Therapy 8 (12):1429–38, 1997.
144. Hamada K, Vannier E, Sacheck JM, Witsell AL, Roubenoff R. Senescence of human skeletal muscle impairs the local inflammatory cytokine response to acute eccentric exercise. FASEB Journal 1919; 264-266.
145. Conboy IM, Conboy MJ, Wagers AJ, Girma ER, Weissman IL, Rando TA. Rejuvenation of aged progenitor cells by exposure to a young systemic environment. Nature 433 (7027):760–4, 2005.
146. Coggan AR, Spina RJ, King DS, Rogers MA, Brown M, Nemeth PM, Holloszy JO. Histochemical and enzymatic comparison of the gastrocnemius muscle of young and elderly men and women. Journal of Gerontology 47 (3):B71–6, 1992.
147. Croley AN, Zwetsloot KA, Westerkamp LM, Ryan NA, Pendergast AM, Hickner RC, Pofahl WE, Gavin TP. Lower capillarization, VEGF protein, and VEGF mRNA response to acute exercise in the vastus lateralis muscle of aged vs. young women. Journal of Applied Physiology 99 (5):1872–9, 2005.
148. Parizkova J, Eiselt E, Sprynarova S, Wachtlova M. Body composition, aerobic capacity, and density of muscle capillaries in young and old men. Journal of Applied Physiology 31 (3):323–5, 1971.
149. Amelink GJ, Koot RW, Erich WB, Van Gijn J, Bar PR. Sex-linked variation in creatine kinase release, and its dependence on oestradiol, can be demonstrated in an in-vitro rat skeletal muscle preparation. Acta Physiologica Scandinavica 138 (2):115–24, 1990.

150. Amelink GJ, van der Wal WA, Wokke JH, van Asbeck BS, Bar PR. Exercise-induced muscle damage in the rat: the effect of vitamin E deficiency. Pflugers Archiv - European Journal of Physiology 419 (3-4):304–9, 1991.
151. Stupka N, Lowther S, Chorneyko K, Bourgeois JM, Hogben C, Tarnopolsky MA. Gender differences in muscle inflammation after eccentric exercise. Journal of Applied Physiology 89 (6):2325–32, 2000.
152. Feng X, Li GZ, Wang S. Effects of estrogen on gastrocnemius muscle strain injury and regeneration in female rats. Acta Pharmacologica Sinica 25 (11):1489–94, 2004.
153. Stupka N, Tiidus PM. Effects of ovariectomy and estrogen on ischemia-reperfusion injury in hindlimbs of female rats. Journal of Applied Physiology 91 (4):1828–35, 2001.
154. Tiidus PM, Holden D, Bombardier E, Zajchowski S, Enns D, Belcastro A. Estrogen effect on post-exercise skeletal muscle neutrophil infiltration and calpain activity. Canadian Journal of Physiology & Pharmacology 79 (5):400–6, 2001.
155. Jarvis JC, Mokrusch T, Kwende MM, Sutherland H, Salmons S. Fast-to-slow transformation in stimulated rat muscle. Muscle & Nerve 1919; 1469-75, 1996.
156. Salvini TF, Morini CC, Selistre de Araujo HS, Ownby CL. Long-term regeneration of fast and slow murine skeletal muscles after induced injury by ACL myotoxin isolated from Agkistrodon contortrix laticinctus (broad-banded copperhead) venom. Anatomical Record 254 (4):521–33, 1999.

Section IV

Generalized Approaches

23

Principles of Musculoskeletal Tissue Banking

Theodore I. Malinin

Abstract: Transplantation of bone and tissue allografts is a commonly performed surgical procedure made possible by the development of tissue banks and the wide availability of transplants. Knowledge of the principles of tissue banking and understanding the advantages and risks of musculoskeletal allograft transplantation allows surgeons to make rational decisions about whether a particular patient should or should not receive such transplants.

Bone allografts excised aseptically are preserved by freeze-drying, rapid freezing or by controlled velocity freezing in the presence of cryoprotective agents. Bone and tissue allografts excised without aseptic precautions are, in addition, subjected to secondary sterilization by ionizing radiation or by exposure to ethylene oxide gas. Irradiation and, to a lesser degree, ethylene oxide alters biological properties of allografts.

Although disease transmission with tissue allografts has been reported, allografts from adequately screened and studied cadaver donors are safe.

Keywords: Tissue banking, allografts, freeze-drying, cryopreservation, allograft safety, musculoskeletal tissue, allograft biology.

23.1. Introduction

Transplantation of musculoskeletal allografts is now an accepted surgical practice. In the United States it was brought about by the ready availability of allografts from a number of tissue banks [1–4]. This led, at times, to an indiscriminate use of musculoskeletal transplants with surgeons knowing little about where the grafts came from or how they were prepared [5].

Availability of bone grafts obviated the need for the surgeons to prepare these in the operating room, as was the case before the demonstration of

Department of Orthopedics and Rehabilitation, Miller School of Medicine, University of Miami, Miami, FL

From: *Orthopedic Biology and Medicine: Musculoskeletal Tissue Regeneration, Biological Materials and Methods*
Edited by W. S. Pietrzak © Humana Press, Totowa, NJ

practicality of tissue banking by Kreutz [6], Hyatt [7] and their associates and successors.

Once allograft transplantation became accepted by orthopaedic surgeons and others, the demand for bone allografts resulted in a proliferation of tissue banks. These varied in the scope of operation, as well as in the techniques of allograft excision and preparation. Attempts to standardize tissue banking by voluntary membership organizations have, by and large, failed since adherence to the standards was not mandatory. Some tissue banks excised and processed allografts under aseptic conditions in the operating rooms, while others distributed secondarily sterilized tissues excised without aseptic precautions. Criteria to determine the suitability of tissues for transplantation likewise varied, as did the methods of selection and screening of donors. The question of safety and efficacy, thus, became of paramount importance. Some allografts might have been safe and effective, some either effective or safe, and others neither safe nor effective.

There are a number of ways by which bone allografts could be obtained and prepared. Some tissue banks relied on complex methods of selecting donors and excluding unsuitable donors from the donor pool. Under these circumstances the risk of transmitting disease from the donor to the recipient was slight. On the other hand, allografts obtained from donors about whom little was known, and whose medical status had not been ascertained by laboratory studies and by postmortem examination, presented a problem. In the latter cases, secondary sterilization was relied upon to achieve safety of allografts. Because of these problems, and because of incidents of disease transmission with the allografts, the United States Food and Drug Administration took jurisdiction over the regulation of tissue banks in 2005 [8]. Several states (FL, NY, MD, CA) have also promulgated rules for the operation of tissue banks. The American Association of Tissue Banks (AATB) has periodically updated standards and guidelines for tissue banking. However, in spite of all the existing rules and regulations and oversight problems still occur, as exemplified by the Biomedical Tissue Services, Ltd. incident [9]. This dealt with tissues obtained from unsuitable donors, and falsification of records. To this end, and as a service to their patient, surgeons should be familiar with the principles of tissue banking. This is just as important as understanding the biology of bone and tissue allograft transplantation.

Although cadaver tissues have been transplanted with considerable success since the beginning of the last century, and in large numbers for the last three decades, the general sentiment that autografts are superior to allografts still prevails. The sentiment is correct when applied to normal autografts of appropriate sizes. However, generalizations add little to the comfort and confidence of surgeons who transplant allografts. For large defects autografts are simply not available. Furthermore, their harvesting is associated with considerable morbidity. Thus, the decision making process regarding allograft transplantation is a complex one, and it should be based on the understanding of the advantages and limitations. Once familiarity with the subject is gained, the surgeon will be in a position to determine whether or not transplantation of an allograft will be beneficial for a particular patient. To attain this advantage, the knowledge of how allografts were obtained, processed and stored would be of considerable help, as would the knowledge of the types of allografts available and of the principles governing their behavior on transplantation.

23.2. Selection and Assessment of Donors

Safeguarding the transplant recipients from the possible transmission of disease is dependent upon the screening and selection of donors of tissue allografts. Transmissible infectious diseases preclude tissue donation.

The Food and Drug Administration [8], state agencies and the American Association of Tissue Banks [10] have established broad guidelines for donor acceptance. These are now relatively uniform, with FDA requirements providing the minimal standards. Adherence to FDA and State rules is mandatory. These emphasize criteria for excluding donors with potentially transmissible diseases and disorders that may compromise the integrity of the skeleton, malignancies with some exceptions, diseases of unknown etiology and others. Laboratory tests for syphilis, hepatitis B and C, HIV-I/II and HTLV-I, as well as an autopsy are either recommended or required. Microbiologic testing is also required.

Concern with the transmission of disease from the donor to the recipient is not entirely academic. Viral diseases have been transferred with cornea, skin and vital organs. Transmission of HIV and hepatitis infections with frozen bone and tendons has also occurred [11–15].

23.2.1. Acceptance of Donors

The acceptance of musculoskeletal tissue donors begins with obtaining a history. By necessity the history is, of course, based on secondhand information. A review of available records will frequently provide enough information to exclude a potential donor from the donor pool. Both the FDA and AATB require exclusion from the donor pool of individuals in high risk behavior groups for acquiring infections with human immunodeficiency virus. Other diseases which preclude tissue donation are infections with hepatitis B virus, infections with hepatitis C virus and Trepanema pallidum. Individuals suspected of having Creutzfeld-Jacob Disease are also excluded. Prior to tissue donation the next-of-kin not only grants permission for donation, but also provides medical/social history information. The FDA and AATB rely heavily on the information collected in this manner. However, according to a study conducted by Young and Wilkins, much of the information thus obtained might be inaccurate in as much as 50 percent of cases [16]. Because secondhand medical and social history information is frequently unreliable, the FDA lists physical assessment of the cadaver donor and an autopsy as means of detecting relevant communicable disease. An autopsy remains a reliable diagnostic method of uncovering and documenting pathologic conditions present in potential tissue donors.

Both the FDA and AATB do not specifically prohibit transplantation of tissues from donors with malignancies. This is left to the discretion of the Medical Director of the Tissue Bank. However, it stands to reason that transplantation of tissues from donors with malignancies is not consistent with good medical practice and the interests of the recipients. For these reasons donors with malignancies are not taken by many tissue banks.

23.2.2. Serologic Studies

To obtain as much information as possible on a given donor, the serum of the same is subjected to several serological tests. HIV-I and II antibodies are determined, as are antibodies to HTLV-I and II, and to hepatitis C virus. Serologic tests for hepatitis B antigen and for core and surface antibodies are also performed. Polymerase chain reaction (PCR) has been recently added to the armamentarium of laboratory tests designed to detect early HIV and hepatitis infections. Testing of blood for viral nucleic acids has reduced the undetectable window of infectivity [17]. Standard serologic tests for syphilis are also performed.

In view of the worldwide epidemic of acquired immunodeficiency syndrome (AIDS), surgeons as well as patients have become justifiably concerned about the possibility of HIV transmission with the graft. Concern with the AIDS epidemic prompted the American Academy of Orthopaedic Surgeons to be one of the first organizations to acknowledge the problem and form a Task Force on AIDS and Orthopaedic Surgery. The report of the Task Force included recommendations for reducing the likelihood of HIV transmission through bone and tissue allografts [18]. With proper safeguards the risk of such transmission is low. Safeguards include rigorous donor screening, serologic testing and exclusion of donors for logistical reasons. Under these circumstances the risk of possibly obtaining tissues from an undetected HIV-infected donor has been calculated to be less than one in 1 million [19]. With the addition of tests for viral nucleic acids, the risk has been reduced even more.

23.2.3. Microbiologic Studies

Microbiologic studies of cadaver musculoskeletal tissue donors are an essential component in assessing the suitability of allografts for transplantation. Since tissues from cadaver donors may harbor microorganisms, allografts excised from these donors cannot be assumed to be sterile, even if strict antiseptic precautions are used during their excision. If microorganisms are present, it is essential to know what they are and where they were found [20]. This knowledge enables one to determine suitability or unsuitability of tissue for transplantation, as well as its potential for secondary sterilization.

Blood and bone marrow cultures are helpful in predicting contamination of musculoskeletal tissues. Positive blood and bone marrow cultures with similar microbial species correlate with a higher rate of positive cultures from bone (30%) as compared with positive blood (15%) or marrow cultures (11%) alone [20].

The origin of microorganisms in cadaver blood is unclear. Whether blood contamination from the GI tract, the respiratory tree or the mucus membranes occurs concurrently with the events leading to death, or whether it takes place after death, has not been established [21]. The recovery of pathogens from autopsy specimens and the reported discrepancy between antemortem evidence of infection and postmortem culture results lead to the belief that visceral microflora may be subject to agonal and postmortem dissemination. The time and sequence of such dissemination has not been defined [22]. That postmortem microbial contamination does occur within two or more days is unquestionable [23]. Postmortem dissemination within 24 hours is supported by the study, which shows that the only statistically significant difference between clinically uninfected donors from which clostridia were removed and those not harboring these organisms was the interval between death and the excision of tissues [24]. Such being the case, the 24-hour limitation on excision of musculoskeletal tissue imposed by the American Association of Tissue Banks appears logical.

The concern with patient safety and potential transmission of microbial infections stimulated interest in the study of microbiology of cadaver donors. To this end, several studies were conducted by the author and associates [2, 20, 24, 47, 55]. Final results were derived from 1,747 consecutive donors of musculoskeletal tissues. From these 41,434 samples were collected; 4,631 (11%) of these were positive. However, pathogenic microorganisms were recovered from only 2,245 (5.4%) of total samples. These were recovered from 433 (25%) donors. A single species pathogenic microorganism was recovered from 83 percent of these, with the remaining 17 percent yielding two or more pathogenic species. The groups of pathogenic microorganisms recovered from musculoskeletal cadaver donors included ß hemolytic Streptococci, Clostridium sp, Enterococci, group D Streptococci, gram negative anaerobic microorganisms, Staphylococcus aureus and Streptococcus viridans group. One or more positive cultures of skin flora and environmental organisms of low pathogenic potential were recovered from 46 percent of all donors. Entirely negative cultures were obtained from 29 percent of donors. These data also show a statistically significant increase in postmortem microbial contamination with the increase of postmortem interval.

Contamination of musculoskeletal allografts with Clostridium species deserves a special consideration because of the reports of Clostridium sordelli infections associated with allograft transplantation [15]. Extensive microbiological studies of cadaver donors indicate that contamination with C. sordelli is not as rare as once thought. Clostridial contamination occurs in a significant percentage of tissue donors (8.1%), with C. sordelli being the most commonly isolated organism [24].

Clostridial infections associated with allografts have emphasized the need for adequate microbiological assessment of donors. This requires taking multiple samples, including blood and bone marrow samples. Since the percentage of pathogenic microorganisms is relatively small, these can be detected reliably only when an adequate number of samples are obtained. If this is not done, the extent of tissue contamination with dangerous microorganisms can be underestimated, or missed altogether.

23.2.4. Autopsy

Autopsy remains an accurate diagnostic modality for defining pathologic changes in the deceased, including those that might preclude transplantation of tissues. Numerous studies report major discrepancies between the clinical diagnoses and postmortem findings [25–27]. Most studies report discrepancies of about 12 percent. The figure has not improved significantly, despite advances in imaging and other diagnostic techniques. In our experience review of autopsy findings on 4,575 consecutive musculoskeletal donors showed major discrepancies between clinical diagnoses and autopsy findings of around 3 percent. These included unsuspected thyroid, renal, lung, larynx and colon carcinomas with metastases, as well as cases of myocarditis, granulomatous disease, lymphoma, active tuberculosis, active histoplasmosis and Alzheimer's disease, etc. Were it not for autopsy findings which excluded these donors from the donor pool, tissues from some 135 donors with the above enumerated diseases would have been transplanted into recipients. One can predict most patients would not wish to accept this risk.

Autopsies of transplantation donors have unique features, as do autopsies performed for medicolegal reasons, teaching purposes and research. While medical examiners are masters at discovering the sequence of last events and teachers and students of pathology at unraveling the pathophysiology of an illness, the prosector of transplantation donors is responsible for preventing the transmission of disease from a donor to a recipient. It follows that such an autopsy must be an orderly search for both obvious and subtle evidence of disease. The task is important for two reasons. First, the number of recipients of grafts from a multiple organ, cornea, bone and tissue donor often exceeds 30. Second, recognizing potentially dangerous diseases rests with the pathologist. Clinicians and/or coordinators involved in the evaluation of donors screen out unacceptable donors as best they can. However, many potential donors may have diseases such as viral myocarditis, a wide range of cancers, a host of neurologic diseases and diseases of unknown etiology. These may become apparent only upon microscopic examination.

23.3. Excision of Allografts

Tissues must be excised less than 24 hours postmortem if the donor's body has been refrigerated. If it has not been refrigerated, excision of tissues has to be performed within 12 hours of death.

Methods of excision of bone, tendons and other tissues have been described in detail elsewhere [2, 28]. Ideally excision of bone and tissues is performed in an operating room using standard aseptic surgical techniques (Figs. 23.1 and 23.2). Repeated microbiologic monitoring is helpful and multiple samples are advisable.

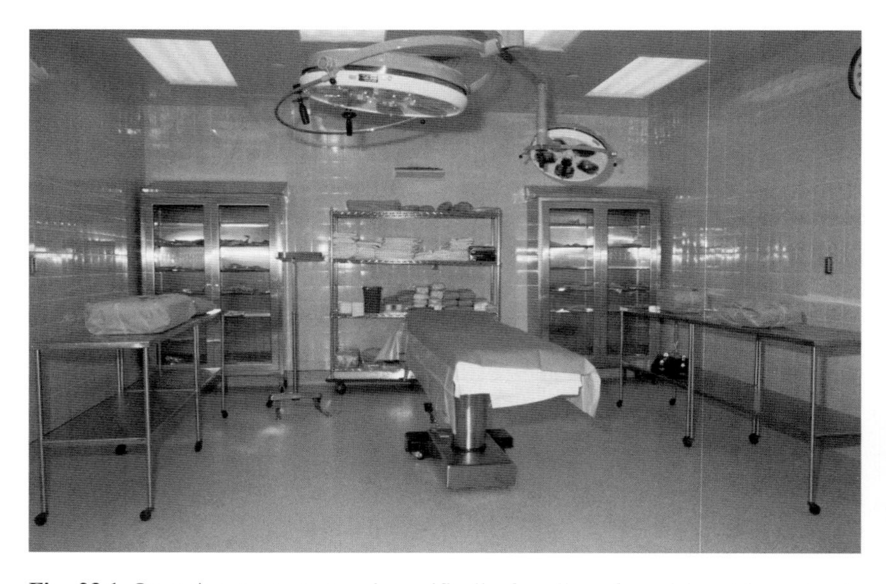

Fig. 23.1 Operating room reserved specifically for allograft excision. Tissue Bank, Dept. of Orthopaedics and Rehabilitation, University of Miami

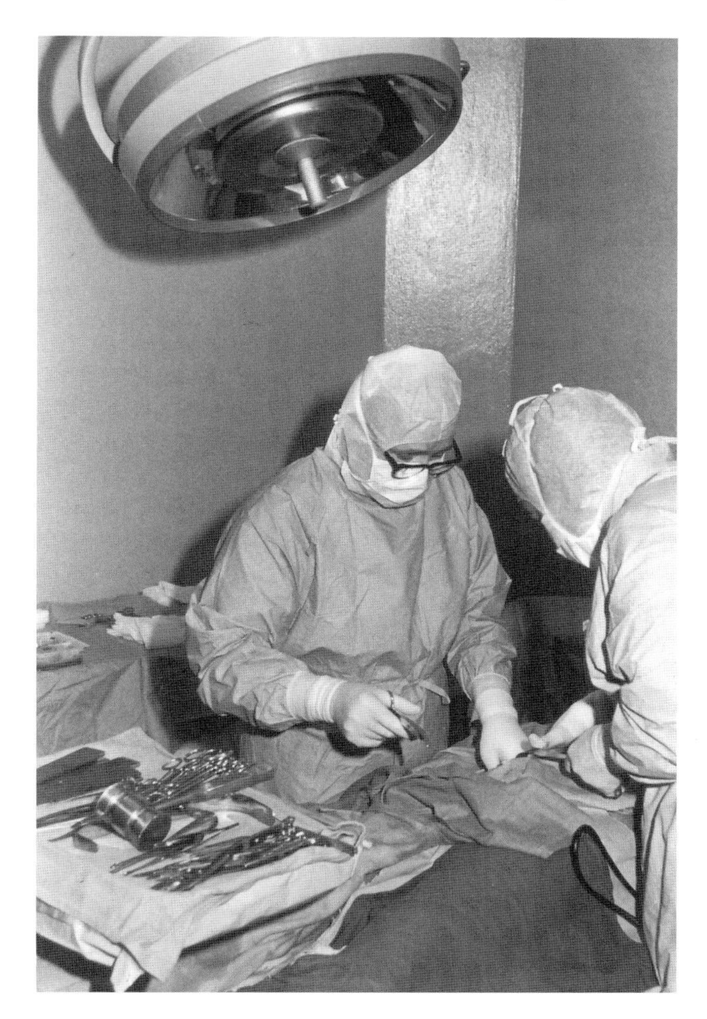

Fig. 23.2 Bone and tissue allografts are excised using aseptic precautions

If an operating room is not available, conventional rooms converted to a temporary operating room setting can produce the necessary aseptic environment.

In addition to the surgeon, at least two operating room technicians or nurses are needed for the recovery. One of these works on the back table, obtains culture samples and wraps and packages the excised allografts.

Tissues are excised with anticipation of their surgical use. The bones can be cleaned of soft tissues, and the ligaments divided either in the operating room or later in a processing facility. The description of techniques is based on several trial and error attempts to excise bone allografts with the utmost efficiency and with as little contamination as possible.

The extremities and the trunk of the donor are prepared by shaving and scrubbing with povidone-iodine soap and rinsing with alcohol. Antiseptic detergents other than povidone-iodine can be used just as effectively. The body is then transferred to an operating room table.

In the operating room the body is prepped with povidone-iodine or other prep. This can be followed with a 70 percent alcohol soak. If alcohol is not used, iodine solution is best left on the body. The operative area is then draped as for major surgery. The perineum is sealed with a towel and/or with a plastic adhesive. The extremities are prepped on the anterior side and the posterior aspects while being held up by a technician.

After the initial skin incisions are made, it is advisable to spray the edges of the skin with an antiseptic solution. It is convenient to obtain blood samples from the great saphenous vein. The vein is isolated and a catheter is passed through it into the inferior vena cava. Alternatively, blood samples can be collected from the jugular or iliac veins, or by heart puncture. A small incision over the iliac crest facilitates collection of a bone marrow sample.

The excision of the tissues and bones of the extremities is usually performed in layers. In the leg, the fascia lata is identified and excised. The gracilis and semitendinosus tendons are exposed by reflecting the sartorius muscle and excised from their origins to the insertions. The peroneus longus, tibialis anterior and tibialis posterior tendons are excised *in toto* after transecting transcrural and cruciate crural ligaments.

The patellar tendon is divided at its origin in the rectus femoris muscle. The suprapatellar bursa is incised and the ligament dissected free and reflected downward to expose the knee joint. The femur shaft is exposed by separating the rectus femoris from the vastus lateralis and by incising the vastus intermedius. The femur may be divided with an osteotomy accomplished at any desired level, or it may be excised with the knee joint and the tibia. It is convenient to remove the Achilles tendon *en-block* with the calcaneus and talus. The fibula is removed by subperiosteal dissection. The ilium is freed up by subperiosteal dissection, usually with curved osteotomes. It is important to divide the sacroiliac ligaments during the dissection. The sacroiliac joint is divided medially. If only the ilium is to be removed, it is osteotomized immediately below the inferior anterior iliac spine. The osteotomized ilium is grasped with bone forceps and rotated. Ligaments preventing this rotation are divided and the ilium removed. To remove the entire hemipelvis, a small incision can be made over the symphysis ossium pubis and the symphysis divided. The dissection of the ischium and the pubis can be performed blindly with scissors through the existing incisions.

Bones of the upper extremity are excised through a standard deltopectoral incision, which can be extended inferiorly to facilitate removal of the elbow and the radius. The deltoid muscle is detached anteriorly, facilitating easy approach to the shoulder joint, disarticulation of the proximal humerus and removal of the rotator cuff.

The elbow is removed *in toto* with the distal humerus, proximal ulna and the radius. The distal radius is removed by extending the incision to about 3 cm above the radial styloid. Further extension of the incision into the wrist may expose the same, and should be avoided if the donor will have an open casket funeral.

The scapulae are excised posteriorly through semicircular incisions along the lateral borders of the scapulae. The ribs are removed last since they have the highest incidence of microbial contamination of all bones. This can probably be explained by the close proximity of the ribs to the skin. Ribs are removed subperiosteally through a standard autopsy incision.

Separate incisions can be used for the removal of any additional bone in the body, exercising standard aseptic precautions. The only bone which cannot be excised aseptically is the mandible.

23.3.1. Reconstruction of the Donor's Body

Reconstruction of the body is of the utmost importance in maintaining the dignity of the deceased. Unless otherwise specified, it is assumed the reconstruction of the body is necessary to enable funeral directors to provide cosmetically acceptable remains. In addition, after the excision of bone allografts, the body is turned over for an autopsy. A reconstructed body facilitates postmortem examination inasmuch as it allows the pathologist to ascertain the gross appearance of the body.

Reconstruction of the extremities is accomplished by replacing excised bone with wooden dowels, hinged plastic or metal rods or similar devices, packing the cavities with gauze and cotton, and tightly closing the incisions.

23.4. Processing of Musculoskeletal Allografts

Bone allografts are usually processed in a separate facility. This allows for orderly processing of allografts and does not interfere with the excision of tissues. However, some tissue banks excise and process allografts in the same room or suite of rooms.

After excision individually packaged allografts are usually refrigerated overnight and processed after the results of serological studies and the gross autopsy, if available, are known. Separate procedures are used for processing frozen allografts, cryopreserved allografts, fresh articular allografts and freeze-dried allografts.

23.4.1. Freezing of Tissue Allografts

Storing tissues in readily available freezers, at temperatures between −15 and −20° C, is easy and popular. However, at this temperature ice crystals continue to grow and eventually destroy the tissue. Therefore, tissues can only be maintained in home-type freezers (about −15° C) for a limited time. No precise data is available to indicate the maximum storage time for tissues maintained at these temperatures. Recommendations vary from three months to one year. Wilson reported a high failure rate with bone grafts stored for over one year at these temperatures [29]. Brown, et al. reported satisfactory incorporation of bone grafts stored in such freezers for six months or less [30].

In addition to mechanical disruption by ice crystals, tissue injury from freezing may be caused by dehydration, metabolic aberrations resulting from storage at temperatures at which some enzymes may continue to function, and by direct chemical injury.

Solid carbon dioxide and mechanical freezers operate at temperatures near −79° C, the melting point of solid carbon dioxide. However, these temperatures are still not low enough to prevent the growth of ice crystals.

For reliable long-term storage, it is necessary to employ very low (cryogenic) temperatures. Only at about −120° C does the gradual growth of ice crystals cease completely. Temperatures below −120° C can be obtained through the use of liquefied (cryogenic) gases, usually liquid nitrogen, or by specially designed low temperature mechanical freezers.

Because of the reliability of liquid nitrogen and the simplicity of liquid nitrogen freezers, liquid nitrogen freezing and storage has been employed by many tissue banks. With the advent of ultra-low mechanical freezers, these too have been used, but their reliability (frequent breakdowns), cost and limited storage space per unit make them considerably less effective than cryogenic gas freezers. The advantage of mechanical freezers is that gas vapors do not obscure vision in the freezing compartments.

Liquid nitrogen, which boils at −196° C at atmospheric pressure, provides a range of cryogenic temperatures at a reasonable cost. Chemical inertness is a major property of liquid nitrogen that is very important. Unlike carbon dioxide or other solvents used for freezing, it does not react with the materials with which it comes in contact. It has no effect on the pH of frozen tissue and vaporizes without leaving a residue.

23.4.2. Cryopreservation

To understand the principles, advantages and limitations of cryopreservation, it is necessary to be familiar with events associated with cooling, freezing, storage at sub-zero temperatures and thawing of tissues. The term cryoreservation is frequently misused. It means controlled velocity cooling of tissue exposed to a cryoprotective agent and storage at cryogenic temperatures.

23.4.2.1. Temperature Shock

When tissues are injured by cooling to near 0° they are considered sensitive to thermal shock. Thermal shock, cold shock and constitutional cold death are terms used interchangeably.

The deleterious effects of cooling are manifested in deterioration of physiological functions of many cell types [31–32]. It has been postulated that most mammalian cells are, to some degree, susceptible to cold shock. Chondrocytes, the preservation of which is of major importance to tissue banks, are not very sensitive to thermal shock. Isolated animal chondrocytes recover from cooling [33], as do cartilage slices [34]. Cartilage on osteochondral constructs, likewise, survives cooling, but not indefinite hypothermic storage [35–36].

23.4.2.2. Consequences of Freezing

The decrease in temperature below normothermia causes a decrease of molecular kinetic energy and produces changes in chemical reaction rates, solubility, diffusion rates and viscosity. These changes can cause irreversible injury, but they are far less damaging than those which take place when tissues are taken below their freezing point. The biochemical changes caused by temperature drop alone do not produce cell death. Cell death occurs with freezing of water, i.e., transformation of available water into ice crystals. Formation of interstitial and intracellular ice subjects the cells not only to direct physical forces, but also exposes them to high concentrations of solutes in unfrozen fluids. Cells and tissues can be damaged by either mechanism. When 90 percent of freezable water is converted to ice, the concentration of sodium chloride increases almost 10-fold. A concentration of sodium chloride of about 8.5 percent has a denaturing effect on the cell membrane lipoprotein components [37]. It follows that the longer cells are exposed to harmful temperatures, the greater the injury. Slow cooling produces longer exposures to concentrated solutes, but paradoxically it also produces better survival than rapid cooling. The presence of electrolytes in the surrounding medium may actually reduce the damage from low temperatures.

The change from the colloidal to the solid state does not occur instantaneously at a particular point in the cooling curve. It may take place within minutes or hours, depending on the volume of the object being frozen and the temperature differential between the specimen and the cooling environment.

When water molecules are transformed from the liquid to the solid state there is a considerable release of energy [38]. As water undergoes crystallization, the energy referred to as "latent heat of fusion" is liberated [39]. Much was made of this phenomenon in designing controlled rate freezing equipment which compensates for the release of latent heat of fusion by rapid cooling of the freezing chamber. This is done to avoid a rise in temperature in the specimen and, thus, prevent its re-warming and reaching the melting point again. The importance of this phenomenon is greatly exaggerated. Release of the latent heat of fusion is a phenomenon demonstrable most readily in aqueous solutions. However, the amount of heat released, i.e., rise in temperature, is dependent on its measurement. If a 5 ml tube with saline is frozen, thermocouples placed near the wall of the vessel will show a transient rise in temperature as cooling proceeds. Thermocouples placed in the center will register only slight temperature elevations [40]. Tomford, et al. achieved the best results with preservation of chondrocytes by cooling the cells to −40° C without compensation for the release of the latent heat of fusion, maintaining cell suspensions at this temperature for five minutes, and then transferring frozen suspensions into a −80° C freezer [41]. However, freezing of chondrocyte suspension is not identical to cryopreservation of organized cartilage. Articular cartilage matrix is high in water content. Since about 75 percent of the wet weight of cartilage is water, alteration of the same during freezing would cause a major disruption of the tissue [42]. If the rate of cooling is slow, the heat can be removed, but from a few growing crystals. Under these conditions the temperature of the material being frozen remains near or at the melting point of the solution. If, on the other hand, the cooling is rapid, the temperature of the specimen falls until sufficient numbers of water crystals are formed to release the heat. Consequently, rapid cooling produces many small crystals. There is no time for translocation of water between the compartments and ice crystals are formed within the cells, as well as in the interstitial fluid.

Many attempts have been made to control ice crystal formation by altering the cooling rates. Parkes applied a two-state freezing technique [43]. It consisted of plunging the ampules with tissue into freezing mixtures at −20° or −30° C and, five to 30 minutes later, transferring them to −79° C. This produced excellent results. However, rapid cooling from +20° C to −79° C yielded poor results. Embryonic rat tibiae cooled rapidly to −20° C survived as often as the controls. If these were cooled below −30° C, none survived. Results were variable between −20° C and −30° C. These experiments demonstrate the rate of freezing's importance, as well as that of the critical temperature below which tissues do not survive except under unusual circumstances. Critical temperatures vary between tissues, probably due to difference in eutectic points of their fluids.

23.4.2.3 Controlled Velocity Freezing

Controlled cooling velocity was devised to minimize destructive effects of crystallization of water. It was empirically determined that the rate of cooling of 1° C per minute yielded the best results.

As usual, an isolated phenomenon in biology does not stand on its own. In addition to cooling rates, thawing rates must also be considered. Early in the development of cryobiology Taylor noted that the best results were obtained when an ampule of frozen tissue was thawed by placing it directly into a +45° C bath [44]. An oscillographic report showed that, for small fragments of tissue, warming from −196° C to 0° C occurred in 0.25 seconds. If the same tissue was thawed in a +20° C bath, the thawing time was increased three-fold. Therefore, thawing of cryopreserved tissues in a +40° to 45° C solution is considered a procedure of choice.

23.4.2.4 Cryoprotective Agents

When cryobiology was first being developed as a discipline, it became apparent that controlling the rate of freezing alone was not enough to avoid freezing damage. To this end, a search was made for chemical agents which would protect against freezing damage. The first such recognized agent was glycerol. Its cryoprotective effect was discovered in 1949 [45].

Glycerol lowers the freezing point of water and, through its hydroscopic properties, facilitates the movement of water out of the cell. One mole of glycerin is capable of binding approximately three moles of water [37]. The glycerin-water complex is an effective cryoprotective agent for cartilage freeze preservation [46]. It has been used extensively for cryopreservation of osteochondral allografts [47].

Since the advent of glycerol as a cryoprotective agent, many other compounds have been tested for their ability to prevent freeze-thaw damage in tissues. The list includes polyvalent alcohols, sugars, sera, ethylene glycol, egg yolk, pyridine N-oxide, polyvinylpyrrolidone, dimethyl sulfoxide and many others. With the exception of dimethyl sulfoxide, none of the tested compounds were found to be as effective as glycerol.

Dimethyl sulfoxide (methyl sulfoxide, methanylsulfonic acid) is very soluble in water because of proton bonding of water molecules to the oxygen atom. Dimethyl sulfoxide boils at 189° C with some decomposition. Its melting point is 6° C. It has relatively low toxicity when tested in animals [48].

Lovelock and Bishop reported in 1959 that dimethyl sulfoxide was, in certain circumstances, a better cryopreservative than glycerol [49]. However, in animal studies no difference was found between glycerol and dimethyl sulfoxide in their cryoprotective effect on cartilage [35]. Marco, et al. showed DMSO to be inferior to glycerol in the cryopreservation of articular cartilage [46].

Ashwood-Smith stated that, unlike glycerin, DMSO passed freely through cell membranes [50]. However, other investigators showed that such may not be the case, as C^{14}-labeled DMSO accumulates at cell membranes and in the interstitial spaces [51]. Cation exchange resin studies showed a strong DMSO-water bond and formation of DMSO.$2H_2O$ complex [52].. Ashwood-Smith also discovered and described radioprotective properties of DMSO [53–54].

23.5. Cryopreserved Osteochondral Allografts

Osteochondral allografts are brought into the processing room after storage in a refrigerator. The allografts are transferred to a room temperature, antibiotic-free tissue culture medium and cleansed of excess soft tissue attachments and bone marrow. After at least one hour of washing in antibiotic-free solution, and during the process of cleaning the allografts, a set of tissue samples is obtained for microbiologic culturing.

Osteoarticular allografts are prepared to meet the requirements for given operations [55]. Femurs are usually osteotomized at the proximal or mid-portion of the diaphysis, humeri and tibiae in the distal one-third. A portion of the knee capsule, along with the collateral and cruciate ligaments, is preserved with the distal femur. The patellar ligament, menisci and cruciate and collateral ligaments must also be preserved with proximal tibiae.

With the exception of the joint capsules, ligaments and tendons that might be used in reconstruction of the recipient's extremity, the periosteum and all other soft tissue attachments are meticulously removed from the allografts (Fig. 23.3). The bone marrow is, likewise, reamed out and washed out. The rotator cuff and capsule are preserved on the humerus. The elbow is preserved with the capsule and all the ligaments, but the capsule is incised to allow for fluid access into the joint space. The distal radius is preserved with as much of the capsule as possible.

Hemipelves include the entire ilium, acetabulum, pubis and ischium. The hip joint capsule is preserved on these specimens (Fig. 23.4).

During processing osteochondral allografts are kept in a tissue culture medium or in a balanced salt solution so that the articular cartilage does not dessicate. After the allograft is prepared, it is washed in cold tissue culture solution and then transferred for 30 to 40 minutes either to a 15 percent glycerol or a 10 to 15 percent dimethyl sulfoxide solution. After exposure to cryoprotective agents, the grafts are placed in the chamber of a liquid nitrogen controlled rate freezing apparatus pre-cooled to 4° C. The allografts are

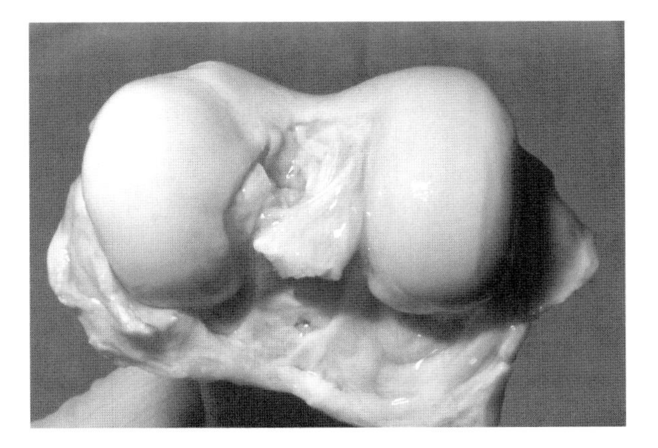

Fig. 23.3 Osteochondral allograft of a distal femur The capsule, collateral and cruciate ligaments are preserved

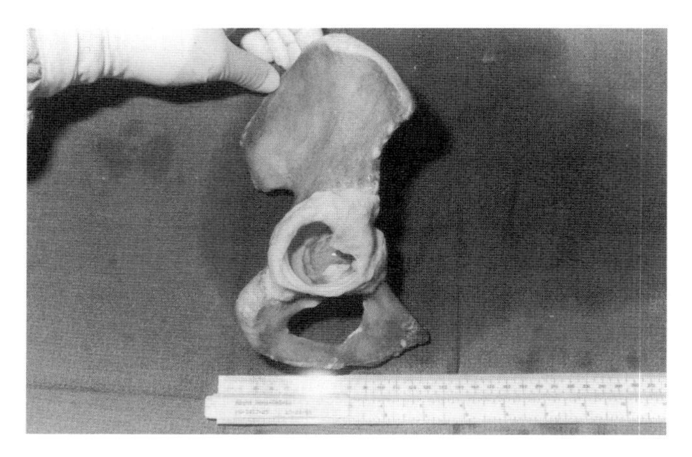

Fig. 23.4 An allograft of a hemipelvis. Capsule which will be used in reconstruction is preserved. All other tissue attachments, including periosteum are removed.

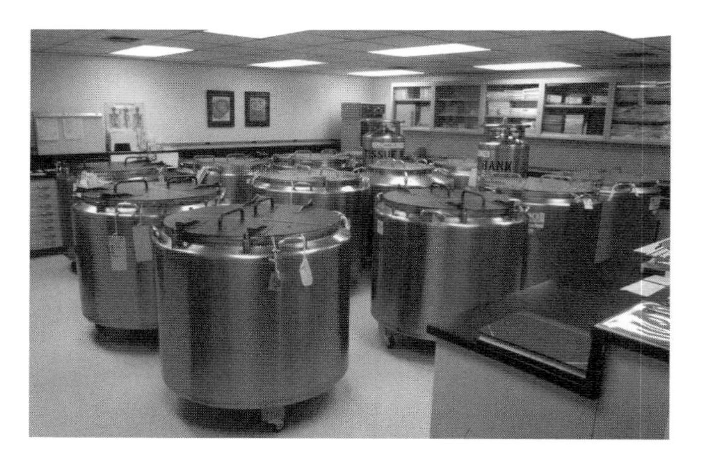

Fig. 23.5 Liquid nitrogen storage facility

cooled to −40° to −60° C at rates from 0.5° to 2.0° C per minute. They are then brought down rapidly to −100° C and are transferred into the vapor phase of liquid nitrogen freezers until the day they are to be used or shipped (Fig. 23.5). Excessive time of exposure to cryoprotective solutions should be avoided, as toxicity is proportional to the time of exposure.

23.6. Fresh Articular Cartilage Allografts

Allotransplantation of articular cartilage for the treatment of isolated articular cartilage defects has become more popular during the last decade [56]. To this end, either fresh allografts or allografts stored in tissue culture media at hypothermia (usually 2° to 10° C) are employed. There has been some confusion regarding the length of time these grafts can be maintained in hypothermic storage and still remain transplantable. Some investigators have advocated transplanting cartilage within 48 hours of excision; others limit storage time to seven to 14 days [57]. However, cold storage for as long as 40 days before transplantation has also been employed. Most experimental studies, as well as current clinical experience, indicate that unfrozen osteoarticular transplants do not do well if maintained in hypothermic storage for much longer than two weeks [36, 58]. Such being the case, and in the absence of a clearly delineated time of hypothermic storage, it seems advisable to remain within the safe limits.

23.7. Freeze-Drying

Freeze-drying of musculoskeletal tissue allografts has now been practiced for over 50 years. Although the process was described before World War II, it was not applied to human tissues until 1951 [6].

Freeze-drying applies the natural phenomenon of sublimation to laboratory and industrial endeavors. If the atmospheric pressure is reduced below that of the vapor pressure of ice, drying will take place without melting the ice. In freeze-drying the water is removed from the ice as vapor. Thus, the ice from a frozen biologic structure disappears and the water vapor is re-solidified in a cold condenser.

Freeze-drying depends on unique properties of water, which has a melting point of 0° C. It is not applicable to other chemical solutions. Thus, unless special devices and methods are employed, freeze-drying will remove only water from a biological object frozen in an aqueous chemical mixture. Other chemicals with boiling points different from that of water will remain as residues. Freeze-drying procedures are lengthy, but freeze-dried tissues can be stored and transported at room temperature. However, changes produced in tissues by freeze-drying are not insignificant. These have been attributed to alterations in protein configuration or the blocking of hydrophilic sites of proteins [59]. On the positive side these alterations are probably responsible for reducing the antigenicity of freeze-dried allografts. The exact mechanisms by which freeze-drying decreases the antigenicity and the sensitizing properties of tissue are unknown.

Most of the initial work on freeze-drying human tissues has been performed by the United States Navy Tissue Bank. Tissue grafts frozen to –76° C were placed in the freeze-dryer chamber and allowed to warm to 0° C within the first 18 hours. The internal condenser was maintained at –45° C. After about 10 years this technique was replaced by a seven-day freeze-drying cycle in which the temperature of the allograft being freeze-dried was increased stepwise from –40° to 0° C over three days. This technique is still employed today. Modern freeze-dryers with external condensers have greatly improved the efficiency of the process [2].

A variation of the technique includes placement into freeze-dryer chambers of tissue grafts frozen in the vapor phase of liquid nitrogen. The condenser temperature is maintained at between –60° and –70° C. The vacuum in the freeze-dryer chamber is about 10 – 20° mtorr. The freeze-drying cycle is maintained from about three to 14 days. The discrepancies on the lengths of freeze-drying cycles depend on the efficiency of the apparatus, the amount of material placed in the chamber, and to different ways of measuring residual moistures [60]. Before opening the chambers the shelves can be warmed to avoid moisture condensation.

Freeze-dried allografts must be rehydrated prior to implantation. The importance of rehydration lies not only in the necessity to retain mechanical strength, but also in the resiliency of the grafts. When tendons are reconstituted, they should not be handled until the tissue becomes entirely pliable. If bent before they are rehydrated, the fibers in these will fracture. Likewise, cross-clamping of tendon grafts will result in their fracture.

23.8. Bone Allografts for Clinical Transplantation

Of a variety of grafting materials available, freeze-dried and frozen allografts are the most common.

When allografts which retain bone morphogenic protein (BMP) are placed in contact with vascularized host bone, they will unite with it and their calcified matrix will be replaced by new bone. The individual peculiarities of the human skeleton are such that each bone has its own requirements for healing, immobilization and bone grafting. Therefore, there is no universal, all-purpose bone allograft, and there is no single way of preparing all bone allografts. To date, in reconstructive surgery of the skeletal system, the most successful bone allografts have been aseptically processed freeze-dried or frozen cortico and corticocancellous grafts which have not been subjected to extensive manipulations, such as exposure to chemical agents, heating, irradiation, etc. [2].

Bone allografts commonly used in orthopaedic reconstructive procedures can be broadly divided into particulate and structural grafts. Particulate grafts can be crushed cancellous or cortical bone (bone chips), ground bone, morselized bone or microparticulate grafts. The latter types of grafts are used for filling defects with largely intact walls. The structural grafts are bone plates (bone struts) and bone blocks of various sizes and shapes which are placed externally or in the medullary canal. When deficits are extreme, bones can be replaced by massive bone allografts.

23.9. Secondary Sterilization

Chemical solution immersion is a simple way to preserve and sterilize bone allografts. Many of these, including ethyl alcohol, have been investigated; none endured the test of time. When alcohol-fixed bone grafts were implanted into rodents, the bone was absorbed, but a few layers of new bone appeared in and around the grafts. Osteoclasts were absent at the periphery of alcohol-fixed grafts. Thus, it became evident that, unlike boiling or autoclaving, the osteoinductive principle of the graft was not destroyed, but to a great degree extracted by alcohol [61]. When this alcoholic extract was injected into rabbits, osteogenesis was induced in about one-third of the animals.

The boiled and alcohol-fixed grafts are mentioned here to demonstrate the differences of the recipient's response to bone transplants prepared in different ways. The aforementioned allografts, as well as allografts sterilized by immersion in other sterilizing solutions, are still in use. Relative paucity of information on the behavior of secondarily sterilized bone allografts transplanted into humans resulted in the empirical development of methods for bone allograft preparation which proceeded largely along empirical lines. Virtually everything was tried, but the only two methods of secondary sterilization which withstood the test of time are irradiation and sterilization with ethylene oxide gas.

23.9.1 Irradiation

The only reason to irradiate bone and soft tissue allografts is to prevent the transmission of infections, including those caused by HIV. Irradiation is ineffective against prions and, thus, cannot prevent transmission of Creutzfeld-Jacob disease. Relatively high doses of irradiation are needed to inactivate HIV in bone, but the actual dose estimates vary. Although a 15 to 25 kGy dose is commonly used, Conway, et al. stated that 15 kGy would not reliably inactivate HIV in bone allografts [62]. Therefore, doubling the dose to 30 kGy may be necessary. Irradiation in this range alters biomechanical integrity of the graft [63] and reduces its osteoinductive potential [64–65]. Therefore, whether or not to implant irradiated allografts is a personal choice. It must be balanced with the choice between reducing the chance of infection transmission and the undesirable effects of irradiation.

23.9.2 Ethylene Oxide Sterilization

Ethylene oxide sterilizes the air, but penetrates other materials such as paper, cloth and cellophane. It has been shown to have bactericidal and virucidal properties [66–69]. However, variation in resistance to ethylene oxide among spore forming organisms has also been noted.

When tissues are sterilized with ethylene oxide, its secondary products, ethylene glycol (EG) and ethylene chlorohydrin (ECH), remain the same. These residues, in high enough concentrations, cause hemolysis and inflammation. For this reason the FDA has published a limit on the quantity of these compounds on the implantable devices. [70]

23.10. Biology of Bone Allografts

Many varieties of preserved bone allografts have been studied experimentally and clinically. Since osteocytes in transplanted bone are dead, the grafts themselves do not contribute cells to osteogenesis. The basis for this complex biologic activity is the stimulation of the mesenchymal cells of the recipient to form new bone, which produces healing of the host-graft interface and gradually replaces the graft itself. For this reason, to be effective, bone allografts must possess osteoinductive potential. Osteoinductive potential is maintained by some methods of preservation and destroyed by others.

One of the earliest methods of preserving bone was by boiling. However, early on it was shown that boiled bone was nonosteogenic and was slowly absorbed. According to Lacroix, seven months posttransplantation boiled bone autografts remained almost intact. Autoclaved bone behaved in like fashion [61].

Morphologic analysis of allogenic bone grafts removed from patients shows the grafts to be acellular, but surrounded by mesenchymal tissue which undergoes metaplasia and ossification. This basically summarizes the entire spectrum of bone allograft interaction with the host. Aside from temporal considerations, no quantitative differences have been noted between the autograft and freeze-dried, and to a lesser degree frozen allograft incorporation as these go through revascularization, osteoclastic resorption, new bone formation and remodeling. The response to allograft implantation is modified by their treatment, which may include irradiation, exposure to chemicals, etc. Exposure to hydrogen peroxide diminishes or abolishes the osteogenic potential of the graft [71].

The general acceptance of frozen or freeze-dried bone allografts is based in part on reduced immunogenicity of these preparations [72]. The reason for the latter is most likely the destruction of the antigen presenting cells which reside in the trabeculae filled within bone marrow [73].

23.10.1. Intercalary Allografts

In comparing the healing pattern of freeze-dried segmental autografts to that of fresh autografts, Burchardt, et al. [74] noted little difference between the two. However, when they compared freeze-dried allogenic cortical grafts to fresh autografts, they noted that the allografts repaired incompletely and failed to establish skeletal continuity. These findings, which were widely publicized, were at variance with the findings by other investigators [75]. The discrepancies can be explained by variation in freeze-drying techniques and by not subjecting transplanted bone segments to rigid internal fixation. In studies in which segmental cortical bone allografts Fig. 23.6 were subjected to freeze-drying regimens designed to produce bone of acceptable dryness [60] and which were subjected to rigid internal fixation, healing of allograft-host junctions and eventual replacement of transplanted bone with new bone were noted [76]. Segments of the radius which were at least three times the diameter of the excised bone were replaced with freeze-dried intercalary allografts. In one group of animals the segmental allografts were press fitted into the gaps in the radius. No internal fixation was used. In another group the same procedure was performed, except the allograft segments were secured in place with stainless steel compression plates and bi-cortical screws.

All animals in the press fit group either dislocated the allografts or developed nonunions. In animals transplanted with freeze-dried intercalary bone allografts secured in place with stainless steel plates, healing occurred (Figs. 23.7 and 23.8).

Healed allografts showed union of the host-graft junction with cancellous bone ingrowth in the ends of the allografts (Fig. 23.9).

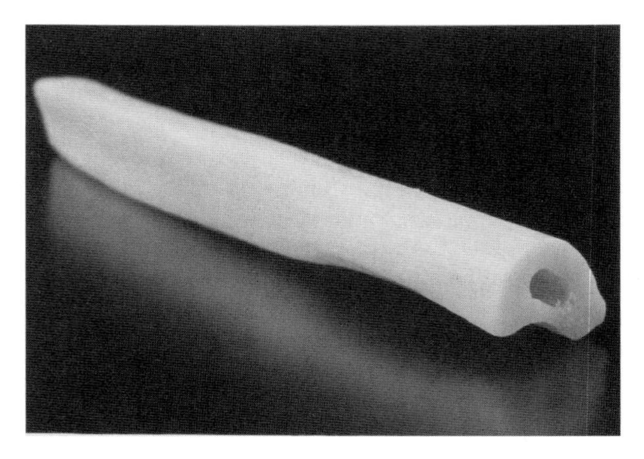

Fig. 23.6 Freeze-dried intercalary allografts

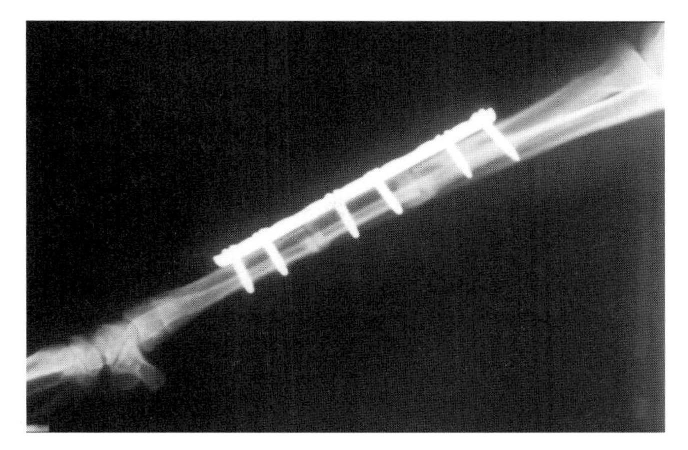

Fig. 23.7 Freeze-dried intercalary allograft in a canine model, four weeks post transplantation. Host graft junctions are visible

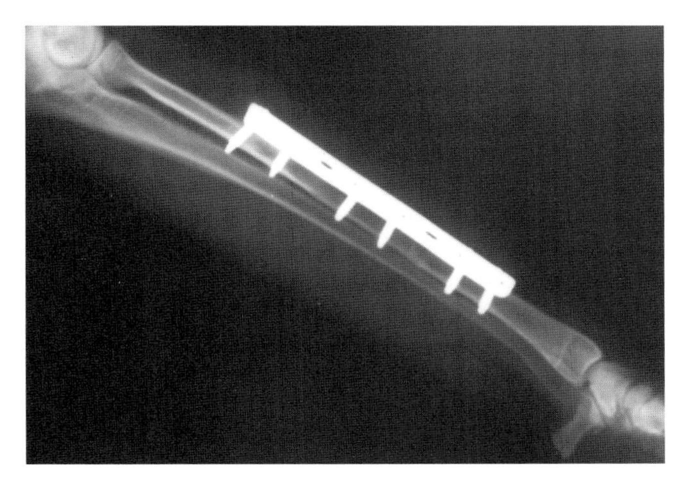

Fig. 23.8 Freeze-dried intercalary allografts (same as in Fig. 23.8) eight weeks posttransplantation. Host-graft junctions have healed completely

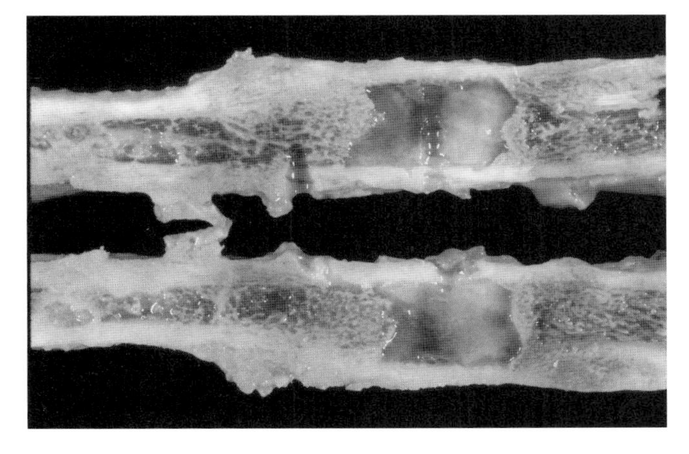

Fig. 23.9 Section through a diaphyseal bone with an intercalary allograft, 12 weeks posttransplantation. Ingrowth of the cancellous bone into the graft is evident

Bone replacement, as evidenced by the uptake of tetracycline, was noted in the cortical portion of the allograft. This was associated with vascular ingrowth into cortical bone and osteoblastic activity.

23.10.2 Onlay Bone Allografts

The loss of structural support for a prosthetic implant reduces the durability of the implant. When bone loss is severe enough to prevent accommodation and containment of the prosthesis, there is a need to restore the bone stock. In many cases this can be accomplished with bone plate allografts, which demonstrate remarkable biologic activity. The use of only cortical plate allografts to repair the wall of the deficient femur and, thus, stabilize the implant in a large group of patients was first reported by Emerson, et al. [4]. Several subsequent studies have confirmed this finding. Bone plate allografts with retained osteoinductive potential unite consistently and reliably, on average by nine months. In animal models healed bone plate allografts restore mechanical strength of the entire bone [76]. Rigidly fixed allografts unite with the underlying host bone by vascularization and formation of a callus-like structure. This occurs prior to the allograft undergoing remodeling. Thus, there is an indication that the allografts are biologically active.

In an attempt to determine the basis for the biological activity of bone plate allografts, bone morphogenetic protein (BMP) was measured in cortical bone allografts in accordance with a technique described by Urist, et al. [77]. The BMP content in these allografts was high. The freeze-drying and allograft processing methods, which included rapid freezing and freeze-drying, may have been important as these allowed for the preservation of BMP. Allografts sterilized by irradiation or ethylene oxide have not produced comparable results.

23.10.3 Particulate Bone Allografts

Particulate bone allografts have been used to fill cavitary and peri-prosthetic defects for the last two decades with considerable clinical success [78–79]. Radiographic assessment of the grafts showed incorporation in over 90 percent of patients. Complications were few. However, despite clinical success with particulate allografts, ideal properties of these grafts are still ill-defined. Consequently, tissue banks prepare particulate allografts in different sizes and by a variety of methods. One of the parameters which warrant attention is the size of the particle graft in relation to osteoinduction and osteoconduction. Osteoinduction depends on the biological property of the graft reflected by its ability to stimulate ingrowth of neovasculature, mobilize the mesenchymal cells of the host and transform these into osteoprogenitor cells. This process is mediated by the release of various growth factors, the principal of which is bone morphogenetic protein (BMP). To be effective BMP must be present in pharmacological quantities [80]. In addition, BMP depends on intraosseous lipid for transport, which must be present in the graft to facilitate delivery of BMP to the site [81]. Ideally allografts, in addition to being osteoinductive, must also be osteoconductive. They must provide direct opposition between the graft and the host and, in addition to mechanical support, allow for ingrowth of newly formed bone. Densely packed bone particles of appropriate sizes may satisfy both of these requirements [82]. Washing of the graft with removal of bone marrow and extraosseous fat allows for compacting of the graft material in the defect [83].

In the experimental nonhuman primate model, bone allografts with particles of different sizes showed clear differences in the healing patterns and osteogenic potential. Particles in the range of 300 to 90 microns produced rapid healing by direct ossification. Particles below 100 microns had a significantly reduced osteoinductive potential. Particles larger than 300 microns were much slower in healing and incorporation than 300 to 90 micron particles. Small-sized powdery bone particles below 75 μ induced little osteogenesis. Small particles of hydroxyapatite inhibit osteoclastic activity [84]. Because of these undesirable properties of powdered preparations, the term "bone powder" should not be applied across the board. Powder means a dry substance composed of minute dust-like particles, precisely the composition which does not enhance osteogenesis. For this reason, and to delineate bone particle sizes most effective in inducing bone healing, the term "microparticulate bone allograft" is more descriptive. It clearly delineates particulate compositions between small granules and powders. Frozen microparticulate allografts lag considerably behind their freeze-dried counterparts in inducing bone healing.

23.10.4. Cancellous and Corticancellous Allografts

The most striking difference between cancellous allografts and autografts is the time sequence of the healing process [85]. Otherwise, freeze-dried or frozen cancellous allografts follow the pattern of healing exhibited by autografts (Fig. 23.10).

23.10.5. Demineralized Bone Allografts

The subject of demineralized bone matrix is dealt with in another chapter in this book. Therefore, it will be mentioned only briefly.

There is considerable confusion with regard to demineralized bone matrix (DBM) and demineralized, or more precisely, partially decalcified bone.

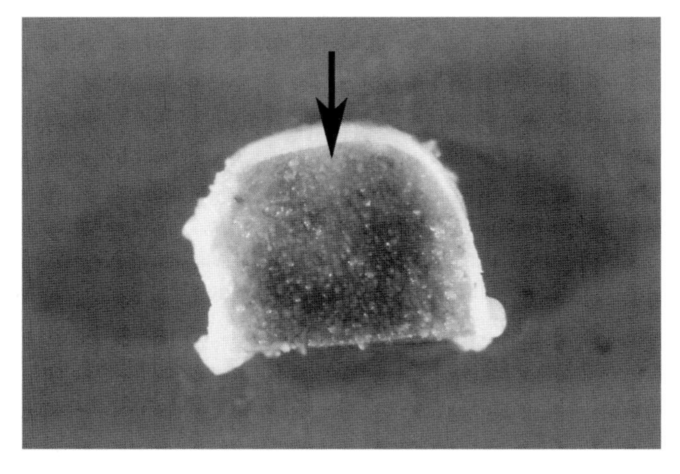

Fig. 23.10 Cancellous bone of the osteoarticular graft (arrow) has been replaced with the bone of the host

The methods of preparation of these allografts are distinct, as are their biological properties. DBM is prepared by simply demineralizing bone in hydrochloric acid (usually 1N HCl) until the calcium content is reduced to less than 2 percent. Since DBM is prepared from particulate bone, the preparation frequently entails freeze-drying the bone, grinding it, demineralizing it and refreeze-drying it again. Thus, in contradistinction to other freeze-dried bone allografts, DBM is freeze-dried twice. DBM is grossly amorphous and soft and does not provide structural support.

Partially demineralized, partially decalcified or surface decalcified bone is exemplified by Urist's chemosterilized, antigen-extracted allogeneic (AAA) bone [86]. Preparation of this allograft is complex and time consuming, but its clinical efficacy has been documented [87].

The calcium content of AAA bone is about 10 to 15 percent. The calcium content of surface demineralized bone allograft is somewhat higher, usually around 20 percent. Both of these types of preparations maintain osteoconductive properties.

23.11. Discussion and Conclusions

Review of the principles of tissue banking was undertaken to familiarize the reader with the developments that led to tissue banking as it is practiced today. These principles evolved from trial and error, observation, laboratory studies and clinical results. These were not conducted in a systematic manner or in a logical sequence. Demand for allografts did not allow for step-wise progression of the development of tissue banking. Instead a trial and error approach was used. Pieces of information from disjointed laboratory studies and clinical experiences, when these became available, influenced the modification and development of the new techniques. Several tissue banks adopted proprietary techniques and methodology for allograft preparation. These were promoted mainly through advertising, without adequate data published in scientific literature substantiating the claims. In preparing this chapter references to unsubstantiated claims and general statements were avoided. Instead, sound, well-established principles and findings were summarized and brought to the reader's attention in hope that this information would help the reader to make up his/her own mind regarding the preparation and transplantation of musculoskeletal tissue allografts. Laboratory studies with bone allografts help to predict the behavior of such grafts transplanted into humans. Experiments with intercalary allografts clearly show the need for rigid internal fixation. Press fitted allografts simply do not heal, even with external immobilization. Incorporating internally fixed allografts relies on the formation of external callus and endosteal replacement of the graft, but vascularization of the cortical portions of the allografts must be associated with biomechanical weakness. This has clinical relevance.

Laboratory studies with onlay cortical plate allografts paved the way for their success in revision surgery of deficient proximal femurs.

Studies with articular cartilage allografts demonstrated latent injury of cryopreserved chondrocytes in intact cartilage. Although viable cells must be present in the cryopreserved cartilage, as demonstrated by tissue culture experiments, the survival of chondrocytes in the intact frozen cartilage is not achieved in quantities sufficient to maintain its normal configuration over the years. Thus, articular hyaline cartilage in cryopreserved osteochondral allografts will be transformed into fibrocartilage.

Limiting the cold storage time of fresh osteoarticular grafts applicable to human transplants also resulted from laboratory endeavors.

These are but a few examples of information used to establish principles of tissue banking. Hopefully, additional information which will have bearing on the preparation and transplantation of a variety of musculoskeletal tissue allografts will be forthcoming in the future.

References

1. Kozak JA, Heilman AE, O'Brien JP. Anterior lumbar fusion options; techniques and graft materials. Clin. Ortho 1994; 200:45–51.
2. Malinin, TI. Acquisition and banking of bone allografts in: Bone Grafts and Bone Substitutes (M. Habal & H. Reddi eds.) W.B. Saunders Co. 1992. Philadelphia. p. 206.
3. Mankin HJ, Doppelt S, Tomford WW. Clinical experience with allograft implantation. Clin Orth & Rel Res 1983;174:69–72.
4. Emerson RH Jr., Malinin TI, Cuellar AD, Head WC and Peters PC. Cortical strut allografts in the reconstruction of the femur in revision total hip arthroplasty. A basic science and clinical study. Clin Orth 1992; 285:35–44.
5. Lavernia CI, Malinin TI, Temple HT, Moreyra CE. Bone and tissue allograft use by orthopaedic surgeons. J. Arthzoplasty. 2004;19:430–433.
6. Kruetz FP, Hyatt GW, Turner TC, Bassett AJ. The preservation and clinical use of freeze-dried bone. J. Bone & Joint Surg. 1951; 33(A): 863–872.
7. Hyatt G, Butler MC. Bone grafting: The procurement, storage and clinical use of bone allografts. AAOS, Instr Course Lect. 1957;14–436.
8. US Food and Drug Administration, 21 CFR, Part 1271, 2004.
9. Centers for Disease Control and Prevention. (Malarkey M et al). Brief Report: Investigation into recalled human tissue for transplantation. United States, 2005–2006, MMWR. 2006:55(20): 564–566.
10. American Association of Tissue Banks. Standards for Tissue Banking. McLean, VA 2005.
11. Eastlund T. Bacterial infection transmitted by human tissue allografts. Cell & Tissue Banking, 2006 (in press).
12. Centers for Disease Control. Invasive Streptococcus pyogenes infection after allograft implantation – Colorado 2003 MMWR, 2003;52:1174–1176.
13. Centers for Disease Control and Prevention. Hepatitis C virus transmission in an antibody-negative organ and tissue donor, US 2000–2002 MMWR 2003; 52:273–274.
14. Simonds RJ, Holmberg SD, Hurwitz RL, Coleman TR, Bottenfield S, Conley LJ, Kohelnberg SH, Castro KG, Dahan BA, Schable CA, Rayfield MA, Rogers MF. Transmission of human immunodeficiency virus type 1 from a seronegative organ and tissue donor. N. Engl. J. Med. 1992;326(11):726–732.
15. Centers for Disease Control and Prevention. Update: Allograft associated bacterial infections. MMWR 2002;5:207–210.
16. Young SE, Wilkins RM. Medical / Social history questionnaires; validating the process. Proc. 19th Ann. Meeting. Am Assoc Tissue Banks, Atlanta, GA. Sept 9–13, 1995, A-38.
17. Strong M, Nelson K, Pierce M, Stramer SL. Preventing disease transmission by deceased tissue donors by testing blood for viral nucleic acid. Cell and Tissue Banking. 2005;6:249–253.
18. American Academy of Orthopaedic Surgeons Task Force on AIDS and Orthopaedic Surgery, AAOS, Park Ridge, IL, 1989.

19. Buck BE, Malinin TI, Brown MD. Bone transplantation and human immunodeficiency syndrome (AIDS). Clin Orthop. 1989;240:129–136.
20. Martinez OV, Buck BE, Hernandez M, Malinin TI. Blood and marrow cultures as indicators of bone contamination in cadaver donors. Clin Orthop 2003;409:317–324.
21. DuMolin G, Love W. The value of autopsy microbiology. Clin Microbiol Newsletter. 1982;10:165–167.
22. Koneman E, Davis M. Postmortem bacteriology 3. The significance of microorganisms recovered at autopsy. Am J Clin Path. 1974;61-28-40.
23. Roberts FJ. Procurement, interpretation and value of postmortem culture. Eur J Clin Microbiol Infec Dis. 1998;17:821–827.
24. Malinin TI, Buck BE, Temple HT, Martinez OV, Fox WP. Incidence of clostridial infection in donors' musculoskeletal tissues. J Bone Joint Surg. 2003;85B:1051–1054.
25. Chacon M, Gazitua R, Paebla C. Clinical correlation between the premortem study and autopsy. Rev Med Chil 1997;125(10):1173–1176.
26. Thurlbeck WM. Accuracy of clinical diagnosis in a Canadian teaching hospital. Can Med Assoc J. 1981;125:443–447.
27. Friedrici HH, Sebastian M. Autopsies in a modern teaching hospital. A review of 2,537 cases. Arch. Pathol Lab Med. 1984; 108(6):518–521.
28. Malinin TI. Allografts for the reconstruction of the cruciate ligaments of the knee: Procurement, sterilization and storage. Sports Med & Arthroscopy Rev. 1993; 1:31–41.
29. Wilson, PD. Follow-up study of the use of refrigerated homologous bone transplants in orthopaedic operations. J Bone & Joint Surg. 1951; 33(A): 307–323.
30. Brown MD, Malinin TI, Davis PB. A roentgenographic evaluation of frozen allografts versus autografts in anterior cervical spine fusions. Clin Orthop 1976; 119:231–236.
31. Sherman JK. Low temperature research on spermatozoa and eggs. Cryobiology. 1964;1:103–129.
32. Malinin TI. Processing and storage of viable human tissue. Public Health Service Publication No 1442, US Government Printing Office, Washington, DC 1966.
33. Tomford WW, Mankin HJ, Friedlaender GE, Doppelt SH, Gebhard MC. Methods of banking bone and cartilage for allograft transplantation. Orthop Clin North Am. 1987; 18:241.
34. Brighton CT, Lane JM, Kohl JK. In vitro rabbit articular cartilage organ model. 11 ^{35}S incorporation in various oxygen tensions. Arthritis Rheum 1984; 17:245–251.
35. Malinin TI, Wagner JL, Pita JC, Lo H. Hypothermic storage and cryopreservation of cartilage. Clin Orthop 1985; 197:15–26.
36. Malinin TI, Temple HT, Buck BE. Transplantation of osteochondral allografts after cold storage. J Bone Joint Surg. 2006; 88A:762–770.
37. Lovelock JE. The denaturation of lipid-protein complexes as a cause of damage by freezing. Proc R Soc Lond Biol Sci 1957;147:427–433.
38. Meryman HT. Preservation of living cells. Fed. Proc. 1963; 22:781–89.
39. Perry VP, Kerby CC, Kowalski FJ, Malinin TI. The freezing of human kidney cell suspensions. Cryobiology. 1975;1:274–284.
40. Luyet BJ. An attempt at systematic analysis of the notion of freezing rates and evaluation of the main contributory factors. Cryobiology. 1966;2:198–205.
41. Tomford WW, Duff GP, Mankin HJ. Experimental freeze preservation of chondrocytes. Clin Orthop 1985; 197:11–14.
42. Pegg DE, Wang L, Vaughn D. Cryopreservation of articular cartilage. Part 2. The mechanism of cryoinjury. Cryobiology. 2006; 52:347–359.
43. Parkes AS. Factors affecting the viability of frozen ovarian tissue. J. Endocrinol. 1958; 17:357–359.

44. Taylor AC. The physical state of transition in the freezing of living cells. Ann N.Y. Acad Sci 1960; 85:595–609.
45. Polge C, Smith AV, Parkes AS. Revival of spermatozoa after vitrification and dehydration at low temperature. Nature. 1949; 164–166.
46. Marco F. Leon C, Lopez-Oliva F, Perez AJ, Sanches-Barba A, Lopez-Duran, Stern L. Intact articular cartilage cryopreservation: In vivo evaluation. Clin Orthop 1992; 283:11–16.
47. Malinin TI, Martinez OV, Brown MD. Banking of massive osteoarticular and intercalary bone allografts—12 years experience. Clin Orthop 1985; 187:44–57.
48. Panuska JA, Malinin TI, Mentz RJ. Effect of dimethyl sulfoxide on cooling rates of unrestrained rats. Cryobiology. 1966; 2:345–350.
49. Lovelock JE, Bishop MWH. Prevention of freezing damage in living cells by dimethyl sulfoxide. Nature. 1959; 183:1394–1395.
50. Ashwood-Smith MJ. Radioprotective and cryoprotective properties of dimethyl sulfoxide in cellular systems. Ann NY Acad Sci. 1967; 141(1):45–62.
51. Malinin GI, Fontana DJ, Baumgart DC. Distribution of C ^{14} labeled dimethyl sulfoxide in tissues in intact animals. Cryobiology. 1969; 5:328–335.
52. Wu NM, Malinin TI. Nuclear magnetic resonance studies of some cation and anion exchange in dimethyl/sulfoxide-water systems. Anal Chem 1980; 52:186–189.
53. Ashwood-Smith MJ. Radioprotective effect of combinations of AET or cysteamine with dimethyl sulphoxide. Int J Radiat Bio. 1962; 5:201–202.
54. Ashwood-Smith MJ. The radioprotective action of dimethyl sulphoxide and various other sulphoxides. Int J Radiat Bio. 1961; 3:41–48.
55. Buck BE, Malinin TI. Human bone and tissue allografts; preparation and safety. Clin Orthop 1994; 303:8–17.
56. Bugbee WD. Alternatives to arthroplasty of the knee: biologic resurfacing. Cur Opinion Orthop 2001; 12:1–7.
57. Czitrom AA, Keating S, Gross AE. The viability of articular cartilage in fresh osteochondral allografts after clinical transplantation. J Bone Joint Surg. 1990; 72:574–581.
58. Ball ST, Amiel D, Williams SK, Tonz W, Chem AC, Sah RL, Bugbee WD. The effects of storage on fresh human osteochondral allografts. Clin Orthop 2004; 418:246–252.
59. Greif D. The important variables in the long-term stability of viruses dried by sublimation of ice in vacuo. Progress in refrigeration science and technology. Proceedings of the XIII International Congress of Refrigeration. Westbort, AVI Publishing Co. 1973; 657–662.
60. Malinin TI, Wu NM, Flores A. Freeze-drying of bone for allotransplantation. In: Osteochondral Allografts. G.E. Friedlander, HJ Mankin, KW Sell eds.) Little Brown & Co., Boston/Toronto 1983 pp 181–192.
61. Lacroix P, L'Organisacion des Os. Editions Desoer, Liege 1949.
62. Conway B, Tomford WW, Hirsch MS, Schooley, RT, Mankin HJ. Effects of gamma radiation on HIV-1 in a bone allograft model. Trans. 36 Annual Meeting, Orth Res Soc. 1990:15–:225.
63. Gibbons MJ, Butler JH, Grood ES, Bylski-Austrow DI, Levy MS, Noyes FR. Effects of gamma irradiation on the initial mechanical and material properties of goat bone-patella tendon-bone allografts. J Orthop Res. 1991; 9:209–218.
64. Buring K, Urist MR. Effect of ionizing radiation on the bone induction principle in the matrix of bone implants. Clin Orthop 1967; 55:225–234.
65. Urist MR, Hernandez A. Excitation transfer in bone. Arch Surg. 1974; 119:486–493.
66. Kerulek K, Gammon RA, Lloyd RS. Microbiological aspects of ethylene oxide sterilization. II. Microbial resistance to ethylene oxide. Appl Microbiol. 1970; 19:152–156.

67. Klaienbeek A, Van Torngen HAE. Virucidal action of ethylene oxide. J Hyg. 1954; 52:525–528.
68. Sidwell RW, Dixon GJ, Westbrook L, Dulmadge EA. Procedure for the evaluation of the virucidal effectiveness of an ethylene oxide gas sterilizer. Appl Microbiol. 1969; 17:790–796.
69. Prolo DJ, Pedrotti PW, White DJ. Ethylene oxide sterilization of bone, dura mater and fascia lata for human transplantation. Neurosurg. 1980; 6:529–539.
70. Gardner S. Ethylene oxide, ethylene chlorohydrin and ethylene glycol. Proposed maximum residue limits and maximum levels of exposure. Fed. Reg. 1978; 43:27474–27483.
71. Carpenter ET, Gendler E, Malinin TI, Temple HT. Effect of hydrogen peroxide on osteoinduction by demineralized bone. Am J Orthop. 2006; 35:562–567.
72. Horowitz MC, Friedlaender GE. Immunologic aspects of bone transplantation: A rationale and future studies. Orthop Clin North Am. 1987; 18:227–233.
73. Czitrom AA, Axelrod, Fernandes B. Antigen presenting cells in allotransplantation. Clin Orthop. 1985; 197:27–31.
74. Burchardt H, Jones H, Glowczewskie F, Rudner C, Enneking WF. Freeze-dried allogenic segmental cortical bone grafts in dogs. J Bone & Joint Surg. 1978; 60(A): 1082–1090.
75. Heiple KG, Chase SW, Herndon CH. A comparative study of the healing process following different types of bone transplantation. J Bone & Joint Surg. 1963; 45A:1593–1616.
76. Malinin TI, Mnaymneh W, Wagner JL, Borja F. Healing of internally fixed intercalary canine allografts of freeze-dried bone. Orthop Trans. 1985; 9:339.
77. Urist MR. Bone transplants and implants. In: Fundamental and clinical bone physiology (MR Urist ed) JB Lippincott Co., Philadelphia, 1980 pp 331–393.
78. Sloof TJ, Buma P, Schreurs BW, Schimmel JW, Huiskes R, Gardeniers J. Acetabular and femoral reconstruction with impacted graft and cement. Clin. Orthop 1996; 324:108–115.
79. Temple HT, Malinin TI, Wang J. Packing of osseous defects with cortical bone powder allografts. Proc.72 Ann. Mtg. AAOS 6:627, 2005.
80. Urist MR, Sato K, Brownell AG, Malinin TI, Lietze A, Huo Y-K, Prolo DJ, Oklund S, Finerman GA, de Lange RJ. Human bone morphogenetic protein (hBMP). Proc Soc Exp Bio Med. 1983; 173:194–199.
81. Urist MR, Benham K, Krendi F, Raskin K, Nguyen TD, Shamie AN, Malinin TI. Lipids closely associated with bone morphogenetic protein (BMP) and induced heterotopic bone formation. Connect Tissue Res. 1997; 36(1) 9–20.
82. Malinin TI, Temple HT. Importance of particle size on healing of bone. Proc. 71 Annual Meeting, Am Acad Orth Surg. 5:633, 2004.
83. Dunlop DG, Brewster NT, Madabhushi SP, Usmani AS, Paukaj P, Howie CR. Techniques to improve the shear strength of impacted bone graft: The effect of particle size and washing of the graft. J Bone Joint Surg. 2003; 85-A:639–646.
84. Sun JS, Liu HC, Chang LH, Li J, Lin FH, Tai HC. Influence of hydroxyapatite particle size on bone cell activities; an in vitro study. J Biomed Materials Res. 39(3):390–397,1998.
85. Heiple KG, Goldberg VM, Powell AE, Bos GD, Zika JM. Biology of cancellous bone repair. In: Osteochondral Allografts. (G.E. Friedlander, HJ Mankin, & KW Sell, eds.) Little, Brown & Co. Boston/Toronto. 1983:37–49.
86. Urist MR, Mikulski A, Boyd SD. A chemosterilized antigen-extracted autodigested alloimplant for bone banks. Arch Surg. 1975; 110:416.
87. Johnson EE, Urist MR. One-stage lengthening of femoral nonunion augmented with human bone morphogenetic protein. Clin Orthop 1998; 347:105–116.

24

Bioabsorbable Polymer Applications in Musculoskeletal Fixation and Healing

William S. Pietrzak

Abstract: Bioabsorbable internal fixation of hard and soft tissue has gained popularity over the past 20 years, especially in the fields of sports medicine, trauma and craniofacial surgery. This technology continues to coexist with metallic fixation and there is no pretense that, in its current form, it will obsolete metallic devices. The development of bioabsorbable technology requires the dedicated effort of a multidisciplinary team of surgeons, materials scientists and engineers. Expertise in one field, however, does not guarantee a working knowledge in other fields. For instance, some surgeons may be unfamiliar with the nuances of bioabsorbable polymers while some engineers and materials scientists may be unfamiliar with biological concepts such as healing and tissue fixation. The purpose was to develop the necessary background of bioabsorbable fixation in a stepwise fashion as a tool toward understanding for the clinician, engineer and scientist alike. Concepts including basic polymer science, bioabsorbable polymer chemistry and material properties, degradation mechanisms, fixation principals, experimental studies, recent clinical results and a look at what the future may hold are included. The field of bioabsorbable fixation is dynamic and much work remains before the technology reaches its full potential. Papers such as this will help to provide synergy among various specialists to help propel this technology forward.

Keywords: Internal fixation, bioabsorbable, biodegradable, polymer, healing.

24.1. Introduction

Tissue fixation has evolved over many centuries, from the earliest use of sutures over 6,000 years ago [1] to the present. State-of-the-art materials in the mid-20th Century for osteosynthesis included metals such as stainless steel

Department of Bioengineering, University of Illinois at Chicago, Chicago, IL, Biomet, Inc., Warsaw, IN

From: *Orthopedic Biology and Medicine: Musculoskeletal Tissue Regeneration, Biological Materials and Methods*
Edited by W. S. Pietrzak © Humana Press, Totowa, NJ

and others [2]. While successful, bone near the metal implant can become osteoporotic due to stress shielding [3]. Other complications include metal sensitivity, palpability, tissue irritation, poor cosmesis, interference with therapeutic irradiation and the potential for growth restriction and transcranial migration in pediatric patients [3]. Although metal implants can be removed after healing, there is additional risk and cost [4].

In the first half of the 20th Century polymers synthesized from glycolic acid and other α-hydroxy acids were initially abandoned because of instability [5–6]. Later, medical application became apparent [5–6]. Osteosynthesis via bioabsorbable rigid internal fixation now compliments metallic osteosynthesis [3, 5, 7]. Advancements in treatment of injured joints has further extended bioabsorbable device use to soft tissue repair, especially in the shoulder and knee [8].

Most clinical bioabsorbable polymers are composed of one or more base monomers that are chemically related, yet small changes in polymer structure and composition can profoundly influence the mechanical, degradation and biological properties [7, 9]. This chapter will help the reader to better understand this subject as well as to make informed decisions regarding clinical use and the future evolution of bioabsorbable technology.

24.2. Basic Science

24.2.1. Polymer Fundamentals

Following are basic concepts that provide a foundation for the understanding of bioabsorbable polymer technology [10–11].

A *polymer* consists of long chains of *mers*, or subunits, covalently bound together. Organic polymers have a backbone of repeating carbon or carbon and oxygen atoms. Typically, synthetic polymers are formed by polymerization of a small number of *monomer* types. A *homopolymer* is comprised of only one monomer type which, if abbreviated by A, may be denoted by A-A-A-A-A-A-A, or poly(A) for short. If comprised of two monomers, e.g., A and B, it would be a *copolymer* and described as poly(xA-co-yB) with x and y the mole fractions, or for convenience, x:y A:B. There are two possible arrangements for two monomers. For a *random copolymer* no long-range repeating pattern exits, e.g., A-A-B-A-B-B-B-A-A-B-B-A-B-B-B-B-A. In the case of a *block copolymer*, there are large alternating domains of the two monomers, e.g., A-A-A-A-A-A-A-B-B-B-B-B-B-B-B-A-A-A-A-A-A. This progression can continue with three types of monomers, in which case a *terpolymer* forms, and so on. If each monomer can only bind to two other monomers, then a *linear polymer* will be created. If, however, some monomers are trifunctional, then side branches can form along the polymer chain, creating a *branched polymer*. If the branches from one chain connect with those from other chains, a *network polymer* forms.

Following polymerization a *statistical distribution of molecular weights* results. Although there are several ways to characterize molecular weight, one common method is based on *inherent viscosity*, which is related to mean molecular weight [12]. A known volume of polymer solution of concentration c at temperature T is allowed to pass through a capillary under gravity, with transit time, t_{soln} recorded, as well as that for pure solvent, t_{solv} (t_{soln}>t_{solv}). The inherent viscosity, η_{inh}, is calculated as:

$$\eta_{inh} = \ln(t_{soln}/t_{solv})/c \quad [1]$$

This method does not work for network polymers since such polymers will swell, but not dissolve.

Two fundamental polymeric structural arrangements exist, i.e., *amorphous* and *crystalline*. In the first case the chains randomly twist and entangle with each other, like a bowl of spaghetti (Fig. 24.1). In the crystalline arrangement the polymer chains fold back and forth to form local regions of order, or crystallites, which are dense and stable (Fig. 24.1). Steric regularity along the polymer chain is required for crystals to form. Thus, homopolymers have a strong propensity to crystallize whereas random copolymers do not. In general, polymers that have the ability to crystallize are *semicrystalline* in which there exist isolated crystalline regions separated by amorphous regions (Fig. 24.1).

In general a solid specimen deforms when it is loaded. For metals and ceramics the response is instantaneous. For polymers, however, the deformation is time-dependent. Polymer chains cannot respond instantly to an applied stress because time is required for them to disentangle from neighboring chains. While stress is applied, deformation will increase over time, e.g, the polymer will *flow*. Hence, polymers are *viscoelastic*, with both solid and liquid properties. For example, if a weight is suspended on a polymer specimen, it will elongate or *creep* over time, and may rupture. Related to creep is *stress relaxation*. This is illustrated by quickly stretching a specimen and then holding its length constant. The force with which the specimen attempts to contract will diminish over time, and may approach zero, as the chains reorient to minimize the internal stresses.

Polymer properties are strongly temperature-dependent. At low temperatures the amorphous chains cannot overcome energy barriers to movement and are, effectively, "frozen" in place, with the polymer behaving as a stiff, brittle glass. As temperature increases over a narrow range, the amorphous chains gain thermal energy, becoming mobile. In the process, the polymer transforms to a rubber, with reduced stiffness or modulus, capable of large deformations

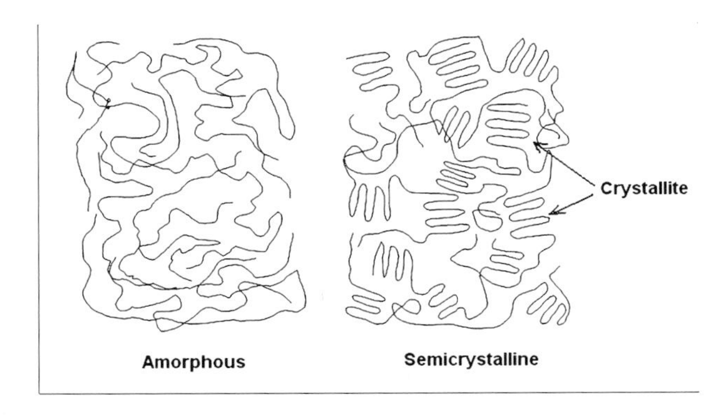

Fig. 24.1 Left: amorphous polymer, Right: semicrystalline polymer

(*ductile* behavior). The midpoint of this temperature range is called the *glass transition temperature*, or T_g, and varies by polymer. Passage through the T_g has no effect on crystalline domains, if they exist. However, as temperature is further increased and passes through the *melt temperature*, T_m, the polymer crystals undergo a true solid–to-liquid change of state.

24.2.2. Bioabsorbable Polymers

24.2.2.1. Chemistry and Nomenclature

Most synthetic bioabsorbable polymers are derivatives of α-hydroxy acids having the structure: HO-CHR-COOH [5, 13]. The simplest is glycolic acid, in which the R group is H. The R group for lactic acid is CH_3. Lactic acid has a chiral carbon atom and, hence, exists in both the D and L enantiomeric forms.

α-hydroxy acid chains can be formed by step-growth polymerization whereby monomers are added one at a time to the growing chain; however, better properties are achieved by first preparing an intermediate purified cyclic dimer and then performing a ring-opening reaction in which repeating units are added in pairs (Fig. 24.2) [6, 13]. The cyclic dimers that correspond to glycolic acid and (D or L) lactic acid are glycolide and (D or L) lactide, respectively. When a subunit adds to the chain, a molecule of water is formed and released as a by-product (condensation reaction). The ester bond that forms makes bioabsorbable polymers polyesters. It is common to refer to the polymers in terms of their basic repeating units, e.g., poly (glycolic acid) or poly (L-lactic acid), which may be abbreviated as PGA and PLLA, respectively. Alternatively, they are also referred to as poly(glycolide), poly(L-lactide), etc.

Other ring-type subunits include e-caprolactone, p-dioxanone and trimethylene carbonate. Figure 24.3 shows the synthesis of the polyesters poly(e-caprolactone) (PCL), poly (p-dioxanone) (PDO) and a copolymer of glycolide and trimethylene carbonate (G/TMC). There are two to five consecutive $-CH_2-$ groups along the backbone of these polymers. Due to the relatively free rotation about the C-C bond, these polymers tend to be quite flexible and have low T_g values.

24.2.2.2. Physical Properties

Table 24.1 lists some physical properties for several common bioabsorbable polymers, showing several relationships. First, copolymers are generally amorphous, having no true melting temperature. Second, polymers containing e-caprolactone, p-dioxanone and trimethylene carbonate are extremely flexible

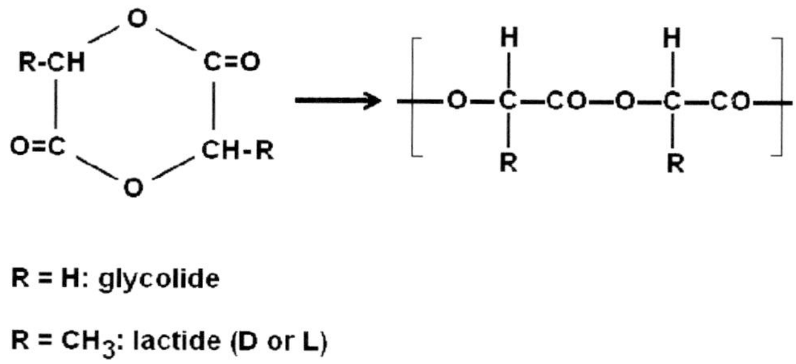

R = H: glycolide

R = CH_3: lactide (D or L)

Fig. 24.2 Ring-opening polymerization of PGA and PLLA

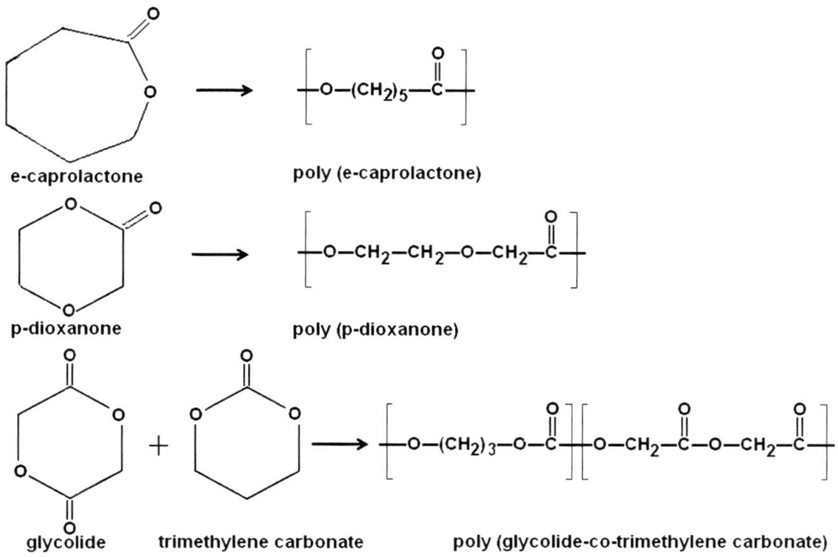

e-caprolactone → poly (e-caprolactone)

p-dioxanone → poly (p-dioxanone)

glycolide + trimethylene carbonate → poly (glycolide-co-trimethylene carbonate)

Fig. 24.3 Polymerization of a) e-caprolactone, b) p-dioxanone and c) glycolide and trimethylene carbonate copolymer

Table 24.1 Selected thermal and mechanical properties for common bioabsorbable polymers [5, 12, 14, 15]

Polymer	T_g(°C)	T_m (°C)	Modulus (GPa)	Elongation (%) R
PGA	35–40	225–230	7.0	15–20
PLLA	58–65	173–184	2.7	5–10
PDLLA	55–60	Amorphous	1.9	3–10
PCL	−65–60	58–63	0.4	300–500
PDO	−16–0	110	1.5	N/A
2:1 PGA-TMC	N/A	N/A	2.4	N/A
82/18 PLLA/PGA	57	N/A	4 (unoriented)	N/A
			7 (oriented)	N/A
85/15 PDLLA	50–55	Amorphous	2.0	3–10
75/15 PDLLA	50–55	Amorphous	2.0	3–10
65/35 PDLLA	45–50	Amorphous	2.0	3–10
50/50 PDLLA	45–50	Amorphous	2.0	3–10
Bone			10–20	
Steel			200	
Titanium alloy (6Al-4V)			110	

(low modulus) and tend to have relatively low T_g and T_m. When implanted they are exposed to an *in vivo* temperature of 37° C and, hence, are above T_g and are in the rubbery domain. The stiffer polymers have T_g's substantially above 37° C and are in the glassy domain *in situ*. PGA has the highest modulus of the listed polymers, however its T_g is around normal body temperature so *in vivo* stiffness may be lower. Third, stainless steel and titanium alloy have moduli an order of magnitude greater than bone, hence their ability to induce stress shielding. The modulus of bioabsorbable polymers is smaller than bone, thus stress shielding is not a concern, but the challenge is to design the implant to be sufficiently strong to withstand biomechanical loading.

Following polymerization there is no preferred direction to the polymer chains and the polymer is *isotropic*, meaning that the mechanical properties are equivalent in every direction. There are processing techniques, however, that allow the polymer chains to acquire a preferred orientation, or direction, in which the mechanical properties become enhanced in certain directions (*anisotropic*). For instance, if a polymer rod is heated to above its T_g (but below the T_m) and drawn through a small orifice, or die, the rod will narrow and lengthen and the chains will orient with the draw direction [3, 16]. If tension remains on the drawn rod as it cools to below T_g, orientation will remain. This is often referred to as *self-reinforcement* or *orientation* [3, 15–16]. This increases the tensile, bending and shear properties of the rod [14–15, 17]. For example, orientation increases the modulus of an 82:18 PLLA:PGA copolymer from 4GPa to 7GPa [15]. Certain loading patterns, however, can cause the oriented polymer to delaminate into fibrils [14]. This process also renders the polymer *birefringent* whereby there is a change in refractive index with direction and manifests as the ability to rotate the plane of polarized light [10]. Under a polarizing microscope oriented polymers may be identified in tissue sections in which the oriented polymer appears with a light-dark pattern [18].

24.2.2.3 Bioabsorption

We will primarily adopt "bioabsorption" and its derivatives to describe the process of strength and mass loss *in vivo*. The terms bioresorption and biodegradation can also be used, although it might be argued that subtle differences in meaning exist [6, 19].

The ester bonds in a bioabsorbable polymer are susceptible to *hydrolysis*. During hydrolysis the bond is cleaved by water and two smaller chains are formed with hydroxyl and carboxylic acid end groups (Fig. 24.4). Most common bioabsorbable polymers undergo *bulk* hydrolysis with the carboxylic acid chain ends acting as autocatalysts [17, 20]. In the case of glycolide- and lactide-based polymers, as well as polydioxanone, the center of the implant can degrade faster than the exterior [17, 20–21]. This is due to accumulation of low molecular weight chains (*oligomers*) containing catalytic acidic end groups that form faster than they can diffuse away.

Many factors influence the rate of hydrolysis. One is the *hydrophilicity* and *hydrophobicity* of the side groups. The R group of PGA is H, so the polar –COO– groups impart overwhelming hydrophilic character to the polymer,

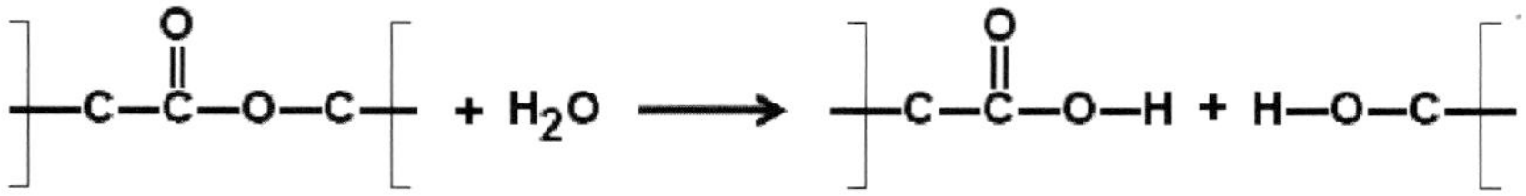

$$\left[-C-\overset{O}{\overset{\|}{C}}-O-C- \right] + H_2O \longrightarrow \left[-C-\overset{O}{\overset{\|}{C}}-O-H \right] + \left[H-O-C- \right]$$

Fig. 24.4 Ester bond hydrolysis

enabling fast hydrolysis [17, 22]. The R group in PLLA is $-CH_3$, which is hydrophobic, attenuating the ability to interact with water, resulting in slower hydrolysis [17, 22]. It is more difficult for water to invade the dense crystalline regions than the amorphous regions, so the latter will hydrolyze more rapidly than the former [6]. During hydrolysis the crystallinity may increase until the latter stages, when these regions undergo delayed hydrolysis [6, 23]. In general, the hydrolysis rate decreases with increasing molecular weight, crystallinity and orientation [6].

In vivo, the implant loses integrity and fragments as mechanical properties deteriorate. This is followed by a macrophage response in which the polymer debris is phagocytized and metabolically cleared [9]. The metabolic pathways are polymer-specific. For instance, L-lactic acid enters the Kreb's cycle and is eliminated as carbon dioxide and water, or may be converted to glycogen in the liver [6, 17]. Glycolic acid may be excreted in the urine or converted to serine and then pyruvate, entering the Kreb's cycle [16–17]. The majority, 94 percent, of the end products of poly (dioxanone) hydrolysis are excreted in the urine, with the balance in the feces or exhaled as carbon dioxide [17].

Controversy exists over the role of enzymes in hydrolysis *in vivo* [6, 12,21]. It has been suggested that enzymes may accelerate degradation of glycolide, lactide and e-caprolactone-based polymers, and that polydioxanone degrades by nonenzymatic hydrolysis [6, 12, 17, 24], however, others view this generally as a nonenzymatic process [9, 20, 22].

Based on the foregoing, *in vivo* bioabsorption can be viewed as occurring in two stages – hydrolysis and metabolism [9]. The effect on the polymer occurs in the following order: molecular weight reduction, strength reduction and mass reduction (Fig. 24.5). Typically, the polymer will reach zero or little strength before the overall mass has substantially declined.

In vitro studies enable the examination of implant degradation under controlled conditions. Typically, the device is submersed in pH 7.4 phosphate buffer at 37° C and tested at intervals. The implant may be placed in buffer alone [15] or may be inserted into a substrate, with the construct placed in the bath, as may be performed to measure the extraction force of suture anchors over time [25]. *In vitro* studies, however, cannot fully approximate the complex mechanical, cellular and metabolic *in vivo* environment. In general, bioabsorbable polymers degrade faster *in vivo* than *in vitro*, which has led to

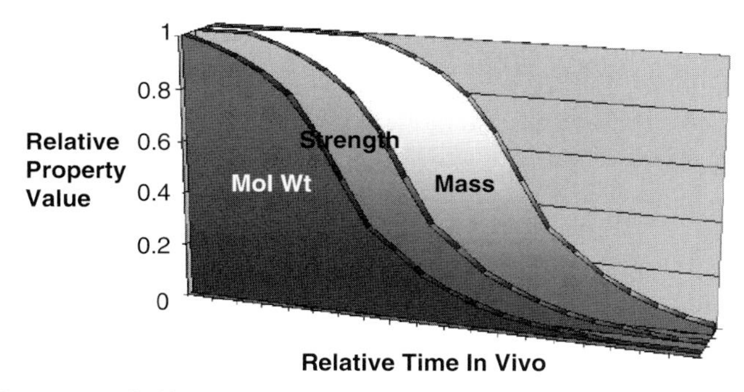

Fig. 24.5 Sequence of effects on polymer of *in vivo* bioabsorption

Table 24.2 Approximate absorption profiles for common bioabsorbable polymers

Polymer	**Strength retention**	**Mass loss**	**Ref.**
PGA	0% at 2–7 weeks	<12 mos	[15,22]
Self-reinforced PLLA	0% at 36 weeks	6 years	[22]
Polydioxanone	0% at 3–8 weeks	6 mos	[15,28]
Polyglyconate (2:1 glycolide:TMC)	0% at 4 weeks	<12 mos	[29,30]
85 L-lactide 15 glycolide	70% at 7 weeks	12 mos	[23]
L-lactide and D,L lactide	70% at 24 weeks	2 years	[23]
70 L-lactide 30 D,L lactide	0% at 18 mos	2 years	[6]
82 L-lactide 18 glycolide (oriented)	40–50% at 12 weeks	12–18 mos	[15,31,32]
82 L-lactide 18 glycolide (unoriented)	25% at 12 weeks	12–18 mos	[26,31,32]

the proposal that enzymes may play a role [12, 17]. An alternative explanation is that most animal studies are performed in species whose body temperature is 38 to 41° C [12]. This increase in temperature over standard *in vitro* conditions (37° C) can account for about a 25 percent increase in hydrolysis of a PLLA/PGA copolymer [12]. Landes, et al. [23] performed a unique human clinical study in which bioabsorbable fixation was placed in mandibles and maxillae, then explanted and analyzed over time. Degradation was slower *in vivo* than *in vitro*. The authors suggested that enzymes may play a greater role in polymer degradation in animals than in humans.

Table 24.2 lists intervals over which strength and mass loss occurs for several common polymers. Values are representative since they depend on polymer details (composition, molecular weight, crystallinity, etc.), implant configuration (method of processing and sterilization, size and shape, degree of orientation), *in vitro* test conditions (temperature, pH, buffer to polymer ratio, frequency of buffer exchange) and *in vivo* conditions (species and implant site) [6, 9, 12, 17, 20, 22–23]. "Half-life" was not cited since the time course of strength and mass loss is often not a simple exponential function [15, 26–27].

Some polymers lose strength in less than one month while others require six months or longer. Also, the time required for complete mass loss (six months to six years) is frequently multiples of that required for complete strength loss. Finally, even within the family of glycolide- and lactide- based polymers, considerable variation exists in strength and mass loss profiles.

24.2.2.4 The Physiological Response to Bioabsorbable Polymer Implants
Following implantation an initial inflammatory reaction is evoked that is part of the normal healing response [9]. As with any foreign material, the body will wall it off with a fibrous capsule. As the material is metabolized its volume diminishes. In a soft tissue environment, tissue will collapse into the volume formerly occupied by the implant with, perhaps, a residue of the fibrous capsule remaining. In the case of an osseous implant, bony or fibrous fill depends on the skeletal site, the hole size, the observational period and implant material. Lajtai, et al. [33] used magnetic resonance imaging (MRI) to

determine that new bone completely filled in the region formerly occupied by a copolymer (85:15 D,L lactide:glycolide) anterior cruciate ligament (ACL) interference screw by five years. Fink, et al. [34], using a PGA/TMC copolymer interference screw, found that the implant was not visible on MRI at one year, however bone had not yet filled in by three years. Bach, et al. [35] also used PGA/TMC copolymer interference screws, finding complete absorption by one year, with fibrous or fibrous/fatty tissue replacement by two years. Following bilateral sagittal split mandibular osteotomies fixed with 82:18 PLLA:PGA screws, Edwards, et al. [36] found near or complete trabecular bone fill in the osseous hole by 18 months, ascertained by radiography as well as by one two-year bone biopsy. In a rabbit model of calvarial bone graft healing using the same copolymer, Eppley and Sadove [37] found that while implants were histologically gone by 12 months, screw hole outlines persisted, indicating lack of bony fill.

Adverse reactions to bioabsorbable implants have been reported, especially in their early clinical history [22]. These included pronounced fibrous encapsulation, local osteolysis and the formation of sterile sinuses [3–5, 7, 9, 22, 38–39]. Two important contributing factors are rapidly hydrolyzing polymers and the presence of degradation-resistant crystals [3, 5, 7, 9, 22, 38–39]. If the degradation rate exceeds the local clearance ability of the tissue, acidic products may accumulate, resulting in sequelae. Also, as the amorphous regions preferentially hydrolyze, the degradation-resistant crystals (if present) may be released to which the body may respond as it does to total joint prosthesis wear particles [9]. Fast absorbing polymers such as PGA have manifest such reactions with as high an incidence as 55 percent within two to four months, while very slowly degrading polymers such as PLLA may require five years or more for such reactions to present, but typically with much lower incidence [22, 38–39]. Ashammakhi, et al. [3] recently reported that incidence of clinically manifest reactions to self-reinforced PLLA in the orthopaedic skeleton is around 0.1 percent. It is important to remember, however, that even stainless steel implants can present similar reactions. Gill, et al. [40] reported a 9 percent incidence of osteolysis using PDO pins to fix chevron osteotomies for bunion procedures, similar to the 7 percent incidence observed using standard K-wires. For the past 10 years or so, bioabsorbable implants have been made almost exclusively from amorphous copolymers and terpolymers derived from glycolide, L-lactide, D-lactide and trimethlylene carbonate, although the homopolymers PDO and PLLA remain in clinical use [5, 20, 41].

Such tissue reactions in animals are uncommon [23]. Consequently, caution must be exercised when extrapolating animal results to anticipated clinical results. General trends associated with a tendency toward clinically relevant tissue reactions include large implants, polymers that either degrade quickly or release degradation-resistant crystals or contain aromatic dyes, use in older (>40 years) patients and placement in poorly vascular regions [7]. Very few studies have reported such reactions in children [42–43].

24.2.2.5 Principles of Bioabsorbable Internal Fixation

Both the implant and the healing union contribute to the overall tissue interface strength, as shown in Fig. 24.6. Typically, the initial stability provided by the implant will be less than that of the native or fully healed structure. Two important biomechanical criteria should be met: 1) the initial stability

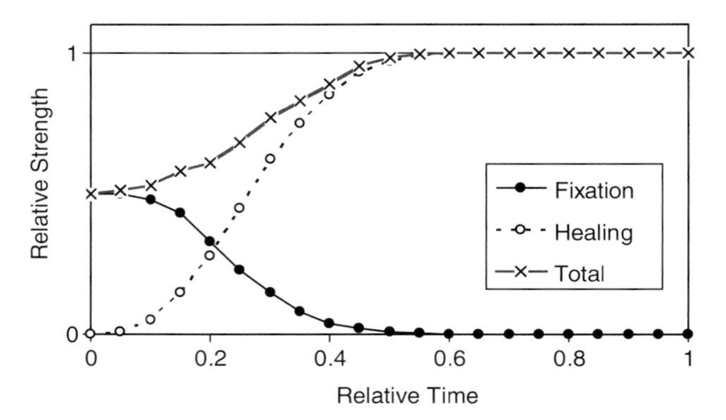

Fig. 24.6 Superposition of hypothetical healing and biological fixation strength curves

must withstand the anticipated *in situ* loads, and 2) the rate of implant strength decline should not exceed the rate of increase of the healing union. Load will gradually transfer from the degrading implant to the surrounding tissue, which may aid the healing response. The healing rate will depend on the tissues involved, extent of injury, age and metabolic status of the patient, diet and lifestyle and comorbidity, illustrating the importance of matching the material to the patient. A healthy pediatric patient may do well with a fast degrading implant, but an elderly, diabetic patient may require a longer strength retention profile to compensate for slower healing.

One key concept of internal fixation is interfragmental osseous compression to enhance stability [44]. With adequate local circulation and proper compression, primary bone union will occur without radiologic signs of callus formation [44]. Compression may be achieved with metal lag screws, compression plates, tension bands or other methods [44]. The polymeric nature of bioabsorbable implants, however, precludes their ability to maintain long-term compression due to stress relaxation and creep [45]. In spongious bone even metal screws may not be able to maintain long-term compression due to stress relaxation of the bone itself [45]. Thus, the inability for bioabsorbable implants to provide compression on a long-term basis does not necessarily preclude their use for certain applications.

Although many bioabsorbable implants resemble their metallic counterparts, some differences exist in application technique [7]. For example, metallic self-tapping screws exist, but bioabsorbable osteosynthesis screws require tapping in all but, perhaps, the softest bone. While metal plates can be adapted with bending instruments, bioabsorbable plates below T_g are brittle and might fracture from excessive bending. They can be intraoperatively heated to above T_g for molding purposes, although a transient change in mechanical properties may occur, including increased toughness [26, 46]. Heating self-reinforced plates is not advised because residual stresses can relax and cause distortion. Oriented, or self-reinforced, plates can be bent at ambient temperature; however, repeated bending can weaken them [3]. Bioabsorbable implants can be conveniently cut using hot-wire cautery [28].

24.3. Review of Preclinical Studies

We will consider preclinical studies to include all *in vitro* and *in vivo* studies required to support clinical use in humans. Many of these types of studies are mandated by the governments of the countries in which the device is to be sold, with the specific requirements varying with device and country. Much of the Basic Science discussed in the preceding section was derived from such studies, with several excellent reviews available [17, 20, 47–49]. For example, Brady, et al. [50] studied elimination pathways by implanting ^{14}C-labelled poly lactic acid into the abdominal walls of rats and measuring excretion and organ distribution after sacrifice. The highest radioactivity was in the kidney and most was eliminated via respiratory CO_2. Li [21] furthered the understanding of the hydrolysis of lactic and glycolic acid-based polymers through *in vitro* studies; in particular, the conditions under which degradation can accelerate from within. Cutright and Hunsuck [51] performed an early osteosynthesis study in rhesus monkeys using poly lactic acid sheets for reconstruction of orbital defects. Powers, et al. [52] performed both *in vitro* and *in vivo* studies to compare the fixation provided by a PGA:TMC (2:1) tack and a PLLA:PGA (82:18) rivet. The *in vitro* strength loss profiles were quite different for the two devices (<4 weeks for tack and >8 weeks for rivet), yet both performed similarly *in vivo* for reattachment of the medial collateral ligament to its tibial insertion site in goats.

The type of preclinical study performed depends on the stage of device development. For instance, basic biocompatibility data will be required for a new polymer. *In vitro* studies of strength loss and *in vivo* studies of mass loss and tissue reaction are also necessary [15, 18]. Process parameters for device fabrication, including sterilization, should be defined to ensure that polymer or device deterioration does not occur [5, 49].

Ideally, the *in situ* loads to which the device will be exposed will be available from the literature; however, that is rarely the case. If preexisting devices for that indication have a successful published clinical history, then they can be tested alongside the new device for comparison. For example, percutaneous K wires commonly provide fixation for proximal interphalengeal joint (PIPJ) arthrodesis to correct hammertoe deformity. A bioabsorbable threaded and barbed PLLA/PGA pin was biomechanically compared to K-wire fixation, *in vitro*, demonstrating equivalent fixation properties and providing evidence of the device's suitability for this application [53].

Fixation implants are designed to gain purchase in tissue and must be evaluated in a suitable substrate. Cadaver bone may be used, but is highly variable [54] and is often derived from the elderly, which might not be representative of younger patients. Reproducible synthetic substrates exist, however, bone is a complex biomaterial and difficult to mimic [53, 55]. Animal bone is another possibility, but may differ from human bone [56]. For soft tissue procedures it might be possible to use dense rubber substrates to simulate insertion into tendons, ligaments and other tissues, but if *in vitro* studies are conducted, it is important that the rubber/implant interface not preclude infiltration by water. Cadaveric human or animal soft tissue is often the best substrate [57–59], but cannot be adapted to *in vitro* studies as it would deteriorate.

Ideally, animal studies should closely approximate the clinical application. Animal models of fixation in the metaphysis, diaphysis or craniofacial skeleton often do correlate well with clinical use [32, 60–61]. For other applications it may be difficult to find a suitable animal model. For instance, due to the large anatomical differences between the human shoulder and that of nonprimates, good animal shoulder models do not exist. For that reason the copolymer rivet in the Powers, et al. [52] study, developed for the shoulder, was compared to a copolymer tack that had extensive clinical history for shoulder fixation. Both were tested in a goat model of medial collateral ligament reattachment, with the assumption that if both performed equivalently (which they did), then the rivet should be suitable for shoulder procedures.

Other preclinical studies involve determination of storage conditions and shelf-life, which includes consideration of material properties and packaging [5].

24.4. Clinical Review

Bioabsorbable fixation usage is procedure-specific, being a function of cost, the limitations of metal implants and clinical outcomes. A brief survey of some common clinical uses follows.

24.4.1. Foot and Ankle

Bioabsorbable fixation is widely used in forefoot procedures such as correction of hallux valgus (bunion) deformity. Successful fixation has been provided by copolymer pins (82:18 PGA:PLLA) [38], PLLA pins [62], polydioxanone pins and PLLA screws [63]. Chevron osteotomies are often performed in the metatarsal head. Cancellous bone, in general, readily heals and this osteotomy is relatively stable [38]. Thus, bioabsorbable fixation provides supplemental stability which may explain the high success rate over a range of implant and polymer types.

Fixation of the tibiofibular syndesmosis with a metal transfixation screw is effective, but screws frequently break from shear stresses resulting from the attempted longitudinal movement of the fibula [39]. As such, these screws are usually removed after six to eight weeks [38]. Several studies attest to the clinical utility of PLLA screws [64–66] and 82:18 PGA:PLLA screws [67] for syndesmotic fixation.

24.4.2. Knee

ACL-deficient knees are typically repaired with bone-patellar tendon-bone or hamstring grafts fixed with interference screws, cross-pins and other devices [68–74]. Bioabsorbable fixation obviates removal of a metal implant during revision surgery [73]. Biomechanically, bioabsorbable implants can provide equivalent fixation to metal devices [70–71] and several randomized, controlled, prospective clinical studies have shown similar outcomes [72–74]. Overall, the complication rate is low, however, bone tunnel widening has been observed for both types of implants that can complicate revision procedures [74–76]. A blend of PLLA and hydroxyapatite may reduce this phenomenon [76]. There have been published case studies of complications resulting from the breakage or migration of bioabsorbable ACL fixation devices [77–79].

Arthroscopic meniscal repair using suture is technically demanding. This has engendered a plethora of bioabsorbable implants for this purpose, including 30:70 D,L-lactic acid darts, absorbable suture with a sliding PLLA component to cinch the repair, PLLA barbed devices, 82:18 PLLA:PGA screws and staples and polydioxanone implants consisting of a curved shaft with two perpendicular crossbars [80–83]. Farng and Sherman [83] recently reviewed the clinical results utilizing these devices. While many showed acceptable outcomes, instances of device-related irritation, breakage and chondylar injury have been reported [83–85]. Due to the wide variance in implant designs, polymer composition and degradation characteristics, generalizations are difficult and each device requires separate evaluation.

24.4.3. Hand and Wrist

Despite complication rates with metal fixation as high as 36 percent, bioabsorbable fixation use in the hand has been limited, possibly due to a lack of controlled studies [86–87]. Waris, et al. [88] reported three cases in which self-reinforced 70:30 L/D,L lactide plates and screws were used in complicated hand injuries, with good results. Scaphoid fractures and nonunions have been successfully treated with self-reinforced PLLA screws, achieving solid union in five of six cases [89]. In a case study of an 82:18 PLLA:PGA copolymer plate and screws to treat a metacarpal fracture in a 19-year-old man, the patient returned with the screws still engaged, but the plate fractured [90]. The patient was "particularly non-compliant," suggesting the importance of patient selection. Waris, et al. [41] summarized several studies using bioabsorbable pins and tacks for hard and soft tissue procedures in the hand.

Metallic distal radius dorsal plating is removed in 12 to 29 percent of cases [91]. In a recent survey 95 percent of patients would prefer bioabsorbable distal radius fixation [92]. Gangopadhyay, et al. [91] used 82:18 PLLA:PGA dorsal distal radius plates and screws in 26 patients presenting with fractures that were dorsally displaced, angulated or both, with a mean follow-up of 17 months. Radiological success was achieved in 22 patients. There were two cases of inflammation between eight and 11 weeks, which were treated with aspiration or debridement, ultimately yielding an excellent result. In one case of severe dorsal comminution, a revision was performed to replace a broken plate, again illustrating the importance of patient selection.

24.4.4. Spine

The spine is one of the most difficult anatomic regions to achieve fusion and, hence, is a stringent test of fixation. Anterior cervical discectomy and fusion is performed to treat anterior degenerative or traumatic instability of the cervical spine [93]. Bioabsorbable anterior cervical plates that provide stability for six to 12 months can reduce or eliminate the complications associated with metal devices [94]. Sheets and screws of 70:30 L/D,L-lactide have been successfully used for graft containment in one- and two-level fusions, with intraoperative heating of the mesh enabling it to be shaped to fit the construct [95]. In that study 25 of 26 patients achieved radiographic fusion by six months, with one patient requiring revision with a titanium plate and screws. Brunon, et al. [96] used poly lactic acid plate and screw placement in the cervical spine in five patients, with good or excellent results in four and an incomplete result in one by 18 months. One inflammatory response was reported. The clinical use of bioabsorbable interbody cages for posterior lumbar interbody fusion has also been reported [94].

24.4.5. Shoulder

Bioabsorbable fixation of soft tissue in the shoulder is common, possibly due to the extreme mobility of this joint and the propensity for metal implants to loosen, migrate or break. Two of the most common procedures are Bankart repair for recurrent anterior instability and rotator cuff repair. McBirnie, et al. [97] performed arthroscopic rotator cuff repair in 53 patients using 2:1 PGA: TMC tacks, with a minimum 24-month follow-up. Eleven patients also had unstable SLAP lesions (superior labral tears) that were also repaired with the tacks. Mean American Shoulder and Elbow Society (ASES) scores, which include a pain and function component, significantly increased from 32.7 (preoperative) to 84.6 (postoperative), and all Short Form 36 Health Survey (SF-36) scores significantly improved as well. There were no complications attributed to the implants. Freedman, et al. [98] performed a meta-analysis of six studies of open or arthroscopic Bankart repair using bioabsorbable tacks or transglenoid sutures, the latter of which has historically been considered the "gold standard" for this procedure. They found no difference in recurrent dislocation or total recurrence (dislocation + subluxation) between the tacks and sutures, although open procedures had significantly better outcomes than those performed arthroscopically. While, in general, bioabsorbable implants are well-suited for shoulder applications, they are not a panacea. Just as with metal implants, they can dislodge and become loose bodies [99], and metal fixation can, at times, result in better outcomes than bioabsorbable fixation, but this is highly dependent on implant design and technique [100].

24.4.6. Craniofacial Skeleton

Modern pediatric craniofacial surgery has undergone a multitude of advancements and innovations in surgical techniques over the past two decades. Early in the development of craniofacial surgery it became apparent that a method of bone fixation was needed to provide both intraoperative stability and postoperative maintenance of the desired change in bone shape and contour. Numerous creative methods of loop suture and stainless steel wire ligatures were initially used, but their lack of three-dimensional stability left these methods wanting. The development of metallic plate and screw fixation, particularly the adaptation to a smaller size, provided rigid bone fixation that was ideal for maintaining new bony configurations. With widespread use, however, certain concerns surfaced due to the young age of the implanted patients and the unique pattern of cranial vault growth [101]. These issues primarily revolve around the potential need for secondary removal due to device loosening, skin irritation and device exposure. Uniquely, intracranial translocation to the endocranial surface and dural violation pose the more grave potential risks of causing secondary headaches and/or creating a seizure focus [102–105]. Of less concern is the potential for growth restriction, although this has been shown to have only a relatively minor local effect which is restricted to the area of the implantation site [106–107].

An ideal system for pediatric craniofacial bone healing would provide rigid fixation during the initial phase of healing while being eliminated from the body through natural processes after it is no longer needed. Plate and screw fixation devices composed of bioabsorbable polymers appear to most closely match the requirements needed for this application and have been under experimental investigation for decades [47]. Craniofaical bioabsorbable bone fixation implants have been clinically available since 1996 and have been implanted in tens of thousands of patients, the vast majority undoubtedly being in the young pediatric patient under two years of age [101, 108]. Long-term experience in large numbers of these patients demonstrates that bioabsorbable PLLA-PGA plate and screw fixation in pediatric cranial vault reconstruction is as safe and effective as metal devices, with no added risks of infection or reconstruction instability [101]. A major advantage is that they eliminate the need for any secondary device-related procedures. There is a very low occurrence of isolated foreign body reactions, which are self-limiting and require no treatment as the material is metabolized [101, 109–110].

The experiences with bioabsorbable craniofacial fixation have been subsequently expanded to include maxillofacial fracture fixation [111–113], elective orthognathic surgical corrections [114] and even as fixation posts in aesthetic forehead/brow repositioning [115]. These clinical experiences have been similar to that of pediatric craniofacial surgery with good stability, no increased rates of infection and relatively few localized reactions during the resorptive process.

24.5. Future Trends and Needs

Bioabsorbable fixation has co-existed with metallic fixation for the past 20 years and will likely continue to do so for the foreseeable future. Bioabsorbable implant usage, however, should continue to grow over the next three to five years in response to several developments. First, as published clinical studies of efficacy accumulate, surgeons in certain specialties will more fully embrace the technology as sports medicine, trauma and craniofacial surgeons have done over the past decade. Second, surgeons will creatively apply existing implants to new applications, ultimately expanding their clinical role. One possibility would be to use cyanoacrylate adhesives to apply fixation plates to regions of thin or soft bone that might not be biomechanically suited to screw or other intraosseous fixation [116]. While this can currently be done, a "thinking outside of the box" approach such as this can expand the clinical role of bioabsorbable fixation. Third, surgeons and implant manufacturers will continue to collaborate on new implant designs for situations in which metal technology cannot be applied. A recent example is the development of bioabsorbable meniscal repair devices for which there is no metallic counterpart. Fourth, "hybrid" fixation devices comprised of bioabsorbable polymers impregnated with bioactive molecules such as antibiotics and growth factors can potentially reduce complications as well as enhance healing [117–118]. Currently, such devices largely remain in the experimental phase, but it is conceivable that some may reach the market within the next several years, following successful completion of regulatory requirements. Fifth, for bioabsorbable implants to further encroach into the realm of metals, the mechanical properties will require enhancement. Efforts are underway to combine bioabsorbable polymers with fillers such as bioceramics, but are also largely experimental at this time [119]. It is possible that some strength-enhanced composite materials will become available within the next few years.

24.6. Conclusions

Bioabsorbable internal fixation of hard and soft tissue has progressively evolved over the past 20 years. The clinical success rate using these devices has improved during this period, a function of better materials, implant designs and instruments, as well as improved understanding of where they may be effectively applied and where it is best to use metallic fixation. As stronger bioabsorbable materials are developed, these devices will further encroach into those applications currently dominated by metallic fixation. Once bioabsorbable implants, combined with bioactive molecules, become clinically available, a whole new chapter in internal fixation will begin.

References

1. Snyder CC. On the history of the suture. Plast Reconstr Surg 1976;58:401–406.
2. Sequin F, Texhammar R. AO/ASIF Instrumentation. Springer-Verlag, New York, p. 1981:27–30.
3. Ashammakhi N, Suuronen R, Tiainen J, Tormala P, Waris T. Spotlight on naturally absorbable osteofixation devices. J Craniofac Surg 2003;14:247–259.
4. Busam ML, Esther RJ, Obremskey WT. Hardware removal: indications and expectations. J Am Acad Orthop Surg 2006;14:113–120.
5. Middleton JC, Tipton AJ. Synthetic biodegradable polymers as orthopedic devices. Biomaterials 2000;21:2335–2346.
6. Hutmacher D, Hurzeler MB, Schliephake H. A review of material properties of biodegradable and bioresorbable polymers and devices for GTR and GRB applications. Int J Oral Maxillofac Implants 1996;11: 667–678.
7. Pietrzak WS. Principles of development and use of absorbable internal fixation. Tissue Eng 2000;6:425–433.
8. Burkart SS. The evolution of clinical applications of biodegradable implants in arthroscopic surgery. Biomaterials 2000;21:2631–2634.
9. Pietrzak WS, Sarver DR, Verstynen ML. Bioabsorbable polymer science for the practicing surgeon. 1997;8: 87–91.
10. Billmeyer FW. Textbook of Polymer Science. Wiley: Hoboken, NJ, 1984, 3rd Edition.
11. Rosen SL. Fundamental principles of polymeric materials. Wiley: Hoboken, NJ, 1993, 2nd Edition.
12. Pietrzak WS, Kumar M, Eppley BL. The influence of temperature on the degradation rate of LactoSorb copolymer. J Craniofac Surg 2003;14:176–183.
13. Vert M, Christel P, Chabot F, Leray J. Bioresorbable plastic materials for bone surgery. In: Macromolecular Biomaterials. Editors: Hastings GW, Ducheyne P, CRC Press, Inc., Boca Raton, 1984,p.119–142.
14. Vainionpaa S, Rokkanen P, Tormala P. Surgical applications of biodegradable polymers in human tissues. Prog Polym Sci 1989;14:679–716.
15. Pietrzak WS, Caminear DS, Perns SV. Mechanical characteristics of an absorbable copolymer internal fixation pin. J Foot Ankle Surg 2002;41:379–388.
16. Tormala P. Ultra-high strength, self-reinforced absorbable polymeric composites for applications in different disciplines of surgery. Clin Mater 1993;13:35–40.

17. Simon JA, Ricci JL, Di Cesare PE. Bioresorbable fracture fixation in orthopedics: A comprehensive review. Part I. Basic science and preclinical studies. Am J Orthop 1996;26:665–671.
18. Eppley BL, Reilly M. Degradation characteristics of PLLA-PGA bone fixation devices. J Craniofac Surg 1997;8:116–120.
19. Hovis WD, Watson JT, Bucholz RW. Biochemical and biomechanical properties of bioabsorbable implants used in fracture fixation. Tech Orthopaedics 1998; 13: 123–129.
20. Athanasiou KA, Agrawal CM, Barber FA, Burkhart SS. Orthopaedic applications for PLA-PGA biodegradable copolymers. Arthroscopy 1998;14: 726–737.
21. Li S. Hydrolytic degradation characteristics of aliphatic polyesters derived from lactic and glycolic acids. J Biomed Mater Res 1999;48:342–353.
22. Viljanen VV, Lindholm TS. Background of the early development of absorbable fixation devices. Tech Orthopaedics 1998; 13:117–122.
23. Landes CA, Ballon A, Roth C. In-patient versus in vitro degradation of P(L/DL)LA and PLGA. J Biomed Mater Res B Appl Biomater 2006:76:403–411.
24. Schakenraad JM, Hardonk MJ, Feijen J, Molenaar I, Nieuwenhuis P. Enzymatic activity toward poly(L-lactic acid) implants. J Biomed Mater Res 1990;24:529–545.
25. Meyer DC, Fucentese SF, Ruffieux K, Jacob HA, Gerber C. Mechanical Testing of absorbable suture anchors. Arthroscopy 2003;19:188–193.
26. Pietrzak WS, Sarver DR, Bianchini SD, D'Alessio K. Effect of simulated heating and shaping on mechanical properties of a bioabsorbable fracture plate material. J Biomed Mater Res 1997;38:17–24.
27. Daniels AU, Chang MKO, Andriano KP, Heller J. Mechanical properties of biodegradable polymers and composites proposed for internal fixation of bone. J Appl Biomater 1990;1:57–78.
28. Rovinsky D, Durkin RC, Otsuka NY. The use of bioabsorbables in the treatment of children's fractures. Tech Orthopaedics 1998; 13: 130–138.
29. Farrar DF, Gillson RK. Hydrolytic degradation of polyglyconate B: the relationship between degradation time, strength and molecular weight. Biomaterials 2002;23:3905–3912.
30. Powers DL, Sonawala M, Woolf SK, An YH, Hawkins R.Comparison of the biomechanics and histology of two soft-tissue fixators composed of bioabsorbable copolymers. J Biomed Mater Res. 2001;58:486–495.
31. Wiltfang J, Merten HA, Schultze-Mosgau S, Schrell U, Wenzel D, Kessler P. Biodegradable miniplates (LactoSorb): long-term results in infant minipigs and clinical results. J Craniofac Surg 2000;11:239–243.
32. An YH, Friedman RJ, Powers DL, Draughn RA, Latour RA Jr. Fixation of osteotomies using bioabsorbable screws in the canine femur. Clin Orthop Rel Res 1998;355:300–311.
33. Lajtai G, Schmiedhuber G, Unger F, Aitzetmuller G, Klein M, Noszian I, Orthner E. Bone tunnel remodeling at the site of biodegradable interference screws used for anterior cruciate ligament reconstruction: 5-year follow-up. Arthroscopy 2001;17:597–602.
34. Fink C, Benedetto KP, Hackl W, Hoser C, Freund MC, Rieger M. Bioabsorbable polyglyconate interference screw fixation in anterior cruciate ligament reconstruction: a prospective computed tomography-controlled study. Arthroscopy 2000;16: 491–498.
35. Bach FD, Carlier RY, Elis JB, Mompoint DM, Feydy A, Judet O, Beaufils P, Vallee C. Anterior cruciate ligament reconstruction with bioabsorbable polyglycolic acid interference screws: MR imaging follow-up. Radiology 2002;225:541–550.
36. Edwards RC, Kiely KD, Eppley BL. The fate of resorbable poly-L-lactic/polyglycolic acid (LactoSorb) bone fixation devices in orthognathic surgery. J Oral Maxillofac Surg 2001;59:19–25.

37. Eppley BL, Sadove AM. A comparison of resorbable and metallic fixation in healing of calvarial bone grafts. Plast Reconstr Surg 1995:96:316–322.
38. Caminear DS, Pavlovich R Jr. Pietrzak WS. Fixation of the chevron osteotomy with an absorbable copolymer pin for treatment of hallux valgus deformity. J Foot Ankle Surg 2005:44:203–210.
39. Larsen MW, Pietrzak WS, DeLee JC. Fixation of osteochondritis dissecans lesions using poly(L-lactic acid)/poly(glycolic acid) copolymer bioabsorbable screws. Am J Sports Med 33:68–76.
40. Gill LH, Martin DF, Coumas JM, Kiebzak GM. Fixation with bioabsorbable pins in chevron bunionectomy. J Bone Joint Surg Am 1997;79:1510–1518.
41. Waris E, Ashammakhi N, Kaarela O, Raatikainen T, Vasenius J. Use of bioabsorbable osteofixation devices in the hand. J Hand Surg 2004;29B:590–598.
42. Bostman O, Makela EA, Sodergard J, Hirvensalo E, Tormala P, Rokkanen P. Absorbable polyglycolide pins in internal fixation of fractures in children. J Pediatr Orthop 1993;13:242–245.
43. Kumar CR, Sood S, Ham S. Complications of bioresorbable fixation systems in pediatric neurosurgery. Childs Nerv Syst 2005;21:205–210.
44. H. Willenegger. AO/ASIF Instrumentation. Springer-Verlag, New York, 1981. p. 19–24.
45. Hofmann GO, Wagner FD. New implant designs for bioresorbable devices in orthopaedic surgery. Clin Mater 1993;14:207–215.
46. Pietrzak WS. Rapid cooling through the glass transition transiently increases ductility of PGA/PLLA copolymers: a proposed mechanism and implications for devices. J Mater Sci Mater Med 2007;18:1753–1763.
47. Eppley BL, Pietrzak WS. Bioabsorbable plate and screw fixation in craniomaxillofacial surgery. In: Biodegradable Polymeric Materials and Their Applications. Vol 2. Applications. Mallapragada S, Narasimhan B, eds. Stevenson Ranch, CA: American Scientific Publishers, 2006, p. 271–306.
48. An YH, Woolf SK, Friedman RJ. Pre-clinical in vivo evaluation of orthopaedic bioabsorbable devices. Biomaterials. 2000:21:2635–2652.
49. Athanasiou KA, Niederauer GG, Agrawal CM. Sterilization, toxicity, biocompatibility and clinical applications of polylactic acid/polyglycolic acid copolymers. Biomaterials 1996;17:93-93–102.
50. Brady JM, Cutright DE, Miller RA, Battistone GC. Resorption rate, route, route of elimination, and ultrastructure of the implant site of polylactic acid in the abdominal wall of the rat. J Biomed Mater Res. 1973;7:155–166.
51. Cutright DE, Hunsuck EE. The repair of fractures of the orbital floor using biodegradable polylactic acid. Oral Surg Oral Med Oral Pathol 1972;33:28–34.
52. Powers DL, Sonawala M, Wolf SK, An YH, Hawkins R, Pietrzak WS. Comparison of the biomechanics and histology of two soft-tissue fixators composed of bioabsorbable copolymers. J Biomed Mater Res 2001;58:486–495.
53. Pietrzak WS, Lessek TP, Perns SV. A bioabsorbable fixation implant for use in proximal interphalangeal joint (hammertoe) arthrodesis: Biomechanical testing in a synthetic bone substrate. J Foot Ankle Saurg 2006;45:288–294.
54. Cristofolini L, Viceconti M, Cappello A, Toni A. Mechanical validation of whole bone composite femur models. J Biomech 1996;29:525–535.
55. Thompson MS, McCarthy ID, Lidgren L, Ryd L. Compressive and shear properties of commercially available polyurethane foams. J Biomech Eng 2003;125:732–734.
56. Nurmi JT, Sievanen H, Kannus P, Jarvinen M, Jarvinen TL. Porcine tibia is a poor substitute for human cadaver tibia for evaluating interference screw fixation. Am J Sports Med 2004;32:765–771.
57. Biomechanical evaluation of a bioabsorbable expansion bolt for hamstring graft fixation in ACL reconstruction: an experimental study in calf tibial bone. Arch Orthop Trauma Surg. 2005;125:577–584.

58. Boenisch UW, Faber KJ, Ciarelli M, Steadman JR, Arnoczky SP. Pull-out strength and stiffness of meniscal repair using absorbable arrows or Ti-Cron vertical and horizontal loop sutures. 1999;27:626–631.
59. Dervin GF, Downing KJ, Keene GC, McBride DG. Failure strengths of suture versus biodegradable arrow for meniscal repair: an in vitro study. Arthroscopy 1997;13:296–300.
60. Eppley BL, Sadove AM. A comparison of resorbable and metallic fixation in healing of calvarial bone grafts. Plast Reconstr Surg 1995;96:316–322.
61. Bos RR, Rozema FR, Boering G, Nijenhuis AJ, Pennings AJ, Jansen HW. Bone-plates and screws of bioabsorbable poly (L-lactide)–an animal pilot study. Br J Oral Maxillofac Surg 1989;27:467–476.
62. Porter MD, Anderson MG. Results of bioabsobable fixation of metatarsal osteotomies. Am J Orthop 2004;33:609–611.
63. Barca F, Busa R. Austin/chevron osteotomy fixed with bioabsorbable poly-L-lactic acid single screw. J Foot Ankle Surg 1997;36:15–20.
64. Kaukonen JP, Lamberg T, Korkala O, Pajarinen J. Fixation of syndesmotic ruptures in 38 patients with a malleolar fracture: a randomized study comparing a metallic and a bioabsorbable screw. J Orthop Trauma 2005;19:392–395.
65. Sinisaari IP, Luthje PM, Mikkonen RH. Ruptured tibio-fibular syndesmosis: comparison of metallic to bioabsorbable fixation. Foot Ankle Int 2002;23:744–778.
66. Hovis WD, Kaiser BW, Watson JT, Bucholz RW. Treatment of syndesmotic disruptions of the ankle with bioabsorbable screw fixation. J Bone Joint Surg Am 2002;84-A(1):26–31.
67. Miller SD, Carls RJ. The bioresorbable syndesmotic screw: application of polymer technology in ankle fractures. Am J Orthop. 2002;31(1 Suppl):18–21.
68. Miller SL, Gladstone JN. Graft selection in anterior cruciate ligament reconstruction. Orthop Clin North Am 2002;33:675–683.
69. Harilainen A, Sandelin J, Jansson KA. Cross-pin femoral fixation versus metal interference screw fixation in anterior cruciate ligament reconstruction with hamstring tendons: results of a controlled prospective randomized study with 2-year follow-up. Arthroscopy 2005;21:25–33.
70. Piltz S, Dieckmann R, Meyer L, Strunk P, Plitz W, Lob G. Biomechanical evaluation of a bioabsorbable expansion bolt for hamstring graft fixation in ACL reconstruction: an experimental study in calf tibial bone. Arch Orthop Truama Surg 2005;125:577–584.
71. Brand JC Jr, Nyland J, Caborn DN, Johnson DL. Soft-tissue interference fixation: bioabsorbable screw versus metal screw. Arthroscopy 2005;21:911–916.
72. Benedetto KP, Fellinger M, Lim TE, Passler JM, Schoen JL, Willems WJ. A new bioabsorbable interference screw: preliminary results of a prospective, multicenter, randomized clinical trial. Arthroscopy 2000;16:41–48.
73. Hackl W, Fink C, Benedetto KP, Hoser C. [Transplant fixation by anterior cruciate ligament reconstruction. Metal vs. bioabsorbable polyglyconate interference screw. A prospective randomized study of 40 patients] Unfallchirung 2000;103:468–474.
74. Kaeding C, Farr J, Kavanaugh T, Pedroza A. A prospective randomized comparison of bioabsorbable and titanium anterior cruciate ligament interference screws. Arthroscopy 2005;21:147–151.
75. Hersekli MA, Akpinar S, Ozalay M, Ozkoc G, Cesur N, Uysal M, Pourbagher A, Tandogan RN. Tunnel enlargement after arthroscopic anterior cruciate ligament reconstruction: comparison of bone-patellar tendon-bone and hamstring autografts. Adv Ther 2004;21:123–131.
76. Robinson J, Huber C, Jaraj P, Colombet P, Allard M, Meyer P. Reduced bone tunnel enlargement post hamstring ACL reconstruction with poly-l-lactic acid/hydroxyapatite bioabsorbable screws. Knee 2006;13:127–131.

77. Baums MH, Zelle BA, Schultz W, Ernstberger T, Klinger HM. Intraarticular migration of a broken biodegradable interference screw after anterior cruciate ligament reconstruction. Knee Surg Sports Traumatol Arthrosc 2006;14:865–868.
78. Krappel FA, Bauer E, Harland U. The migration of a BioScrew® as differential diagnosis of knee pain, locking after ACL reconstruction: a report of two cases. Arch Orthop Trauma Surg 2006;126:615–620.
79. Lembeck B, Wulker N. Severe cartilage damage by broken poly-L-lactic acid (PLLA) interference screw after ACL reconstruction. Knee Surg Sports Traumatol Arthrosc 2005;13:283–286.
80. Barber FA, Herbert MA, Richards DP. Load to failure testing of new meniscal repair devices. Arthroscopy 2004;20:45–50.
81. Oberlander MA, Chisar MA. Meniscal repair using the Polysorb meniscal stapler XLS. Arthroscopy 2005;21:1148e1–1148e5.
82. Barber FA, Johnson DH, Halbrecht JL. Arthroscopic meniscal repair using the BioStinger. Arthroscopy 2005;21:744–750.
83. Farng E, Sherman O. Meniscal repair devices: a clinical and biomechanical literature review. Arthroscopy 2004;20:273–286.
84. Gliatis J, Kouzelis A, Panagopoulos A, Lambiris E. Chondral injury due to migration of a Mitek RapidLoc meniscal repair implant after successful meniscal repair: a case report. Knee Surg Sports Traumatol Arthrosc 2004
85. Chondral injury due to migration of a Mitek RapidLoc meniscal repair implant after successful meniscal repair: a case report. Knee Surg Sports Traumatol Arthrosc 2005;13:280–282.
86. Page SM, Stern PJ. Complications and range of motion following plate fixation of metacarpal and phalangeal fractures. J Hand Surg 1998;28:827–832.
87. Hughes TB. Bioabsorbable implants in the treatment of hand fractures: an update. Clin Orthop Relat Res 2006;445:169–174.
88. Waris E, Ninkovic M, Harpf C, Ninkovic M, Ashammakhi N. Self-reinforced bioabsorbable miniplates for skeletal fixation in complex hand injury: three case reports. J Hand Surg [Am] 2004;29:452–457.
89. Kujala S, Raatikainen T, Kaarela O, Aschammakhi N, Ryhanen J. Successful treatment of scaphoid fractures and nonunions using bioabsorbable screws: report of six cases. J Hand Surg [Am] 2004;29:68–73.
90. Lionelli GT, Korentager RA. Biomechanical failure of metacarpal fracture resorbable plate fixation. Ann Plast Surg 2002;49:202–206.
91. Gangopadhyay S, Ravi K, Packer G. Dorsal plating of unstable distal radius fractures using a bio-absorbable plating system and bone substitute. J Hand Surg [Br] 2005;31:93–100.
92. Mittal R, Morley J, Dinopoulos H, Drakoulakis EG, Vermani E, Giannoudis PV. Use of bio-absorbable implants for stabilization of distal radius fractures: the United Kingdom patients' perspective. Injury 2005;36:333–338.
93. Vaccaro AR, Carrino JA, Venger BH, Albert T, Kelleher PM, Hilibrand A, Singh K. Use of a bioabsorbable anterior cervical plate in the treatment of cervical degenerative and traumatic disc disruption. J Neurosurg 2002;97(4 Suppl):473–480.
94. Vaccaro AR, Singh K, Haid R, Kitchel S, Wuisman P, Taylor W, Branch C, Garfin S. The use of bioabsorbable implants in the spine. Spine J 2003;3:227–237.
95. Park MS, Aryan HE, Ozgur BM, Jandial R, Taylor WR. Stabilization of anterior cervical spine with bioabsorbable polymer in one- and two-level fusions. Neurosurgery 2004;54:631–635.
96. Brunon J, Duthel R, Fotso MJ, Tudor C. [Anterior osteosynthesis of the cervical spine by phusiline bioresorbable screws and plates. Initial results apropos of 5 cases] Neurochirugie 1994;40:196–202.
97. McBirnie JM, Minianci A, Miniaci SL. Arthroscopic repair of full-thickness rotator cuff tears using bioabsorbable tacks. Arthroscopy 2005;21:1421–1427.

98. Freedman KB, Smith AP, Romeo AA, Cole BJ, Bach BR. Open Bakart repair versus arthroscopic repair with transglenoid sutures or bioabsorbable tacks for recurrent anterior instability of the shoulder. A meta-analysis. Am J Sports Med 2004;32:1520–1527.
99. Magee T, Shapiro M, Hewell G, Williams D. Complications of rotator cuff surgery in which bioabsorbable anchors are used. Am J Roentgenol 2003;181:1227–1231.
100. Cummins CA, Strickland S, Appleyard RC, Szomor ZL, Marshall J, Murrell GAC. Arthroscopy 2003;19:239–248.
101. Eppley BL, Morales L, Wood R, Pensler J, Goldstein J, Havlik RJ, Habal M, Losken A, Williams JK, Burnstein F, Rozzelle AA, Sadove AM. Resorbable PLLA-PGA plate and screw fixation in pediatric craniofacial surgery: clinical experience in 1883 patients. Plast Reconstr Surg 2004;114:850–856.
102. Papay FA, Hardy S, Morales L Jr., Walker M, Enlow D. "False" migration of rigid fixation appliances in pediatric craniofacial surgery. J Craniofac Surg 1995;6: 309–313.
103. Beck J, Parent A, Angel MF. Chronic headache as a sequela of rigid fixation for craniosynostosis. J Craniofac Surg 2002;13:327–330.
104. Duke BJ, Mouchantat RA, Ketch LL, Winston KR. Transcranial migration of microfixation plates and screws. Case report. Pediatr Neurosurg 1996;25:31–34.
105. Goldberg DS, Bartlett S, Yu JC, Hunter JV, Whitaker LA. Critical review of microfixation in pediatric craniofacial surgery. 1995;6:301–307.
106. Berryhill WE, Rimell FL, Ness J, Marentette L, Haines SJ. Fate of rigid fixation in pediatric craniofacial surgery. Otolaryngol Head Neck Surg 1999;121:269–273.
107. Barone CM, Jimenez DF. Special considerations in pediatric cranial fixation: a technical overview. J Craniomaxillofac Trauma 1996;2:42–47.
108. Pietrzak WS, Verstynen ML, Sarver DR. Bioabsorbable fixation devices: status for the craniomaxillofacial surgeon. J Craniofac Surg 1997;8:92–96.
109. Eppley BL. Use of resorbable plate and screw fixation in pediatric craniofacial surgery. Operative Tech Plast Surg 2003;9:36–45.
110. Eppley BL, Li M. Long spanning resorbable plates in cranial vault reconstruction. J Craniofac Surg 2003;14:89–91.
111. Eppley BL. Repair of midfacial fractures using resorbable plates and screws. Operative Tech Otolaryngology Head-Neck Surg 2002;13:287–292.
112. Eppley BL. Zygomaticomaxillary fracture repair with resorbable plates and screws. J Craniofac Surg 2000;11:377–385.
113. Eppley BL. Use of a resorbable fixation technique for maxillary fractures. J Craniofac Surg 1998;9:317–321.
114. Edwards RC, Kiely KD, Eppley BL. Fixation of bimaxillary osteotomies with resorbable plates and screws: initial experience in 20 consecutive cases. J Oral Maxillofac Surg 2001;59:271–276.
115. Eppley BL, Coleman JJ 3rd, Sood R, Ha RY, Sadove AM. Resorbable screw fixation technique for endoscopic brow and midfacial lifts. Plast Reconstr Surg 1998;102:241–243.
116. Ahn DK, Sims CD, Randolf MA, O'Connor D, Butler PE, Amarante MT, Yaremchuk MJ. Craniofacial skeletal fixation using biodegradable plates and cyanoacrylate glue. Plast Reconsr Surg 1997;99:1508–1515.
117. Makinen TJ, Veiranto M, Knuuti J, Jalava J, Tormala P, Aro HT. Efficacy of bioabsorbable antibiotic containing bone screw in the prevention of biomaterial-related infection due to Staphylocuccus aureus. Bone 2005;36:292–299.
118. Tieline L, Puolakkainen P, Pohjonen T, Rautavuori J, Tormala P, Rokkanen P. The effect of transforming growth factor-beta1, released from a bioabsorbable self-reinforced polylactide pin, on a bone defect. Biomaterials 2002;23:3817–3823.
119. Bleach NC, Nazhat SN, Tanner KE, Kellomaki M, Tormala P. Effect of filler content on mechanical and dynamic mechanical properties of particulate biphasic calcium phosphate–polylactide composites. Biomaterials 2002;23:1579–1585

25

Tissue Adhesives: Science, Products and Clinical Use

William D. Spotnitz

Abstract: The field of tissue adhesives is a new and rapidly developing area of surgical technology. Since the approval of the first such agent, fibrin sealant in the Unites States in 1998, five distinct families of agents have emerged with a wide variety of Food and Drug Administration (FDA) approved indications. These indications include hemostasis, colon sealing, skin closure, lung sealing, vascular sealing and dural sealing. These materials are not only useful in many different surgical specialties including cardiac, thoracic, vascular, general, plastic, transplant, trauma and neurologic surgery, but can also be used in a variety of experimental applications such as drug delivery and tissue engineering. The object of this chapter is to review the five new families of tissue adhesives and hemostats with particular emphasis on the relevant chemistry, available products and clinical uses, as well as future experimental and clinical applications. The chemical reactions basic to these materials, commercially available products, clinical algorithms for use and potential future developments will be described.

The five families are fibrin sealants, cyanoacrylates, bovine gelatin and human thrombin, polyethylene glycol polymers and albumin cross-linked with glutaraldehyde. Multiple commercially approved products now exist within these families and represent novel additions to the traditional surgical armamentarium of ligatures, sutures, clips and staples. As the technical challenges of the modern surgical environment continue to increase with the widespread use of minimally invasive procedures, the need for surgical tissue adhesives will continue to grow and this remains an important area of future research and development.

Keywords: Hemostats, sealants, tissue adhesives, algorithms, fibrin sealant, cyanoacrylates, gelatin and thrombin, polyethylene glycol (PEG) polymers, albumin, glutaraldehyde.

Surgical Therapeutic Advancement Center, Department of Surgery, University of Virginia Health System, Charlottesville, VA

From: *Orthopedic Biology and Medicine: Musculoskeletal Tissue Regeneration, Biological Materials and Methods*
Edited by W. S. Pietrzak © Humana Press, Totowa, NJ

25.1. Introduction

The field of tissue adhesives, including hemostats and sealants is rapidly growing. Since the approval of fibrin sealant by the Food and Drug Administration (FDA) in 1998, new products are now being developed on an almost yearly basis. These materials are designed to work in clinical situations where traditional surgical techniques such as sutures, clips or cautery may not be effective. As more minimally invasive surgical approaches are implemented, the technical challenges for the surgeon continue to increase. Laparoscopic, thoracoscopic, endoscopic and robotic approaches are just a few of the new ways by which patient care is being enhanced. These modern methods are improving patient care by allowing for smaller incisions and less morbidity, but are simultaneously increasing the skills required by the surgeon. In this setting tissue adhesives are entering the armamentarium as additional weapons capable of helping the surgeon in this rapidly changing 21st Century surgical environment.

A comparison of surgeons and master carpenters is helpful in understanding the usefulness of tissue adhesives. A master carpenter would not think of creating fine cabinets without saws, nails and glues. On the other hand, surgeons have had scalpels and sutures to help in surgical procedures, but have not had effective surgical glues. Thus, the development of efficacious tissue adhesives is the solution to a significant surgical need. An additional comparison includes the fact that carpenters actually have a wide variety of glues that are used in specific environments such as the bonding of wood, metal and plastic. A variety of surgical tissue adhesives are also now either available or under development. Each has specific indications and usefulness. Presently approved indications include hemostasis and skin closure, as well as sealing of colon, blood vessels and dura. In this chapter the methods of action, available products and clinical indications for the present five families of tissue adhesives will be reviewed. These families are fibrin sealants, cyanoacrylates, gelatin and thrombin, polyethylene glyclol (PEG) polymers and albumin cross-linked with glutaraldehyde.

It would be remiss to proceed without mentioning a framework for evaluating tissue adhesives. There are five criteria which can be used to judge these materials, including efficacy, safety, usefulness, cost and regulatory approvability. No one agent can be expected to work in all situations, but the ideal agent would have certain specific characteristics. It would be effective in its use and might be expected to even have applications in multiple surgical specialties. Thus, a cardiac surgeon might desire a quickly acting agent to rapidly stop bleeding, while a plastic surgeon might want a more slowly polymerizing material which would allow for positioning of skin flaps and grafts before achieving final fixation. In addition the product should be safe with no risk of infectious, inflammatory, immunologic or carcinogenic side effects. Its ease of use is also important. Complex preparation or reconstitution of adhesive components is not desirable in modern operating rooms where personnel time is at a premium. Application of the tissue adhesives needs to be as easy and as technically tailored as possible. The material itself must be straightforward to use so that it can be easily spread and controlled. Also, a wide variety of applicators capable of dripping and spraying the agents during different procedures such as endoscopic and laparoscopic surgery should be available. The cost of these materials is also not a trivial issue. Hospital administrators and operating room supervisors are carefully monitoring costs and reimbursement for all items used in the operating room. Cost-benefit analysis for tissue adhesive use is important and these materials will gain wider acceptance if they have clearly demonstrated financial as well as clinical benefits. Cost benefits as well as efficacy and safety should be considered in randomized multicenter clinical trials. Finally, the approvability of these agents is not an insignificant matter. Fibrin sealant was approved for clinical use in Europe 25 years before its first approval in the United States in 1998. Thus, developing materials that can reasonably traverse the regulatory approval process by the FDA is an important requirement.

It is also useful to understand the learning environment of the surgeon-in-training when discussing new technologies. Surgeons learn not only by reading and studying, but by experience. In many ways the training of a surgeon is an apprenticeship. Thus, new tissue adhesives should not only be easy to use, but should be integrated elements of surgical training programs in the operating room, just as established methods such as dissection and suturing are today. As the capabilities of tissue adhesives are improved, surgeons will use them more and more. However, clear and easily obtained educational programs for their effective and safe use remain important.

Finally, it is important to emphasize that tissue adhesives have both on- and off- label surgical uses. All of the on-label FDA-approved applications of these materials will be discussed in this chapter. However, many off-label unapproved indications will also be mentioned when supported by the literature and personal experience. Clinical reviews of the use of these materials exist in many specialties as diverse as cardiac [1] and plastic surgery [2].

25.2. Methods of Action and Products

25.2.1. Fibrin Sealants

Fibrin sealants were approved for use in the United States in 1998 for hemostasis in cardiac surgery [3], and were the first family of available tissue adhesives in the United States. Fibrin sealant is a two component biologic material (Fig. 25.1) based on the interaction of pooled plasma blood products, fibrinogen and thrombin. In the setting of trace elements of factor XIII and calcium, fibrin is formed which may require stabilization by antifibrinolytic agents. The sealant polymerizes in 30 seconds to three minutes. The two presently approved commercial products are Tisseel VH® (Baxter, Westlake Village, CA) and Evicel™ (Johnson & Johnson, Somerville, NJ). Both of these products are manufactured abroad. Tisseel is made by Baxter Immuno (Vienna, Austria) and Evicel is manufactured by Omrix Biopharmaceuticals (Ramat-Gan, Israel). Fibrin sealants are made by deriving fibrinogen and thrombin from pooled plasma obtained from screened human donors. Thus, they have at least a theoretical risk of viral or prion (Jakob Creutzfeldt) disease transmission. Viral inactivation techniques are used in these products. Tisseel employs cryoprecipitation, adsorption, vapor heating and freeze-drying. Evicel uses cryoprecipitation, pasteurization, solvent detergent cleansing and nanofiltration to reduce the risk of viral disease transmission. Tisseel requires an antifibrinolytic agent, bovine aprotinin (Trasylol, Bayer, West Haven, CN). Aprotinin carries a risk of immunologic responses including allergy and

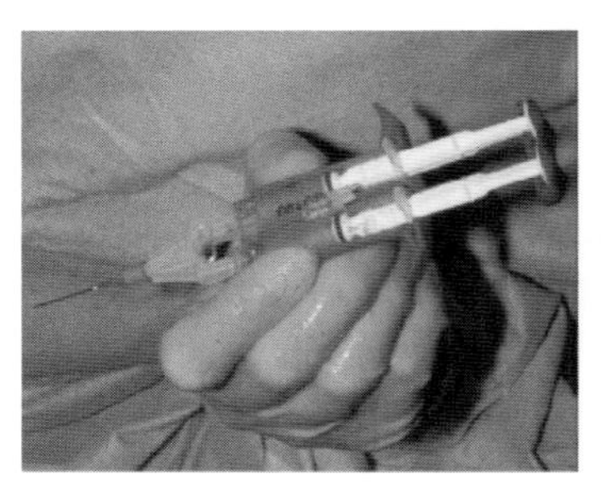
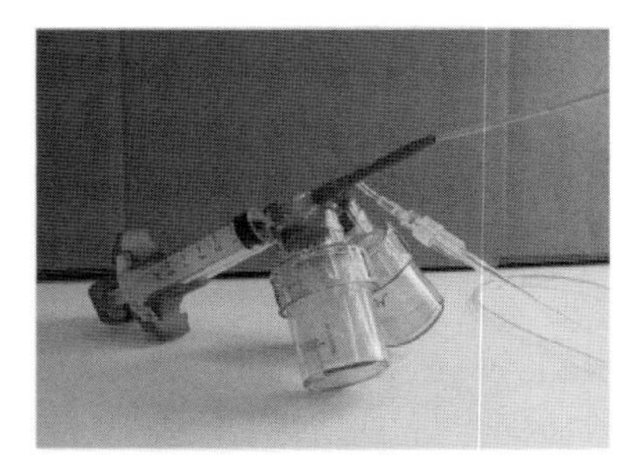

Fig. 25.1 Applicators for Tisseel and Crosseal fibrin sealants showing a system for drip application (left) and spray application (right)

anaphylaxis. Evicel was recently developed and approved for sale and does not require any antifibrinolytic for stabilization because it is plasminogen-reduced. Thus, the contraindications related to possible seizure activity (as a result of gamma aminobutyric acid inhibition) associated with earlier forms of fibrin sealant (Crosseal™, Johnson & Johnson, Somerville, NJ) containing tranexamic acid have now been eliminated.

Tisseel is approved for hemostasis in cardiac surgical and splenic trauma procedures to achieve hemostasis. It is also approved for sealing of a colon anastomosis at the time of colostomy closure. It contains fibrinogen (75–115 mg/ml), thrombin (500 IU/ml), aprotinin (3,000 KIU/ml) and calcium (40 μmol/ml). The manufacturer provides Tisseel in 0.5, 1, 2 and 5 ml kits. A variety of needle and spray devices, as well as applicators for laparoscopic and endoscopic use, can be obtained. Storage is recommended in a refrigerator, but it can be stored at room temperature for up to six months.

Evicel is approved for hemostasis in liver surgery. It consists of two elements, a biologically active component (BAC), containing fibrinogen (50 mg/ml) and a separate thrombin (1,000 IU/ml) component. Calcium (5.9 mg/ml) is also contained in Evicel. The product is provided in 1, 2 and 5 ml kits which are designed for needless transfer. The fibrin sealant is supplied with a triple lumen applicator to avoid clogging, which is capable of both drip and spray application. Evicel can be stored frozen for two years, in the refrigerator for 30 days and at room temperature for 24 hours.

One additional commercial form of fibrin sealant is available and is distributed under the name Vitagel™ (formerly Costasis®) by Angiotech (Herndon, VA). This product allows for the patient's own blood to be centrifuged to obtain plasma which can be used in combination with bovine thrombin and collagen (included in the kit) to make a low fibrin concentration form of collagen augmented fibrin sealant. The primary risk of this material is related to the bovine thrombin and includes potential coagulopathy from human antibodies to impurities, bovine factor V and bovine thrombin which can cross-react with human clotting proteins and cause bleeding [4].

A product related to fibrin sealant is platelet gel [5]. Devices are commercially available which can produce platelet gel from a patient's own blood (Magellan™ Autologous Platelet Separator System, Medtronic, Memphis, TN). Platelet gel consists of platelet-rich plasma combined with bovine thrombin and has the risks of coagulopathy, as mentioned above for Vitagel. Its advantages are the absence of pooled fibrinogen reducing the risk of blood-borne disease transmission, and the presence of platelets rich in growth factors which are thought to aid in the healing process of wounds. The combination of platelet-rich plasma and bovine thrombin to make the final product of platelet-rich gel has not been evaluated by the FDA as a commercial product.

Finally, there are a variety of blood bank methods including cryoprecipitation [6] to make concentrated fibrinogen which, in combination with commercially available bovine thrombin (Thrombin-JMI®, King Pharmaceuticals, Bristol, Tennessee), can produce a noncommercial form of fibrin sealant. Devices (Cryoseal®, Thermogenesis, Rancho Cordova, CA) to aid in the cryoprecipitation of plasma to make concentrated fibrinogen are commercially available.

An extensive literature of several thousand papers exists detailing the clinical uses of fibrin sealant in large numbers of different surgical specialties [7].

25.2.2. Cyanoacrylates

Cyanoacrylates are approved for use as adjuncts to wound closure when the skin is not under tension, and have also been approved for use as a wound bacterial barrier. They have been used extensively for closure of traumatic lacerations and small surgical incisions in wounds without hair or mucosal surfaces [8]. Placement of deep dermal sutures in addition to topical skin application of cyanoacrylates is recommended to minimize the tension on the wound. Cyanoacrylates work by bonding to the superficial layers of the skin for several days before these layers are naturally exfoliated in the normal process of skin regeneration. Thus, there is no need to remove the adhesive as it is normally sloughed in about seven days. However, because the closure is only as strong as the bond of the superficial layers of skin to the deeper dermis, there is a risk of wound dehiscence if these products are not used with deep dermal or subcuticular sutures.

Cyanoacrylates have strong internal and adherence bonding strength. They achieve significant strength within 30 seconds of application and function by polymerizing during an exothermic reaction in the presence of hydroxyl groups in tissues. Cyanoacrylates undergo biodegradation in a reaction which results in the formation of cyanoacetate and formaldehyde, which can both be toxic. The inflammatory or carcinogenic [9] potential of cyanoacrylates, as well as their degradation rates, are inversely proportional to the length of their alkoxycarbonyl (-COOR) side chains. Thus, the longer the side chains the slower the breakdown and formation of toxic degradation products. Therefore, 2-octyl cyanoacrylate (Dermabond™, Johnson & Johnson, Somerville, NJ) and n-butyl-2-cyanoacrylate (Indermil®, United States Surgical, Norwalk, CT) with longer side chains have had safety profiles satisfactory for human topical application and regulatory approval by the FDA.

These agents can be stored at room temperature, although long-term storage may be better at refrigerator temperatures between 2° C and 5° C. They come

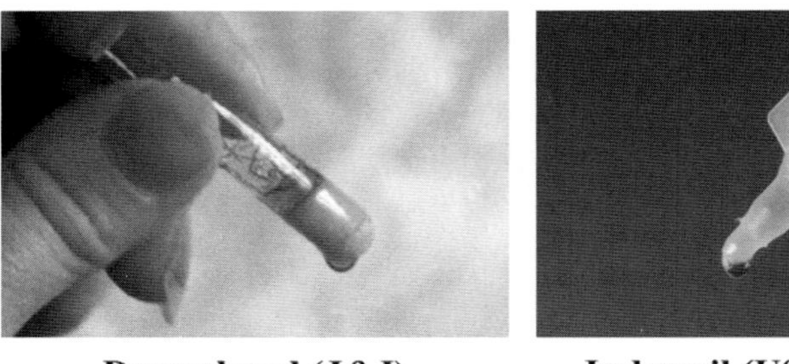

Fig. 25.2 Container applicators for Dermabond (left) and Indermil (right) cyanoacrylate tissue adhesives which are indicated for the closure of low tension skin wounds, preferably with deep dermal or subcuticular sutures

in small container 0.5 ml ampoule applicators (Fig. 25.2) which allow the liquids to be painted on to skin wounds. A higher viscosity form of Dermabond is now available in a pen-like applicator which makes the liquid less likely to run quickly to dependent body areas. Wounds should be carefully cleaned and dried with excellent hemostasis prior to application of these tissue adhesives. The manufacturer recommends applying three layers to the skin of the wound, separated by 30 seconds, with a one centimeter band width of application to each side of the wound. The material is particularly effective for reducing pain and the emotional trauma of wound closure in children. The material produces a cosmetic appearance equivalent to wounds closed with sutures alone. This method avoids the need for suture removal following wound healing. During application, some patients are aware of a sensation of heat release due to the exothermic reaction. The biggest risk is inadvertent application to the eye lids resulting in tight closure during facial surgical procedures. Wound dehiscence is another complication of this material.

25.2.3. Gelatin and Thrombin

This material is a particularly effective hemostatic agent [10]. It combines the passive and active biologic hemostatic effects of gelatin swelling (20% within 10 minutes) and thrombin clotting, respectively, with the ability to apply manual pressure which is usually the first mainstay of achieving hemostasis in surgery. The gelatin and thrombin mixture is prepared within minutes using a pre-filled gelatin containing syringe, as well as liquid thrombin. This mixture has the consistency of toothpaste or cream of wheat and stays where it is placed, even when there is active bleeding (Fig. 25.3). The agent can be used in conjunction with manual pressure from a moist operating room gauze or a lap pad as the gelatin and thrombin are only activated on contact with the fibrinogen contained in the blood of an actively bleeding wound. Thus, the hemostatic agent will not stick to the non-bloody moist surfaces of a gauze or lap pad. The agent can also be re-applied by using the applicator to place additional material in close proximity to the source of bleeding. Hemostasis is usually achieved within two minutes.

Gelatin and Thrombin

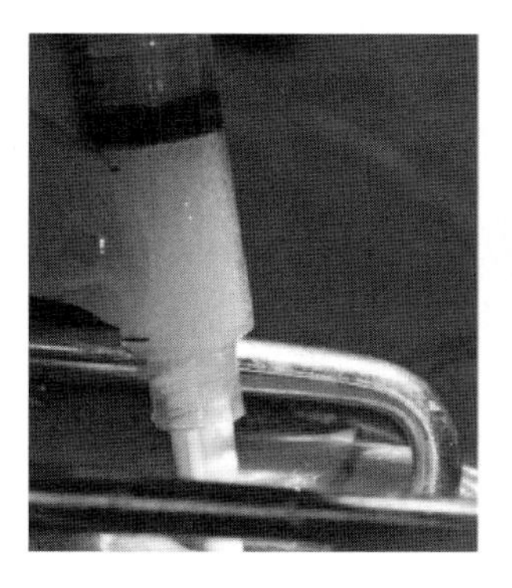

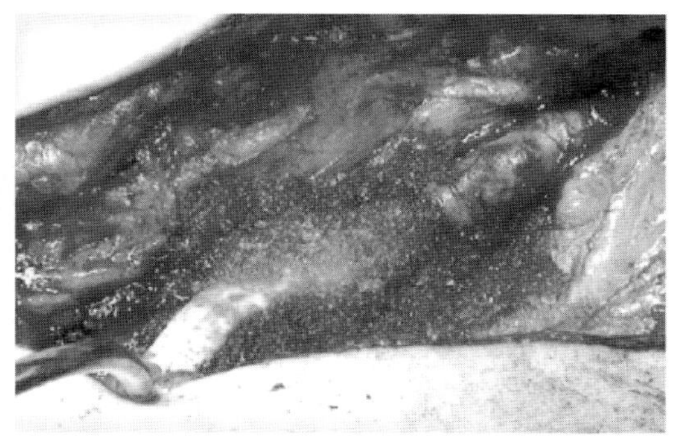

Floseal (Baxter)

Fig. 25.3 The applicator and appearance of Floseal gelatin and thrombin, which can be used as an effective hemostatic material

Gelatin and thrombin is supplied commercially as Floseal™ (Baxter, Fremont, CA) and comes in kits containing gelatin and human thrombin (500 IU/ml) reaching a final volume of 5 ml after mixing. The manufacturer has replaced bovine thrombin previously used in this material with virally inactivated pooled human thrombin to avoid the risks of coagulopathy associated with bovine thrombin [4] which were discussed in a previous section. The kits are stored at room temperature. Curved stainless steel as well as longer endoscopic applicators are available and can be sterilized for repeated use. The material is biodegraded within six to eight weeks. Risks beyond those associated with human pooled plasma thrombin are those of allergic reaction to bovine gelatin.

An alternative form of this product is provided as Surgiflo™ (Johnson & Johnson, Somerville, NJ). This product consists of gelatin in a syringe applicator set which allows the gelatin to be combined with saline or thrombin. The only approved source of stand-alone thrombin in the United States at the time of this writing is bovine thrombin (Thrombin-JMI, King Pharmaceuticals, Bristol, TN) and its use may be associated with the antibody-induced coagulopathy previously discussed for bovine thrombin in the fibrin sealant section.

25.2.4. Polyethylene Glycol (PEG) Polymers

These synthetic products are hydrogels which are highly absorptive of water. PEG polymers were first used as a commercially available tissue adhesive in Focalseal®-L (Genzyme, Cambridge, MA) lung sealant. This product required a primer, a hydrogel which was activated by light, and a light source. It was relatively cumbersome to use and is no longer available for sale.

Presently two PEG polymer hydrogels [11, 12] are available commercially (Fig. 25.4). Coseal™ (Baxter, Fremont, CA) for vascular sealing and Duraseal® (Confluent Surgical, Waltham, MA) for dural sealing are FDA-approved.

Coseal is made from two PEG polymers which are activated upon mixing and polymerize significantly by 60 seconds. The material swells by 400

PEG Polymers

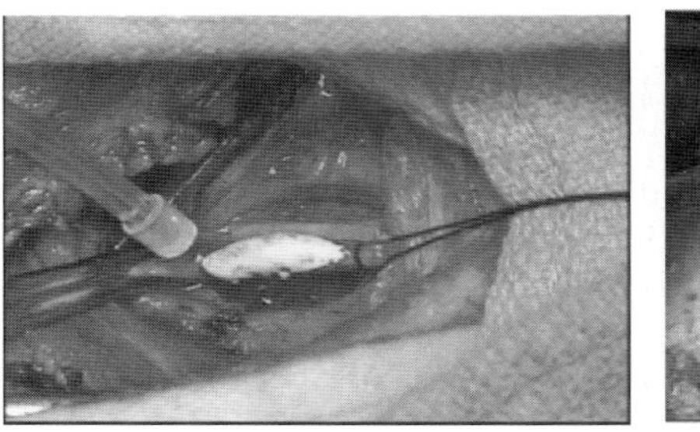

Coseal (Baxter)

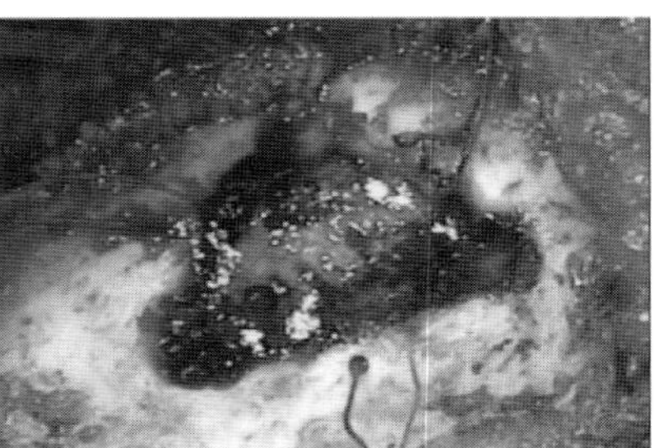

Duraseal (Confluent)

Fig. 25.4 Coseal (left) and Duraseal (right) are PEG polymer hydrogels approved for vascular and dural sealing, respectively

percent over 24 hours. It is storable at room temperature and is provided in 2, 4 and 8 ml kits. The kits include an applicator which mixes the two PEG components from separate syringes and sprays the material onto a vascular anastomosis. It is recommended for application to dry tissues at a distance of 3 cm and for use within three hours of preparation. Coseal is absorbed in about four weeks.

Duraseal is a single PEG polymer sealant which is provided in dual syringes. One contains the polyethylene glycol polymer ester (clear) and the other contains trilysine amine solution with FD&C Blue #1 dye. The dual syringe applicator allows for spraying 4 ml of the material from a distance of 2 to 4 cm onto the dural closure site and the material swells by approximately 50 percent. Duraseal is hydrolyzed in four to eight weeks. It should be used within one hour of preparation.

The risk profiles of these synthetic products are relatively benign.

25.2.5. Albumin Cross-linked with Glutaraldehyde

This material is composed of purified bovine serum albumin (BSA) and glutaraldehyde. The glutaraldehyde creates covalent bonds within the albumin as well as between the albumin and adjacent tissues allowing for the strong adhesive effect. The aldehyde groups of glutaraldehyde react with amine groups, specifically lysine, of albumin and tissue surfaces creating a strong internal adhesive as well as adhesive to surface adherence bonds. Bioglue® (Cryolife, Kennesaw, GA) is approved for vascular sealing of large blood vessels [13]. The BSA is treated with heat precipitation and chromatographic techniques to remove viruses and bovine spongiform encephalitis causative agent. It is also terminally sterilized with gamma irradiation. The material is supplied for use in either an applicator gun (Fig. 25.5) containing 5 ml, or by a syringe applicator in 2, 5 and 10 ml sizes. Applicator tips are available in a variety of lengths. Bioglue polymerizes in 30 seconds to two minutes and biodegrades over a period of months. Complications associated with the adhesive include nerve dysfunction, microemboli [14] and limitation of anastomotic growth. It has been a particularly useful agent in aortic dissection procedures.

Albumin & Glutaraldehyde

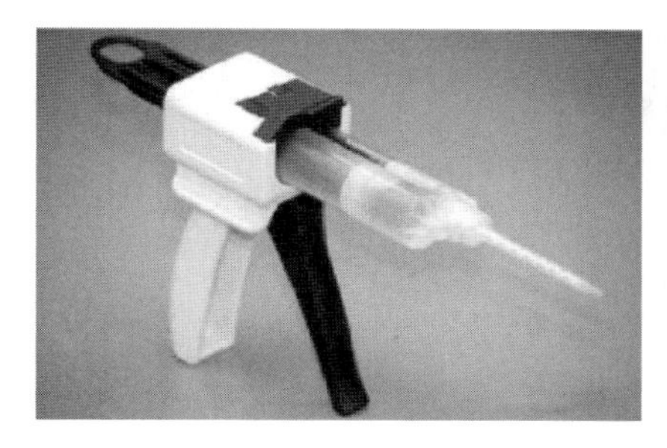

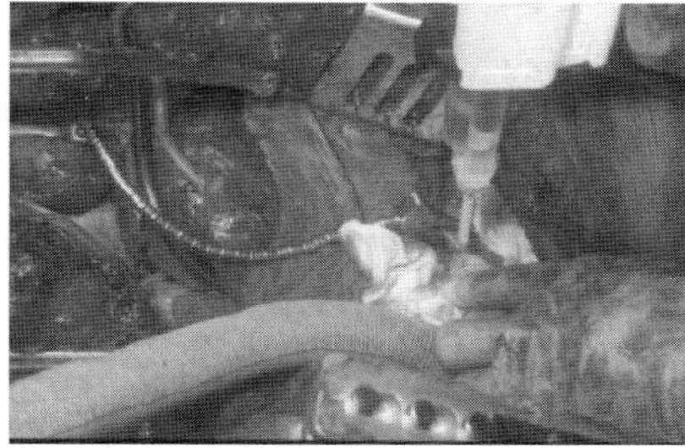

Bioglue (Cryolife)

Fig. 25.5 Bioglue gun applicator (left) and application in large vessel vascular surgery (right)

25.3. Clinical Use

The following discussion of algorithms is based on my own surgical experience, as well as my own clinical synthesis of the literature. Clearly, each surgeon may prefer to develop his or her own algorithms to fit their personal practice. In addition, the previous sections have included only the FDA-approved indications for these materials. In the following sections, additional off-label indications will be added, based on literature and my clinical experience.

25.3.1. Hemostasis Algorithm

The materials which have been reviewed with respect to hemostatic efficacy are fibrin sealant (Tisseel and Evicel) and gelatin and thrombin (Floseal). Neither is a substitute for excellent surgical technique or an appropriate use of sutures or cautery. Also, these agents will not be effective for massive bleeding possibly requiring sutures or patches. However, for bleeding not appropriately treated with sutures or cautery, these two products are very useful. The effectiveness of these agents depends on the source (arterial or venous) and the location (localized or diffuse) of bleeding. Decisions about which material to use in any given setting can be mapped in an algorithm (Fig. 25.6). For localized arterial bleeding, gelatin and thrombin is an excellent choice because it is not easily dislodged by a stream of blood (toothpaste-like consistency) and it can be combined with manual pressure by the surgeon. It can also be used for more diffuse arterial bleeding, but it is not easily spread over a large surface area. Fibrin sealant, on the other hand, is initially a liquid and can be washed away from the operative field by a stream of arterial blood before it ever polymerizes. Thus, fibrin sealant for arterial bleeding of a localized or diffuse nature should be used with a carrier sponge which can be used to deliver the sealant to the bleeding site and also allows application of pressure to the sponge by the surgeon. A similar set of recommendations exists for localized venous bleeding. The only difference is that when there is diffuse bleeding such as that from surgical adhesions, spray application of fibrin sealant can be

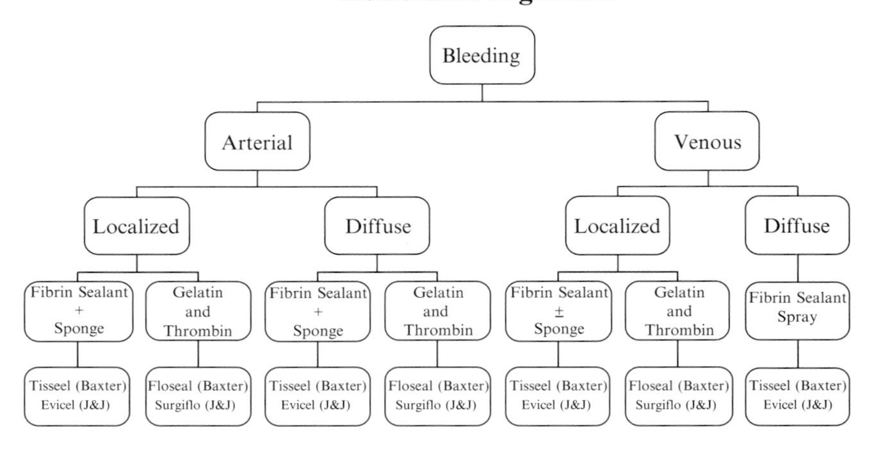

Fig. 25.6 Algorithm for the application of active hemostatic agents, fibrin sealant and gelatin and thrombin, to bleeding sites

very effective since it can be distributed nicely over a large area with excellent mixing of the two sealant components. The liquid sealant is not rapidly washed away by slow diffuse venous bleeding, thereby allowing time for the sealant to fully polymerize. Gelatin and thrombin is not an effective means for prophylactic prevention of bleeding since it will not be activated in the absence of blood fibrinogen. However, since Fibrin sealant contains both fibrinogen and thrombin, it can be used as a preventive sealant because it polymerizes without a source of active bleeding.

25.3.2. Tissue Adherence Algorithm

The available materials for this application can be used for bonding the skin edges of surgical wounds as well as for connecting tissue flaps (Fig. 25.7). Cyanoacrylates (Dermabond and Indermil) can be used to approximate the epidermis after placement of deep dermal or subcuticular sutures and also serve as a bacterial barrier. Good application technique is important including use of the recommended three layers. Cyanoacrylates can also be used with skin staples to prevent leakage of serous fluids from wounds. However, at the time of this writing these materials are only approved for topical skin application. Fibrin sealant (Tisseel and Evicel), on the other hand, can be used for internal application. Fibrin sealant is a much weaker adhesive than cyanoacrylate and, thus, cannot hold skin edges together. It can be used successfully to attach broad flaps of tissue and eliminate potential spaces where seroma or other fluids may accumulate. The literature on this application of fibrin sealant is contradictory [15]. This is because the successful use of fibrin sealant in this application is technique- and time-dependent [16]. If the sealant spray is applied and flaps are quickly approximated so that the sealant polymerizes with the flaps in contact, then an excellent seal is created. However, if there is a time delay between the spray application of the sealant and the contact of

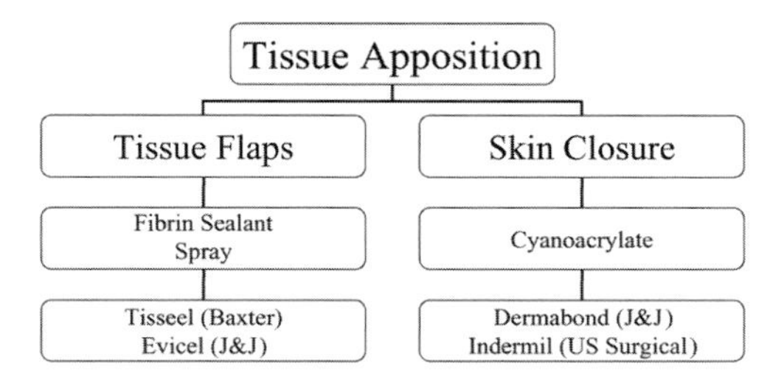

Fig. 25.7 Tissue adherence algorithm for skin closure using cyanoacrylates and tissue flap apposition using fibrin sealant

the two flaps so that the sealant is fully polymerized prior to tissue–to-tissue apposition, then the sealant actually functions as a relatively good anti-adhesive and will increase seroma formation. A similar effect will occur if the flaps are properly attached by rapid apposition after the spray application of fibrin sealant, but the bond of the flaps is later disrupted by some mechanical force such as raising the flap to place skin or subcutaneous sutures. Thus, it is important to: 1) pre-place a lattice work of monofilament sutures prior to spraying the sealant which can later be tightened so that no additional suture placement is required after flap apposition, and 2) quickly apply pressure to the flaps so that excellent apposition is achieved for a period of two minutes while the sealant polymerizes.

Similarly, spray fibrin sealant is an excellent way to attach partial thickness skin grafts to underlying beds and can eliminate the need for pressure dressings as well as anchoring peripheral sutures or staples. In fact, there are regions of difficult graft attachment, such as the head and neck where the only way to assure graft take may be to use fibrin sealant. It is important to avoid too thick a layer of sealant as this prevents diffusion of nutrients from the underlying tissue bed to the graft and can reduce graft survival.

25.3.4. Sealing Algorithms

25.3.4.1. Vascular

The sealing of blood vessels following vascular anastomosis is an important application of tissue adhesives and sealants. The algorithm (Fig. 25.8) is based on the use of fibrin sealant (Tisseel, Evicel), gelatin and thrombin (Floseal), dual PEG polymer (Coseal) and albumin crosslinked with glutaraldehyde (Bioglue). The clinical application is divided into sealing the vascular anastomosis before and after allowing blood to re-enter the vessel. This re-entrance of blood, after removal of vascular clamps placed for proximal and distal control, creates a pressure-filled anastomosis. Prior to pressurization, sealant materials are effective in sealing the anastomosis, provided that time is allowed for full polymerization of the individual agents. The strongest material is albumin crosslinked with glutaraldehyde and this material also tends to strengthen the tissues themselves, allowing for safer placement of primary sutures in a vascular dissection or additional sutures in a straightforward anastomosis. However, this agent also has a higher risk profile than the others with some evidence that

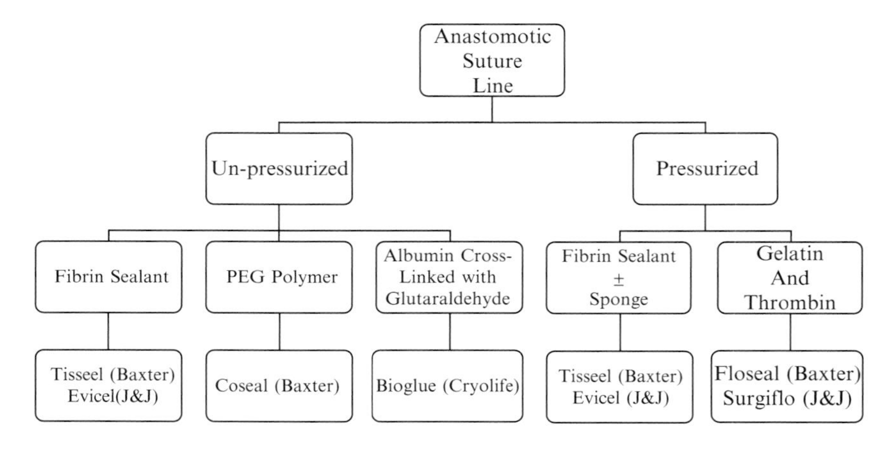

Fig. 25.8 Vascular sealing can be achieved with on-label vascular sealants such as PEG polymer and albumin cross-linked with glutaraldehyde and in the presence of active bleeding with the on-label established hemostatic agents, fibrin sealant and gelatin and thrombin

microemboli and false aneurysms may occur. The synthetic dual PEG polymer has the largest safety margin, but its strength is not equivalent to albumin crosslinked with glutaraldehyde. Fibrin sealant is also useful in this setting for sealing needle holes such as those created in synthetic grafts when using polypropylene sutures to achieve an anastomosis between graft and blood vessel. However, fibrin sealant may not be strong enough to prevent bleeding from significant anastomotic gaps in large blood vessel anastomoses.

Once the vessel is pressurized, neither the dual PEG polymer nor albumin cross-linked with glutaraldehyde (pure sealants) are indicated, because neither has an inherent hemostatic capability. In this setting the appropriate agents are those with an inherent hemostatic capacity. Thus, the application of gelatin and thrombin or fibrin sealant with a carrier sponge to the site of active bleeding (Fig. 25.6) is indicated.

With all of these agents the dryer the blood vessel walls the better the adherence strength of the reinforcing materials. The agents should not be used as a substitute for a well-placed suture.

25.3.4.2. Dural

There are two choices which have been shown to be effective in sealing the dura during neurosurgical operations to prevent cerebrospinal fluid (CSF) leakage. These are the blue PEG polymer and fibrin sealant (Fig. 25.9). The synthetic PEG is relatively strong, easily visible, and has an improved safety profile. Thus, it would appear to be an excellent option in this FDA-approved setting and may even be useful in other off-label indications. Application of fibrin sealant in this setting is supported by the literature [17], but is not an on-label indication. It is worthwhile noting how critically important satisfactory dural closure is in this setting. If there is a leak, there is no inherent clotting

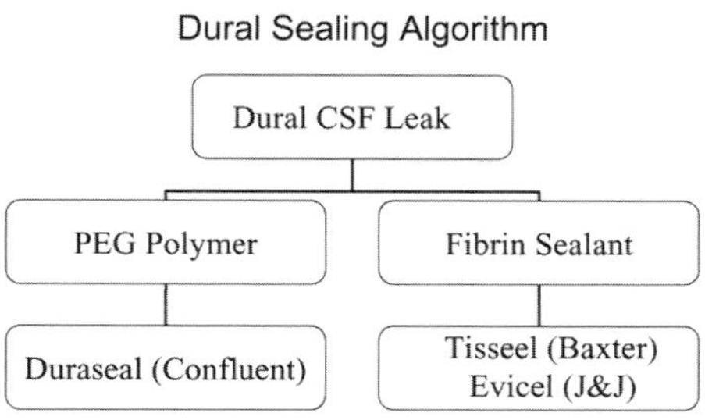

Dural Sealing Algorithm

Dural CSF Leak

PEG Polymer

Fibrin Sealant

Duraseal (Confluent)

Tisseel (Baxter)
Evicel (J&J)

Fig. 25.9 Dural sealing can be facilitated by both PEG polymer and fibrin sealant

mechanism in the CSF to help with closure and a CSF fistula may be established which can lead to infection and life-threatening complications. Thus, a reliable adjunct to suture closure of the dura which can eliminate CSF leakage is an important role for tissue adhesives and sealants.

25.3.4.3. Pulmonary

There is no FDA-approved agent now marketed for pulmonary application (Focalseal is no longer available from the distributor). However, several agents may be useful for sealing of the pulmonary parenchyma or bronchial tree (Fig. 25.10) and have literature or anecdotal reports supporting their use. Agents which may be useful include fibrin sealant, both the dual and blue PEG polymers, and albumin crosslinked with glutaraldehyde. This clinical application is particularly challenging for a tissue adhesive because it requires good internal and adherence bonding strength, as well as elasticity so that the material can change shape and contour as the lung inflates and deflates. Prevention of pulmonary air leak at staple lines of the lung or bronchus can prevent significant morbidity and mortality from prolonged fistulas. As lung volume reduction surgery on fragile emphysematous lung is performed more frequently, this application becomes even more important.

25.3.4.4. Colonic

Fibrin sealant is FDA-approved for sealing colonic anastomosis at the time of colostomy closure (Fig. 25.11). A relatively small clinical trial on low colonic anastomoses demonstrated a smaller rate of leakage associated with the use of fibrin sealant. In this setting, the bowel wall must be as dry as possible to achieve the best adherence of the sealant.

25.3.5. Lymphostasis Algorithm

The fibrin sealant literature supports the spray application of this material to eliminate lymphatic leaks [18] and the potential spaces for serous or lymphatic fluid accumulation (Fig. 25.12). The literature, with respect to seroma accumulation, is controversial for the reasons discussed above under the use of fibrin sealant for tissue flap apposition. Timing and surgical technique are critical in this situation. Delayed flap apposition or destruction of established bonds can actually make the sealant function as a good anti-adhesive and may make fluid accumulations worse than they might be if the sealant had not been used. Control of lymphatic leaks can be particularly important in thoracic surgery in proximity to the thoracic duct,

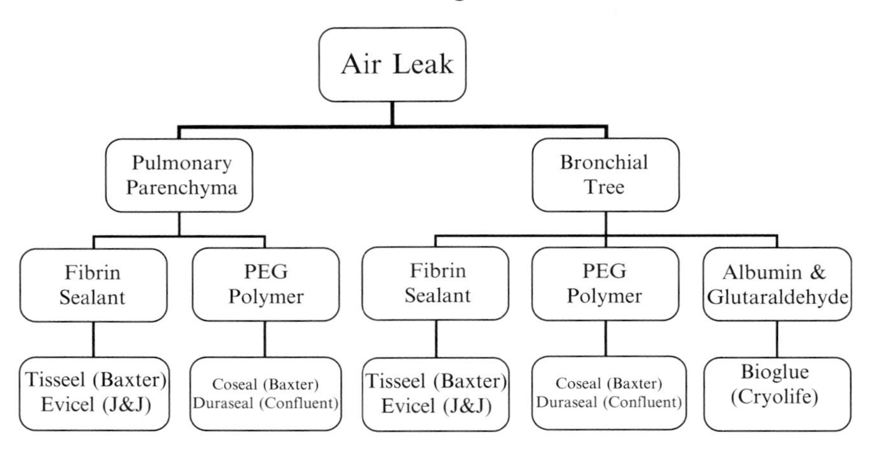

Fig. 25.10 None of the presently available materials used in this algorithm are approved by the FDA for pulmonary or bronchial sealing

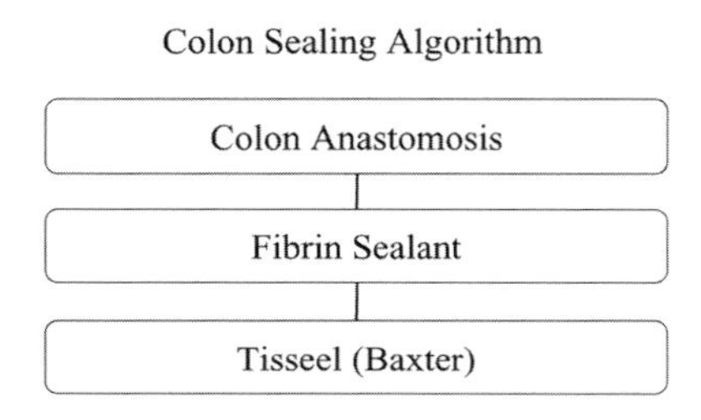

Fig. 25.11 One of the two commercially available fibrin sealant products is approved by the FDA for colonic sealing, as shown in this algorithm

as well as in tumor resection surgery involving large lymphatic beds in the head and neck, axilla and groin.

25.4. Trends and Future Needs

Excellent progress has been made in this field even though no commercial FDA-approved products existed in the United States prior to 1998. There are now five families of new adhesives. In the future new refinements, including more efficacious and safer materials, will be seen within these families. Also, there will be new families of agents which will enter the marketplace and improve the quality of surgical care. There will also be additional uses for these adhesives beyond the traditional concept of glue. For example, these materials can be used as drug delivery mechanisms and may be useful in new tissue engineering applications.

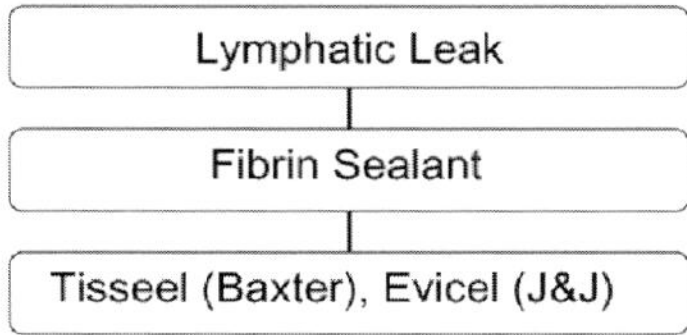

Fig. 25.12 The literature supports the use of fibrin sealant to achieve lymphostasis

25.5. Conclusion

In this chapter the five major families of new hemostats, sealants and tissue adhesives have been described with respect to the science of their methods of action, the available commercial products and some algorithms for their clinical use. The literature descriptions are not all inclusive as the body of accumulated knowledge of these materials now exceeds several thousand papers. The purpose of this chapter is to give the reader enough information to develop an enthusiasm for the potential of these materials and a basis for further review of this topic. This area is continuing to develop and new materials and applications are being introduced even at this very moment.

Acknowledgments: The author wishes to thank Kirk Barbieri and Phil Lang of the Heart and Vascular Center of the University of Virginia Health System for their timely technical assistance in the preparation of this chapter.

References

1. Spotnitz WD, Burks S. Use of tissue sealants in cardiac surgery. In Franco KL and Verrier ED (eds): "Advanced Therapy in Cardiac Surgery", Second Edition, Hamilton, Ontario, Canada, B.C. Decker, Inc., 2003:1–12.
2. Spotnitz WD, Burks S. The tissue adhesive decision; algorithms for successful clinical use. In Saltz R and Toriumi DM (eds): "Tissue Glues in Cosmetic Surgery", St. Louis, Missouri, Quality Medical, Inc, 2003:46–67.
3. Rousou J, Gonzalez-Lavin L, Cosgrove D, Weldon C, Hess P, Joyce L, Bergsland J, Gazzaniga A. Randomized clinical trial of fibrin sealants in patients undergoing resternotomy or reoperation after cardiac operations. J Thorac Cardiovasc Surg 1989;97:194–203.
4. Ortel TL, Mercer MC, Thames EH, Moore KD, Lawson JH. Immunologic impact and clinical outcomes after surgical exposure to bovine thrombin. Ann Surg 2001;233:88–96.
5. Hill AG, Hood AG, Reeder GD, Potter PS, Iverson LIG, Keating RF, Speir AM, Lefrak, EA. Perioperative autologous sequestration II: A differential centrifugation Technique for autologous component therapy: Methods and results. Am Acad Cardiovasc Perfus 1993:14;122–1225.
6. Spotnitz WD, Mintz PD, Avery N, Bithell TC, Kaul S, Nolan SP. Fibrin glue from stored human plasma: An inexpensive and efficient method for local blood bank preparation. Am Surg 1987;53:460–464.

7. Spotnitz WD, Prabhu R, Welker R, Burks SG. Clinical uses of fibrin sealant. In Mintz PD (ed): "Transfusion Therapy: Clinical Principles and Practice", Second Edition, Bethesda, Maryland, AABB Press, 2004:437–477.
8. Quinn J, Drzewiecki A, Li M, Stiell I, Sutcliffe T, Elmslie T, Wood W. A randomized, controlled trial comparing a tissue adhesive with suturing in the repair of pediatric facial lacerations. Ann Emerg Med 1993;22:1130–1135.
9. Samson D, Marshall D. Carcinogenic potential of isobutyl-2-cyanoacrylate. J Neurosurg 1986;65:571–572.
10. Oz MC, Cosgrove DM Badduke BR, Hill JD, Flannery M, Palumbo R. Topic N, and The Fusion Matrix Study Group. Controlled clinical trial of a novel hemostatic agent in cardiac surgery. Ann Thorac Surg 2000;69:1376–1382.
11. Glickman M, Gheissari A, Money S, Martin J, Ballard JL. Coseal Multicenter Vascular Surgery Group. A polymeric sealant inhibits anastomotic suture hole bleeding more rapidly than Gelfoam/thrombin: Results of a randomized controlled trial. Arch Surg 2001;137:326–331.
12. Grotenhuis JA. Costs of postoperative cerebrospinal fluid leakage: 1-year, retrospective analysis of 412 consecutive nontrauma cases. Surg Neurol 2005;64: 490–493.
13. Hewitt CW, Marra SW, Kann BR, Tran HS, Puc MM, Chrizanowski FA Jr, Tran JL, Lenz SD, Cilley JH Jr, Simonetti VA, DelRossi AJ. Bioglue surgical adhesive for thoracic aortic repair during coagulopathy: Efficacy and histopathology. Ann Thorac Surg 2001;71:1609–1612.
14. LeMaire SA, Carter SA, Won T, Wang X, Conklin LD, Coselli JS. The threat of adhesive embolization: BioGlue leaks through needle holes in aortic tissue and prosthetic grafts. Ann Thorac Surg. 2005;80:106–110.
15. Carless PA, Henry DA. Systematic review and meta-analysis of the use of fibrin sealant to prevent seroma formation after breast cancer surgery. Br J Surg. 2006;93:810–9.
16. Moore M, Burak W Jr, Nelson E, Kearney T, Simmons R, Mayers L, Spotnitz W. Fibrin sealant reduces the duration and amount of fluid drainage following axillary dissection: A randomized prospective clinical trial. J Am Coll Surg 2001;192: 591–599.
17. Shaffrey, CI, Spotnitz WD, Shaffrey ME, Jane JA. Neurosurgical applications of fibrin glue: Augmentation of dural closure in 134 patients. Neurosurgery 1990;26:207–210.
18. Yoshimura Y, Kondoh T. Treatment of chylous fistula with fibrin glue and clavicular periosteal flap. Br J Oral Maxillofac Surg. 2002;40:138–139.

26

Platelet-Rich Plasma in Orthopedics

Jennifer E. Woodell-May[1] and William S. Pietrzak[2]

Abstract: Autologous platelet-rich plasma (PRP) has become a popular clinical treatment in a variety of soft tissue and hard tissue applications. Clinicians use PRP to harvest the platelets' natural ability to promote hemostasis and to release cytokines into the wound bed with hopes of stimulating the rate of healing and improving tissue quality. Platelet-derived growth factor, transforming growth factor β1, vascular endothelial growth factor, basic fibroblast growth factor, epidermal growth factor, insulin-like growth factor and connective tissue growth factor are among the more notable cytokines released from platelets. To understand the utility of PRP in orthopedics, a review of the preclinical studies with PRP reveals a wide breadth of models where PRP enhances the outcomes. However, it is apparent that PRP is most successful when paired with the appropriate matrices and/or cell therapies for optimal results. Reviews of peer-reviewed clinical studies, ranging from Level I evidence clinical trials to Level IV case series reports, also reveal a wide range of clinical utility for PRP. Future clinical trials should attempt to refine the clinical application of PRP for each indication for use. These studies must be designed with the appropriate outcome measures and follow-up time-points to capture the benefits of PRP. Given the data published to date, PRP appears to be a powerful autologous therapy for surgeons looking to enhance bone and soft tissue formation. Future investigations will further define PRP's optimal role in medicine.

Keywords: Platelet-rich plasma, PRP, platelet concentrate, platelet gel, AGF, growth factors, platelets, PDGF, TGF-β, orthopedics, wound healing.

[1] Biomet, Inc., Warsaw, IN
[2] Department of Bioengineering, University of Illinois at Chicago, Chicago, IL, Biomet, Inc., Warsaw, IN

From: *Orthopedic Biology and Medicine: Musculoskeletal Tissue Regeneration, Biological Materials and Methods*
Edited by W. S. Pietrzak © Humana Press, Totowa, NJ

26.1. Introduction

The healing response to injury has evolved over millions of years to promote survival of a species. While humans possess sufficient healing potential to survive a variety of injuries, healing may take a long time to complete or the regenerated tissue may consist primarily of nonfunctional scar. A complex healing process at a tissue injury site is initiated by platelets, which are responsible for arresting bleeding and providing hemostasis. These same platelets, upon activation by mediators at the injury site, release bioactive proteins that signal wound healing cells to clean the wound and form new tissue. Recent attempts have been made to increase the healing rate and functionality of deposited tissue by augmenting the natural healing process and harnessing the healing potential of platelets.

An emerging clinical technology attempts to harvest the body's natural healing capacity by collecting platelets from a patient, concentrating them in a small amount of plasma and administering the platelets to the patient at the injury site. This concentrated platelet product is known as platelet-rich plasma (PRP). Other names include platelet concentrate and autologous growth factor (AGF). Once activated to form a gel, it can also be called platelet gel or autologous platelet gel.

PRP has been used in many fields of surgery. Applications in orthopedics include spine, joint arthroplasty, dental, craniomaxillofacial, sports medicine and foot and ankle procedures [1–6]. PRP has also been useful in other fields such as cardiovascular, plastic surgery and ulcer wound healing [7–9]. While many of these studies attempt to determine if an autologous platelet approach does enhance wound healing mechanisms, a definitive conclusion has not been reached. First, many nuances in the production of PRP include the level of platelet concentration and the ability to not prematurely activate the platelets and lose the active factors during the platelet processing [10]. Second, many of the commercially available PRP systems have not been well characterized, which makes interpretation of results difficult [11]. Finally, few prospective, randomized clinical studies have been performed from which to draw unambiguous conclusions.

Despite these limitations, a growing body of evidence – taken collectively – seems to support a clinical role for PRP in wound healing. The purpose of this chapter is to provide a basic background of platelets, their role in wound healing, methods of concentration and administration and an objective summary of animal and human studies that investigate the role of PRP in wound healing for orthopedics.

26.2. Basic Science

26.2.1. Platelet Biology

Platelets are fragments of large bone marrow cells called megakaryocytes and are formed during hematopoiesis. They are approximately 2 to 4 μm in diameter with a volume of 10×10^{-9} mm^3 [12, 13]. Platelets lack a nucleus, but do contain organelles such as mitochondria, dense bodies, α-granules and lysosomal granules. The dense bodies contain adenosine diphosphate (ADP), adenosine triphosphate (ATP), Ca^{2+}, serotonin, histamine, dopamine and catecholamines [14]. The α-granules, which number about 50 to 80 per platelet, contain adhesive proteins, coagulation factors, fibrinolytic factors, antiproteases, mitogenic growth factors, cytokines and bactericidal proteins [10, 14]. The phospholipid bilayer platelet membrane is covered with glycoprotein receptors that mediate interactions with surfaces, bioactive molecules and other platelets [13, 14]. Conformational changes in platelets, which are integral to their function, are mediated by actin and myosin fibers within the platelets [14].

Normal human platelet concentration is 200,000 to 400,000 platelets per microliter, and they typically circulate for a 10-day lifespan [10, 12]. Platelet physiologic function is two-fold: 1) hemostasis and 2) initiation of wound healing [10].

26.2.2. Hemostasis

Platelets maintain hemostasis by formation of a platelet plug and by modulating fibrin formation via the coagulation cascade [13]. When a blood vessel is injured, collagen becomes exposed. The exposed collagen interacts with the glycoprotein receptors of the platelet membrane, resulting in a signal transduction cascade that causes the platelets to adhere to each other and to undergo conformational change [13]. These conformational changes, including pseudopodia formation, are associated with release of internal stores of Ca^{2+} within the platelet, which in turn stimulates the released of the contents of the α-granules and dense granules outside of the platelet [12]. This process is known as platelet activation (Fig. 26.1) [15]. The substances released from

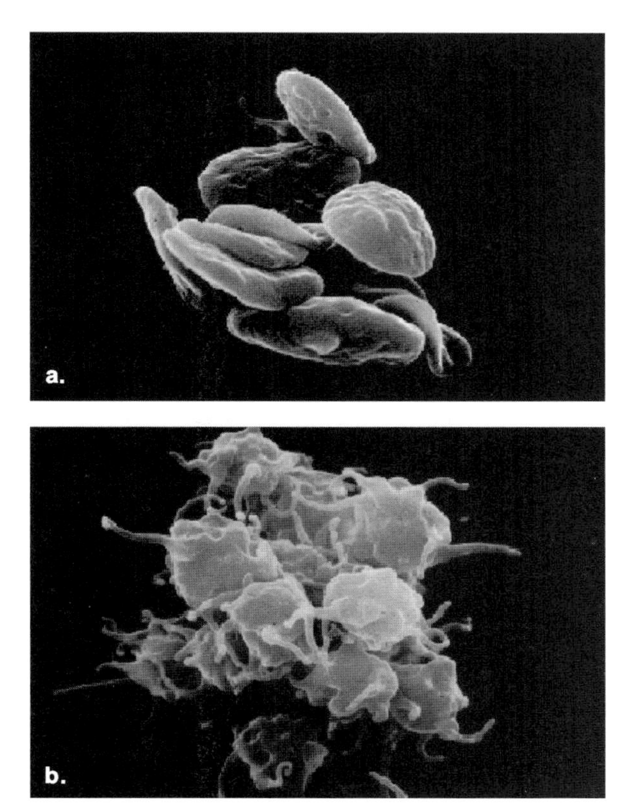

Fig. 26.1 (a) Schematic of resting platelets; (b) Schematic of platelets activated by thrombin. Permission to reproduce image from Thieme publishers (Gawaz, 2002 [15])

the activated platelets and into the surrounding plasma, specifically ADP and thrombin, activate adjacent platelets. These activated platelets aggregate together, forming the platelet plug [12, 13].

Along with the platelet plug formation, another major component of a blood clot is the fibrin mesh, which is derived through the coagulation cascade. The coagulation cascade is the process through which a series of normally inactive plasma proteins become activated, either by the intrinsic pathway through interactions with a surface, or extrinsically by the presence of tissue factor [16]. These activated factors continue a feed-forward loop that results in the formation of a three-dimensional fibrin matrix.

Both pathways converge at the activation of Factor X, which prompts the conversion of prothrombin to thrombin. Thrombin catalyzes the formation of fibrin from fibrinogen, which first forms a fibrin thread and then ultimately cross-links into a stable three-dimensional mesh [13]. The fibrin matrix, platelet plug and trapped white and red blood cells together make up the thrombus, a clot that stops bleeding at an injured site. Figure 26.2 details the schematic of the coagulation cascade and illustrates the multiple levels within the coagulation cascade during which activated platelets can directly participate in the process.

As can be seen from Fig. 26.2 several steps in the cascade require the presence of calcium ions. The presence of calcium forms the basis for citrate-based anticoagulants, or blood preservatives, such as citrate-phosphate-dextrose (CPD) and acid-citrate-dextrose (ACD) [10]. The added citrate ions chelate the calcium ions, essentially disabling the calcium ion-dependent steps of the cascade, which can be reversed by adding a calcium salt, e.g., $CaCl_2$.

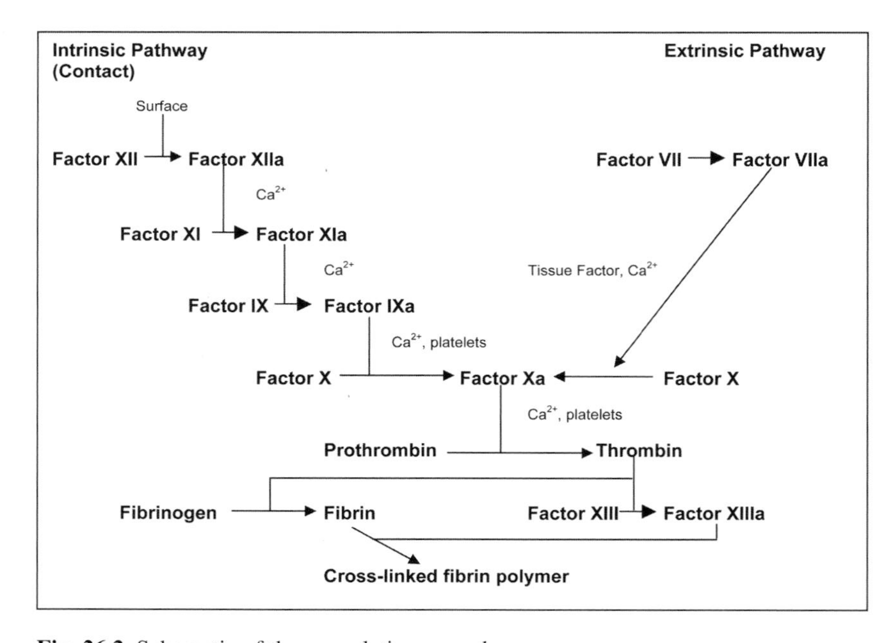

Fig. 26.2 Schematic of the coagulation cascade

26.2.3. Wound Healing

The wound healing cascade is a temporal series of events that begins within seconds of the injury and continues with remodeling for months following the event. The basic nature of the cascade is similar, whether the injury occurs in hard or soft tissue, with local signaling of precursor cells to ensure the appropriate tissue-specific phenotype modulation. The general healing process can be divided into three stages, including inflammatory, proliferative and remodeling phases [10, 17, 18].

The inflammatory phase (beginning immediately after the injury) includes initial hemostasis that involves platelet activation, aggregation and formation of a fibrin matrix, as described above. During degranulation, or release of the α-granule contents during platelet activation, platelets initiate the coagulation cascade and release cytokines that are responsible for cueing the wound healing process. The cytokines released are chemotactic for circulating white blood cells (WBC), recruiting them to marginate out of nearby blood vessels and migrate into the wound bed. Neutrophils, the first WBC responders, start cleaning the site by removing bacteria and cell debris [17, 18].

During the proliferative phase (days) an influx of monocytes migrates to the site, signaled by the growth factors released from the platelets. These circulating monocytes differentiate into macrophages. As the platelets are removed from the wound site, the activated macrophages take over the signaling-modulation role from the platelets. Macrophages remove debris by phagocytosis and also secrete factors that promote further wound healing events. Following the macrophages, fibroblasts begin to lay down collagen granulation tissue. New capillaries begin to feed the repair area, marking the start of angiogenesis. During this time undifferentiated stem cells migrate to the injury site. Depending on the signals present in the wound, the stem cells can differentiate into tissue-specific cells such as bone, cartilage or new blood vessels [17, 18].

The final phase of wound healing is the remodeling phase (months). During this phase the collagen tissue contracts, bringing the edges of the wound together. Cell density and vascularity decrease, excess repair matrix is removed and the collagen fibers orient along lines of stress to maximize strength [10]. The granulation tissue itself accumulates and remodels into scar tissue or is turned over to specific tissue types like skin or bone [17, 18]. In general, soft tissue heals by scar formation, although some components of the original tissue may have re-formed within the scar. Bone is unique in that it typically heals without scar; that is, healed bone cannot be distinguished from uninjured bone [10].

26.2.4. Growth Factors Released from Platelets

The cytokines released from activated platelets signal wound healing events to occur. Among the releasate is platelet-derived growth factor (PDGF) (isoforms AA, AB, BB), transforming growth factor β (TGF-β1 and TGF-β2), vascular endothelial growth factor (VEGF), basic fibroblast growth factor (bFGF), epidermal growth factor (EGF), insulin-like growth factor (IGF), connective tissue growth factor (CTGF) and others [10, 14; 19; 20]. Several of these signaling proteins, in particular PDGF and TGF-β, are transformed into active states during platelet degranulation by the addition of histones and carbohydrate side chains [10]. Table 26.1 gives an example of a growth factor profile in whole blood and delivered in a commercial PRP preparation [19].

Since platelets modulate wound healing in every tissue in the body, it is not expected that tissue-specific morphogens would be contained within platelet releasate. Specifically, large amounts of bone morphogenetic proteins, capable of differentiating mesenchymal stem cells into osteoblasts and chondrocytes, are not found in platelets. However, small amounts of BMP-2, BMP-4 and BMP-6 have been identified in washed platelet releasate, detected by western blot [21]. In our laboratory we were able to detect, using the enzyme linked immunosorbant assay method (ELISA), small amounts of BMPs from PRP releasate, i.e., 23 pg/ml of BMP-2 and 46 pg/ml of BMP-4 (unpublished data). No detectable amount of BMP-7 was found. These are negligible amounts compared to the BMP content of human demineralized bone matrix (DBM), where we found, on average per gram of DBM powder, 21 ng of BMP-2, 5 ng of BMP-4 and 84 ng of BMP-7 [22].

The effects of many growth factors on cell behavior and wound healing have been studied. Release of PDGF into a wound bed can have a chemotatic effect on monocytes, neutrophils, fibroblasts, mesenchymal stem cells and osteoblasts. PDGF is also a powerful mitogen for fibroblasts and smooth muscle cells, and is involved in all three phases of wound healing, including angiogenesis, formation of fibrous tissue and reepithelilization [23]. In a clinical study pressure ulcers that were treated daily (100 μg/g or 300 μg/g) with a PDGF-BB wound healing gel showed significantly decreased ulcer volume, compared to ulcers treated with a gel lacking PDGF-BB [24].

TGF-β1 is a mitogen for fibroblasts, smooth muscle cells and osteoblasts. Additionally, it promotes angiogenesis and extracellular matrix production [23, 25]. In a rat tibial fracture model, injections of TGF-β (4 and 40 ng) every other day for 40 days resulted in a dose-dependent increase in bone thickness, with the 40 ng dose additionally increasing mechanical strength [26]. As with many growth factors, dosing is critical. Broderick, et al. injected a much higher dose (335 μg of TGF-β) in a canine humeral model and found a decrease in bone mineralization [27].

Additionally, actions of other growth factors present in platelet releasate have been described. VEGF promotes angiogenesis and can promote healing of chronic wounds and facilitate endochondral ossification [25, 28]. However, as seen with high doses of TGF-β, high doses of VEGF (0.5 μg into rat segmental defect) inhibited bone formation [29]. EGF, another platelet-derived

Table 26.1 Example of growth factor profile delivered in a PRP (average of n=10 patients) [19]

	Whole blood	PRP	Fold increase
Platelets	197,000 platelets/μl	1,600,000 platelets/μl	8.1X
PDGF-BB	3.3 ng/ml	17 ng/ml	5.2X
TGF-β1	35 ng/ml	120 ng/ml	3.4X
VEGF	155 pg/ml	955 pg/ml	6.2X
EGF	129 pg/ml	470 pg/ml	3.6X

growth factor, is a mitogen for fibroblasts, endothelial cells and keratinoctyes, and is also useful in healing chronic wounds [25]. IGF, also found in platelets, regulates bone maintenance, is an important modulator of cell apoptosis and, in combination with PDGF, can promote bone regeneration [30, 31]. CTGF, found in concentrations 20-fold higher than other growth factors, promotes angiogenesis, cartilage regeneration, fibrosis and platelet adhesion [20].

Furthermore, many synergistic effects between these growth factors have been found. In a rabbit limb ischemia model the combined administration of VEGF and bFGF significantly increased angiogenesis in the ischemic limb over either factor given alone [32]. Another synergistic mitogenic effect was seen *in vitro* with the addition of bFGF, TGF-β and IGF-2 to osteoblasts [33], while chemotactic effects were seen with the addition of TGF-β1 and PDGF-BB to osteoblasts [34]. Additionally, in a porcine wound healing model, increased collagen content and maturity, increased angiogenesis and increased connective tissue volume were found without an increase in inflammation when PDGF was used in combination with IGF-1 or with TGF-α [35].

These factors are actively secreted from the α-granules within 10 minutes of clotting, with more than 95 percent of the presynthesized growth factors secreted within the first hour [10]. In addition the secreted growth factors remain bound to the fibrin clot and are slowly released during clot degradation. Therefore, the platelets local to the wound site continue to directly signal and modulate wound healing for several days.

26.2.5. PRP Procurement Methods

Normal whole blood contains approximately 94 percent red blood cells (RBC), 0.06 percent white blood cells (WBC), and 5.9 percent platelets, by number. A typical PRP can alter this concentration, as an example, to 52.1 percent RBC, 0.26 percent WBC and 47.6 percent platelets. These elements are collected in the buffy coat, a layer of WBC and platelets that form between the RBC and plasma during centrifugation. The buffy coat is suspended in a volume of plasma and delivered back to the patient. Depending on the system used to prepare the PRP, the concentration of platelets can typically range from four to eight times greater than the levels in whole blood (11;36). In addition, many systems allow the collection of a plasma layer, called the platelet poor plasma (PPP). The platelet poor plasma (PPP) can also be delivered to the patient as an autologous fibrin product for topical hemostasis [1].

Several commercial systems to produce PRP are commercially available. These systems can be divided into three basic categories: the apheresis technique, the single-spin tabletop technique and the double-spin tabletop technique. The first and oldest technology is the creation of a PRP from the output of an apheresis device (plateletpheresis). In these systems, whole, anticoagulated blood is introduced into a bowl that is spinning inside of a centrifuge. The blood separates along the walls of the bowl into the fractions described above. Each layer is then transferred to different collection bags. In many cases the PRP apheresis devices further concentrate the PRP with additional centrifugation and/or filtration to remove water. These systems usually process an entire unit of blood, so the volume of PRP produced is typically greater than with the other methods. Additionally, the RBCs can typically be re-infused to the patient.

The other two types of systems are considered tabletop devices requiring only 50 to 100 cc or less of blood. With the double-spin technologies, whole blood is introduced into a disposable unit and placed into a centrifuge. The first centrifugation spin, called the soft spin, runs for a relatively short time at low revolutions per minute (rpm). This spin divides the blood into the components of RBC, buffy coat and plasma. Depending on the device, the plasma and buffy coat are transferred, manually or automatically, into a new chamber for the second centrifugation cycle, or hard spin. The hard spin runs for a longer time period and at a higher rpm. This spin will create a platelet pellet at the bottom of the chamber which, once re-suspended in plasma, becomes the PRP.

Single-spin technologies only use one centrifugation cycle that separates the blood into RBC, buffy coat and plasma. These devices then have methods to capture the buffy coat from this disposable, such as a tuned density buoy that captures the buffy coat and allows it to be extracted from the device.

Table 26.2 summarizes these three types of devices, comparing the amount of blood drawn for processing, the volume of PRP produced, whether the packed cell layer can be re-infused into the patient, the fold-increase in platelet concentration in the PRP over baseline and the percent platelet recovery, which refers to the percentage of all platelets present in the initial blood draw that are contained in the final PRP produced. As can be seen, within a given class of device, a wide range in values exists for most of these characteristics, especially the fold-increase in platelet concentration and the percent platelet recovery.

The following table provides several parameters to consider when comparing platelet concentration devices, divided into parameters associated with the quality of the PRP product produced, the ease of use of the system and options available with the system.

Quality of Product	Ease of Use	Options
• Platelet concentration	• Time of preparation	• Operator input
• Growth factor profile delivered	• Number of steps	• Volume of blood draw
• Volume of PRP produced	• Sterile barrier steps	• PPP collection availability
• Percent recovery of platelets		• RBC re-infusion capability
• Concentration of white blood cells		• Cost
• Reproducibility of product		
• Activation of platelets during processing		

One of the main challenges in characterizing a PRP is to accurately determine the platelet concentration since levels can be much higher than most hematology analyzers are designed to count. Woodell-May, et al. devised a protocol for validating high PRP platelet counts made with a hematology analyzer (Cell-Dyn 3700, Abbott Labs) using manual counts for reference, and established a general method to ensure accuracy of the platelet count [11]. While utilization of PRP is still being investigated, the addition of a

Table 26.2 Methods to produce a PRP

Device	Blood draw (cc)	Volume of PRP (cc)	Re-infuse RBC?	PRP (fold increase)	Percent platelet recovery
Apheresis Technology [36,37]	450–550	48–83	Yes	1.6–2.6X	14–48%
Single-spin technology [11,19,36,37]	60	5.5–6	No	4.1–8X	43–85%
Double-spin technology [36–38]	50–110	7–9.3	No	1.6–6X	12–77%

means to expeditiously and accurately determine platelet counts can bolster the relevance of future study conclusions [39].

The last step in platelet application is to prepare the delivery system. Typically, activation solution must be made, which generally consists of a solution of thrombin in 10 percent $CaCl_2$ solution [10]. When added to PRP, calcium ions reverse the effects of the citrate-based anticoagulant, as explained above, while the thrombin activates the platelets as well as catalyzes the formation of the fibrin mesh. The most common delivery system uses a dual syringe spray apparatus [1]. The PRP is drawn into a 10 cc syringe and the activation solution is drawn into a 1 cc syringe. Both are connected, in tandem, to the dual spray apparatus (Fig. 26.3). Both syringe plungers are advanced in unison, with the solutions mixed in a 1:10 volume ratio and a combined spray exiting a single orifice. In this way the PRP becomes activated as it is applied to the wound. The PPP can be delivered in a similar fashion. In bone grafting applications, PRP can be mixed with bone grafting material such as demineralized bone matrix, allograft bone chips or synthetic bone void fillers.

26.3. Review of Preclinical Studies

PRP has been studied in a variety of preclinical models including orthopedics, spine, dental, craniomaxillofacial and sports medicine. A summary of selected published preclinical studies using PRP can be found in Table 26.3. A (+) was assigned to the study if any positive result was seen with the PRP, a (**o**) was given if no difference was found between the test and control groups, and a (−) was given when the PRP caused an inhibitory effect.

The varied studies described in Table 26–3 illustrate the nonspecific response of the body to PRP application, with the local tissue environment modulating the effect to ensure that the appropriate site-specific tissue is regenerated. Although open to interpretation, 15 of the 18 studies (83%) appear to show a positive influence of PRP on wound healing and tissue regeneration, two (11%) show a neutral effect, and one (6%) shows an inhibitory effect Upon closer inspection, however, it can be seen that some of the studies that reported positive PRP results used PRP in conjunction with osteoconductive matrices, so the effects of PRP in isolation may not have been tested. This is not necessarily a limitation, however, since a multifaceted approach is often required to attempt to match the combined osteoconductivity, osteoinductivity and osteogenicity of the "gold standard" autograft in bone healing applications.

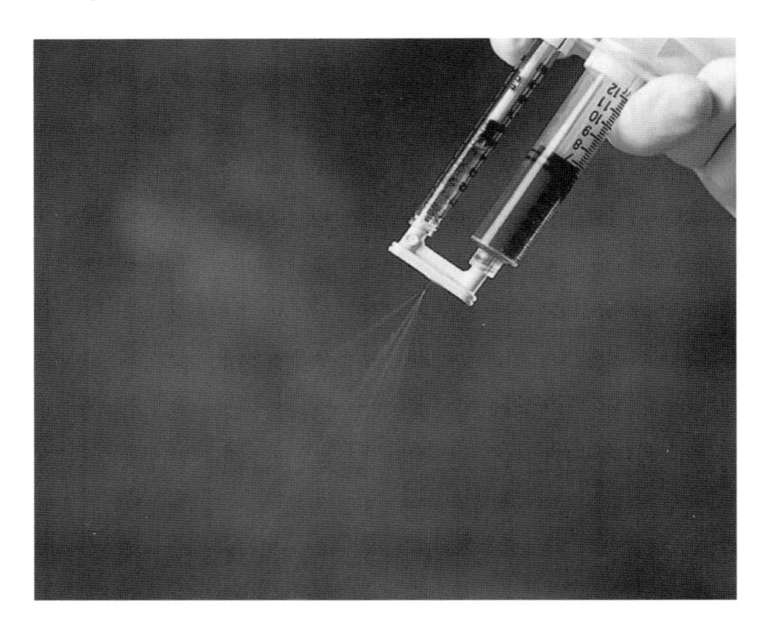

Fig. 26.3 Dual spray showing the PRP treatment in the 10 cc syringe and activation solution in the 1 cc syringe connected in tandem with a dual-tip spray connection

Table 26.3 Summary of PRP preclinical studies (+) = positive result; (**o**) = no difference between the test and control groups; (–) inhibitory effect

Ref.	Study	Results	PRP?
Orthopedics			
[40]	PRP in gelatin-hydrogel carrier in rabbit ulna defect (4 weeks)	PRP-gelatin hydrogel had increased bone formation by x-ray while controls had little to none	+
[41]	PRP with selected marrow cells on DBM and cancellous chips (CC) in a canine segmental defect (16 weeks)	The PRP with selected marrow cells and DBM-CC demonstrated 100% fusion along with the autograft group, and histologically showed more mature bone than the autograft group	+
[42]	PRP, concentrated marrow, and allograft, alone and in combination, in a critically sized defect in rabbit femurs (2, 4 and 12 weeks)	PRP in combination with marrow or with allograft healed faster than any of the variables tested individually. The fastest healing rate was seen when all 3 were combined into one treatment	+
[43]	PRP with cultured stem cells with allograft bone in a segmental defect in sheep (4 months)	PRP and stem cells had better bone formation and increased vascular invasion and remodeling of the graft over allograft only group	+
[44]	PDGF or PRP with DBM in nude-mouse 56-day intramuscular implantation	PRP reduced osteoinductivity of DBM with high activity and had no effect on DBM with low activity	–
[45]	PRP on coralline HA in a bone chamber rat model (4 weeks)	PRP treated groups had significantly higher bone ingrowth scores over untreated groups	+
[46]	PRP around self-tapping screw in rabbits (4 weeks)	Increased bone formation with PRP concentrations of 1,000,000 platelets/μl, but inhibitory with higher concentrations	+
[47]	PRP and allograft in gap model around titanium implant in canine (3 weeks)	PRP and PRP with allograft had no significant effect on implant fixation, but autograft did have increased push out strength	**o**

(continued)

Table 26.3 (continued)

Ref.	Study	Results	PRP?
[48]	Fracture model in a rat comparing non-diabetic, diabetic, and diabetic with PRP healing of fracture	The PRP group had improved early cellular proliferation and chondrogenesis and late mechanical strength over diabetic fracture healing without PRP	+
Dental and Craniomaxillofacial			
[49]	PRP and particulate dentin-plaster of paris around dental implants in a dog (6 and 12 weeks)	Groups with dentin-plaster of paris and PRP had higher percentage of bone contact than control groups	+
[50]	PRP with DBM compared to autograft in a cranial defect in a domestic pig (2,3,12,and 26 weeks)	PRP enhanced production of bone matrix proteins at 2-week time-point	+
[51]	Comparison of autograft, PRP, PRP with cultured mesenchymal stem cells, and Bio-oss® in teeth extraction sites in dogs (2,4,8,and 12 weeks)	The PRP with MSCs and autograft groups had significantly higher hardness values and mature bone formation seen by histology compared to the control groups	+
[52]	PRP with freeze-dried bone in cranium defect in rabbit compared to bone alone (1, 2 and 4 months)	PRP groups tended toward increased bone density and increased bone area, but the values were not significant	o
[53]	Bovine bone with and without PRP in calvarial defects in rabbit	Groups with PRP had greater bone density	+
[54]	PRP, autograft, and PRP mixed with cultured mesenchymal stem cells in a canine mandible defect (8 weeks)	The newly formed bone was statistically significant in the autograft (61%) and PRP/MSC (67%) with respect to the untreated defects	+
Spine			
[55]	Comparison of PRP with coralline HA, autograft, autograft with PRP, and coralline HA with PRP and marrow in a sheep posterolateral spine fusion	At six months, the stiffness of the coralline with PRP and marrow was statistically the same as the autograft group, but lower in ultimate load. This group also had 100% bilateral fusion	+
Sports Medicine			
[56]	PRP injected into a 3 mm resection of the Achilles tendon in a rat (28 days)	The PRP treated group had increased strength and improved histology scores over buffer solution control	+
[57]	PRP-collagen implant into central third of a canine ACL defect (compared to empty) (3 and 6 weeks)	PRP-collagen treated groups had higher strength and increased tissue fill	+

It appears that the mixture of PRP with an osteoconductive carrier, such as allograft bone or ceramic bone void fillers, can enhance bone formation over the carrier alone [45, 49, 52–53, 55]. However, in more challenging models for bone formation, such as in a gap model around an implant or in a posterolateral spine fusion, PRP mixed with an osteoconductive matrix could not significantly improve the outcome [47, 55]. To overcome these challenges, adding bone marrow aspirate or cultured mesenchymal stem cells to the graft in addition to the PRP performed as well as autograft [41–43, 51, 54–55].

In vitro support of the combination of PRP with bone marrow was shown with a dose-dependent increase in stem cell proliferation with the addition of PRP [43]. This composite approach avoids the donor site morbidity associated with autograft harvest.

Applications that take advantage of the angiogenic effect of PRP are illustrated by the increased tissue repair seen after injection of PRP into an ACL or Achilles tendon [56, 57]. Additionally, adding PRP to a bone repair model with compromised vascularity, such as in a diabetic animal, improved fracture healing [48]. In a critically sized segmental defect model, increased vascular invasion was seen in groups implanted with PRP, cultured stem cells and allograft bone, over groups implanted with the allograft alone [43].

The proliferative and angiogenic growth factors delivered in PRP, when combined with DBM, might be expected to accelerate bone healing compared to DBM alone. Ranly, et al. added the single growth factor, PDGF, to DBM powder in an ectopic bone formation model in a nude mouse [44]. An insignificant increase in DBM osteoinductivity was seen with the lowest dose, 0.1 μg PDGF/10 mg DBM implant, but there was an inhibition of osteoinductivity with the two higher doses of 1 μg PDGF/10 mg DBM implant and 10 μg PDGF/10 mg DBM implant. The low dose compares to that which may be present in a typical 6 cc PRP preparation [19] (approximately 100 ng), while the inhibitory doses are one and two orders of magnitude greater than that found in a typical PRP. In the same study, PRP was added to DBM. After a 56-day implantation no difference in the bone induction histology score appeared with or without PRP, but an increase in DBM resorption with the addition of PRP was detected. Ossicles formed in this model will remodel over time, so it may be expected that the addition of PRP would accelerate the natural remodeling process, which would include the resorption of the DBM particles. In a similar study a more physiologic dose of 50 ng of PDGF was added to 25 mg of DBM in an aged rat ectopic model and was implanted for 14 days [58]. The PDGF addition to the DBM increased mRNA production of collagen Type II, alkaline phosphatase activity and calcium content, which are all indicative of bone formation. These studies illustrate the complex nature of the effect of PRP on osseous healing, and that important study design considerations include the animal model, dosage, outcome measures and time intervals.

While the *in vivo* ectopic osteoinduction model has become a standard method and enables comparison among studies, an orthotopic model may be more predictive of expected clinical outcomes. When DBM was mixed with PRP in a porcine cranial defect and healing was compared to autograft, PRP enhanced bone formation compared to autograft at the earliest time-point of two weeks. However, at later time-points PRP had no effect on mineralization [50].

Animal studies utilize species-specific PRP. Since blood cell size varies from species to species, it is possible that the ability for PRP systems to concentrate platelets might also be species-dependent. In the majority of animal studies, the actual platelet dose was not quantified, which can confound attempts to compare studies. In our laboratory we compared the platelet concentration and growth factor profile in various species, and compared it to humans using a single-spin, table-top platelet concentration system that had been previously characterized for processing human blood [19]. Table 26.4 (unpublished data) summarizes the multi-species results.

Table 26.4 PRP preparations in different animal species

	Platelet counts			Growth factors		
Species	**Baseline (×10³ platelets/μl)**	**PRP (×10³ platelets/μl)**	**Fold increase**	**Baseline (ng/ml)**	**PRP (ng/ml)**	**Fold increase**
Human n=10	197±42	1600±330	8.1	PDGF = 3.3 TGF-β = 35	PDGF = 17 TGF-β = 120	PDGF = 5.2 TGF-β = 3.4
Horse n=27	171±81	929±196	5.4	PDGF = 1.7 TGF-β =7.3	PDGF = 10.9 TGF-β = 13.5	PDGF = 6.6 TGF-β = 1.9
Pig n=3	286±53	1528±5	5.3	PDGF = 3.8 TGF-β = 0.1	PDGF = 14.7 TGF-β = 0.5	PDGF = 3.3 TGF-β = 3.7
Dog n=2	298	2160	7.3	ND	ND	
Sheep n=3	354±48	3022±114	8.5	ND	ND	
Cow n=153	328±69	2645±680	8.1	ND	ND	

Whole blood platelet counts for all species were essentially within the normal range of human platelet counts of 200,000 platelets/μl to 400,000 platelets/μl [12]. However, the ability of the platelet concentration system to collect platelets varied five to eight times over baseline, depending on species. This is probably due to variances in cell size and density. Similarly, the amount of the growth factors PDGF and TGF-β1 also varied with the different species preparations. It is interesting to note that the fold increase in growth factors did not necessarily match the corresponding fold increase in platelet concentration, a result also noted by others [19]. We were unable to count goat platelets accurately because there is less size difference between red blood cells and platelets than for other species, which limits usefulness of the goat model.

From the vast range of preclinical studies using PRP in orthopedic applications, the results appear to predict that PRP used in clinical orthopedic applications will be successful. The next section will address the clinical use of PRP to date.

26.4. Clinical Review

The best evidence to support clinical use of PRP is prospective, randomized and controlled studies (Level of Evidence I (blinded) or II (not-blinded)) [59]. A search has revealed only one Level I study and five Level II studies published in orthopedic applications, with the balance being retrospective and case studies (Level III (retrospective, controlled studies) and Level IV (case series with no controls)) as summarized in Table 26.5. As with the preclinical studies a (+) was assigned to the study if any positive result was seen with the PRP, a (**o**) was given if no difference was found between the test and control groups and a (–) indicates when the PRP caused an inhibitory effect.

As seen in the preclinical studies, PRP as an adjuvant to other treatments has resulted in excellent clinical outcomes. For example, a case series of patients treated with PRP and cultured mesenchymal stem cells in distraction osteogenesis had successful outcomes without taking an autograft harvest [61]. PRP has also been used with autograft and has increased bone maturation

Table 26.5 Summary of PRP clinical studies (+) = positive result; (**o**) = no difference between the test and control groups; (–) inhibitory effect

Ref.	Study	Level of Evidence	Results	PRP?
Orthopedics				
[1]	PRP on wound closure following a TKA (81 with PRP, 72 without). Follow up was 6 weeks	III	PRP patients left the hospital sooner, had higher range of motion, received less transfused RBCs, and had less of a hemoglobin drop	+
[60]	PRP with bone chips in a tibial osteotomy for genu varus. (5 chips+PRP, 5 chips alone). Biopsies were taken at 45 days postop	III	PRP with chips appeared to accelerate healing expressed by new vessel formation and new bone formation	+
[61]	Case report of 3 patients using PRP with cultured mesenchymal stem cells in distraction osteogenesis	IV	Target lengths were obtained with injecting PRP and MSCs into the distraction callus	+
[62]	Case reports of 19 patients undergoing orthopedic reconstruction with PRP used with hydroxyapatite	IV	At 12.9 months follow-up, all patients had improved osteoblast reaction and bone reconstruction was observed	+
Spine				
[63]	Retrospective look at patients (76 with AGF, 76 without) that underwent instrumented lumbar fusion with autograft mixed with PRP	III	No difference in autograft nonunion rate with or without PRP	**o**
[64]	Prospective analysis in 1 and 2 level instrumented TLIF procedures with autograft (22 with PRP and 62 without)	III	The PRP group had a 19% decrease in pseudoarthrodesis, but it was not significant	**o**
[65]	Patients (23) with instrumented TLIF with autograft and PRP compared to historic control	II	AGF patients fused faster, but no significant difference in pseudoarthrosis rates	**o**
[4]	A prospective, randomized study of anterior-posterior interbody lumbar fusion with autograft (22) and PRP and allograft (15)	II	Allograft with AGF had the same rate of fusion and pseudoarthrodesis rates as the autograft group	+
[66]	A retrospective analysis of anterior intradisc fusion in 19 patients with PRP, autograft, and coralline HA with a disc spacer	III	No pseudoarthrosis was seen and solid fusions were seen in five patients	+
[67]	A retrospective analysis of patients undergoing single-level intertransverse lumbar fusion with autograft (27) and autograft with PRP (32)	III	Fusion in the control group was 91% and in the PRP group was 62%	–
[68]	Combination of PRP with autograft for either interbody fusions or posterolateral intertransverse fusions	IV	Patients (58 of 60) had solid or maturing fusions	+
Foot and Ankle				
[69]	Case studies (4) of Charcot's foot in diabetic patients treated with bone graft soaked in PRP	IV	All 4 had successful fusion with return to normal footwear	+
[2]	PRP with autograft in syndesmosis fusion with total ankle implantation (66 with PRP, 48 without)	III	PRP group had statistically significant improvement in fusion rates and a significant reduction in delayed unions and nonunions	+

(continued)

Table 26.5 (continued)

Ref.	Study	Level of Evidence	Results	PRP?
[70]	PRP mixed with autograft in fusion of tibiofibular joint in 20 patients	IV	Follow-up (6 month) had 100% fusion compared to historic control of only 62% fusion	+
[71]	PRP as adjuvant in high-risk foot and ankle surgery on 62 patients (123 procedures)	IV	Overall union rate was 94%, achieved at 41 days with PRP and 45 days with autograft	+
Sports Medicine				
[72]	Buffered PRP injected into chronic elbow tendinosis (15 with PRP, 5 with bupivacaine)	II	At eight weeks the PRP group had 60% improvement in pain versus 16% in the control group. At six months the PRP group had 81% improvement, and at final follow-up (25.6 months) had 93% reduction in pain	+
[5]	PRP used to aide in attachment of a non-traumatic articular cartilage avulsion of a soccer player	IV	Complete articular cartilage healing was achieved with return to symptom-free activity	+
Dental and Craniomaxillofacial				
[73]	PRP with bovine bone and GTR membrane periodontal intrabony defect fill (n=18/group)	III	Groups with PRP and bone had significantly more fill than GTR membrane alone	+
[3]	PRP with bovine bone in periodontal intrabony defects (13 bilateral defects)	I	PRP mixed with the bone significantly increased defect fill over bone alone	+
[74]	PRP with autograft in resorbed maxilla to improve dental implant fixation (19 patients, 76 implants with PRP, 76 without PRP)	II	Resonance frequency analysis at one year showed that implants were significantly more stable in groups with PRP	+
[75]	Bilateral sinus graft cases (3) using PRP with bovine bone (PRP on one side)	III	No difference in vital bone production or interfacial bone contact on implants	o
[76]	Case studies of alveolar ridge and/or sinus augment with allograft with PRP (15)	IV	89% of the implant fixtures were considered clinically successful	+
[77]	PRP mixed with autograft in mandibular reconstruction (44 with PRP and autograft, 44 with autograft alone)	III	PRP plus autograft groups had radiographic graft maturity of 1.6–2.1 times greater than without PRP, and also had 25% more bone density determined by histomorphometry	+
[78]	PRP with HA (35) compared to HA (35) alone for intrabony defects	II	PRP group had statistically significant improvement in probe depth and attachment gain	+
[6]	Sinus floor augmentation with β-TCP with and without PRP (22 with PRP, 23 without)	II	New bone formation was 8–10% higher in PRP with β-TCP group. Resorption of the β-TCP was not present	+

TKA = total knee arthroplasty, TLIF = transforminal lumbar interbody fusion, GTR= guided tissue regeneration, HA = hydroxyapatite, β-TCP = β tricalcium phosphate over autograft alone [2, 70, 74, 77]. However, more surprisingly, PRP in combination with allograft has demonstrated clinical outcomes equivalent to autograft in a spine fusion study [4]. PRP, in combination with osteoconductive matrices, has also improved the clinical results compared to the osteoconductive material alone [3, 6, 60, 73, 78]. In the only Level I evidence trial using PRP, PRP mixed with xenograft in periodontal intrabony defects significantly increased defect fill over the xenograft alone [3].

While many favorable outcomes with PRP have been demonstrated clinically, not all published results support the use of PRP. Specifically, in clinically challenging spine fusion cases, three studies have published no difference between PRP and the control groups [63–65], and one study found increased bone resorption when PRP was used [67]. However, two of these studies did show a decrease in pseudoarthrodesis and a faster fusion rate in the PRP groups, though the results were not significant [64–65]. The comparisons between PRP and control groups were compared at a 24-month follow-up time in the Hee, et al. [65] study, and at 34 months in the Castro, et al. [64] study. Given that the effects of PRP are suggested to speed up healing processes, it should be expected that groups compared at this late follow-up time-point would be equal. Similarly, in the Carreon, et al. study, no difference was found with the addition of PRP mixed with autograft with instrumented lumbar spine fusion at 32- to 37-month follow-up [63]. Any effect the PRP had on healing would more likely be seen early on in the healing process, but not in the overall amount of bone formation once the fusion is complete. In the Weiner and Walker study the fusion rate was much lower in the PRP with autograft group than the autograft alone [67]. As this procedure was uninstrumented, it was a very challenging spine fusion model. Without instrumentation, micromotion can occur more freely at the fusion site. Since PRP contains angiogenic growth factors, one might expect that micromotion would increase fibrosis tissue formation preferentially over bone, increasing the pseudoarthrodesis. In contrast, a case series published with PRP mixed with autograft in an instrumented spine fusion demonstrated 58 out of 60 patients fusing [68], and yet another case series with PRP and autograft in an instrumented spine fusion showed no pseuodoarthrosis [66].

In a prospective, randomized trial (Level II) comparing PRP and allograft to autograft in spine fusions, the groups were compared at six months post-operation and found to be equivalent [4]. These results are promising in that PRP might find clinical utility as an adjuvant with other matrices to reduce the need for a painful autograft harvest. However, both preclinical and clinical results suggest that PRP can enhance biologic repair and, in conjunction with adequate bone matrices and/or cells, can be effective in spine fusion at a much lower cost, both in terms of material costs when compared to recombinant BMPs, and in morbidity of the donor site when compared to an autograft harvest.

In the field of dental and craniomaxillofacial surgery, many procedures are bilateral. This permits PRP to be added unilaterally, allowing each patient to be his or her own control. As mentioned earlier, in the only published Level I evidence trial (with double-blinding), PRP mixed with xenograft in periodontal intrabony defects significantly increased defect fill over the xenograft alone [3]. In several other studies PRP showed enhanced results over control groups in bilateral intrabony defects [3, 73–74]. Only in one series of three patients in a bilateral defect did PRP show no difference when mixed with xenograft in a sinus lift [75]. However, in a prospective, randomized study comparing PRP with a synthetic bone void filler (β-TCP) in a sinus lift, PRP was shown to increase bone formation [6].

In the only soft tissue application reviewed, PRP injections improved chronic elbow tendinosis (or tennis elbow) [72]. Mishra and Pavelko found statistically significant improvement in visual analog pain scores in patients that received injections of buffered PRP into the tendon area of maximum tenderness. The treatment groups received PRP that was 5.4-fold higher concentration than their whole blood. The control groups received the same injection technique with bupivacaine, but did not see the improvement that the PRP group did. It can, therefore, be concluded that the injection into the tendon alone was not enough to stimulate healing. The authors hypothesize that the concentrated growth factors in PRP work together to initiate the healing response. Tendon improvement could be due to increased collagen Type I production from the tendon fibroblasts [79], or from increased angiogenesis into the site [80].

As with the preclinical studies, the actual dose of platelets delivered or the concentration of growth factors is not always reported in the clinical studies. This makes it difficult to determine the correct platelet dose for each surgical application. *In vitro* experiments have shown a dose-dependent increase in stem cell proliferation with a dose of up to a 10-fold increase in platelets over baseline [81–82]. Combined with DBM in an ectopic implantation model, a dose-dependent inhibition of bone formation was seen with recombinant PDGF [44]. However, as mentioned earlier, at doses normally found in a PRP, a slight increase in bone formation was seen. Many growth factors exhibit this biphasic response, with stimulatory effects on bone formation at lower doses and inhibitory effects at high doses [25–29].

One study evaluated the dose-dependent response of bone formation with PRP around an implant in a rabbit model [46]. In this study, three levels of platelet concentration were compared. The lowest concentration was 164,000 to 373,000 platelets/μl (0.5–1.5X fold increase over whole blood), an intermediate dose was 503,000 to 1,729,000 platelets/μl (2-6X fold increase over whole blood) and a high dose was 1,845,000 to 3,200,000 platelets/μl (9–11X fold increase over whole blood). At four weeks only the intermediate group had significant increase of bone. From this study the authors draw the conclusion that the optimum dose of PRP concentration is 1,000,000 platelets/μl [46].

26.5. Future Trends and Needs

Clinical utilization of PRP will continue to evolve. Future devices will provide PRP faster and more efficiently, with more customization of end level products such as fibrinogen concentration or output volume. Development of better delivery devices and methods to combine PRP with various matrices will also continue to emerge. Concurrently, more Level I and Level II evidence studies will need to be completed to further refine the uses of PRP, matching clinical indications with the right matrix and cell technologies. Additionally, designing these studies with the appropriate follow-up time-points will be critical to capture the clinical benefits of PRP. It is clear from the review of the studies to date that a one-size-fits-all solution for all PRP applications does not exist.

The choice of the appropriate matrix and, when required, fixation technique, will need to be coupled to each application that PRP finds utility. In addition to defining the clinical utilizations, better characterization of the PRP products should be included in the studies to help elucidate the correct platelet concentration for each application.

26.6. Conclusions

PRP has demonstrated numerous clinical benefits to patients [1, 3–4, 6]. Better matching of clinical indication to the right matrices and/or requirement of cell delivery will need to be determined in future evaluations. Better characterization of the product delivered and further refinement in clinical utility will better elucidate the dose of platelets that is optimal for each application. The working hypothesis is that the optimal platelet dose is 1,000,000 platelets/μl [46]. This number was determined from one clinical indication. It is reasonable to consider that this type of dosing study would be needed for each new indication for use, and that each indication would have a discrete optimal platelet dose.

PRP remains a potentially powerful autologous therapy for surgeons that want to enhance bone formation. The addition of growth factors such as PDGF, TGF-β1 and VEGF will promote cellular bioactivity by increasing cell proliferation, chemotaxis and angiogenesis. The benefits seen to date with PRP's use will continue to encourage researchers to actively investigate the use of PRP in orthopedics and in other fields of medicine [72].

Reference

1. Berghoff WJ, Pietrzak WS, Rhodes RD. Platelet-rich plasma application during closure following TKA: A retrospective study. Orthopedics 2006; 29(7):590–606.
2. Coetzee JC, Pomeroy GC, Watts JD, Barrow C. The use of autologous concentrated growth factors to promote syndesmosis fusion in the Agility total ankle replacement. A preliminary study. Foot Ankle Int 2005; 26(10):840–846.
3. Hanna R, Trejo PM, Weltman RL. Treatment of intrabony defects with bovine-derived xenograft alone and in combination with platelet-rich plasma: a randomized clinical trial. J Periodontol 2004; 75(12):1668–1677.
4. Jenis LG, Banco RJ, Kwon B. A prospective study of Autologous Growth Factors (AGF) in lumbar interbody fusion. Spine J 2006; 6(1):14–20.
5. Sanchez M, Azofra J, Anitua E et al. Plasma rich in growth factors to treat an articular cartilage avulsion: a case report. Med Sci Sports Exerc 2003; 35(10):1648–1652.
6. Wiltfang J, Schlegel KA, Schultze-Mosgau S, Nkenke E, Zimmermann R, Kessler P. Sinus floor augmentation with beta-tricalciumphosphate (beta-TCP): does platelet-rich plasma promote its osseous integration and degradation? Clin Oral Implants Res 2003; 14(2):213–218.
7. Khalafi RS, Bradford DW. Effect of autologous platelet rich plasma application on postoperative complication rates following a median sternotomy. Regenerate World Congress on Tissue Engineering and Regenerative Medicine . 2006. 4-25-0006.
8. Margolis DJ, Kantor J, Santanna J, Strom BL, Berlin JA. Effectiveness of platelet releasate for the treatment of diabetic neuropathic foot ulcers. Diabetes Care 2001; 24(3):483–488.
9. Welsh WJ. Autologous platelet gel-clinical function and usage in plastic surgery. Cosmetic Dermatology 2000;13–18.

10. Pietrzak WS, Eppley BL. Platelet rich plasma: biology and new technology. J Craniofac Surg 2005; 16(6):1043–1054.
11. Woodell-May JE, Ridderman DN, Swift MJ, Higgins J. Producing Accurate Platelet Counts for Platelet Rich Plasma: Validation of a Hematology Analyzer and Preparation Techniques for Counting. J Craniofac Surg 2005; 16(5):749–756.
12. Venkataraman BV, Naga Rani MA. Platelets and antiplatelet drugs. Indian Journal of Pharmacology 1992; 24:188–193.
13. Hanson SR, Harker LA. Blood coagulation and blood-materials interactions. In: Ratner BD, Hoffman AS, Schoen FJ, Lemons JE, editors. Biomaterials Science. An Introduction to Materials in Medicine. San Diego: Academic Press, 1996: 193–199.
14. Anitua E, Andia I, Ardanza B, Nurden P, Nurden AT. Autologous platelets as a source of proteins for healing and tissue regeneration. Thromb Haemost 2003;(91):4–15.
15. Gawaz M. Blood Platelets. Stuttgart, Germany: Thieme Medical Publishers, 2002.
16. Bhanot S, Alex JC. Current Applications of Platelet Gels in Facial Plastic Surgery. Facial Plastic Surgery 2002; 18(1):27–33.
17. Clark RAF. Overview and general considerations of wound repair. In: Clark RAF, editor. The Molecular and Cellular Biology of Wound Repair. New York: Plenum Press, 1996: 3–50.
18. Lorenz HP, Longaker MT. Wounds: Biology, Pathology, and Management. In: Norton JA, Bollinger RR, Chang AE, Lowry SF, Mulvihill SJ, Pass HI et al., editors. Surgery : Basic Science and Clinical Evidence. New York: Springer-Verlag, 2001: 77–88.
19. Eppley BL, Woodell JE, Higgins J. Platelet quantification and growth factor analysis from platelet-rich plasma: implications for wound healing. Plast Reconstr Surg 2004; 114(6):1502–1508.
20. Kubota S, Kawata K, Yanagita T, Doi H, Kitoh T, Takigawa M. Abundant retention and release of connective tissue growth factor (CTGF/CCN2) by platelets. J Biochem (Tokyo) 2004; 136(3):279–282.
21. Sipe JB, Zhang J, Waits C, Skikne B, Garimella R, Anderson HC. Localization of bone morphogenetic proteins (BMPs)-2, –4, and –6 within megakaryocytes and platelets. Bone 2004; 35(6):1316–1322.
22. Pietrzak WS, Woodell-May J, McDonald N. Assay of Bone Morphogenetic Protein-2, –4, and –7 in Human Demineralized Bone Matrix. J Craniofac Surg 2006; 17(1):84–90.
23. Hosgood G. Wound healing. The role of platelet-derived growth factor and transforming growth factor beta. Vet Surg 1993; 22(6):490–495.
24. Rees RS, Robson MC, Smiell JM, Perry BH. Becaplermin gel in the treatment of pressure ulcers: a phase II randomized, double-blind, placebo-controlled study. Wound Repair Regen 1999; 7(3):141–147.
25. Bennett SP, Griffiths GD, Schor AM, Leese GP, Schor SL. Growth factors in the treatment of diabetic foot ulcers. Br J Surg 2003; 90(2):133–146.
26. Nielsen HM, Andreassen TT, Ledet T, Oxlund H. Local injection of TGF-beta increases the strength of tibial fractures in the rat. Acta Orthop Scand 1994; 65(1):37–41.
27. Broderick E, Infanger S, Turner TM, Sumner DR. Inhibition of bone mineralization following high dose TGF-b1 application. Transactions of the 49th Annual Meeting of the Orthpaedic Research Society, New Orleans, LA 28, 144. 2003. 2-2-2003.
28. Maes C, Carmeliet P, Moermans K et al. Impaired angiogenesis and endochondral bone formation in mice lacking the vascular endothelial growth factor isoforms VEGF164 and VEGF188. Mech Dev 2002; 111(1–2):61–73.

29. Harten RD, Svach DJ. Vascular endothelial growth factor inhibits DBM induced bone formation. Transactions of the 49th Annual Meeting of the Orthpaedic Research Society, New Orleans, LA 28, 51. 2003. 2-2-2003.
30. Schliephake H. Bone growth factors in maxillofacial skeletal reconstruction. Int J Oral Maxillofac Surg 2002; 31(5):469–484.
31. Spencer ME, Tokunaga A, Hunt TK. Insulin-like growth factor binding protein-3 is present in the alpha-granules of platelets. Endocrinology 1993; 132(3): 996–1001.
32. Asahara T, Bauters C, Zheng LP et al. Synergistic effect of vascular endothelial growth factor and basic fibroblast growth factor on angiogenesis in vivo. Circulation 1995; 92(9 Suppl):II365–371.
33. Kasperk CH, Wergedal JE, Mohan S, Long DL, Lau KH, Baylink DJ. Interactions of growth factors present in bone matrix with bone cells: effects on DNA synthesis and alkaline phosphatase. Growth Factors 1990; 3(2):147–158.
34. Lind M. Growth factor stimulation of bone healing. Effects on osteoblasts, osteomies, and implants fixation. Acta Orthop Scand Suppl 1998; 283:2–37.
35. Lynch SE, Colvin RB, Antoniades HN. Growth factors in wound healing. Single and synergistic effects on partial thickness porcine skin wounds. J Clin Invest 1989; 84(2):640–646.
36. Kevy SV, Jacobson MS. Comparison of methods for point of care preparation of autologous platelet gel. J Extra Corpor Technol 2004; 36:28–35.
37. Waters JH, Roberts KC. Database review of possible factors influencing point-of-care platelet gel manufacture. J Extra Corpor Technol 2004; 36(3):250–254.
38. Weibrich G, Kleis WK, Hitzler WE, Hafner G. Comparison of the platelet concentrate collection system with the plasma-rich-in-growth-factors kit to produce platelet-rich plasma: a technical report. Int J Oral Maxillofac Implants 2005; 20(1):118–123.
39. Wan DC, Longaker MT. Discussion Re: Woodell-May et al.: producing accurate platelet counts for platelet rich plasma: validation of a hematology analyzer and preparation techniques for counting. J Craniofac Surg 2005; 16(5):757–759.
40. Hokugo A, Ozeki M, Kawakami O et al. Augmented bone regeneration activity of platelet-rich plasma by biodegradable gelatin hydrogel. Tissue Eng 2005; 11(7–8):1224–1233.
41. Brodke D, Pedrozo HA, Kapur TA et al. Bone grafts prepared with selective cell retention technology heal canine segmental defects as effectively as autograft. J Orthop Res 2006; 24(5):857–866.
42. Dallari D, Fini M, Stagni C et al. In vivo study on the healing of bone defects treated with bone marrow stromal cells, platelet-rich plasma, and freeze-dried bone allografts, alone and in combination. J Orthop Res 2006; 24(5):877–888.
43. Lucarelli E, Fini M, Beccheroni A et al. Stromal stem cells and platelet-rich plasma improve bone allograft integration. Clin Orthop Relat Res 2005;(435):62–68.
44. Ranly DM, McMillan J, Keller T et al. Platelet-derived growth factor inhibits demineralized bone matrix-induced intramuscular cartilage and bone formation. A study of immunocompromised mice. J Bone Joint Surg Am 2005; 87-A(9):2052–2064.
45. Siebrecht MAN, De Rooij PP, Arm DM, Olsson ML, Aspenberg P. Platelet concentrate increases bone ingrowth into porous hydroxyapatitie. Orthopedics 2002; 25:169–172.
46. Weibrich G, Hansen T, Kleis W, Buch R, Hitzler WE. Effect of platelet concentration in platelet-rich plasma on peri-implant bone regeneration. Bone 2004; 34(4):665–671.
47. Jensen TB, Rahbek O, Overgaard S, Soballe K. Platelet rich plasma and fresh frozen bone allograft as enhancement of implant fixation. An experimental study in dogs. J Orthop Res 2004; 22(3):653–658.
48. Gandhi A, Dumas C, O'Connor JP, Parsons JR, Lin SS. The effects of local platelet rich plasma delivery on diabetic fracture healing. Bone 2005; 38:540–546.

49. Kim SG, Chung CH, Kim YK, Park JC, Lim SC. Use of particulate dentin-plaster of paris combination with/without platelet-rich plasma in the treatment of bone defects around implants. Int J Oral Maxillofac Implants 2002; 17(1):86–94.
50. Thorwarth M, Wehrhan F, Schultze-Mosgau S, Wiltfang J, Schlegel KA. PRP modulates expression of bone matrix proteins in vivo without long-term effects on bone formation. Bone 2006; 38(1):30–40.
51. Ito K, Yamada Y, Nagasaka T, Baba S, Ueda M. Osteogenic potential of injectable tissue-engineered bone: a comparison among autogenous bone, bone substitute (Bio-oss), platelet-rich plasma, and tissue-engineered bone with respect to their mechanical properties and histological findings. J Biomed Mater Res A 2005; 73A(1):63–72.
52. Aghaloo TL, Moy PK, Freymiller EG. Evaluation of platelet-rich plasma in combination with freeze-dried bone in the rabbit cranium. Clin Oral Implants Res 2005; 16(2):250–257.
53. Kim ES, Park EJ, Choung PH. Platelet concentration and its effect on bone formation in calvarial defects: an experimental study in rabbits. J Prosthet Dent 2001; 86(4):428–433.
54. Yamada Y, Ueda M, Naiki T, Takahashi M, Hata K, Nagasaka T. Autogenous injectable bone for regeneration with mesenchymal stem cells and platelet-rich plasma: tissue-engineered bone regeneration. Tissue Eng 2004; 10(5–6):955–964.
55. Walsh WR, Loefler A, Nicklin S et al. Spinal fusion using an autologous growth factor gel and a porous resorbable ceramic. Eur Spine J 2004; 13(4):359–366.
56. Aspenberg P, Virchenko O. Platelet concentrate injection improves Achilles tendon repair in rats. Acta Orthop Scand 2004; 75(1):93–99.
57. Murray MM, Spindler KP, Devin C et al. Use of a collagen-platelet rich plasma scaffold to stimulate healing of a central defect in the canine ACL. J Orthop Res 2006; 24(4):820–830.
58. Howes R, Bowness JM, Grotendorst GR, Martin GR, Reddi AH. Platelet-derived growth factor enhances demineralized bone matrix-induced cartilage and bone formation. Calcif Tissue Int 1988; 42(1):34–38.
59. Phillips B, Ball C, Sackett D et al. Levels of evidence and grades of recommendation. Centre for Evidence-Based Medicine, www.cebm.net/levels_of_evidence.asp#levels. 1998.
60. Savarino L, Cenni E, Tarabusi C et al. Evaluation of bone healing enhancement by lyophilized bone grafts supplemented with platelet gel: A standardized methodology in patients with tibial osteotomy for genu varus. J Biomed Mater Res B Appl Biomater 2006; 76(2):364–372.
61. Kitoh H, Kitakoji T, Tsuchiya H et al. Transplantation of marrow-derived mesenchymal stem cells and platelet-rich plasma during distraction osteogenesis–a preliminary result of three cases. Bone 2004; 35(4):892–898.
62. Franchini M, Dupplicato P, Ferro I, De GM, Aldegheri R. Efficacy of platelet gel in reconstructive bone surgery. Orthopedics 2005; 28(2):161–163.
63. Carreon LY, Glassman SD, Anekstein Y, Puno RM. Platelet gel (AGF) fails to increase fusion rates in instrumented posterolateral fusions. Spine 2005; 30(9): E243–E246.
64. Castro FP, Jr. Role of activated growth factors in lumbar spinal fusions. J Spinal Disord Tech 2004; 17(5):380–384.
65. Hee HT, Majd ME, Holt RT, Myers L. Do autologous growth factors enhance transforaminal lumbar interbody fusion? Eur Spine J 2003; 12(4):400–407.
66. Lowery GL, Kulkarni S, Pennisi AE. Use of autologous growth factors in lumbar spinal fusion. Bone Supplement 1999; 25 No.2:47S–50S.
67. Weiner BK, Walker M. Efficacy of autologous growth factors in lumbar intertransverse fusions. Spine 2003; 28(17):1968–1971.
68. Bose B, Balzarini MA. Bone graft gel: autologous growth factors used with autograft bone for lumbar spine fusions. Adv Ther 2002; 19(4):170–175.

69. Grant WP, Jerlin EA, Pietrzak WS, Tam HS. The utilization of autologous growth factors for the facilitation of fusion in complex neuropathic fractures in the diabetic population. Clin Podiatr Med Surg 2005; 22(4):561–584.
70. Barrow CR, Pomeroy GC. Enhancement of syndesmotic fusion rates in total ankle arthroplasty with the use of autologous platelet concentrate. Foot Ankle Int 2005; 26(6):458–461.
71. Bibbo C, Bono CM, Lin SS. Union rates using autologous platelet concentrate alone and with bone graft in high-risk foot and ankle surgery patients. J Surg Orthop Adv 2005; 14(1):17–22.
72. Mishra A, Pavelko T. Treatment of chronic elbow tendinosis with buffered platelet-rich plasma. Am J Sports Med 2006; In Press.
73. Camargo PM, Lekovic V, Weinlaender M, Vasilic N, Madzarevic M, Kenney EB. Platelet-rich plasma and bovine porous bone mineral combined with guided tissue regeneration in the treatment of intrabony defects in humans. J Periodontal Res 2002; 37(4):300–306.
74. Thor A, Wannfors K, Sennerby L, Rasmusson L. Reconstruction of the severely resorbed maxilla with autogenous bone, platelet-rich plasma, and implants: 1-year results of a controlled prospective 5-year study. Clin Implant Dent Relat Res 2005; 7(4):209–220.
75. Froum SJ, Wallace SS, Tarnow DP, Cho S-C. Effect of platelet-rich plasma on bone growth and osseointegration in human maxullary sinus grafts: three bilateral case reports. J Periodontol 2002; 22(1):45–53.
76. Kassolis JD, Rosen PS, Reynolds MA. Alveolar ridge and sinus augmentation utilizing platelet-rich plasma in combination with freeze-dried bone allograft: case series. J Periodontol 2000; 71(10):1654–1661.
77. Marx RE, Carlson ER, Eichstaedt RM, Schimmele SR, Strauss JE, Georgeff KR. Platelet-rich plasma: Growth factor enhancement for bone grafts. Oral Surg Oral Med Oral Pathol Oral Radiol Endod 1998; 85(6):638–646.
78. Okuda K, Tai H, Tanabe K et al. Platelet-rich plasma combined with a porous hydroxyapatite graft for the treatment of intrabony periodontal defects in humans: a comparative controlled clinical study. J Periodontol 2005; 76(6):890–898.
79. Klein MB, Yalamanchi N, Pham H, Longaker MT, Chang J. Flexor tendon healing in vitro: effects of TGF-beta on tendon cell collagen production. J Hand Surg [Am] 2002; 27(4):615–620.
80. Kisucka J, Butterfield CE, Duda DG et al. Platelets and platelet adhesion support angiogenesis while preventing excessive hemorrhage. Proc Natl Acad Sci U S A 2006; 103(4):855–860.
81. Haynesworth SE, Kadiyala S, Liang L, Bruder SP. Mitogenic stimulation of human mesenchymal stem cells by platelet releasate suggest a mechanism for enhancement of bone repair by platelet concentrates. 48th Annual Meeting of the Orthopeadic Research Society, Dallas, TX 27, 462. 2002.
82. Lucarelli E, Beccheroni A, Donati D et al. Platelet-derived growth factors enhance proliferation of human stromal stem cells. Biomaterials 2003; 24(18):3095–3100.

27

Gene Therapy Approaches for Musculoskeletal Tissue Regeneration

Renny T. Franceschi

Abstract: Safe, effective methods for bone and cartilage regeneration are needed to reverse bone loss caused by trauma, disease, tumor resection and osteoarthritis. Unfortunately, all current or emerging therapies have serious limitations. As will be developed in this chapter, gene therapy offers a promising approach for musculoskeletal regeneration because it can mimic the natural biological processes of bone development and fracture healing. This chapter will provide an overview of normal skeletal development and fracture repair, and describe how gene therapy in combination with tissue engineering can model critical aspects of these natural processes. Current gene therapy approaches for bone and cartilage regeneration will then be summarized, as well as recent work where combinatorial gene therapy is used to express groups of molecules that synergistically interact. Lastly, proposed new directions will be described that incorporate regulated gene expression and cells seeded in precise three-dimensional configurations on synthetic scaffolds to control both temporal and spatial distribution of regenerative factors. These and related approaches may eventually allow us to achieve the ultimate goal of bone tissue engineering: to reconstruct entire bones with associated joints, ligaments or sutures.

Keywords: Bone, cartilage, gene expression, tissue engineering.

27.1. Introduction

Developing effective therapies for bone and cartilage regeneration is one of the most clinically important long-term goals of research in the mineralized tissue field. Trauma, neoplasia, reconstructive surgery, congenital defects and osteoarthritis are all major worldwide health problems that would greatly benefit from progress in this field. The magnitude of health care burden associated with some of these disorders can begin to be appreciated from the following

University of Michigan School of Dentistry, Ann Arbor, MI

From: *Orthopedic Biology and Medicine: Musculoskeletal Tissue Regeneration, Biological Materials and Methods*
Edited by W. S. Pietrzak © Humana Press, Totowa, NJ

statistics. Of the approximately 6.2 million fractures that occur annually in the United States, 5 to 10 percent (0.3 to 0.6 million) fail to heal properly due to nonunion or delayed union [1], while osteoarthritis affects as many as 21 million people and accounts for over 50 percent of the total joint replacements (Arthritis Foundation website: *http://www.arthritis.org*).

As will be developed in this chapter, future improvements in regeneration therapy will require new molecular biology and tissue engineering-based technologies, including gene therapy. This chapter will summarize major developments in gene therapy related to bone and articular cartilage regeneration, and propose a new paradigm where gene therapy will be used to mimic natural processes occurring during bone development and repair. This will be accomplished by using regulated gene expression for the controlled delivery of regenerative factors coupled with custom-designed scaffolds that serve as a platform for gene and cell delivery. This chapter will cover the following topics: i) a discussion of the limitations of current approaches for bone and cartilage regeneration, ii) an overview of skeletal development and fracture repair and discussion of how these natural processes might be mimicked using gene therapy, iii) a description of gene therapy vectors and tissue engineering scaffolds, iv) a summary of studies that used gene therapy to express single regenerative molecules and v) a description of recent work using gene therapy to express unique combinations of regenerative molecules to enhance osteogenic activity, as well as studies incorporating regulated gene expression to control the timing of regenerative factor synthesis. Lastly, possible future directions for this exciting field will be discussed.

27.2. Limitations of Current Methods for Bone and Cartilage Regeneration

The successful regeneration of musculoskeletal tissues poses a number of challenges to the clinician. Nonunion or delayed union fracture sites are often inflamed and associated with significant scarring that may limit the availability of growth factors and osteogenic precursors. The articular cartilage of joints is devoid of a vasculature. Chondrocytes, which are embedded in an extensive extracellular matrix, receive nutrients only via diffusion from the synovial fluid. These cells consequently have a limited potential to proliferate or synthesize new proteoglycans [2]. Sites of osteoarthritis are also chronically inflamed, which further restricts regeneration [3]. In both cases the regeneration site shares similarities with other chronic wounds that are known to be deficient in growth/differentiation factors and to contain substantial proteolytic activity that likely contributes to rapid growth/differentiation factor degradation [4]. The regeneration of complex bone structures such as joints, craniofacial structures or even entire bones poses vastly more complex problems involving specification of three-dimensional shape as well as type of tissue formed.

For a regeneration therapy to be successful, inhibitory influences of inflammation must be overcome, appropriate precursor cells must be either recruited to or implanted at the regeneration site and cells must be given the appropriate signals and/or environmental cues to grow and differentiate. Current bone regenerative therapies include bone grafts, allogenic and xenograft bone matrix and, more recently, recombinant growth/differentiation factors. Autogenous bone grafts, still considered the gold standard for bone regeneration, contain all the components necessary for regeneration, including viable cells as well as growth/differentiation factors. However, bone regeneration after grafting is variable probably because of differences in the quality of the grafted bone [5–6]. In addition, severe morbidity/trauma can occur at both donor and graft sites. Allogenic bone matrix provides a bone-like extracellular matrix and is a crude source of bone-associated factors including bone morphogenetic proteins (BMPs). These factors have the potential to attract appropriate precursor cells to the regeneration site and stimulate their differentiation to bone. However, allogenic bone matrix has inconsistent osteoinductive activity principally because it contains low levels of regenerative molecules that are further inactivated during processing. There is also a potential risk of disease transmission if this material is not appropriately processed (for review, see [7]).

Recombinant bone morphogenetic proteins (BMPs) have the unique ability to stimulate the differentiation of mesenchymal cells to chondrocytes and osteoblasts and can induce formation of new bone. BMPs 2 and 7 will heal controlled segmental defects in a number of organisms including nonhuman primates [8], and have been successfully used in clinical trials for treatment of fibular and tibial nonunion fractures, maxillofacial reconstructions and spinal fusion (for reviews, see [9–10]. BMPs have been applied clinically in the United States for select applications such as spinal fusions and nonunions. However, clinical outcomes with BMP devices are, at best, no better than bone grafts. Furthermore, BMPs must be used at very high concentrations to be effective, and fail in a significant number of cases [11–12].

Current clinical approaches for articular cartilage regeneration involve drilling or abrasion to introduce mesenchymal chondrogenic precursors from the vascularized subchondral regions into the joint. However, the resulting cartilage contains a high proportion of fibrous elements and provides only temporary relief from osteoarthritic symptoms as a stopgap measure before total joint replacement [13]. Somewhat better outcomes have been reported with osteochondral grafts, but this approach is associated with the same concerns related to donor site morbidity mentioned for bone allografts [14]. Also, perichondral and periosteal grafts harvested from non-weight bearing areas and implantation of cultured chondrocytes have been assessed in limited clinical studies [15–16]. Although some success has been achieved with these approaches, they are limited by the availability of donor graft sites.

In summary, the science of musculoskeletal regeneration is clearly in the early stages of development with all current or emerging therapies having significant limitations. While there are a number of partial explanations for this including inconsistency of graft materials (bone/cartilage grafts or allogenic bone matrix) or, in the case of recombinant proteins, problems with stability or mode of delivery, an underlying problem is that no current regeneration strategies attempt to mimic events occurring during normal bone regeneration where multiple regenerative factors interact in a defined temporal and spatial sequence. An appreciation for the elegance of these natural processes can be gained from a brief review of the mechanisms of bone development and fracture repair.

27.3. Basic Science

27.3.1. Limb Development and Fracture Repair as Models for Regeneration

27.3.1.1. Limb Development

There are two broad phases of skeletal development: an initial commitment phase, when cells that will eventually form bone are specified in time and space, and a differentiation phase where cellular phenotypes necessary to form cartilage and bone are induced. Limb development provides a good example of the types of interactions necessary for skeletal morphogenesis. A number of soluble factors including fibroblast growth factors (FGFs), Wnt proteins, angiogenic factors and BMPs participate in a complex series of events that first define embryologic zones for future endochondral bone development and subsequently induce cartilage and bone of precisely defined morphologies (for reviews, see [17–19]). Limb formation is initiated by expression of FGF10 in presumptive limb regions of the lateral plate mesoderm. FGF10 induces FGF8 and FGF4 in ectodermal layers destined to become the apical ectodermal ridge (AER) of the limb bud and sonic hedgehog in the underlying mesoderm destined to become the zone of polarizing activity (ZPA). FGF 2, 4, 8 and 9 secreted by the AER stimulate proliferation of mesenchymal cells in the progress zone (PZ) of the limb bud immediately under (proximal to) the AER. Cells in the PZ continue to proliferate as undifferentiated mesenchymal cells while more proximal cells form condensations first of the more proximal bones (i.e., humerus) followed by the segmentation into more distal bones of the forearm and hand. Sonic hedgehog (SHH) secreted from the ZPA is responsible for anterior-posterior asymmetry of the limb. SHH is an upstream regulator of BMPs 2, 4 and 7 during limb development, and manipulation of the pattern of SHH expression alters BMP distribution [20–21]. SHH is able to specify the anterior-posterior positioning of mesenchymal condensations destined to become skeletal elements (e.g., specification of the individual digits of the hand) possibly by controlling the location of BMPs [22]. Mesenchymal condensations form a cartilage anlagen that is subsequently replaced by bone via an endochondral process. Vascular invasion, mediated at least in part by vascular endothelial growth factor (VEGF), represents a crucial step in the transition of the cartilage anlagen to bone. Consistent with this concept, mutant mice expressing a VEGF isoform with limited activity have multiple endochondral and intramembraneous bone defects [23]. Also, in endochondral bone formation, VEGF couples hypertrophic cartilage remodeling, ossification and angiogenesis [24–25]. Angiogenesis associated with bony collar formation provides nutrients, oxygen and growth/differentiation factors that may affect mesenchymal stem cell differentiation into bone cells [26]. Blood vessels may also be a source of osteogenic precursors via pericytes associated with the vascular smooth muscle layer [27–28] and/or by delivering blood-borne precursors [29].

Specific transcription factors control the differentiation of mesenchymal precursors down chondrocytic and osteoblast lineages. RUNX2, an essential transcription factor for osteoblast and hypertrophic chondrocyte differentiation, is expressed at early times in limb development coincident with the formation of mesenchymal condensations [30–32]. Two additional factors, SOX9 and Osterix (OSX), have more selective roles in chondrocyte and osteoblast differentiation, respectively. RUNX2, OSX and SOX9 are all induced by BMPs. However, OSX also requires RUNX2 in that it is not present in *Runx2* –/– mice [33–34]. Both *Runx2* and *Sox9* have the ability to convert mesenchymal cells into osteoblasts or chondrocytes and are, therefore, considered master genes for these pathways [35–37].

27.3.1.2. Fracture Healing

Fracture repair, which can be considered a recapitulation of endochondral bone formation, requires multiple factors that are expressed in a defined temporal sequence [38–39]. After a bone fractures, an initial inflammatory response recruits activated macrophages and polymorphonuclear neutrophils (PMNs) that together endocytose microdebris and microorganisms. This is followed by formation of a hematoma under the control of platelet-derived growth factor (PDGF), insulin-like growth factors (IGFs), transforming growth factor β (TGF-β) and FGF2 produced by macrophages [40–41]. Subsequent blastema formation is associated with proliferation of granulation tissue fibroblasts. BMPs, TGF-β and FGF2 induce osteoprogenitors to differentiate into chondrocytes (endochondral bone only) and osteoblasts. Generally, FGFs, IGFs and PDGFs act as mitogenic factors that are widely distributed in the soft callus early in fracture repair, while BMPs are more associated with chondrocytes and osteoblasts later in the healing process. However, individual BMPs also exhibit unique temporal expression patterns, with BMP2 mRNA being highest during the initial inflammatory phase and BMPs 3a, 4, 7 and 8 highest during late chondrogenic and osteogenic phases of fracture repair [42]. The requirement for angiogenesis in fracture healing and bone regeneration is particularly striking. VEGF is up regulated at early times as a result of hypoxia in the fracture callus. This induction is mediated by hypoxia-inducible factor (HIF-1), a transcription factor controlling genes necessary for survival in hypoxic conditions [43]. Consistent with angiogenesis playing an essential role in fracture healing, adenovirus-mediated overexpression of VEGF shortens the endochondral phase of fracture healing [44]. Furthermore, pharmacological inhibition of angiogenesis or treatment with soluble VEGF receptor (soluble Flt1) blocks fracture healing and BMP2 induction of bone formation [45–47].

27.3.2. Cooperative Interactions Between Osteogenic Factors

A common thread linking all the biological systems discussed above is the involvement of multiple bioactive factors in bone induction. In some cases each factor makes a separate contribution to the osteogenic response. For example, growth factors like FGFs, PDGF and VEGF stimulate osteogenic precursor proliferation and angiogenesis while BMPs initiate overt bone formation. Combinations of bioactive factors can synergistically stimulate bone regeneration. For example, the combined application of FGF4 and BMP2 synergistically interact to promote bone formation when implanted in a suitable matrix [40, 48–49]. In some cases osteogenic factors form oligomeric complexes with enhanced biological activity. This concept is best illustrated for the BMPs. Although homodimers of BMPs 2, 4 and 7 all have osteoinductive activity, there is now good evidence that these factors act in combination. BMPs 2, 4 and 7 are expressed in overlapping patterns during limb development [50–51] and overlapping expression of BMPs 2, 3a, 4, 7 and 8 is observed at various times during fracture healing [42]. Although most bone induction studies with BMPs used homodimeric molecules, BMP 2/7 and 4/7 heterodimers can be detected when cDNAs encoding these molecules are coexpressed in cell culture. Furthermore, BMP heterodimers have greater biological activity than their constituent homodimers [50–53].

27.3.3. Use of Gene Therapy to Mimick the Natural Process of Bone Formation

Given the complexity of the natural processes of bone development and fracture healing, it is unlikely that current regenerative therapies involving single bioactive factors or implantation of single cell types will be able to realize the overall goal of bone tissue engineering, which is to reconstruct entire bones with associated joints, sutures and precise three-dimensional morphology. Such complex types of regeneration will require control over the types of factors produced and their temporal sequence of release while at the same time providing the appropriate target precursor cell populations, all within a precisely defined three-dimensional lattice.

Scaffold systems are currently under development that allow controlled release of proteins from artificial matrices [54–57]. However, as currently devised, these systems control only the rate of release and cannot be turned on or off at specific times. Furthermore, they normally release only a single factor at a time. Although none of these limitations are necessarily insurmountable, at the present time protein-based delivery devices do not provide the best means of examining the interplay between multiple factors at a regeneration site.

Gene therapy approaches, in contrast, have the potential to provide control over the timing, distribution and level of multiple regenerative factors that can be either simultaneously or sequentially expressed in a tissue-specific manner. A wide range of viral and non-viral vectors are now available to allow efficient gene transfer into a number of cell types including osteogenic precursors and stem cells. Considerable progress has also been made in the design of tissue engineering scaffolds that can be fabricated into precise three-dimensional configurations to support the growth of genetically modified cells. Lastly, several regulated gene expression systems have been developed for the efficient activation and inhibition of gene expression. The remainder of this chapter will explore each of these areas, review recent progress in the use of gene therapy for bone regeneration and outline future directions for this promising field.

27.3.4. Gene Therapy Vectors and Tissue Engineering Scaffolds

27.3.4.1. Gene Therapy Vectors

A number of vector systems have been developed for gene therapy applications including adenoviruses, adeno-associated viruses, retroviruses, lentiviruses and unmodified plasmid DNA. Each vector system has its own advantages and disadvantages.

Adenoviruses have highly evolved mechanisms to deliver DNA to cells and, unlike retroviruses, are not dependent on cell replication for infection. Adenoviruses infect cells by binding of the viral fiber capsid protein by coxsackievirus and adenovirus receptor (CAR), and binding of the viral penton base by α_v integrins on the cell surface. The broad distribution of these receptors explains why adenoviruses can be used to infect such a wide range of cell types [58–59]. After infection adenoviruses do not normally integrate into the host genome and, instead, remain in the nucleus as an episome that is gradually degraded as cells divide [60]. Most gene therapy studies conducted to date used first generation adenoviruses. These vectors have been genetically modified to be replication incompetent, but still contain most of the viral genome including genes encoding the major coat proteins. Because of this, cells infected with first generation adenovirus vectors will secrete viral proteins and elicit an immune response that will eventually result in their clearance from the body. The combined effects of episomal localization and immunogenicity cause transgene expression from first generation adenoviruses to be quite brief. As an example, we recently determined that the *in vivo* duration of BMP expression from fibroblasts transduced with Ad-BMP2 was less than two weeks [61]. This short period of BMP production has advantages and disadvantages; it can prevent bone formation from exceeding the boundaries of the desired regeneration site, but it can also restrict osteogenesis so much that it is no longer therapeutically useful. Because of these problems, second generation adenovirus-based vectors that lack genes for most or all viral proteins have been developed [62–63]. These vectors have the advantage of being able to package up to 30 kb of foreign DNA. However, they can only be propagated in the presence of helper viruses that contain the missing viral genes necessary to form a viable capsid. In spite of these limitations, first generation adenoviruses continue to be extremely useful for defining which regenerative factors or groups of factors can best stimulate bone regeneration.

Retroviruses are the most widely used vectors for gene therapy applications. Unlike adenoviruses, these RNA viruses use reverse transcriptase to make a double-stranded copy of their genome that is randomly integrated into the host and then replicated as the cell divides [60]. Most gene therapy clinical trials to correct genetic diseases used replication-incompetent murine leukemia virus (MLV), which is non-pathogenic in humans and unlikely to recombine with other human viruses [64]. After integration MLV exists in the host cell as a DNA copy that is not able to transcribe genes encoding viral coat proteins. For this reason the integrated virus cannot elicit an immune response. However, there are two negative aspects to viral integration. First, the integrated retrovirus can disrupt normal cell function by insertional mutagenesis, an event that, unfortunately, was recently observed in patients [65–66]. Second, since retroviral genomes are replicated as cells divide, they remain a permanent part of the host cell, and any transgenes they carry must be under the control of a regulated promoter if they are to be turned off after regeneration has been achieved. Also, retroviruses only infect replicating cells. For this reason MLV vectors are most suitable for *ex vivo* gene therapy applications.

Lentiviruses are a specialized family of retroviruses that include human immunodeficiency virus 1 (HIV-1). Unlike the oncogenic retroviruses described in the preceding paragraph, lentiviral vectors can infect nondividing cells including hematopoietic progenitor cells and marrow-derived stromal cells [67–68]. While lentiviruses integrate into the host cell genome, sites of integration may be more restricted than for traditional retroviruses. This characteristic may explain why lentiviral vectors give more stable gene expression after integration into cells, and also reduces the probability of causing disease through insertional mutagenesis [69]. These features have prompted considerable interest in this family of viruses as vectors for gene therapy. However, because of the lethal nature of many of the parent viruses used to develop lentiviral vectors, a considerable effort has been made to produce modified viruses that are safe for clinical use. Strategies for improving the safety of lentiviral vectors include altering the viral genome to minimize the likelihood of recombinations that could produce replication competent viruses, and elimination of all viral genes that are not necessary for gene transfer.

Like gutted adenovirus vectors, adeno-associated virus (AAV) gene therapy vectors do not express viral proteins and are, therefore, non-immunogenic. These vectors have the further advantage of being non-pathogenic in humans, yet are able to infect a wide range of dividing and nondividing cells without integrating into the genome [60]. Although only a small number of studies examined AAV in gene therapy applications for bone regeneration, Luk and co-workers recently showed that AAV encoding the BMP4 gene could stimulate bone formation after injection into an intramuscular site [70]. AAV vectors show considerable promise for eventual use in the clinic. However, because they are still quite difficult to construct, for research purposes it is probably more appropriate that critical genetic interactions first be studied with more traditional adeno- or retrovirus vectors.

Non-viral vectors that contain only naked DNA and a carrier to facilitate cell uptake have several advantages over viral vectors including ease of manufacture, stability, low immunogenicity and low likelihood of being able to insert into the host cell genome [60]. This class of vector can be injected directly into tissues as naked DNA, adsorbed to liposomes or attached to microprojectiles of gold or tungsten that are injected into cells by high pressure gas or an electrical discharge [71–72]. Although recent advances involving condensation of DNA with liposomes or other carriers have the potential to enhance the uptake of non-viral DNA by cells [73], as currently formulated, cellular uptake of non-viral vectors is an extremely inefficient process, estimated to be 10^{-9} that of viral vectors [74].

27.3.4.2. Tissue Engineering Scaffolds

Tissue engineering scaffolds are critical for the success of any gene therapy strategy. Since they will be discussed elsewhere in this book, they will only be briefly mentioned here. Scaffolds have the potential to control release rates of gene therapy vectors and/or provide a suitable three-dimensional environment for the growth and differentiation of osteoprogenitor and mesenchymal stem cells (for reviews on various aspects of scaffold design, see [54, 75, 76]). Through the use of computer-aided design and three-dimensional printing technologies, scaffolds can also be fabricated into precise geometries. This is particularly important for craniofacial applications where it is critical for the morphology of regenerated bone to be precisely controlled. Using this technology a three-dimensional reconstruction of the specific region targeted for regeneration can be generated from computer-aided tomography (CAT) scans (for an example of this approach, see [77]). In an interesting recent permutation of this technology, it is also possible to print cells suspended in gel droplets to form specific three-dimensional arrays [78]. Furthermore, recent developments in polymer chemistry have made it possible to extensively modify both the surface properties and microporosity of polymer scaffolds to provide a wide range of structures and bioactive surfaces. Such scaffolds have the potential to provide environments conducive to the growth of specific cell types. For example, surface modification of alginate scaffolds can provide a supportive environment for growth of osteoblasts [79].

27.4. Review of Preclinical Studies

27.4.1. Expression of Single Regenerative Factors Using Gene Therapy

The use of gene therapy to stimulate the regeneration of bone and cartilage has been extensively explored over the past decade. Both viral and non-viral vectors were used to direct the constitutive expression of individual factors. Two strategies were used to deliver genes to sites targeted for regeneration (see Fig. 27.1); vectors were either directly administered to *in vivo* sites (*In Vivo* Gene Therapy), or used to transduce cells in tissue culture that were subsequently implanted into animals (*Ex Vivo* Gene Therapy). In both cases cells can be engineered to produce the molecule of interest for sustained periods by transduction with an appropriate vector, thereby avoiding problems associated with protein degradation and delivery from implanted matrices. Because several recent reviews are available on this subject [80–83], only a few illustrative examples will be discussed.

27.4.1.1. Bone Regeneration

Both *in vivo* and *ex vivo* gene therapy approaches have been applied to bone regeneration using adenovirus as well as other vector systems. *In vivo* gene

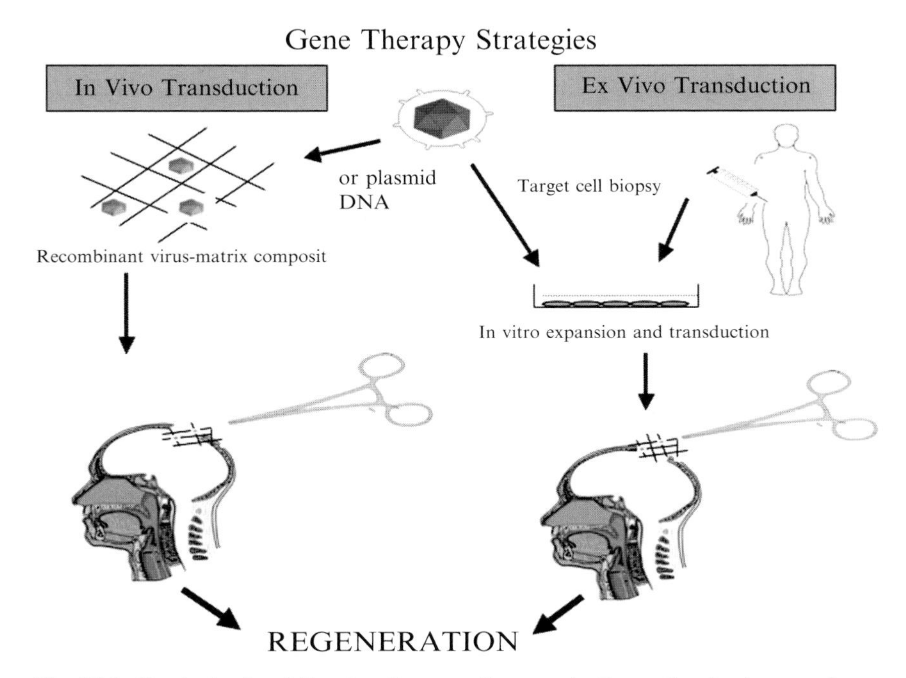

Fig. 27.1 Strategies for delivering therapeutic genes to tissue sites *In vivo* transduction involves direct delivery of a viral or non-viral gene therapy vector to the target tissue of interest using a suitable carrier matrix *Ex vivo* gene therapy first requires transduction of syngeneic cells in tissue culture followed by implantation at the regeneration site of the patient (adapted from [118] courtesy of S. Karger AG, Basel)

therapy using adenovirus expressing BMPs 2, 4, 6, 7 and 9 was shown to induce ectopic bone formation in subcutaneous and/or intramuscular sites [74, 84–86]. This approach has also been successfully used to partially heal segmental femoral defects in both rabbits and rats using an adenovirus encoding BMP2 (AdBMP2) [87–88]. For these experiments muscle surrounding the defect was used to create a closed chamber between the cut ends of the bone and adenovirus was directly injected into this site without the use of a carrier. Direct application of AdBMP7 has also been used to stimulate healing of alveolar bone around titanium dental implants [89]. In this study the AdBMP7 was suspended in a Type I collagen matrix before implantation. An *in vivo* gene therapy approach was also developed using direct transfer of plasmid DNAs encoding BMP4 and a parathyroid hormone fragment that were mixed with a Type I collagen carrier [90–91]. This gene activated matrix or GAM could partially heal a canine femur segmental defect after 52 weeks. A common feature of all these *in vivo* strategies was the need to use very large amounts of the gene therapy vector (2×10^{10} adenovirus particles or 100 mg plasmid DNA). This requirement is likely explained by degradation and clearance of adenovirus vectors by the immune system and the inefficient uptake of plasmid DNA by cells.

Ex vivo approaches have also been extensively examined. Although this approach involves the additional step of first isolating and culturing cells from the host for *ex vivo* transduction, it has the advantage of being able to target the gene therapy to a specific cell population under controlled *in vitro* conditions before implantation into the regeneration site. Two different types of *ex vivo* gene therapy will be discussed; studies using cultured fibroblasts or mesenchymal stem cells (MSCs) as the target cell population.

Cultured dermal or gingival fibroblasts transduced with AdBMP7 *ex vivo* are able to form bone after implantation into subcutaneous and orthotopic sites [92–93]. This response was largely explained by secretion of BMP7 by implanted cells that then acted on neighboring host cells with a lesser amount of bone formation being attributed to direct differentiation of the implanted cells. When implanted into either calvaria or long bone critical size defects (defect size selected to be unable to spontaneously heal), AdBMP7-transduced fibroblasts were also able to stimulate bone regeneration. For the cranial model a 9-mm calvarial defect was created in Lewis rats using a trephine [92]. Cells transduced with either lacZ control adenovirus or Ad-BMP7 were adsorbed to gelatin sponges before placement in defects. The Ad-BMP7-transduced cells induced sufficient bone formation in four weeks to largely close the calvarial defect. For the long bone model, a 2 to 3 mm osteotomy was created in femurs of Fisher rats previously immobilized using an external fixator [93]. Histological and radiological examination of defects revealed significant bone healing by Ad-BMP7-transduced cells after six weeks. Both bone and cartilage formation was seen.

Marrow stromal cells (MSCs) have also been used as targets for *ex vivo* gene transfer. These cells are derived from the tissue culture plastic adherent, non-hematopoietic fraction of marrow. A subfraction of MSCs have stem cell-like properties and the capability to differentiate along all four mesenchymal lineages (bone, cartilage, muscle, fat) [94]. In addition to being a source of BMPs after transduction, these cells directly respond to BMPs and participate in osteogenesis after implantation [95]. This may be particularly important in regenerative sites where the supply of endogenous osteogenic precursors is limiting. MSCs transduced with adenoviruses encoding BMPs were shown to stimulate bone regeneration in a number of experimental models. For example, Ad-BMP2-transduced MSCs can heal femoral segmental defects in rats [96–97], bilateral maxillary defects and calvarial defects in swine [98–99] and induce spine fusion in rabbits and rats [100–101]. Cell populations with mesenchymal stem cell-like properties have also been isolated from muscle and adipose tissue [102–103] and can induce bone formation after transduction with BMP2 or BMP4 vectors [46, 104]. In a recent report a lentivirus vector was also used to express BMP2 in marrow stromal cells that were shown to stably express BMP2 for at least eight weeks *in vitro*. Furthermore, virally infected cells formed bone after implantation into muscle pouches of immunodeficient mice [105].

27.4.1.2. Regeneration of Articular Cartilage

As noted above, the regeneration of cartilage poses particular challenges due to the lack of vascularity and low metabolic activity of this tissue. Two different gene therapy strategies have been used to combat the articular cartilage loss associated with osteoarthritis, approaches to stimulate new cartilage formation and approaches to suppress cartilage loss associated with chronic joint inflammation.

Gene therapy has been used to deliver several growth/differentiation factors associated with cartilage including TGF-β1 [106], IFG-1 [107], BMP2 [108–109], BMP4 [110], BMP7 [111] and FGF2 [112–114]. For these studies full- or partial-thickness defects were created in the patellar groove of the anterior surface of the distal femur using mechanical abrasion, followed by either direct *in vivo* gene therapy or *ex vivo* approaches using various cell types. Defects were then evaluated for amount and histological quality of new cartilage formed. Varying degrees of cartilage regeneration were observed depending on the particular regenerative molecule used, mode of delivery (*in vivo* or *ex vivo*) or type of cell implanted into defects. For example, Di Cesare, et al. showed that plasmid DNA encoding BMP2 as well as recombinant BMP2 protein adsorbed to a Type I collagen matrix could partially heal a femoral trochlea defect, although complete bridging of margin defects was not seen [108]. Also, direct application of adeno-associated virus expressing FGF2 to full-thickness distal femur defects was shown to selectively transduce synoviocytes with high efficiency and heal defects after eight or 12 weeks [113–114]. Using an *ex vivo* approach Lee and co-workers reported complete bridging of a full-thickness cartilage defect in rabbits implanted with NIH3T3 fibroblasts transduced with a retrovirus expressing TGF-β1[106]. In this study the regenerated cartilage was continuous with existing articular cartilage and persisted in the defect for up to 12 weeks. Marrow and other mesenchymal stem cell-like populations have also been examined in *ex vivo* gene therapy studies with BMPs [109–110]. These studies suggested that bone marrow stromal cells and muscle-derived stem cells exhibit a greater chondrogenic response to BMPs than stem cells derived from fat. However, none of these cells completely healed defects.

Inflammation and excessive mechanical loading are both thought to contribute to osteoarthritis. These processes are associated with inflammatory cytokines such as IL-1 leading to the release of matrix metalloproteinases. Gene therapy approaches have been designed to block both these processes.

For example, in a number of studies intra-articular expression of IL-1 receptor agonist protein (IL-1Ra) was shown to inhibit IL-1 activity and arthritis [3, 115–116]. In an interesting application of this approach, Pan and coworkers took advantage of the observation that the inflammatory mediator, lipopolysaccharide (LPS), is able to activate IL-1Ra expression driven by a cytomegalovirus promoter. Because IL-1Ra is secreted with each new inflammatory challenge, this approach was able to suppress joint degeneration that normally occurs in an animal model of rheumatoid arthritis [116]. The use of retroviral expression of human tissue inhibitor of metalloproteinases 1 (TIMP-1) in chondrocytes was also explored as a means of suppressing IL-1-induced cartilage degradation. Compared with control samples, TIMP-1 expressing cartilage resisted the catabolic actions of IL-1, as measured by reduced metalloproteinase activity and degradation of Type II collagen [117].

These studies demonstrate the power of single factor gene therapy in clinically relevant models of bone/cartilage regeneration, and provide strong evidence for the feasibility of this approach as a clinical alternative to protein therapy.

27.4.2. Combinatorial Gene Therapy and Regulated Gene Expression

While the gene therapy approaches currently under investigation offer a promising alternative to protein therapy and may lead to the eventual development of therapeutics, they only partially achieve the potential of this approach as outlined earlier in this chapter. Specifically, gene therapy has the potential to provide control over the types and combinations of regenerative factors produced, as well as the timing, duration and tissue localization of factor synthesis. The following paragraphs will summarize initial studies designed to exploit some of these new gene therapy approaches. Specifically, the discussion will focus on the use of gene therapy to express combinations of interacting regenerative molecules and to control the timing of factor delivery. We will specifically focus on: (i) the osteogenic activity of combinations of BMPs, (ii) interactions between angiogenic and osteogenic signals, (iii) use of an osteogenic transcription factor to increase osteoblast differentiation and BMP responsiveness of MSCs and (iv) the development of inducible gene expression systems to control the timing and duration of osteogenic factor synthesis.

27.4.2.1. Cooperative Interactions between BMPs

As noted above (see Section 2.2, Cooperative Interactions between Osteogenic Factors), multiple BMPs are coexpressed during development and fracture healing and may exist in nature as heterodimers. Furthermore, BMP 2/7 and 4/7 heterodimers have greater biological activity than their constituent homodimers. Taken together, these studies suggest that there may be certain advantages to using combinations of BMPs for bone regeneration. To begin addressing this possibility we examined the ability of combinations of adenoviruses expressing BMPs 2, 4 and 7 to induce *in vitro* osteoblast differentiation and *in vivo* bone formation [61, 118]. For *in vitro* studies mesenchymal cell lines were transduced with AdBMP2, 4 or 7 or virus combinations. Significantly, combined transduction of Ad-BMP2 plus Ad-BMP7, or Ad-BMP4 plus Ad-BMP7, resulted in a synergistic stimulation of osteoblast differentiation. This synergy was explained by formation of BMP2/7 and BMP4/7 heterodimers. To test *in vivo* biological activity, fibroblasts were transduced with specific virus combinations and subcutaneously implanted into C57BL6 mice. Consistent

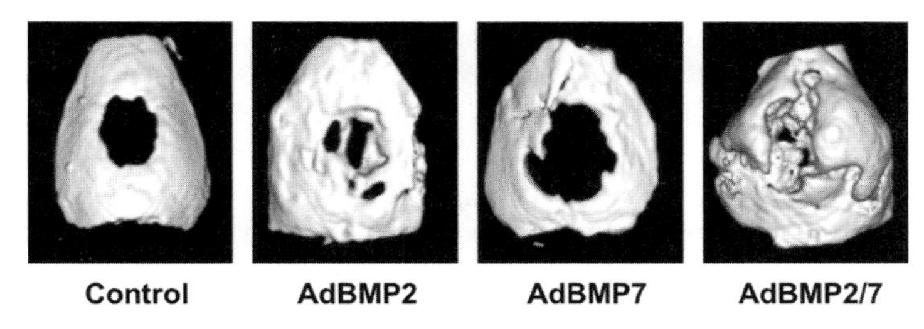

Fig. 27.2 Cooperative interactions between AdBMP2 and AdBMP7 in stimulating healing of a calvarial defect BLK fibroblasts were transduced with equal titers of control vector (AdlacZ), AdBMP2, AdBMP7 or AdBMP2 plus AdBMP7 and adsorbed to collagen sponges for implantation into 7 mm defects in the calvaria of C57BL6 mice Calvaria were harvested after six weeks for analysis by micro-computed tomography Note dramatic enhancement of bone formation in the AdBMP2 plus AdBMP7-treated group (unpublished result, Koh J-T, Zhao M, Wang Z, Krebsbach PH and Franceschi RT)

with *in vitro* results, strong synergy was observed using combined Ad-BMP2/BMP7 treatment which induced two to three-fold more bone than would be predicted, based on the activity of individual Ad-BMPs. We also recently evaluated the osteogenic activity of AdBMP2/7 cotransduction in a cranial defect model, and also observed dramatically enhanced bone healing relative to defect treated with equal titers of AdBMP2 or 7 (Fig. 27-2). These studies show that dramatic enhancement of osteogenesis can be achieved using gene therapy to express specific combinations of interacting regenerative molecules. Because of their increased biological activity, such vector formulations can achieve bone regeneration at much lower viral titers, thereby minimizing possible toxicity and/or immune responses. In related studies Zhu and co-workers used a similar approach to induce *in vitro* osteoblast differentiation and *in vivo* spinal fusion with combinations of Ad-BMP2 and Ad-BMP7 [119].

27.4.2.2. Synergies between Angiogenic and Osteogenic Signals

Normal bone development will not occur in the absence of blood vessel formation (see Section 2). To examine possible interactions between BMP and angiogenic signals, Peng and co-workers used retroviral gene transfer to establish stable muscle-derived stem cell (MDSC) lines expressing BMP4, vascular endothelial growth factor (VEGF) or the VEGF antagonist, soluble Flt1, that were subsequently examined, alone or in combination, for osteogenic activity [46]. VEGF by itself was devoid of osteogenic activity. However, it was able to act synergistically with BMP4 to increase mesenchymal stem cell recruitment and survival, as well as stimulate bone formation in a calvarial defect. Effects of VEGF on bone healing were shown to be critically dependent on the ratio of VEGF to BMP, with excessive VEGF/BMP ratios shown to actually inhibit osteogenesis. Furthermore, the specificity of this response was established by showing that the VEGF response was totally blocked by soluble Flt1 antagonist. In related studies, Huang and co-workers observed enhanced osteogenesis by human MSCs when they were adsorbed to poly(lactic-co-glycolic acid) scaffolds containing combinations of condensed plasmid DNA encoding BMP-4 and VEGF [120]. These studies emphasize the importance of vascularization in the overall process of bone regeneration, and show how the coexpression of angiogenic and osteoinductive factors can enhance bone formation.

27.4.2.3. Use of the RUNX2 Transcription Factor to Stimulate BMP Responsiveness and Osteogenic Activity of Marrow Stromal Cells

MSCs contain stem cells capable of forming all mesenchymal tissues, including bone and cartilage [94]. However, osteogenic cells only represent a small fraction of the total MSC population [121]. Several approaches have been used to enhance this osteogenic activity, including *ex vivo* transduction with AdBMP4 (see Section 4). One problem with this approach is that BMPs are secreted from transduced MSCs to affect host cells as well as implanted MSC differentiation, which may spread the osteogenic response beyond the area targeted for regeneration. As an alternative strategy several groups have explored the use of the osteogenic transcription factor, RUNX2, to enhance the osteogenic potential of MSCs. As discussed in Section 2, *Runx2* is a master gene controlling bone and hypertrophic cartilage differentiation. Expression of RUNX2 in undifferentiated mesenchymal cell lines induces osteoblast differentiation *in vitro* and bone formation after implantation into immunodeficient mice [35–36]. Furthermore RUNX2-expressing cells exhibited enhanced responsiveness to BMPs resulting in further stimulation of osteoblast differentiation [122].

Transduction of primary MSC cultures with Ad-RUNX2 increased RUNX2 protein expression, stimulated osteoblast differentiation/mineralization and increased responsiveness to BMP2 [122–123]. To assess *in vivo* osteogenic activity, Ad-RUNX2 and control (Ad-LacZ) cells were adsorbed to two different carrier scaffolds and subcutaneously implanted into C57BL6 mice. In both cases MSCs expressing RUNX2 formed substantially more bone than cells transduced with the control vector. In related studies stable transduction of primary skeletal myoblasts with a retrovirus encoding RUNX2 has been shown to stimulate *in vitro* osteoblast differentiation and osteogenic activity [124–125]. In these studies RUNX2-expressing cells also exhibited enhanced responsiveness to BMP2. Lastly, Zheng and co-workers showed that Ad-RUNX2-transduced marrow stromal cells could partially heal a calvarial defect in BALB/c mice under conditions where non-transduced MSCs failed to form bone [126].

Taken together, these results show that the responsiveness of osteoprogenitor cell populations to BMPs can be enhanced *in vitro* and *in vivo* by factors like RUNX2 that are major regulators of the osteoprogenitor lineage. In addition they suggest possible therapeutic benefits that may be derived from using bone and cartilage-related transcription factors to enhance BMP responsiveness in osteoprogenitor populations.

27.4.2.4. Regulated Gene Expression

As discussed in Section 1, current approaches to bone regeneration are limited by the lack of control over timing of factor delivery and the use of single regenerative factors. This is markedly different from the natural processes of limb development and fracture healing where growth, angiogenic, chondrogenic and osteogenic factors are expressed in a defined temporal sequence, allowing each factor to target different cell populations. The role of timing and sequence of factor delivery cannot be addressed with the gene delivery approaches discussed so far in this chapter that all used constitutively active promoters to drive transgene expression. To address this issue a number of groups have begun exploring the use of regulated gene expression systems for bone regeneration. Regulated gene expression systems have been developed using tetracycline-regulated promoters to control BMP2 or BMP4 expression. Moutsatsos and co-workers described a Tet-OFF system (inhibited by tetracycline) for controlled expression of BMP2 that was engineered in the C3H10T1/2 cell line and shown to induce repair of a segmental long bone defect [127]. Peng, et al. developed a Tet-ON system (induced by tetracycline) for expression of BMP4 using muscle stem cells, and showed that it could stimulate regeneration of a cranial defect [128]. Because tetracycline/doxycycline are bone-seeking drugs they have the potential to be sequestered in bone and may interfere with regulated expression. Also, the Tet regulated systems, in some cases, exhibited low levels of BMP expression and bone formation in the uninduced state [128–129]. For these reasons, we recently developed a stringent dimerizer-regulated system for BMP2 that is induced by rapamycin and its non-immunosuppressive analogs(130). This system does not express detectable BMP in the uninduced state but, when induced, can partially heal a cranial defect in mice. Using such systems it may be possible to control the temporal sequence of release for groups of interacting factors, thereby gaining greater control over the regenerative response. In this way it should be possible to coordinate regenerative factor synthesis with the presence of the appropriate target cell population. For example, FGF2 has potent anabolic actions on bone *in vivo* and can stimulate bone regeneration when implanted in a suitable matrix [49, 131–132]. However, because a major function of FGFs is to stimulate precursor cell proliferation, they can be antagonistic to differentiation factors like BMPs if both factors are simultaneously presented to cells [133]. However, using regulated gene expression, a regeneration strategy might be envisioned where early FGF2 expression could be used to expand precursor cells present in the early fracture callous, followed by induction of a BMP to stimulate these cells to differentiate to chondrocytes and osteoblasts.

27.5. Clinical Review

Safety concerns and lack of basic knowledge concerning vector clearance from the body have, until now, precluded the initiation of clinical gene therapy protocols for bone or cartilage regeneration. However, it is likely that clinical trials for limited gene therapy applications are likely to take place in the near future (see next section).

27.6. Future Trends and Needs

As outlined in this chapter, gene therapy offers a number of advantages as a skeletal regeneration strategy. In addition to being able to deliver more sustained levels of regenerative factors than can be achieved by protein therapy, it has the potential to easily deliver combinations of factors and to control the timing and duration of factor delivery. Nevertheless, a number of issues must be addressed before gene therapy can become a useful clinical procedure for regenerating bone and cartilage.

As was discussed in Section 3, the two most commonly used gene therapy vectors, adenoviruses and retroviruses, both have serious safety concerns related to immunogenicity and insertional mutagenesis. While these vectors continue to be very useful for experimental validation of gene therapy approaches, their future use in humans will be very limited, especially for elective procedures. Newer vectors such as AAV and, possibly, lentiviruses show greater promise for clinical use, but still must be carefully evaluated. Although direct delivery of naked DNA is currently still a very inefficient process, further improvements in transfection efficiency may ultimately make this the method of choice for certain gene therapy applications. A second issue is related to control of the regeneration response. Most studies to date have used vectors containing constitutively active promoters that will continue to drive regenerative factor expression until the vector or transduced cell is cleared from the body. For example, uncontrolled BMP2 production leads to bone overgrowth that can be attenuated only by also expressing Noggin, a BMP inhibitor [129]. Regulated gene expression may be the eventual method of choice for restricting osteogenic responses of this type. However, certain constitutively active vectors may be cleared from the regeneration site rapidly enough to prevent overgrowth. This needs to be carefully examined on a tissue-by-tissue basis before clinical trials can be considered. It is anticipated that both these issues will be addressed for more straightforward types of regeneration, such as articular cartilage repair and nonunion fractures, in the next few years and that clinical trials, possibly using constitutively active AAV vectors, will commence within the next one to three years.

More advanced gene therapy approaches involving combinations of regenerative factors, control of timing and sequence of factor delivery, as well as cell orientation, will require more basic studies to define optimal factor interactions over time and the development of approaches to seed cells on artificial matrixes in specific orientations. As was developed in this chapter, in the long-term, these approaches hold the greatest promise for regeneration of complex structures containing bone and cartilage such as joints and the regeneration of bones with specific three-dimensional structures. However, several years of basic studies will be required before these technologies can be brought into the clinic.

27.7. Conclusions

Gene therapy has proven to be an effective method for regenerating bone and cartilage in animal models of nonunion fractures, craniofacial defects and osteoarthritis. Its advantages over current protein-based therapies include sustained delivery of regenerative factors, ability to deliver therapeutic factors to specific cell types that can be implanted in the regeneration site, potential to express unique combinations of regenerative factors and ability to regulate the timing, duration and sequence of factor delivery. In spite of these advantages concerns still remain regarding the safety of gene therapy vectors and the uncontrolled nature of gene expression from vectors containing constitutively active promoters. Many of these issues are likely to be resolved within the next few years, with clinical applications first being developed for more straightforward types of regeneration such as articular cartilage repair and fracture healing, while more complex induction of new bone and cartilage will require basic advances in regulated factor delivery and increased understanding of interactions between regenerative factors.

Acknowledgments: Work from the author's laboratory cited in this chapter was supported by NIH/NIDCR grants DE13386, DE 11723 and DE12211.

References

1. Bostrom MP, Saleh KJ, and Einhorn TA. Osteoinductive growth factors in preclinical fracture and long bone defects models. Orthop Clin North Am 1999;30:647–658.
2. Buckwalter JA. Articular cartilage injuries. Clin Orthop Rel Res 2002(402):21–37.
3. Bandara G, Mueller GM, Galea-Lauri J, Tindal MH, Georgescu HI, Suchanek MK, et al. Intraarticular expression of biologically active interleukin 1-receptor-antagonist protein by ex vivo gene transfer. Proc Natl Acad Sci USA 1993;90:10764–10768.
4. Crombleholme TM. Adenoviral-mediated gene transfer in wound healing. Wound Repair Regen 2000;8:460–472.
5. Enneking WF and Mindell ER. Observations on massive retrieved human allografts. J Bone Joint Surg Am 1991;73:1123–1142.
6. Albertson KS, Medoff RJ, and Mitsunaga MM. The use of periosteally vascularized autografts to augment the fixation of large segmental allografts. Clin Orthop Relat Res 1991:113–119.
7. Cook SD, Baffes GC, Wolfe MW, Sampath TK, Rueger DC, and Whitecloud TS, 3rd. The effect of recombinant human osteogenic protein-1 on healing of large segmental bone defects. J Bone Joint Surg Am 1994;76:827–838.
8. Cook SD, Wolfe MW, Salkeld SL, and Rueger DC. Effect of recombinant human osteogenic protein-1 on healing of segmental defects in non-human primates. J Bone Joint Surg Am 1995;77:734–750.
9. Einhorn TA. Clinical applications of recombinant human BMPs: early experience and future development. J Bone Joint Surg Am 2003;85-A Suppl 3:82–88.
10. Groeneveld EH and Burger EH. Bone morphogenetic proteins in human bone regeneration. Eur J Endocrinol 2000;142:9–21.
11. Govender S, Csimma C, Genant HK, Valentin-Opran A, Amit Y, Arbel R, et al. Recombinant human bone morphogenetic protein-2 for treatment of open tibial fractures: a prospective, controlled, randomized study of four hundred and fifty patients. J Bone Joint Surg Am 2002;84-A:2123–2134.
12. Winn SR, Hu Y, Sfeir C, and Hollinger JO. Gene therapy approaches for modulating bone regeneration. Adv Drug Deliv Rev 2000;42:121–138.
13. Hunziker EB. Articular cartilage repair: are the intrinsic biological constraints undermining this process insuperable? Osteoarthritis Cartilage 1999;7:15–28.
14. Hunziker EB. Articular cartilage repair: basic science and clinical progress. A review of the current status and prospects.[see comment]. Osteoarthritis Cartilage 2002;10:432–463.
15. Bruns J and Steinhagen J. Transplantation chondrogener Gewebe zur Behandlung von Gelenkknorpeldefekten. Orthopade 1999;28:52–60.
16. Peterson L, Brittberg M, Kiviranta I, Akerlund EL, and Lindahl A. Autologous chondrocyte transplantation. Biomechanics and long-term durability. Am J Sports Med 2002;30:2–12.
17. Karaplis A. Embryonic development of bone and the molecular regulation of intramembranous and endochondral bone fomration. In: *Principles of Bone Biology* (2nd ed.), edited by Bilezikian J, Raisz L and Rodan G. San Diego: Academic Press, 2002:33–58.
18. Mariani FV and Martin GR. Deciphering skeletal patterning: clues from the limb. Nature 2003;423:319–325.
19. Tickle C. Molecular basis of vertebrate limb patterning. Am J Med Genet 2002;112:250–255.
20. Bitgood MJ and McMahon AP. Hedgehog and Bmp genes are coexpressed at many diverse sites of cell-cell interaction in the mouse embryo. Dev Biol 1995;172:126–138.

21. Francis PH, Richardson MK, Brickell PM, and Tickle C. Bone morphogenetic proteins and a signalling pathway that controls patterning in the developing chick limb. Development 1994;120:209–218.
22. Dahn RD and Fallon JF. Interdigital regulation of digit identity and homeotic transformation by modulated BMP signaling. Science 2000;289:438–441.
23. Zelzer E, McLean W, Ng YS, Fukai N, Reginato AM, Lovejoy S, et al. Skeletal defects in VEGF(120/120) mice reveal multiple roles for VEGF in skeletogenesis. Development 2002;129:1893–1904.
24. Gerber HP and Ferrara N. Angiogenesis and bone growth. Trends Cardiovasc Med 2000;10:223–228.
25. Gerber HP, Vu TH, Ryan AM, Kowalski J, Werb Z, and Ferrara N. VEGF couples hypertrophic cartilage remodeling, ossification and angiogenesis during endochondral bone formation. Nat Med 1999;5:623–628.
26. Bouletreau PJ, Warren SM, Spector JA, Peled ZM, Gerrets RP, Greenwald JA, et al. Hypoxia and VEGF up-regulate BMP-2 mRNA and protein expression in microvascular endothelial cells: implications for fracture healing. Plastic Reconst Surg 2002;109:2384–2397.
27. Doherty MJ, Ashton BA, Walsh S, Beresford JN, Grant ME, and Canfield AE. Vascular pericytes express osteogenic potential in vitro and in vivo. J Bone Miner Res 1998;13:828–838.
28. Steitz SA, Speer MY, Curinga G, Yang HY, Haynes P, Aebersold R, et al. Smooth muscle cell phenotypic transition associated with calcification: upregulation of Cbfa1 and downregulation of smooth muscle lineage markers. Circ Res 2001;89:1147–1154.
29. Olmsted-Davis EA, Gugala Z, Camargo F, Gannon FH, Jackson K, Kienstra KA, et al. Primitive adult hematopoietic stem cells can function as osteoblast precursors. Proc Natl Acad Sci USA 2003;100:15877–15882.
30. Komori T, Yagi H, Nomura S, Yamaguchi A, Sasaki K, Deguchi K, et al. Targeted disruption of Cbfa1 results in a complete lack of bone formation owing to maturational arrest of osteoblasts. Cell 1997;89:755–764.
31. Otto F, Thornell AP, Crompton T, Denzel A, Gilmour KC, Rosewell IR, et al. Cbfa1, a candidate gene for cleidocranial dysplasia syndrome, is essential for osteoblast differentiation and bone development [see comments]. Cell 1997;89:765–771.
32. Ducy P, Zhang R, Geoffroy V, Ridall AL, and Karsenty G. Osf2/Cbfa1: a transcriptional activator of osteoblast differentiation [see comments]. Cell 1997;89:747–754.
33. Nakashima K, Zhou X, Kunkel G, Zhang Z, Deng JM, Behringer RR, et al. The novel zinc finger-containing transcription factor osterix is required for osteoblast differentiation and bone formation. Cell 2002;108:17–29.
34. Yagi K, Tsuji K, Nifuji A, Shinomiya K, Nakashima K, DeCrombrugghe B, et al. Bone morphogenetic protein-2 enhances osterix gene expression in chondrocytes. J Cell Biochem 2003;88:1077–1083.
35. Yang S, Wei D, Wang D, Phimphilai M, Krebsbach PH, and Franceschi RT. In vitro and in vivo synergistic interactions between the Runx2/Cbfa1 transcription factor and bone morphogenetic protein-2 in stimulating osteoblast differentiation. J Bone Miner Res 2003;18:705–715.
36. Byers BA, Pavlath GK, Murphy TJ, Karsenty G, and Garcia AJ. Cell-type-dependent up-regulation of in vitro mineralization after overexpression of the osteoblast-specific transcription factor Runx2/Cbfal. J Bone Miner Res 2002;17:1931–1944.
37. Healy C, Uwanogho D, and Sharpe PT. Regulation and role of Sox9 in cartilage formation. Dev Dyn 1999;215:69–78.
38. Gerstenfeld LC, Cullinane DM, Barnes GL, Graves DT, and Einhorn TA. Fracture healing as a post-natal developmental process: molecular, spatial, and temporal aspects of its regulation. J Cell Biochem 2003;88:873–884.
39. Khan SN, Bostrom MP, and Lane JM. Bone growth factors. Orthop Clin North Am 2000;31:375–388.

40. Nakajima F, Ogasawara A, Goto K, Moriya H, Ninomiya Y, Einhorn TA, et al. Spatial and temporal gene expression in chondrogenesis during fracture healing and the effects of basic fibroblast growth factor. J Orthop Res 2001;19:935–944.
41. Radomsky ML, Thompson AY, Spiro RC, and Poser JW. Potential role of fibroblast growth factor in enhancement of fracture healing. Clin Orthop 1998:S283–293.
42. Cho TJ, Gerstenfeld LC, and Einhorn TA. Differential temporal expression of members of the transforming growth factor beta superfamily during murine fracture healing. J Bone Miner Res 2002;17:513–520.
43. Komatsu DE and Hadjiargyrou M. Activation of the transcription factor HIF-1 and its target genes, VEGF, HO-1, iNOS, during fracture repair. Bone 2004;34:680–688.
44. Tarkka T, Sipola A, Jamsa T, Soini Y, Yla-Herttuala S, Tuukkanen J, et al. Adenoviral VEGF-A gene transfer induces angiogenesis and promotes bone formation in healing osseous tissues. J Gene Med 2003;5:560–566.
45. Mori S, Yoshikawa H, Hashimoto J, Ueda T, Funai H, Kato M, et al. Antiangiogenic agent (TNP-470) inhibition of ectopic bone formation induced by bone morphogenetic protein-2. Bone 1998;22:99–105.
46. Peng H, Wright V, Usas A, Gearhart B, Shen HC, Cummins J, et al. Synergistic enhancement of bone formation and healing by stem cell-expressed VEGF and bone morphogenetic protein-4. J Clin Invest 2002;110:751–759.
47. Street J, Bao M, deGuzman L, Bunting S, Peale FV, Jr., Ferrara N, et al. Vascular endothelial growth factor stimulates bone repair by promoting angiogenesis and bone turnover. Proc Natl Acad Sci U S A 2002;99:9656–9661.
48. Kubota K, Iseki S, Kuroda S, Oida S, Iimura T, Duarte WR, et al. Synergistic effect of fibroblast growth factor-4 in ectopic bone formation induced by bone morphogenetic protein-2. Bone 2002;31:465–471.
49. Lisignoli G, Fini M, Giavaresi G, Nicoli AN, Toneguzzi S, and Facchini A. Osteogenesis of large segmental radius defects enhanced by basic fibroblast growth factor activated bone marrow stromal cells grown on non-woven hyaluronic acid-based polymer scaffold. Biomaterials 2002;23:1043–1051.
50. Lyons KM, Hogan BL, and Robertson EJ. Colocalization of BMP 7 and BMP 2 RNAs suggests that these factors cooperatively mediate tissue interactions during murine development. Mech Dev 1995;50:71–83.
51. Nishimatsu S and Thomsen GH. Ventral mesoderm induction and patterning by bone morphogenetic protein heterodimers in Xenopus embryos. Mech Dev 1998;74:75–88.
52. Israel DI, Nove J, Kerns KM, Kaufman RJ, Rosen V, Cox KA, et al. Heterodimeric bone morphogenetic proteins show enhanced activity in vitro and in vivo. Growth Factors 1996;13:291–300.
53. Tsuji K, Ito Y, and Noda M. Expression of the PEBP2alphaA/AML3/CBFA1 gene is regulated by BMP4/7 heterodimer and its overexpression suppresses type I collagen and osteocalcin gene expression in osteoblastic and nonosteoblastic mesenchymal cells. Bone 1998;22:87–92.
54. Richardson TP, Murphy WL, and Mooney DJ. Polymeric delivery of proteins and plasmid DNA for tissue engineering and gene therapy. Crit Rev Eukaryot Gene Expr 2001;11:47–58.
55. Tabata Y. Tissue regeneration based on growth factor release. Tissue Eng 2003;9 Suppl 1:S5–15.
56. Lutolf MP, Weber FE, Schmoekel HG, Schense JC, Kohler T, Muller R, et al. Repair of bone defects using synthetic mimetics of collagenous extracellular matrices. Nat Biotechnol 2003;21:513–518.
57. Sheridan MH, Shea LD, Peters MC, and Mooney DJ. Bioabsorbable polymer scaffolds for tissue engineering capable of sustained growth factor delivery. J Control Release 2000;64:91–102.
58. Bergelson JM, Cunningham JA, Droguett G, Kurt-Jones EA, Krithivas A, Hong JS, et al. Isolation of a common receptor for Coxsackie B viruses and adenoviruses 2 and 5. Science 1997;275:1320–1323.

59. Neumann R, Chroboczek J, and Jacrot B. Determination of the nucleotide sequence for the penton-base gene of human adenovirus type 5. Gene 1988;69:153–157.
60. Oligino TJ, Yao Q, Ghivizzani SC, and Robbins P. Vector systems for gene transfer to joints. Clin Orthop 2000:S17–30.
61. Zhao M, Zhao Z, Koh J-T, Jin T, and Franceschi RT. Combinatorial gene therapy for bone regeneration: cooperative interactions between adenovirus vectors expressing bone morphogenetic proteins 2, 4 and 7. J Cell Biochem 2005;95:1–16.
62. Armentano D, Zabner J, Sacks C, Sookdeo CC, Smith MP, St George JA, et al. Effect of the E4 region on the persistence of transgene expression from adenovirus vectors. J Virol 1997;71:2408–2416.
63. Hartigan-O'Connor D, Amalfitano A, and Chamberlain JS. Improved production of gutted adenovirus in cells expressing adenovirus preterminal protein and DNA polymerase. J Virol 1999;73:7835–7841.
64. Danos O and Heard JM. Recombinant retroviruses as tools for gene transfer to somatic cells. Bone Marrow Transplant 1992;9 Suppl 1:131–138.
65. Hacein-Bey-Abina S, von Kalle C, Schmidt M, Le Deist F, Wulffraat N, McIntyre E, et al. A serious adverse event after successful gene therapy for X-linked severe combined immunodeficiency. N Engl J Med 2003;348:255–256.
66. Noguchi P. Risks and benefits of gene therapy. N Engl J Med 2003;348:193–194.
67. Zhang XY, La Russa VF, Bao L, Kolls J, Schwarzenberger P, and Reiser J. Lentiviral vectors for sustained transgene expression in human bone marrow-derived stromal cells. Mol Ther 2002;5:555–565.
68. Miyoshi H, Smith KA, Mosier DE, Verma IM, and Torbett BE. Transduction of human CD34+ cells that mediate long-term engraftment of NOD/SCID mice by HIV vectors. Science 1999;283:682–686.
69. Vigna E and Naldini L. Lentiviral vectors: excellent tools for experimental gene transfer and promising candidates for gene therapy. J Gene Med 2000;2:308–316.
70. Luk KD, Chen Y, Cheung KM, Kung HF, Lu WW, and Leong JC. Adeno-associated virus-mediated bone morphogenetic protein-4 gene therapy for in vivo bone formation. Biochem Biophys Res Commun 2003;308:636–645.
71. Klein RM, Wolf ED, Wu R, and Sanford JC. High-velocity microprojectiles for delivering nucleic acids into living cells. 1987. Biotechnology 1992;24:384–386.
72. Yang NS, Burkholder J, Roberts B, Martinell B, and McCabe D. In vivo and in vitro gene transfer to mammalian somatic cells by particle bombardment. Proc Natl Acad Sci U S A 1990;87:9568–9572.
73. Kwok KY, Yang Y, and Rice KG. Evolution of cross-linked non-viral gene delivery systems. Curr Opin Mol Ther 2001;3:142–146.
74. Franceschi RT, Wang D, Krebsbach PH, and Rutherford RB. Gene therapy for bone formation: In vitro and in vivo osteogenic activity of an adenovirus expressing BMP7. J Cell Biochem 2000;78:476–486.
75. Alsberg E, Hill EE, and Mooney DJ. Craniofacial tissue engineering. Crit Rev Oral Biol Med 2001;12:64–75.
76. Liu X and Ma PX. Polymeric scaffolds for bone tissue engineering. Ann Biomed Eng 2004;32:477–486.
77. Chang SC, Liao YF, Hung LM, Tseng CS, Hsu JH, and Chen JK. Prefabricated implants or grafts with reverse models of three-dimensional mirror-image templates for reconstruction of craniofacial abnormalities. Plast Reconstr Surg 1999;104:1413–1418.
78. Mironov V, Boland T, Trusk T, Forgacs G, and Markwald RR. Organ printing: computer-aided jet-based 3D tissue engineering.[erratum appears in Trends Biotechnol. 2004 Jun;22(6):265]. Trends in Biotechnology 2003;21:157–161.
79. Alsberg E, Anderson KW, Albeiruti A, Franceschi RT, and Mooney DJ. Cell-interactive alginate hydrogels for bone tissue engineering. J Dent Res 2001;80:2025–2029.

80. Baltzer AW and Lieberman JR. Regional gene therapy to enhance bone repair. Gene Ther 2004;11:344–350.
81. Wu D, Razzano P, and Grande DA. Gene therapy and tissue engineering in repair of the musculoskeletal system. J Cell Biochem 2003;88:467–481.
82. Evans CH, Ghivizzani SC, and Robbins PD. The 2003 Nicolas Andry Award. Orthopaedic gene therapy. Clin Orthop Rel Res 2004:316–329.
83. Martinek V, Ueblacker P, and Imhoff AB. Current concepts of gene therapy and cartilage repair. J Bone Joint Surg - Br 2003;85:782–788.
84. Musgrave DS, Bosch P, Ghivizzani S, Robbins PD, Evans CH, and Huard J. Adenovirus-mediated direct gene therapy with bone morphogenetic protein-2 produces bone. Bone 1999;24:541–547.
85. Kang Q, Sun MH, Cheng H, Peng Y, Montag AG, Deyrup AT, et al. Characterization of the distinct orthotopic bone-forming activity of 14 BMPs using recombinant adenovirus-mediated gene delivery. Gene Ther 2004;11:1312–1320.
86. Li JZ, Li H, Sasaki T, Holman D, Beres B, Dumont RJ, et al. Osteogenic potential of five different recombinant human bone morphogenetic protein adenoviral vectors in the rat. Gene Ther 2003;10:1735–1743.
87. Baltzer AW, Lattermann C, Whalen JD, Ghivizzani S, Wooley P, Krauspe R, et al. Potential role of direct adenoviral gene transfer in enhancing fracture repair. Clin Orthop 2000:S120–125.
88. Baltzer AW, Lattermann C, Whalen JD, Wooley P, Weiss K, Grimm M, et al. Genetic enhancement of fracture repair: healing of an experimental segmental defect by adenoviral transfer of the BMP-2 gene. Gene Ther 2000;7:734–739.
89. Dunn CA, Jin Q, Taba M, Jr., Franceschi RT, Bruce Rutherford R, and Giannobile WV. BMP gene delivery for alveolar bone engineering at dental implant defects. Mol Ther 2005;11:294–299.
90. Bonadio J, Smiley E, Patil P, and Goldstein S. Localized, direct plasmid gene delivery in vivo: prolonged therapy results in reproducible tissue regeneration [see comments]. Nat Med 1999;5:753–759.
91. Fang J, Zhu YY, Smiley E, Bonadio J, Rouleau JP, Goldstein SA, et al. Stimulation of new bone formation by direct transfer of osteogenic plasmid genes. Proc Natl Acad Sci U S A 1996;93:5753–5758.
92. Krebsbach PH, Gu K, Franceschi RT, and Rutherford RB. Gene therapy-directed osteogenesis: BMP-7-transduced human fibroblasts form bone in vivo. Hum Gene Ther 2000;11:1201–1210.
93. Rutherford RB, Moalli M, Franceschi RT, Wang D, Gu K, and Krebsbach PH. Bone morphogenetic protein-transduced human fibroblasts convert to osteoblasts and form bone in vivo. Tissue Eng 2002;8:441–452.
94. Jiang Y, Jahagirdar BN, Reinhardt RL, Schwartz RE, Keene CD, Ortiz-Gonzalez XR, et al. Pluripotency of mesenchymal stem cells derived from adult marrow. Nature 2002;418:41–49.
95. Musgrave DS, Bosch P, Lee JY, Pelinkovic D, Ghivizzani SC, Whalen J, et al. Ex vivo gene therapy to produce bone using different cell types. Clin Orthop 2000:290–305.
96. Lieberman JR, Daluiski A, Stevenson S, Wu L, McAllister P, Lee YP, et al. The effect of regional gene therapy with bone morphogenetic protein-2-producing bone-marrow cells on the repair of segmental femoral defects in rats. J Bone Joint Surg Am 1999;81:905–917.
97. Lieberman JR, Le LQ, Wu L, Finerman GA, Berk A, Witte ON, et al. Regional gene therapy with a BMP-2-producing murine stromal cell line induces heterotopic and orthotopic bone formation in rodents. J Orthop Res 1998;16:330–339.
98. Chang SC, Chuang HL, Chen YR, Chen JK, Chung HY, Lu YL, et al. Ex vivo gene therapy in autologous bone marrow stromal stem cells for tissue-engineered maxillofacial bone regeneration. Gene Ther 2003;10:2013–2019.

99. Chang SC, Wei FC, Chuang H, Chen YR, Chen JK, Lee KC, et al. Ex vivo gene therapy in autologous critical-size craniofacial bone regeneration. Plast Reconstr Surg 2003;112:1841–1850.
100. Riew KD, Wright NM, Cheng S, Avioli LV, and Lou J. Induction of bone formation using a recombinant adenoviral vector carrying the human BMP-2 gene in a rabbit spinal fusion model. Calcif Tissue Int 1998;63:357–360.
101. Wang JC, Kanim LE, Yoo S, Campbell PA, Berk AJ, and Lieberman JR. Effect of regional gene therapy with bone morphogenetic protein-2-producing bone marrow cells on spinal fusion in rats. J Bone Joint Surg Am 2003;85-A:905–911.
102. Lee JY, Qu-Petersen Z, Cao B, Kimura S, Jankowski R, Cummins J, et al. Clonal isolation of muscle-derived cells capable of enhancing muscle regeneration and bone healing. J Cell Biol 2000;150:1085–1100.
103. Morizono K, De Ugarte DA, Zhu M, Zuk P, Elbarbary A, Ashjian P, et al. Multilineage cells from adipose tissue as gene delivery vehicles. Hum Gene Ther 2003;14:59–66.
104. Gimble J and Guilak F. Adipose-derived adult stem cells: isolation, characterization, and differentiation potential. Cytotherapy 2003;5:362–369.
105. Sugiyama O, An DS, Kung SP, Feeley BT, Gamradt S, Liu NQ, et al. Lentivirus-mediated gene transfer induces long-term transgene expression of BMP-2 in vitro and new bone formation in vivo. Mol Ther 2005;11:390–398.
106. Lee KH, Song SU, Hwang TS, Yi Y, Oh IS, Lee JY, et al. Regeneration of hyaline cartilage by cell-mediated gene therapy using transforming growth factor beta 1-producing fibroblasts. Human Gene Ther 2001;12:1805–1813.
107. Madry H, Cucchiarini M, Terwilliger EF, and Trippel SB. Recombinant adeno-associated virus vectors efficiently and persistently transduce chondrocytes in normal and osteoarthritic human articular cartilage. Human Gene Ther 2003;14:393–402.
108. Di Cesare PE, S RF, Carlson CS, Fang C, and Liu C. Regional gene therapy for full-thickness articular cartilage lesions using naked DNA with a collagen matrix. J Orthop Res 2006;24:1118–1127.
109. Park J, Gelse K, Frank S, von der Mark K, Aigner T, and Schneider H. Transgene-activated mesenchymal cells for articular cartilage repair: a comparison of primary bone marrow-, perichondrium/periosteum- and fat-derived cells. J Gene Med 2006;8:112–125.
110. Kuroda R, Usas A, Kubo S, Corsi K, Peng H, Rose T, et al. Cartilage repair using bone morphogenetic protein 4 and muscle-derived stem cells.[see comment]. Arthritis Rheum 2006;54:433–442.
111. Mason JM, Breitbart AS, Barcia M, Porti D, Pergolizzi RG, and Grande DA. Cartilage and bone regeneration using gene-enhanced tissue engineering. Clin Orthop Rel Res 2000:S171–178.
112. Kaul G, Cucchiarini M, Arntzen D, Zurakowski D, Menger MD, Kohn D, et al. Local stimulation of articular cartilage repair by transplantation of encapsulated chondrocytes overexpressing human fibroblast growth factor 2 (FGF-2) in vivo. J Gene Med 2006;8:100–111.
113. Hiraide A, Yokoo N, Xin KQ, Okuda K, Mizukami H, Ozawa K, et al. Repair of articular cartilage defect by intraarticular administration of basic fibroblast growth factor gene, using adeno-associated virus vector. Human Gene Ther 2005;16:1413–1421.
114. Cucchiarini M, Madry H, Ma C, Thurn T, Zurakowski D, Menger MD, et al. Improved tissue repair in articular cartilage defects in vivo by rAAV-mediated overexpression of human fibroblast growth factor 2. Mol Ther 2005;12:229–238.
115. Roessler BJ, Allen ED, Wilson JM, Hartman JW, and Davidson BL. Adenoviral-mediated gene transfer to rabbit synovium in vivo. J Clin Invest 1993;92:1085–1092.
116. Pan RY, Chen SL, Xiao X, Liu DW, Peng HJ, and Tsao YP. Therapy and prevention of arthritis by recombinant adeno-associated virus vector with delivery of interleukin-1 receptor antagonist. Arthritis Rheum 2000;43:289–297.

117. Kafienah W, Al-Fayez F, Hollander AP, and Barker MD. Inhibition of cartilage degradation: a combined tissue engineering and gene therapy approach. Arthritis Rheum 2003;48:709–718.
118. Franceschi RT, Yang S, Rutherford RB, Krebsbach PH, Zhao M, and Wang D. Gene therapy approaches for bone regeneration. Cells Tissues Organs 2004;176:95–108.
119. Zhu W, Rawlins BA, Boachie-Adjei O, Myers ER, Arimizu J, Choi E, et al. Combined bone morphogenetic protein-2 and −7 gene transfer enhances osteoblastic differentiation and spine fusion in a rodent model. J Bone Miner Res 2004;19:2021–2032.
120. Huang YC, Kaigler D, Rice KG, Krebsbach PH, and Mooney DJ. Combined angiogenic and osteogenic factor delivery enhances bone marrow stromal cell-driven bone regeneration. J Bone Miner Res 2005;20:848–857.
121. Friedenstein AJ, Chailakhyan RK, and Gerasimov UV. Bone marrow osteogenic stem cells: in vitro cultivation and transplantation in diffusion chambers. Cell Tissue Kinet 1987;20:263–272.
122. Phimphilai M, Boules H, Roca H, and Franceschi R. BMP signals are indispensable for RUNX2-dependent osteoblast differentiation. J Bone Miner Res 2006;21:637–646.
123. Zhao Z, Zhao M, Xiao G, and Franceschi RT. Gene transfer of the Runx2 transcription factor enhances osteogenic activity of bone marrow stromal cells in vitro and in vivo. Mol Ther 2005;12:247–253.
124. Gersbach CA, Byers BA, Pavlath GK, and Garcia AJ. Runx2/Cbfa1 stimulates transdifferentiation of primary skeletal myoblasts into a mineralizing osteoblastic phenotype. Exp Cell Res 2004;300:406–417.
125. Gersbach CA, Byers BA, Pavlath GK, Guldberg RE, and Garcia AJ. Runx2/Cbfa1-genetically engineered skeletal myoblasts mineralize collagen scaffolds in vitro. Biotechnol Bioeng 2004;88:369–378.
126. Zheng H, Guo Z, Ma Q, Jia H, and Dang G. Cbfa1/osf2 transduced bone marrow stromal cells facilitate bone formation in vitro and in vivo. Calcif Tissue Int 2004;74:194–203.
127. Moutsatsos IK, Turgeman G, Zhou S, Kurkalli BG, Pelled G, Tzur L, et al. Exogenously regulated stem cell-mediated gene therapy for bone regeneration. Mol Ther 2001;3:449–461.
128. Peng H, Usas A, Gearhart B, Young B, Olshanski A, and Huard J. Development of a self-inactivating tet-on retroviral vector expressing bone morphogenetic protein 4 to achieve regulated bone formation. Mol Ther 2004;9:885–894.
129. Peng H, Usas A, Hannallah D, Olshanski A, Cooper GM, and Huard J. Noggin improves bone healing elicited by muscle stem cells expressing inducible BMP4. Mol Ther 2005;12:239–246.
130. Koh J-T, Ge C, and Franceschi RT. Use of a stringent dimerizer-regulated gene expression system for controlled BMP2 delivery. Mol Ther 2006;14:684–691.
131. Liang H, Pun S, and Wronski TJ. Bone anabolic effects of basic fibroblast growth factor in ovariectomized rats. Endocrinology 1999;140:5780–5788.
132. Pun S, Dearden RL, Ratkus AM, Liang H, and Wronski TJ. Decreased bone anabolic effect of basic fibroblast growth factor at fatty marrow sites in ovariectomized rats. Bone 2001;28:220–226.
133. Terkeltaub RA, Johnson K, Rohnow D, Goomer R, Burton D, and Deftos LJ. Bone morphogenetic proteins and bFGF exert opposing regulatory effects on PTHrP expression and inorganic pyrophosphate elaboration in immortalized murine endochondral hypertrophic chondrocytes (MCT cells). J Bone Miner Res 1998;13:931–941.

28

Paradigms of Tissue Engineering with Applications to Cartilage Regeneration

Benjamin D. Elder and Kyriacos A. Athanasiou

Abstract: Tissue engineering has been widely explored as an option for regeneration of various musculoskeletal tissues. This chapter examines the tissue engineering paradigm, or approach, with a focus on its application to cartilage tissue engineering. Since understanding the tissue engineering approach will require an understanding of cartilage physiology, a brief review of cartilage structure and function is provided. A discussion of current studies of the four parameters of the paradigm, namely scaffolds, cell sources, bioactive agents and bioreactors is presented, along with the latest technologies that incorporate manipulation of several parameters in a single approach.

Keywords: Tissue engineering, scaffolds, growth factors, chondrocytes, bioreactors, cartilage.

28.1. Introduction

Tissue engineering approaches currently are studied to repair many musculoskeletal tissues, including bone, vertebrae, knee meniscus, tendon, ligament, temporomandibular joint (TMJ) cartilage and articular cartilage. This approach aims for functional tissue restoration and involves the use of cells, scaffolds, bioactive agents and mechanical forces. The goal of tissue engineering is to create tissue with biomechanical and biochemical properties that match those of the native tissue.

Cartilage degeneration from injury or from osteoarthritis is one of the greatest challenges in orthopedics, and is the second most common chronic condition reported in the United States [1]. According to the website www.arthritis.org, [2] approximately 21 million people in the United States are afflicted with

Department of Bioengineering, Rice University, Houston, TX

From: *Orthopedic Biology and Medicine: Musculoskeletal Tissue Regeneration, Biological Materials and Methods*
Edited by W. S. Pietrzak © Humana Press, Totowa, NJ

osteoarthritis, resulting in total annual costs of approximately $5,700 per person living with osteoarthritis. Due to the prevalence of articular cartilage pathologies and the need for more effective methods to repair cartilage, tissue engineering has emerged as a promising approach for cartilage regeneration. This chapter will provide an overview of the paradigms of tissue engineering, predominantly exemplified by exploring the strategies currently used to engineer articular cartilage. To gain a better understanding of how tissue engineering approaches are applied to articular cartilage regeneration, a brief discussion of articular cartilage structure and function is provided.

28.2. Background

28.2.1 Structure and Function of Articular Cartilage

Articular cartilage is a specialized form of hyaline cartilage that is essential for the proper function of diarthrodial joints. The main function of articular cartilage is to distribute forces between the subchondral bones. It also provides synovial fluid, lubrication, friction reduction and wear resistance for the joint.

Articular cartilage is avascular, aneural and alymphatic, and is sparsely populated by cells called chondrocytes. Articular cartilage is considered to consist primarily of a solid phase and a fluid phase [3]. Water is the primary component of the fluid phase and accounts for 75 to 80 percent of the wet weight of the tissue. Additionally, electrolytes such as Na^+, Ca^{2+} and Cl^- are found in the fluid phase. The solid phase is characterized by the extracellular matrix (ECM), consisting predominantly of collagen and proteoglycans, which surrounds the chondrocytes and provides structural support to the tissue. The ECM is composed of approximately 50 to 75 percent collagen, and 30 to 35 percent proteoglycans [4–5].

Collagen is the primary constituent of the ECM of articular cartilage. As reviewed elsewhere [5], collagen II accounts for 90 to 95 percent of the collagen in the matrix and is often used as a marker for chondrogenic differentiation in tissue engineering studies. The collagen II fibrils are largely responsible for the tensile strength of the tissue. Other types of collagen are present in the matrix in much smaller amounts and serve varying roles. Collagen XI contributes to fiber formation with collagen II, while collagen VI, IX and X contribute to the ECM structure.

Proteoglycans are glycoproteins that are characterized by long, unbranched and highly charged glycosaminoglycan (GAG) chains [6]. Aggrecan, the most common proteoglycan in articular cartilage, is responsible for the compressive strength of the tissue. In addition to collagen II, the expressions of GAG and aggrecan are also used as specific markers for chondrogenic differentiation.

Mature articular cartilage has a distinct zonal arrangement in vertical sections (Fig. 28.1). Beginning with the articulating surface, it consists of the superficial, middle, deep and calcified zones. These zones exhibit great differences in their properties [7]. The superficial zone comprises the first 10 to 20 percent of the thickness of the tissue, and is characterized by densely packed collagen II fibrils oriented in the direction of shear stress, along with flattened chondrocytes. The middle zone comprises the next 40 to 60 percent of the tissue thickness, and consists of randomly arranged collagen fibers and chondrocytes with a more rounded morphology. It also serves as a transition

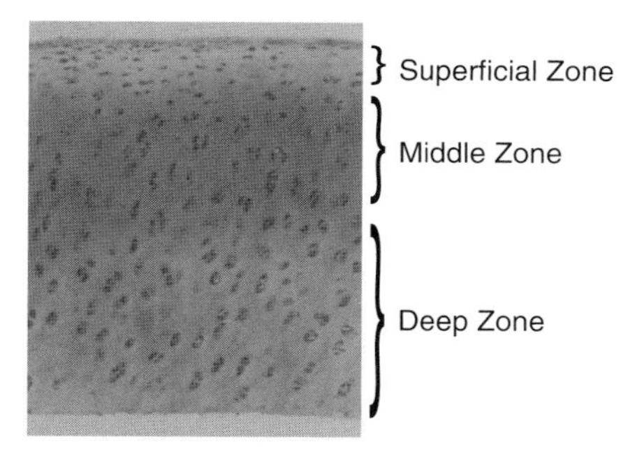

Fig. 28.1 Zonal arrangement of articular cartilage.

between the superficial and deep zones. The deep zone contains collagen fibers that extend into the calcified zone to reinforce the bond between cartilage and bone. The cells of the deep zone appear more ellipsoid in shape and are aligned with the collagen fibers. A distinct tidemark separates the deep zone from the calcified zone. This tidemark is considered the boundary between cartilage and bone. The calcified zone is composed of chondrocytes that are trapped in a calcified matrix.

Chondrocytes sparsely populate cartilage, comprising less than 10 percent of the volume of the tissue [8]. Chondrocytes differentiate from mesenchymal stem cells (MSCs) and are responsible for the maintenance and regulation of the ECM through the enzymatic degradation of existing ECM, the synthesis of new ECM and the production of various bioactive agents such as growth factors. In healthy articular cartilage chondrocytes do not proliferate. Since the tissue is relatively avascular, the chondrocytes exist in a low oxygen tension environment and must obtain oxygen and nutrients from the synovial fluid through diffusion.

28.2.2. Biomechanics of Articular Cartilage

As mentioned above, the aggrecan content of cartilage is largely responsible for its compressive properties. Aggrecan is negatively charged, leading to osmotic swelling and hydration of the tissue from the Donnan osmotic pressure [9]. When cartilage is compressed the interstitial fluid pressure initially supports most of the applied load. The water is then pushed out of the matrix and into the synovial cavity; therefore, it moves from a loaded region to an unloaded region. The frictional force between the exiting water and the matrix leads to dissipation of the applied force, and the load eventually equilibrates. Upon removal of the load fluid comes back into the aggrecan network. This process allows for the cushioning of an applied load without damage to the chondrocytes or ECM. The interaction between the matrix and the interstitial fluid of cartilage is modeled by Mow, et al.'s [3] biphasic theory. Applying the biphasic theory to articular cartilage in studies of creep indentation yields three material properties: the aggregate modulus, the Poisson's ratio and the permeability of the porous solid phase, which measure the stiffness, the apparent compressibility and the resistance to fluid flow, respectively [3]. The mechanical properties of articular cartilage vary with the anatomic location of the joint. A review by Hu, et al. [5] indicated that the aggregate modulus ranges from 0.53 MPa to 1.34 MPa, the Poisson's ratio from 0.00–0.14 and the permeability from 0.90×10^{-15} m^4/Ns to 4.56×10^{-15} m^4/Ns.

Articular cartilage is exposed to a wide variety of forces including hydrostatic pressure, compression and shear forces. As reviewed elsewhere [10], the force exerted on the knee is approximately 3.5 times the body's weight, while the ankle and shoulder experience loads of 2.5 times body weight and 1.5 times body weight, respectively. In addition, contact pressures between 3 to 18 MPa have been observed in the human hip joint [11]. During loading of articular joints synovial fluid inside the joint capsule generates hydrostatic pressure by transmitting force throughout the tissue. Compressive forces are generated in articular cartilage as a result of direct contact between the articulating surfaces. Likewise with compressive forces, shear forces are generated in the knee joint during loading as a result of direct contact between the articulating cartilage surfaces, as the two surfaces attempt to move past each other.

28.2.3. Repair of Articular Cartilage

As reviewed elsewhere [12], injuries of articular cartilage can be classified as 1) chondral damage without visible tissue disruption, 2) cartilage damage alone such as chondral flaps and tears and 3) cartilage damage accompanied by underlying bone damage (osteochondral fracture). As a result of the relatively nonexistent vascular supply, scarcity of chondrocytes in the tissue and the lack of chondrocyte proliferation, the articular cartilage's ability to repair itself is intrinsically limited. As reviewed elsewhere [13], in a chondral injury, the chondrocytes surrounding the defect show a limited ability to proliferate to repair the damaged site. In an osteochondral injury MSCs from the bone marrow can migrate to the site for tissue repair. However, in both cases, the defect is repaired with fibrocartilage formation, which is predominantly collagen I, and lacks the mechanical integrity of articular cartilage, thus leading to its relatively rapid degradation with normal loading of the joint [14].

The current clinical options for treating patients with damaged articular cartilage are relatively limited. According to a recent review [15], the most successful treatment options for restoring native hyaline cartilage have involved tissue grafting, where cartilage is removed from a less load bearing region and is grafted to the defect site. However, this approach involves significant donor site morbidity and the result is often short-lived, as fibrocartilage fills the donor site and the area surrounding the graft. Autologous chondrocyte implantation is another treatment strategy that entails harvesting a limited supply of cartilage cells from the individual, expanding the cells in culture and injecting them in the defect site. The area is then covered with a periosteal flap. As reviewed elsewhere [15], this procedure was intended to treat focal defects of the knee in the United States; however, it has also been used to treat focal defects in the ankle, shoulder, elbow, hip and wrist. Although this procedure has yielded promising results [16], 25 percent of the patients experienced graft failure, 22 percent experienced delamination and 18 percent experienced tissue hypertrophy [17]. In addition to the reported clinical complications, a major drawback to this procedure and any other currently available is that it has only been used to treat focal defects, not entire osteoarthritic joints.

28.2.4. Tissue Engineering

Due to articular cartilage's poor ability to heal itself, and the limited clinical treatment options, tissue engineering may offer the most promising approach to articular cartilage regeneration, potentially providing engineered tissue that is indistinguishable from native cartilage. As reviewed elsewhere [18–19], the biomechanical characteristics of engineered constructs are the most important quantitative indicators of the approximation of the regenerated tissue to native tissue, but biochemical analyses of the collagen and GAG content also yield important information. Tissue engineering aims to accomplish the regeneration of articular cartilage by manipulating four parameters: scaffold material, cell sources, bioactive agents (growth factors/cytokines) and mechanical forces (Fig. 28.2). Although significant steps have been made in the study of each parameter, complete tissue regeneration likely will require the complex task of optimizing these parameters in combination.

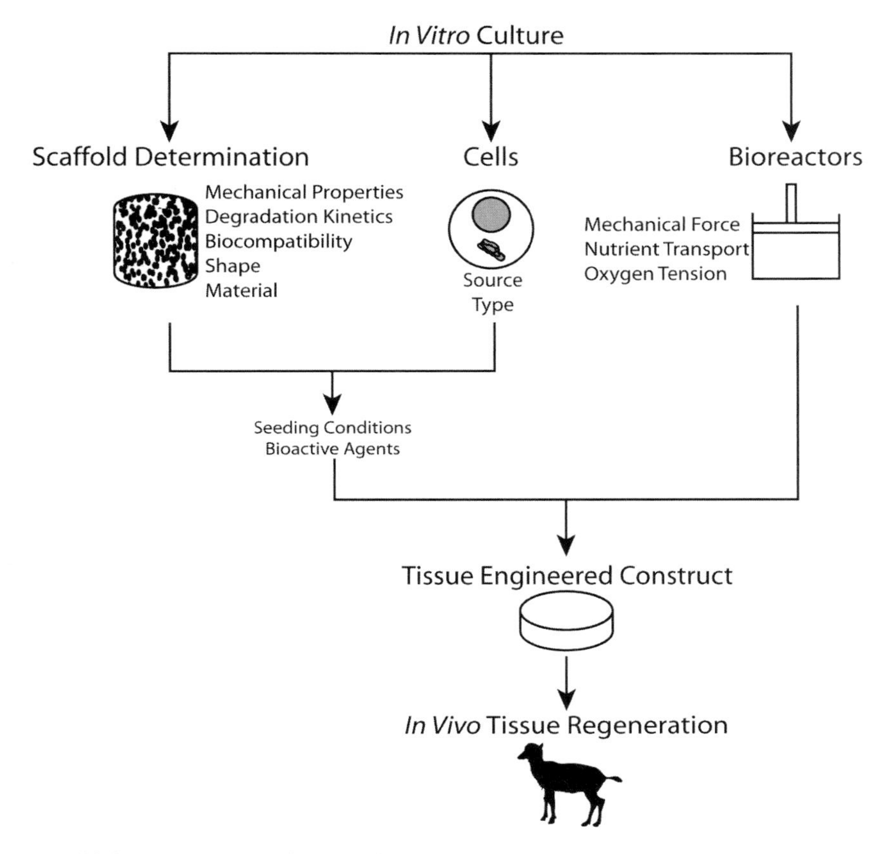

Fig. 28.2 Tissue engineering paradigm.

28.3. Tissue Engineering Paradigms

28.3.1. Scaffolds

The main function of a scaffold in tissue engineering is to provide support and a temporary structure to cells as they begin to secrete and form an ECM. The engineered construct will eventually replace the scaffold as it slowly degrades over time. There are two approaches to employing a scaffold: immediate implantation of the cell seeded scaffold or *in vitro* culture of the scaffold before implantation, and each of these approaches has different design concerns. A scaffold used *in vivo* for cartilage tissue engineering should contain internal channels that allow for diffusion of nutrients and room for tissue growth [20]. Also, it should have adequate biocompatibility to prevent the release of toxic by-products and a large immune response, and should exhibit biodegradation kinetics that match the rate of new tissue formation. In addition a scaffold should have sufficient mechanical properties to allow for its immediate use *in vivo*, as the cells will not have had enough time to synthesize an ECM that will eventually replace the scaffold. Finally, the scaffold should allow for the attachment, proliferation and differentiation of cells seeded on its surface [20]. However, if a scaffold will be cultured *in vitro* rather than implanted immediately, the inherent mechanical properties of the scaffold are not nearly as important, as the degrading scaffold will be replaced by an engineered construct with its own mechanical properties before implantation.

In general scaffold materials can be divided into two groups: natural and synthetic materials. Also, composite scaffolds, which are composed of multiple materials, have been used in tissue engineering. The use of these scaffold materials will be discussed further, with a particular emphasis on successful approaches in cartilage tissue engineering.

28.3.1.1 Natural Polymers

Natural polymers have several properties that are conducive for use as scaffolds. They often have excellent adhesion properties, adequate biocompatibility and decreased toxicity during scaffold degradation [21]. Collagen, fibrin, chitosan, hyaluronan, alginate and agarose have all been investigated with varying degrees of success in cartilage tissue engineering.

Collagen gels have been used extensively as a scaffold material, as collagen is a fundamental component of the ECM of cartilaginous tissues as well as various other connective tissues; therefore, collagen gels are expected to have low immunogenicity although, like all natural polymers, they must be purified before their use. In addition, as a widely abundant ECM component, collagen allows for excellent incorporation of both endogenous and exogenous cells from joint tissue, thus making it an excellent candidate for success in both *in vitro* cell seeding and *in vivo* integration. Nehrer, et al. [22] compared Type I and Type II collagen gels, and found that chondrocyte-seeded Type II collagen gels maintained the chondrocyte phenotype and had increased expression of GAGs. Although some success has been observed with collagen gels, as with all natural scaffolds, concerns regarding pathogen transfer have been expressed. Specifically, the increased incidence of prion diseases such as bovine spongiform encephalopathy has hindered the use of collagen from bovine sources [23].

Fibrin has been used as both a delivery device and a stand-alone scaffold [23]. This material has the advantage of being injectable, which would allow for its noninvasive delivery. Passaretti, et al. [24] demonstrated that chondrocytes expanded through passage one and seeded in a fibrin polymer that was injected subcutaneously in nude mice made an ECM resembling that of native cartilage. However, fibrin has poor mechanical properties and may lead to a host immune response [23].

Chitosan is a polymer derived from the N-deacetylation of chitin, which is abundant in the exoskeleton of arthropods. The properties of chitosan make it extremely useful as a scaffold material. It has excellent biocompatibility [25], is easily synthesized [26] and its mechanical properties and degradation rates can easily be manipulated.

Hyaluronan, alginate, agarose, as well as various synthetic polymers are all used to create hydrogels, which are highly water-soluble polymers that can be cross-linked covalently or physically. They are highly swollen with water, usually containing >90 percent water. Often, hydrogels have excellent biocompatibility, but weak mechanical properties. The main advantage of hydrogels is that as low viscosity, fluid-like solutions, they are injectable and can fill irregularly shaped defect sites. Once the defect site has been filled with a cell/polymer suspension, the hydrogel can be cross-linked, for example, by transdermal photopolymerization [27], thus causing a fluid-solid transition to occur. This procedure permits the researcher to avoid many of the problems involving cell seeding, and provides the clinician with a minimally invasive treatment for chondral defects that avoids surgical intervention. Another advantage of hydrogels is that they are excellent at maintaining the chondrogenic phenotype; this is probably because embedding the chondrocytes in the hydrogel preserves their round morphology. Furthermore, embedding the cells in a hydrogel is extremely useful when using mechanical stimulation, as it allows for uniform force transfer to the cells without the stress shielding that may be caused by other scaffold materials.

Hyaluronan is a naturally occurring polysaccharide that is an important component of articular cartilage. Burdick, et al. [28] recently demonstrated that the mechanical properties and degradation rates of hyaluronan scaffolds could easily be manipulated to encompass a wide range of desirable values which have the potential for clinical use.

Alginate is a polysaccharide derived from algae that has excellent biocompatibility. As a hydrogel alginate can be delivered with an injection, which allows for minimally invasive treatment of chondral defects. Alginate has also proven effective for maintaining or even inducing the chondrogenic phenotype. This is probably because the chondrocytes are embedded in the alginate hydrogel, which enables them to maintain their round morphology. Another exciting attribute of alginate hydrogels is their ability to be formed into different shapes [29], which would allow for the production of a geometrically customized construct prior to implantation. However, the major downside of alginate hydrogels is the inability to modulate their long degradation time *in vivo*, which can hinder the growth of new tissue [20].

Agarose is a polysaccharide derived from seaweed with properties similar to alginate. Like alginate, agarose has excellent biocompatibility, and helps to maintain the chondrogenic phenotype by preserving chondrocytes' round morphology. Agarose has been used extensively in *in vitro* studies [23], although it shares the slow degradation kinetics of alginate. Another problem with agarose is that it may elicit a foreign body giant cell immune response *in vivo* [30].

28.3.1.2. Synthetic Polymers

Synthetic polymers are fabricated in a laboratory, and offer several advantages over natural polymers. Their physical and mechanical properties can easily be modulated, thus allowing for degradation kinetics and mechanical properties that are optimized for a specific application. In addition, since they are not derived from organisms, there is no concern regarding pathogen transmission, and they can easily be synthesized in large quantities. Also, synthetic polymer scaffolds can undergo surface modifications, with peptides or bioactive molecules, that can enhance their biocompatibility and integration in defects. However, unless they are sufficiently small or synthesized to form a hydrogel, they must be surgically implanted into the recipient.

The most widely used materials are the poly(α-hydroxy esters), including polyglycolic acid (PGA), polylactic acid (PLA) and their copolymer poly(lactic-co-glycolic acid) (PLGA) [31–33]. The biocompatibility of each polymer has been extensively studied and allows for their use in various implantation applications.

PLA and PGA are often extruded into long polymer strands that are used to form a highly porous, nonwoven fibrous mesh. The porous nature of the scaffold allows for cell-to-cell communication and nutrient diffusion, but leads to poor mechanical properties until tissue formation occurs. Many studies have demonstrated the efficacy of these polymers in cartilage ECM synthesis and the maintenance of the chondrocyte phenotype [20], as well as efficacy in *in vivo* studies [23].

Copolymers of PLA/PGA are advantageous as they allow for more control over the degradation kinetics by varying the ratios of monomers that are used. PLGA scaffolds have shown promising results in *in vivo* studies [23], but an exciting new approach has been to construct hydrogels out of the copolymer. Mercier, et al. [34] created hydrogels out of PLGA microspheres that, when seeded with chondrocytes and injected in athymic mice, allowed for the production of cartilaginous ECM.

Recently, composite scaffolds have been created using multiple scaffold materials together in an effort to harness the advantages of each component. For example, Caterson, et al. [35] demonstrated the efficacy of a PLA/alginate amalgam for the chondrogenic differentiation of MSCs.

28.3.1.3. "Scaffold-less" Approaches

Despite the promising results obtained using the various aforementioned scaffold materials, there are problems associated with using a scaffold. For example, scaffolds can hinder cell–to-cell communication, contribute to stress shielding and alter the chondrogenic phenotype. Furthermore, they may be toxic or produce toxic by-products during degradation, and their degradation rate must be modulated to coordinate with new tissue formation [36]. As a result of these inherent problems, novel approaches to tissue engineering have been developed that do not employ the use of a scaffold. These approaches include pellet culture [37], aggregate culture [38] and, a more recent approach, the self-assembling process [36].

In the self-assembling process calf articular chondrocytes were seeded at high density in 5 mm diameter and 10 mm deep agarose wells. After 24 hours of culture the cells formed constructs that were not attached to the walls of the agarose wells. After four weeks of culture the constructs were transferred to large wells, and following 12 weeks of culture, this process resulted in tissue engineered constructs of clinically relevant dimensions, at ~15 mm in diameter and 1 mm in thickness. The constructs resembled native articular cartilage morphologically, and had levels of collagen II and GAG approaching that of native tissue, with no collagen I production. Perhaps the most exciting result was that the self-assembled constructs reached over one-third the stiffness of native tissue. The self-assembling process has also been coupled with mechanical stimulation [39]. Hydrostatic pressure application under a treatment of 1 Hz and 10 MPa for four hours/day was shown to stimulate collagen production and aid in the retention of GAGs within constructs compared to static culture. Although more work still needs to be done in the characterization and optimization of the method, the self-assembling process is a promising approach towards functional tissue engineering of articular cartilage.

28.3.2. Cell Sources

An ideal cell source must satisfy several criteria: be easily accessible or available, demonstrate self-renewal or the ability to be expanded extensively, have the capacity to differentiate into the cell lineage of interest upon induction or remain differentiated in the cell lineage of interest and exhibit minimal immunogenicity or tumorigenicity [40]. Progenitor cells such as MSCs and embryonic stem (ES) cells, as well as fully differentiated chondrocytes, have all been used as cell sources for engineered cartilage constructs. Certain advantages and disadvantages are inherent to approaches involving each cell type.

Primary chondrocytes from native cartilage are the most obvious cell source for tissue engineering of cartilaginous tissues. Immature chondrocytes are often used for studies due to their higher metabolic activity [41]. Chondrocytes can easily be isolated from freshly excised articular cartilage following an enzymatic digestion with collagenase. However, a large number of cells must be obtained to be seeded onto a three-dimensional scaffold. Since over-harvesting chondrocytes can lead to further problems at the harvest site, serial passage of chondrocytes on monolayers is required to acquire the large cell density needed for seeding on a three-dimensional scaffold. Chondrocytes passaged in monolayer "dedifferentiate" and become more fibroblast-like in appearance and ECM production: they lose their round morphology and become more spindle-shaped, switch their collagen production from primarily Type II collagen to Type I collagen, and they regain their ability to divide [42–44]. This loss of chondrogenic potential is associated with the suppressed activation of key signaling proteins in the Ras-mitogen-activated protein kinase pathway, which leads to apoptosis [45]. In a recent study it was found that passaged articular chondrocytes in monolayer showed phenotype changes as early as one passage, and their chondrogenic phenotype could not be rescued even with 3-D culture in alginate beads [46]. Despite these limitations, primary chondrocytes continue to be used in clinical applications as several culture conditions, such as culture in agarose gels [47] which allow for the re-expression of the chondrocyte phenotype.

The study of stem cells has gained prominence in cartilage tissue engineering as new chondrocytes originating from host MSCs [48] repair osteochondral defects. Adult MSCs are multipotent cells that can be induced to differentiate down multiple cell lineages such as chondrogenic, osteogenic and adipogenic lineages. MSCs are advantageous as they are able to self-renew, and they can be obtained relatively noninvasively from tissues such as bone marrow aspirates [49–54], adipose tissue [55–60], synovial tissue [61], as well as several other tissues. The chondrogenic phenotype is often characterized by the expression and synthesis of collagen II and proteoglycans, as well as by the upregulation of genes such as sox-9 which are markers of cartilage ECM production. MSCs used in cartilage engineering have been differentiated through the application of members of the transforming growth factor-β (TGF-β) family, as well as dexamethasone. MSCs used in research studies so far have primarily come from bone marrow. Several studies have indicated that a 3-D culture environment is important for chondrogenic differentiation, as it may help to maintain a rounded cell shape. An exciting finding from a study by Yoo, et al. [51] was that the addition of TGF-β1 and dexamethasone maintained the chondrogenic potential of bone marrow-derived MSCs through 20 passages. This is an important finding as *in vitro* expansion through several passages often is required to generate sufficient cells for implantation. Human adipose-derived adult stem (hADAS) cells show great promise for cartilage tissue engineering as they can be isolated from various easily accessible sources such as from the inguinal fat pad [62], infrapatellar fat pad [63] and subcutaneous adipose tissue [52]. hADAS cells express markers characteristic of articular cartilage when cultured with TGF-β1, dexamethasone and ascorbate [57–58, 60, 62]. Although adult stem cells represent a promising cell source for articular cartilage engineering, more work needs to be performed to understand the developmental processes involved in differentiation so that these processes may be further manipulated to optimize *in vitro* cell expansion while maintaining chondrogenic differentiation; then, it may be possible to develop *in vivo* approaches for construct delivery and host integration.

As with the study of several other tissues, the use of embryonic stem cells is increasing in cartilage tissue engineering [64–67]. ES cells are derived from the inner cell mass of the embryonic blastocyst and are pluripotent. Following aggregation into embryoid bodies *in vitro*, they can differentiate into tissue of all three germ layers. ES cells are capable of virtually infinite proliferation while remaining in an undifferentiated state. Because of their pluripotency and their provision of an unlimited cell source, their use is promising for many tissue engineering applications. Although ES cells appear to be an extremely promising cell source, their differentiation pathways must be better elucidated to manipulate them further for cartilage tissue engineering. In addition, the ethical and legal concerns regarding the source and means of collecting ES cells significantly complicate their use.

Finally, an exciting new cell source may derive from dermal fibroblasts which can be triggered to differentiate by culture on cartilage matrix proteoglycans [68–70]. This cell source could be extremely useful as the cells are both easily accessible and widely available.

28.3.3. Growth Factors

Growth factors are used in tissue engineering to modulate cellular differentiation and proliferation, as well as to modulate ECM synthesis. Articular cartilage displays dramatic changes when exposed to growth factors that are naturally present in the native environment. The effects of many of these growth factors alone, and in combination, have been studied for cartilage tissue engineering, including the transforming growth factor beta (TGF-β) family, insulin-like growth factor (IGF), fibroblast growth factors (FGFs), hepatocyte growth factor (HGF) and platelet-derived growth factor (PDGF). As reviewed elsewhere [71], growth factor studies generally are conducted *in vitro* in which the growth factor is delivered as a soluble factor in the media; therefore, the concentration and frequency of delivery can easily be manipulated. Growth factor effects have also been studied *in vivo*, albeit with variable results as it is far more difficult to control the interactions within the body as well as the concentrations [71]. However, as scaffold delivery vehicles and gene therapy approaches continue to improve, delivery of growth factors at more controlled doses and temporal increments may become a more achievable task.

Members of the TGF-β family are probably the most widely used growth factors to date. For cartilage tissue engineering, the notable members of the TGF-β family include TGF-β1, TGF-β3 and bone morphogenetic proteins (BMPs). TGF-β1 [51–53, 56] and TGF-β3 [50, 72] are both widely used as chondrogenic differentiation factors for MSCs and embryonic stem cells. In addition to uses in chondrogenic differentiation, TGF-β1 has been shown to upregulate ECM synthesis although there are conflicting reports on its effects. Several studies have shown that TGF-β1 increases collagen II expression in monolayer [73] and in 3-D scaffolds [74], while other studies have shown no effects on the gene expression of ECM proteins [75]. Possible explanations for the different observed effects of TGF-β1 include variable effects of TGF-β1 on the zonal populations of chondrocytes, as well as variations in the temporal application of the growth factor. The main effect of BMPs in cartilage tissue engineering is chondrogenic differentiation or the maintenance of differentiation. They have also been used extensively in bone tissue engineering for osteogenic differentiation and increased matrix synthesis. As reviewed elsewhere [71], although other BMPs have been studied, BMP-2 has been the most commonly used BMP for studies involving cartilage. BMP-7 is another BMP that is beginning to be used in cartilage tissue engineering, and has also been used recently as a chondrogenic differentiation factor [76].

Several other growth factors show potential for use in cartilage tissue engineering. IGF-I has a profound anabolic effect on chondrocytes *in vitro* [77–79], and has been shown to increase GAG production, as well as aggrecan and collagen II gene expression in articular chondrocytes grown on monolayer [80]. Perhaps the most exciting *in vivo* effect of IGF-I use is the autoinductive autocrine/paracrine transcriptional response, which could potentially be harnessed to extend and amplify the effects of IGF-I on cartilage repair [81]. Basic fibroblast growth factor (bFGF) has been shown to stimulate chondrocyte proliferation and synthesis [82–84], although it has also been used for fibrochondrocyte studies involving the knee meniscus and the temporomandibular joint [33]. FGF-18 has recently been shown to promote chondrogenic differentiation of limb bud mesenchymal cells [85]. HGF has been minimally studied in cartilage tissue engineering, but preliminary studies indicate that it may enhance or modulate chondrocyte proliferation [86–87]. The effects of PDGF on proliferation and ECM synthesis have been minimally reported, but it has been shown to have an effect on chondrocyte proliferation [88].

Although many growth factors show promising results when used alone, their use in combination has yielded exciting results, as synergism between many growth factors has been observed in several studies. BMP-2 and TGF-β1 work in concert for the chondrogenesis of periosteal cells; it was suggested that BMP-2 induces neochondrogenesis, while TGF-β1 modulates the terminal differentiation in BMP-2-induced chondrogenesis [89]. Combined treatments with TGF-β3 and BMP-6, or TGF-β3 and IGF-I were shown to be the most effective combinations for chondrogenic induction of bone marrow MSCs [90]. However, growth factor combinations do not always interact synergistically. For example, the addition of IGF-I and TGF-β in combination did not improve the histologic features or mechanical performance of tissue engineered cartilage constructs [91].

Perhaps the most exciting new results have come from studying the synergism between growth factor application and mechanical stimulation. Bonassar, et al. [92] found that the combination of IGF-I and dynamic compression led to a 290 percent increase in proteoglycan synthesis, a degree greater than that achieved by either stimulus alone. Also, Mauck, et al. [93] showed that the combination of dynamic deformational loading with either TGF-β1 or IGF-I increased the stiffness of engineered constructs by 277 percent or 245 percent, respectively, with respect to untreated free-swelling controls.

Growth factor treatment has been extremely useful for cartilage tissue engineering by allowing and maintaining chondrogenic differentiation [75, 94–95], and has increased production of ECM proteins in studies of articular cartilage [80, 92], knee meniscus [96–97] and the TMJ [33, 98]. However, there are still properties of the growth factors that need to be investigated. In addition to the need to better characterize the roles of each growth factor, their effects on different cell types, the correct dosage frequency and concentrations must be elucidated to optimize their use in tissue engineering.

28.3.4. Mechanical Loading

To serve its function as a biomechanical structure articular cartilage is exposed to a wide variety of forces including hydrostatic pressure, compression and shear forces. Chondrocytes are directly connected to their microenvironment by focal adhesions which are discrete regions of the cell's plasma membrane that bind to extracellular material [21]. In addition to their involvement in the structural integrity of the chondrocyte, focal adhesions are involved in the process of mechanotransduction, in which cells regulate transcriptional activities based on mechanical signals received at their surface. Although the exact mechanisms of mechanotransduction in the chondrocyte have not been completely elucidated, evidence suggests that elements of the cytoskeleton and integrins allow the coordination of mechanical forces and transcriptional changes.

Several studies have suggested that mechanical stimulation is necessary for maintaining and possibly improving the biomechanical function of articular cartilage. For example, during immobilization, articular cartilage undergoes changes characterized by a loss of function [99–100]. Also, in a canine study, articular cartilage in the knee became significantly stiffer following loading in physiologic ranges as a result of running on a treadmill [101]. To investigate these issues further many studies subjected cartilage explants to mechanical stimulation, and determined that mechanical stimulation served to maintain and even upregulate the production of ECM, and it was determined that *in vitro* loading conditions within the physiologic range of native hyaline cartilage were most beneficial [102]. Several methods have been used to deliver mechanical stimulation to articular cartilage; these include hydrostatic pressure, direct compression and shear, and are the predominant forces present in the knee.

28.3.4.1. Hydrostatic Pressure

During loading of diarthrodial joints, synovial fluid inside the joint capsule generates hydrostatic pressure that is transmitted to cartilage. Direct compression of cartilage also generates hydrostatic pressure, as the majority of the force is absorbed by the water in the cartilage matrix. As the fluid tries to leave the cartilage matrix it experiences resistance to its flow and, therefore, cannot easily leave as a result of the relative impermeability of cartilage. Since the water is somewhat "trapped" in the tissue, a uniform normal load or hydrostatic pressure is applied to the individual chondrocytes in the tissue as a result of the interstitial fluid pressure. However, since the cartilage matrix is not completely impermeable, the water is eventually forced out of the tissue and into the synovial cavity. The energy of the applied load is then dissipated as water leaves the tissue and encounters resistance as it moves through the cartilage matrix. In diarthrodial joints during normal activity, the magnitude of this interstitial pressure is usually between 7 and 10 MPa [103]. Also, a normal adult cadence corresponds to frequencies of 0.6 to 1.1 Hz loading per leg during walking [104], and >1.5 Hz during running [105].

Two approaches have been used to combine the application of hydrostatic pressure with culturing techniques for tissue engineering [106]. In the first approach the application of hydrostatic pressure is separated from culturing. The cells are grown in static culture and are moved to a specialized chamber (Fig. 28.3A) at certain times to apply hydrostatic pressure. Following application of hydrostatic pressure, the cells are returned to their static culture conditions and this process is repeated per the desire of the researcher. This approach is beneficial because it allows for the application of hydrostatic pressure only at certain times and for certain durations, rather than applying a continuous load. However, the major drawback of this approach is that there is an increased risk of contamination while transferring the cells between the static culture and hydrostatic pressure chamber. The second approach uses a semicontinuous perfusion system; a single device allows for medium to be delivered to the cells while hydrostatic pressure is applied. This approach is advantageous because it minimizes the possibility of contamination, and it can be automated; however, the downside of this approach is that fluid shear is also introduced into the system.

When using hydrostatic pressure stimulation the parameters that may be varied include the frequency of loading, the duration and magnitude of loading, as well as the time-points at which the cells are subjected to loading.

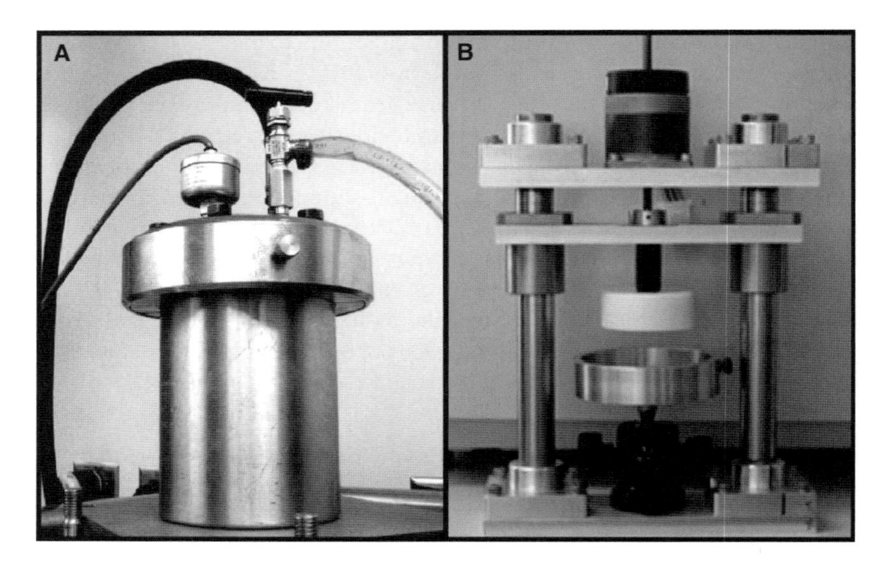

Fig. 28.3 (A) Hydrostatic pressure chamber. (B) Dived compression device.

As reviewed elsewhere [106], loads near the physiological range, between 0.1 and 15 MPa, and frequencies between 0.05 and 1 Hz, have yielded the most favorable results, although the majority of the hydrostatic pressure studies conducted so far have tested explants or monolayers. Research involving the use of hydrostatic pressure in 3-D culture of chondrocytes, especially at longer time-points, is lacking. However, a recent study using hydrostatic pressure at previously tested ranges was shown to have beneficial effects on 3-D constructs [39]. In the study 3-D self-assembled articular chondrocyte constructs (as described previously) were subjected to 10 MPa hydrostatic pressure at 1 Hz for four hours per day and five days per week for up to eight weeks, which led to a significant increase in collagen content while preventing a decrease in GAG content relative to the unstimulated control group. However, no significant difference in mechanical properties was observed between the treatment groups.

Hydrostatic pressure does not always produce beneficial results. For example, several studies that investigated constant hydrostatic pressure found little or no improvement in ECM composition [107–109]. Also, when hydrostatic pressure is above the physiological range, it may actually harm the cells, as decreased ECM production and expression of inflammatory mediators have been observed with these higher pressures [108].

Although the results of using hydrostatic pressure stimulation seem promising at this point, far more work must be undertaken to elucidate the precise application conditions for optimizing biomechanical and biochemical properties, particularly in 3-D engineered articular cartilage constructs.

28.3.4.2. Direct Compression

During normal joint loading in a healthy person compressive forces are generated in articular cartilage as a result of direct contact between the articulating surfaces and once hydrostatic pressure in the interstitial fluid subsides, as water is forced out of the loaded cartilage matrix. If no pathologic processes are present, articular cartilage is able to withstand compression many times per day without injury. In general, cartilage experiences deformation or strain in the range of 2 to 10 percent, which was determined under a load of five times body weight in the human hip [110].

As with hydrostatic pressure, the application of direct compression is usually a two-step approach in which the application of force is separated from culturing. The cells are grown in a static culture and are moved to a specialized device (Fig. 28-3B) at certain times to apply direct compression. These devices are generally designed so that a flat surface compresses the top of the construct at a specific load or displacement. Following application of the force, the cells are returned to their static culture conditions, and this process is repeated as desired.

When using direct compression the parameters that may be varied include strain or magnitude, frequency and the time-points at which the constructs are subjected to loading. As reviewed elsewhere [106], most studies have examined frequencies in the range of 0.0001 to 3 Hz, strains from 0.1 to 25 percent, loads from 0.1 to 24 MPa, and durations lasting hours to weeks, although these parameters are often limited by the equipment used.

As with constant hydrostatic pressure loading, cartilage responds negatively to static loading, most likely as a result of limited mass transport [106]. Therefore, studies using dynamic compression have produced the most positive results. Mauck, et al. [111] found a 33 percent increase in GAG production and an aggregate modulus on the same order of magnitude as in native cartilage when subjecting cartilage constructs to 3 percent strain at 1 Hz and three times of one hour on, one hour off per day, five days per week, for four weeks. Also, in dynamic compression, the loading frequency is an extremely important parameter to be studied. Lee, et al. [112] subjected constructs to compression at frequencies from 0.3 to 3 Hz and 15 percent strain, and found that GAG synthesis was significantly higher in the constructs subjected to 1 Hz compression. Interestingly, in addition to improved biochemical properties, dynamic compression has recently been shown to enhance the chondrogenic differentiation of MSCs, again indicating that mechanical loading plays an important role in cartilage repair [113].

28.3.4.3. Bioreactors and Shear Forces

The purpose of a bioreactor is to create an environment that will aid in the development of the desired tissue properties. In tissue engineering the major uses of bioreactors have been in the application of shear forces or in examining the effects of media perfusion and gas exchange on constructs.

As with compressive forces, shear forces are generated in the knee joint during loading as a result of direct contact between the articulating cartilage surfaces, as the two surfaces attempt to move past each other. Although a thin layer of synovial fluid provides lubrication between the cartilage surfaces, shear forces continue to occur as the surface-to-surface contact is not completely frictionless. Several studies (see reference [106]) have shown how applying shear to cartilage constructs is beneficial. The most widely used bioreactors in cartilage tissue engineering have been spinner flasks, perfusion bioreactors and rotating wall bioreactors.

Spinner flasks are perhaps the simplest bioreactors used, as a magnetic stir bar mixes oxygen and nutrients throughout the medium. Their primary use has been for cell seeding of scaffolds, as mixing in spinner flasks has proven extremely useful for uniformly seeding cells on scaffolds at high yields [114]. This approach involves attaching scaffolds to needles suspended from a stopper at the top of the flask. Cells in the medium are mixed in the flask due to the stir bar, and eventually are seeded onto the scaffold. Bueno, et al. [115] recently used a modified spinner flask, called a wavy-walled bioreactor, which is designed to enhance the mixing of the medium while minimizing the shear. They found that the kinetics of chondrocyte aggregation were significantly improved over a spinner flask when using a wavy-walled bioreactor.

In a direct perfusion bioreactor a scaffold is surrounded tightly by a medium chamber consisting of a hollow tube, and medium is forced through the fixed scaffold, from one end of the tube to the other. This design allows for a more uniform shear force and a more uniform concentration of nutrients to be delivered to the construct, as the cells located in the entire scaffold thickness are exposed both to convective solute transport and to a flow-induced mechanical stimulus [116]. Also, as used in some of the hydrostatic pressure systems, these bioreactors prevent the need to change the medium and, therefore, reduce the risk of contamination. Janssen, et al. [117] recently used a direct perfusion bioreactor in the production of engineered bone constructs of clinically relevant dimensions. A further modification to these systems can allow for the recycling of used medium along with the addition of fresh medium, which allows beneficial proteins such as ECM constituents to be maintained in the medium.

The use of rotating wall bioreactors has been a promising approach. The main improvement over a direct perfusion bioreactor is that a low shear environment is created without sacrificing the high diffusion in the perfusion systems. Essentially this device consists of two concentric cylinders separated by a space containing medium and scaffolds. The rotation rates of the cylinders can be modulated so as to create different flow and shear environments within the fluid. For example, to produce a low shear force, both cylinders are rotated slowly at the same rate or nearly the same rate. This technique has been coupled with other parameters, such as in the investigation of the effects of oxygen tension on cartilage constructs [118]. Since cartilage tissue is avascular and chondrocytes are exposed to a low oxygen tension environment *in vivo*, Saini and Wick [118] investigated the effects of oxygen tension on developing chondrocytes in a concentric cylinder bioreactor. They found that 5 percent oxygen tension led to constructs with double the GAG content of constructs cultured in 20 percent oxygen, with no effect on chondrocyte proliferation or collagen production. Interestingly, Wang, et al. [58] found that 5 percent oxygen tension was also an extremely effective inducer of chondrogenesis in hADAS cells, as it led to increased protein, collagen and GAG synthesis, with an inhibition of cell proliferation. This is a significant finding, as it may provide additional means of controlling the growth and metabolism of undifferentiated progenitor cells. However, culture in a rotating wall bioreactor has not always proven beneficial; a recent TMJ disc tissue engineering study found little or no benefit when using a rotating wall bioreactor, compared to static culture [119].

The use of bioreactors in tissue engineering has yielded exciting results and possibilities. Future directions of bioreactor use will likely involve the combination of the hydrodynamic flow chambers with other sources of mechanical stimulation [120], as well as with growth factor addition in the medium. As these technologies improve and the processes of growth factor addition and mechanical stimulation are optimized, it may become possible to create a large scale cartilage bioreactor for mass production of engineered constructs.

28.4. Future Trends and Needs

Successful tissue engineering approaches that will be used in the clinic likely will require optimization of the four parameters of the tissue engineering paradigm. Scaffolds will need to exhibit adequate biocompatibility and mechanical properties, and allow for diffusion of nutrients to the seeded cells, or a "scaffold-less" approach such as the self-assembling process will need to be employed. Stem cells, both adult and embryonic, represent a promising cell source for articular cartilage engineering; however, more work needs to be performed to understand the developmental processes involved in differentiation so that these processes may be further manipulated to optimize *in vitro* cell expansion while maintaining chondrogenic differentiation. Growth factor application must also be optimized for tissue engineering through further characterization of the roles of each growth factor and their effects on different cell types, as well as elucidation of the correct dosage frequency and concentrations. Finally, as scaffolds, cell sources, growth factor application and mechanical stimulation are optimized, mass production of tissue engineered constructs may become possible through the creation of large scale bioreactors.

Current tissue engineering approaches strive to obtain a construct with mechanical, biochemical and histological properties as close as possible to native tissue. However, since relatively few constructs have seen clinical use to date, it is unclear how closely the properties of the construct must mimic those of native tissue to prove clinically functional. It is likely that, as the parameters of the tissue engineering paradigm are optimized to produce constructs that approach native tissue properties, constructs with a wide spectrum of properties will be produced along the way. Then, implantation studies may be performed to determine the optimal properties a construct must possess for *in vivo* use.

28.5. Conclusions

Damaged cartilage has a limited ability to heal itself and clinical treatment is unable to fully restore tissue function. Therefore, tissue engineering is an ideal approach for successful cartilage regeneration through the interaction of the selected scaffold, cell source, growth factors and mechanical stimulation. Although many promising results have been attained thus far, tissue engineering still has hurdles to overcome as successful regeneration of cartilage cannot be realized until the four parameters of the tissue engineering paradigm have been optimized. Nonetheless, this is an exciting time as we are rapidly approaching widespread clinical use of tissue engineered cartilage constructs for treatment of articular cartilage, knee meniscus and TMJ pathologies.

References

1. Benson V, Marano MA. Current estimates from the National Health Interview Survey, 1995. Vital Health Stat 10 1998(199):1–428.
2. Osteoarthritis Fact Sheet. In. http://www.arthritis.org/ conditions/Fact_Sheets/OA_Fact_Sheet.asp.
3. Mow VC, Kuei SC, Lai WM, Armstrong CG. Biphasic creep and stress relaxation of articular cartilage in compression: Theory and experiments. J Biomech Eng 1980;102(1):73–84.
4. Buckwalter JA, Hunziker EB, Rosenberg LC, Coutts R, Adams M, Eyre D. Articular Cartilage: Composition and Structure. 2nd ed. Park Ridge: American Academy of Orthopedic Surgeons; 1979.
5. Hu JC, Athanasiou KA. Structure and Function of Articular Cartilage. In: An YH, Martin KL, eds. Handbook of Histology Methods for Bone and Cartilage. 1st ed. Totowa, NJ: Humana Press Inc.; 2003:73–95.
6. Ruoslahti E. Structure and biology of proteoglycans. Annu Rev Cell Biol 1988;4:229–55.
7. Darling EM, Hu JC, Athanasiou KA. Zonal and topographical differences in articular cartilage gene expression. J Orthop Res 2004;22(6):1182–7.
8. Jeffery AK, Blunn GW, Archer CW, Bentley G. Three-dimensional collagen architecture in bovine articular cartilage. J Bone Joint Surg Br 1991;73(5):795–801.
9. Lai WM, Mow VC, Zhu W. Constitutive modeling of articular cartilage and biomacromolecular solutions. J Biomech Eng 1993;115(4B):474–80.
10. Mow VC, Flatow EL, Ateshian GA. Biomechanics. In: Buckwalter JA, Einhorn TA, Simon SR, eds. Orthopaedic Basic Science: Biology and Biomechanics of the Musculoskeletal System: American Academy of Orthopaedic Surgeons; 2000: 140–2.
11. Hodge WA, Carlson KL, Fijan RS, et al. Contact pressures from an instrumented hip endoprosthesis. J Bone Joint Surg Am 1989;71(9):1378–86.
12. Buckwalter JA. Articular cartilage injuries. Clin Orthop Relat Res 2002(402):21–37.
13. Hunziker EB. Articular cartilage repair: are the intrinsic biological constraints undermining this process insuperable? Osteoarthritis Cartilage 1999;7(1):15–28.
14. Buckwalter JA. Articular cartilage: injuries and potential for healing. J Orthop Sports Phys Ther 1998;28(4):192–202.
15. Alford JW, Cole BJ. Cartilage restoration, part 2: techniques, outcomes, and future directions. Am J Sports Med 2005;33(3):443–60.
16. Erggelet C, Browne JE, Fu F, Mandelbaum BR, Micheli LJ, Mosely JB. [Autologous chondrocyte transplantation for treatment of cartilage defects of the knee joint. Clinical results]. Zentralbl Chir 2000;125(6):516–22.
17. Wood JJ, Malek MA, Frassica FJ, et al. Autologous cultured chondrocytes: adverse events reported to the United States Food and Drug Administration. J Bone Joint Surg Am 2006;88(3):503–7.
18. Darling EM, Athanasiou KA. Biomechanical strategies for articular cartilage regeneration. Ann Biomed Eng 2003;31(9):1114–24.
19. Leipzig ND, Athanasiou KA. Cartilage Regeneration. In: Bowlin GL, Wnek G, eds. Encyclopedia of Biomaterials and Biomedical Engineering: Marcel Dekker, Inc. ; 2004:283–91.
20. Darling EM, Athanasiou KA. Bioactive Scaffold Design for Articular Cartilage. In *Biomedical Technology and Devices Handbook*. In: Moore J, Zouridakis G, eds. Biomedical Technology and Devices Handbook New York: RC Press; 2003: Ch 21 (1–16).
21. Athanasiou KA, Shah AR, Hernandez RJ, LeBaron RG. Basic science of articular cartilage repair. Clin Sports Med 2001;20(2):223–47.
22. Nehrer S, Breinan HA, Ramappa A, et al. Canine chondrocytes seeded in type I and type II collagen implants investigated in vitro. J Biomed Mater Res 1997;38(2):95–104.

23. Frenkel SR, Di Cesare PE. Scaffolds for articular cartilage repair. Ann Biomed Eng 2004;32(1):26–34.
24. Passaretti D, Silverman RP, Huang W, et al. Cultured chondrocytes produce injectable tissue-engineered cartilage in hydrogel polymer. Tissue Eng 2001;7(6):805–15.
25. Lahiji A, Sohrabi A, Hungerford DS, Frondoza CG. Chitosan supports the expression of extracellular matrix proteins in human osteoblasts and chondrocytes. J Biomed Mater Res 2000;51(4):586–95.
26. Nettles DL, Elder SH, Gilbert JA. Potential use of chitosan as a cell scaffold material for cartilage tissue engineering. Tissue Eng 2002;8(6):1009–16.
27. Elisseeff J, Anseth K, Sims D, et al. Transdermal photopolymerization of poly(ethylene oxide)-based injectable hydrogels for tissue-engineered cartilage. Plast Reconstr Surg 1999;104(4):1014–22.
28. Burdick JA, Chung C, Jia X, Randolph MA, Langer R. Controlled degradation and mechanical behavior of photopolymerized hyaluronic acid networks. Biomacromolecules 2005;6(1):386–91.
29. Thornton AJ, Alsberg E, Albertelli M, Mooney DJ. Shape-defining scaffolds for minimally invasive tissue engineering. Transplantation 2004;77(12):1798–803.
30. Rahfoth B, Weisser J, Sternkopf F, Aigner T, von der Mark K, Brauer R. Transplantation of allograft chondrocytes embedded in agarose gel into cartilage defects of rabbits. Osteoarthritis Cartilage 1998;6(1):50–65.
31. Athanasiou KA, Agrawal CM, Barber FA, Burkhart SS. Orthopaedic applications for PLA-PGA biodegradable polymers. Arthroscopy 1998;14(7):726–37.
32. Almarza AJ, Athanasiou KA. Seeding techniques and scaffolding choice for tissue engineering of the temporomandibular joint disk. Tissue Eng 2004;10(11–12): 1787–95.
33. Detamore MS, Athanasiou KA. Evaluation of three growth factors for TMJ disc tissue engineering. Ann Biomed Eng 2005;33(3):383–90.
34. Mercier NR, Costantino HR, Tracy MA, Bonassar LJ. A novel injectable approach for cartilage formation in vivo using PLG microspheres. Ann Biomed Eng 2004;32(3):418–29.
35. Caterson EJ, Li WJ, Nesti LJ, Albert T, Danielson K, Tuan RS. Polymer/alginate amalgam for cartilage-tissue engineering. Ann NY Acad Sci 2002;961:134–8.
36. Hu JC, Athanasiou KA. A self-assembling process in articular cartilage tissue engineering. Tissue Eng 2006;12(4):969–79.
37. Furukawa KS, Suenaga H, Toita K, et al. Rapid and large-scale formation of chondrocyte aggregates by rotational culture. Cell Transplant 2003;12(5):475–9.
38. Stewart MC, Saunders KM, Burton-Wurster N, Macleod JN. Phenotypic stability of articular chondrocytes in vitro: the effects of culture models, bone morphogenetic protein 2, and serum supplementation. J Bone Miner Res 2000;15(1):166–74.
39. Hu JC, Athanasiou KA. The effects of intermittent hydrostatic pressure on self-assembled articular cartilage constructs. Tissue Eng 2006.
40. Song L, Baksh D, Tuan RS. Mesenchymal stem cell-based cartilage tissue engineering: cells, scaffold and biology. Cytotherapy 2004;6(6):596–601.
41. Takemitsu Y. The effect of age upon sulfate-S35 fixation of chondroitin sulfate in cartilage and bone of the normal white rats and S35-autoradiographic study of these tissues. Kyushu J Med Sci 1961(12):251–81.
42. Benya PD, Nimni ME. The stability of the collagen phenotype during stimulated collagen, glycosaminoglycan, and DNA synthesis by articular cartilage organ cultures. Arch Biochem Biophys 1979;192(2):327–35.
43. Benya PD, Padilla SR, Nimni ME. The progeny of rabbit articular chondrocytes synthesize collagen types I and III and type I trimer, but not type II. Verifications by cyanogen bromide peptide analysis. Biochemistry 1977;16(5):865–72.
44. Benya PD, Padilla SR, Nimni ME. Independent regulation of collagen types by chondrocytes during the loss of differentiated function in culture. Cell 1978;15(4):1313–21.

45. Schulze-Tanzil G, Mobasheri A, de Souza P, John T, Shakibaei M. Loss of chondrogenic potential in dedifferentiated chondrocytes correlates with deficient Shc-Erk interaction and apoptosis. Osteoarthritis Cartilage 2004;12(6):448–58.
46. Darling EM, Athanasiou KA. Rapid phenotypic changes in passaged articular chondrocyte subpopulations. J Orthop Res 2005;23(2):425–32.
47. Benya PD, Shaffer JD. Dedifferentiated chondrocytes reexpress the differentiated collagen phenotype when cultured in agarose gels. Cell 1982;30(1):215–24.
48. Shapiro F, Koide S, Glimcher MJ. Cell origin and differentiation in the repair of full-thickness defects of articular cartilage. J Bone Joint Surg Am 1993;75(4):532–53.
49. Butnariu-Ephrat M, Robinson D, Mendes DG, Halperin N, Nevo Z. Resurfacing of goat articular cartilage by chondrocytes derived from bone marrow. Clin Orthop Relat Res 1996(330):234–43.
50. Mauck RL, Yuan X, Tuan RS. Chondrogenic differentiation and functional maturation of bovine mesenchymal stem cells in long-term agarose culture. Osteoarthritis Cartilage 2006;14(2):179–89.
51. Yoo JU, Barthel TS, Nishimura K, et al. The chondrogenic potential of human bone-marrow-derived mesenchymal progenitor cells. J Bone Joint Surg Am 1998;80(12):1745–57.
52. Huang JI, Kazmi N, Durbhakula MM, Hering TM, Yoo JU, Johnstone B. Chondrogenic potential of progenitor cells derived from human bone marrow and adipose tissue: a patient-matched comparison. J Orthop Res 2005;23(6):1383–9.
53. Hegewald AA, Ringe J, Bartel J, et al. Hyaluronic acid and autologous synovial fluid induce chondrogenic differentiation of equine mesenchymal stem cells: a preliminary study. Tissue Cell 2004;36(6):431–8.
54. Gronthos S, Zannettino AC, Hay SJ, et al. Molecular and cellular characterisation of highly purified stromal stem cells derived from human bone marrow. J Cell Sci 2003;116(Pt 9):1827–35.
55. Nathan S, Das De S, Thambyah A, Fen C, Goh J, Lee EH. Cell-based therapy in the repair of osteochondral defects: a novel use for adipose tissue. Tissue Eng 2003;9(4):733–44.
56. Betre H, Ong SR, Guilak F, Chilkoti A, Fermor B, Setton LA. Chondrocytic differentiation of human adipose-derived adult stem cells in elastin-like polypeptide. Biomaterials 2006;27(1):91–9.
57. Awad HA, Wickham MQ, Leddy HA, Gimble JM, Guilak F. Chondrogenic differentiation of adipose-derived adult stem cells in agarose, alginate, and gelatin scaffolds. Biomaterials 2004;25(16):3211–22.
58. Wang DW, Fermor B, Gimble JM, Awad HA, Guilak F. Influence of oxygen on the proliferation and metabolism of adipose derived adult stem cells. J Cell Physiol 2005;204(1):184–91.
59. Li X, Lee JP, Balian G, Greg Anderson D. Modulation of chondrocytic properties of fat-derived mesenchymal cells in co-cultures with nucleus pulposus. Connect Tissue Res 2005;46(2):75–82.
60. Lin Y, Luo E, Chen X, et al. Molecular and cellular characterization during chondrogenic differentiation of adipose tissue-derived stromal cells in vitro and cartilage formation in vivo. J Cell Mol Med 2005;9(4):929–39.
61. Nishimura K, Solchaga LA, Caplan AI, Yoo JU, Goldberg VM, Johnstone B. Chondroprogenitor cells of synovial tissue. Arthritis Rheum 1999;42(12):2631–7.
62. Huang JI, Beanes SR, Zhu M, Lorenz HP, Hedrick MH, Benhaim P. Rat extramedullary adipose tissue as a source of osteochondrogenic progenitor cells. Plast Reconstr Surg 2002;109(3):1033–41; discussion 42–3.
63. Wickham MQ, Erickson GR, Gimble JM, Vail TP, Guilak F. Multipotent stromal cells derived from the infrapatellar fat pad of the knee. Clin Orthop Relat Res 2003(412):196–212.
64. Keller G. Embryonic stem cell differentiation: emergence of a new era in biology and medicine. Genes Dev 2005;19(10):1129–55.

65. Kramer J, Hegert C, Guan K, Wobus AM, Muller PK, Rohwedel J. Embryonic stem cell-derived chondrogenic differentiation in vitro: activation by BMP-2 and BMP-4. Mech Dev 2000;92(2):193–205.
66. Levenberg S, Huang NF, Lavik E, Rogers AB, Itskovitz-Eldor J, Langer R. Differentiation of human embryonic stem cells on three-dimensional polymer scaffolds. Proc Natl Acad Sci U S A 2003;100(22):12741–6.
67. Levenberg S, Burdick JA, Kraehenbuehl T, Langer R. Neurotrophin-induced differentiation of human embryonic stem cells on three-dimensional polymeric scaffolds. Tissue Eng 2005;11(3–4):506–12.
68. French MM, Rose S, Canseco J, Athanasiou KA. Chondrogenic differentiation of adult dermal fibroblasts. Ann Biomed Eng 2004;32(1):50–6.
69. Yates KE, Mizuno S, Glowacki J. Early shifts in gene expression during chondroinduction of human dermal fibroblasts. Exp Cell Res 2001;265(2):203–11.
70. Mizuno S, Glowacki J. Chondroinduction of human dermal fibroblasts by demineralized bone in three-dimensional culture. Exp Cell Res 1996;227(1):89–97.
71. French MM, Athanasiou KA. Differentiation Factors and Articular Cartilage Regeneration. In: Ashammakhi N, Ferretti P, eds. Topics in Tissue Engineering; 2003:1–19.
72. Ahn JI, Terry Canale S, Butler SD, Hasty KA. Stem cell repair of physeal cartilage. J Orthop Res 2004;22(6):1215–21.
73. Galera P, Vivien D, Pronost S, et al. Transforming growth factor-beta 1 (TGF-beta 1) up-regulation of collagen type II in primary cultures of rabbit articular chondrocytes (RAC) involves increased mRNA levels without affecting mRNA stability and procollagen processing. J Cell Physiol 1992;153(3):596–606.
74. Blunk T, Sieminski AL, Gooch KJ, et al. Differential effects of growth factors on tissue-engineered cartilage. Tissue Eng 2002;8(1):73–84.
75. Park Y, Sugimoto M, Watrin A, Chiquet M, Hunziker EB. BMP-2 induces the expression of chondrocyte-specific genes in bovine synovium-derived progenitor cells cultured in three-dimensional alginate hydrogel. Osteoarthritis Cartilage 2005;13(6):527–36.
76. Knippenberg M, Helder MN, Zandieh Doulabi B, Wuisman PI, Klein-Nulend J. Osteogenesis versus chondrogenesis by BMP-2 and BMP-7 in adipose stem cells. Biochem Biophys Res Commun 2006;342(3):902–8.
77. Tyler JA. Insulin-like growth factor 1 can decrease degradation and promote synthesis of proteoglycan in cartilage exposed to cytokines. Biochem J 1989;260(2):543–8.
78. Guenther HL, Guenther HE, Froesch ER, Fleisch H. Effect of insulin-like growth factor on collagen and glycosaminoglycan synthesis by rabbit articular chondrocytes in culture. Experientia 1982;38(8):979–81.
79. Luyten FP, Hascall VC, Nissley SP, Morales TI, Reddi AH. Insulin-like growth factors maintain steady-state metabolism of proteoglycans in bovine articular cartilage explants. Arch Biochem Biophys 1988;267(2):416–25.
80. Darling EM, Athanasiou KA. Growth factor impact on articular cartilage subpopulations. Cell Tissue Res 2005;322(3):463–73.
81. Nixon AJ, Saxer RA, Brower-Toland BD. Exogenous insulin-like growth factor-I stimulates an autoinductive IGF-I autocrine/paracrine response in chondrocytes. J Orthop Res 2001;19(1):26–32.
82. Arevalo-Silva CA, Cao Y, Weng Y, et al. The effect of fibroblast growth factor and transforming growth factor-beta on porcine chondrocytes and tissue-engineered autologous elastic cartilage. Tissue Eng 2001;7(1):81–8.
83. Toolan BC, Frenkel SR, Pachence JM, Yalowitz L, Alexander H. Effects of growth-factor-enhanced culture on a chondrocyte-collagen implant for cartilage repair. J Biomed Mater Res 1996;31(2):273–80.
84. Fujimoto E, Ochi M, Kato Y, Mochizuki Y, Sumen Y, Ikuta Y. Beneficial effect of basic fibroblast growth factor on the repair of full-thickness defects in rabbit articular cartilage. Arch Orthop Trauma Surg 1999;119(3-4):139–45.

85. Davidson D, Blanc A, Filion D, et al. Fibroblast growth factor (FGF) 18 signals through FGF receptor 3 to promote chondrogenesis. J Biol Chem 2005;280(21):20509–15.
86. Amano O, Koshimizu U, Nakamura T, Iseki S. Enhancement by hepatocyte growth factor of bone and cartilage formation during embryonic mouse mandibular development in vitro. Arch Oral Biol 1999;44(11):935–46.
87. Grumbles RM, Howell DS, Wenger L, Altman RD, Howard GA, Roos BA. Hepatocyte growth factor and its actions in growth plate chondrocytes. Bone 1996;19(3):255–61.
88. Kieswetter K, Schwartz Z, Alderete M, Dean DD, Boyan BD. Platelet derived growth factor stimulates chondrocyte proliferation but prevents endochondral maturation. Endocrine 1997;6(3):257–64.
89. Hanada K, Solchaga LA, Caplan AI, et al. BMP-2 induction and TGF-beta 1 modulation of rat periosteal cell chondrogenesis. J Cell Biochem 2001;81(2):284–94.
90. Indrawattana N, Chen G, Tadokoro M, et al. Growth factor combination for chondrogenic induction from human mesenchymal stem cell. Biochem Biophys Res Commun 2004;320(3):914–9.
91. Kaplan BA, Gorman CR, Gupta AK, Taylor SR, Iezzoni JC, Park SS. Effects of transforming growth factor Beta and insulin-like growth factor 1 on the biomechanical and histologic properties of tissue-engineered cartilage. Arch Facial Plast Surg 2003;5(1):96–101.
92. Bonassar LJ, Grodzinsky AJ, Frank EH, Davila SG, Bhaktav NR, Trippel SB. The effect of dynamic compression on the response of articular cartilage to insulin-like growth factor-I. J Orthop Res 2001;19(1):11–7.
93. Mauck RL, Nicoll SB, Seyhan SL, Ateshian GA, Hung CT. Synergistic action of growth factors and dynamic loading for articular cartilage tissue engineering. Tissue Eng 2003;9(4):597–611.
94. Darling EM, Athanasiou KA. Retaining zonal chondrocyte phenotype by means of novel growth environments. Tissue Eng 2005;11(3–4):395–403.
95. Sailor LZ, Hewick RM, Morris EA. Recombinant human bone morphogenetic protein-2 maintains the articular chondrocyte phenotype in long-term culture. J Orthop Res 1996;14(6):937–45.
96. Pangborn CA, Athanasiou KA. Effects of growth factors on meniscal fibrochondrocytes. Tissue Eng 2005;11(7–8):1141–8.
97. Pangborn CA, Athanasiou KA. Growth factors and fibrochondrocytes in scaffolds. J Orthop Res 2005;23(5):1184–90.
98. Almarza AJ, Athanasiou KA. Evaluation of three growth factors in combinations of two for temporomandibular joint disc tissue engineering. Arch Oral Biol 2006;51(3):215–21.
99. Helminen HJ, Saamanen AM, Jurvelin J, et al. [The effect of loading on articular cartilage]. Duodecim 1992;108(12):1097–107.
100. Palmoski MJ, Colyer RA, Brandt KD. Joint motion in the absence of normal loading does not maintain normal articular cartilage. Arthritis Rheum 1980;23(3):325–34.
101. Jurvelin J, Kiviranta I, Tammi M, Helminen HJ. Effect of physical exercise on indentation stiffness of articular cartilage in the canine knee. Int J Sports Med 1986;7(2):106–10.
102. Hall AC, Urban JP, Gehl KA. The effects of hydrostatic pressure on matrix synthesis in articular cartilage. J Orthop Res 1991;9(1):1–10.
103. Hall AC, Horwitz ER, Wilkins RJ. The cellular physiology of articular cartilage. Exp Physiol 1996;81(3):535–45.
104. Waters RL, Lunsford BR, Perry J, Byrd R. Energy-speed relationship of walking: standard tables. J Orthop Res 1988;6(2):215–22.
105. Schwab GH, Moynes DR, Jobe FW, Perry J. Lower extremity electromyographic analysis of running gait. Clin Orthop Relat Res 1983(176):166–70.

106. Darling EM, Athanasiou KA. Articular cartilage bioreactors and bioprocesses. Tissue Eng 2003;9(1):9–26.
107. Lammi MJ, Inkinen R, Parkkinen JJ, et al. Expression of reduced amounts of structurally altered aggrecan in articular cartilage chondrocytes exposed to high hydrostatic pressure. Biochem J 1994;304 (Pt 3):723–30.
108. Takahashi K, Kubo T, Arai Y, et al. Hydrostatic pressure induces expression of interleukin 6 and tumour necrosis factor alpha mRNAs in a chondrocyte-like cell line. Ann Rheum Dis 1998;57(4):231–6.
109. Parkkinen JJ, Lammi MJ, Pelttari A, Helminen HJ, Tammi M, Virtanen I. Altered Golgi apparatus in hydrostatically loaded articular cartilage chondrocytes. Ann Rheum Dis 1993;52(3):192–8.
110. Armstrong CG, Bahrani AS, Gardner DL. In vitro measurement of articular cartilage deformations in the intact human hip joint under load. J Bone Joint Surg Am 1979;61(5):744–55.
111. Mauck RL, Soltz MA, Wang CC, et al. Functional tissue engineering of articular cartilage through dynamic loading of chondrocyte-seeded agarose gels. J Biomech Eng 2000;122(3):252–60.
112. Lee DA, Noguchi T, Frean SP, Lees P, Bader DL. The influence of mechanical loading on isolated chondrocytes seeded in agarose constructs. Biorheology 2000;37(1–2):149–61.
113. Angele P, Schumann D, Angele M, et al. Cyclic, mechanical compression enhances chondrogenesis of mesenchymal progenitor cells in tissue engineering scaffolds. Biorheology 2004;41(3–4):335–46.
114. Vunjak-Novakovic G, Obradovic B, Martin I, Bursac PM, Langer R, Freed LE. Dynamic cell seeding of polymer scaffolds for cartilage tissue engineering. Biotechnol Prog 1998;14(2):193–202.
115. Bueno EM, Bilgen B, Carrier RL, Barabino GA. Increased rate of chondrocyte aggregation in a wavy-walled bioreactor. Biotechnol Bioeng 2004;88(6):767–77.
116. Raimondi MT, Boschetti F, Falcone L, Migliavacca F, Remuzzi A, Dubini G. The effect of media perfusion on three-dimensional cultures of human chondrocytes: integration of experimental and computational approaches. Biorheology 2004;41(3–4):401–10.
117. Janssen FW, Oostra J, Oorschot A, van Blitterswijk CA. A perfusion bioreactor system capable of producing clinically relevant volumes of tissue-engineered bone: in vivo bone formation showing proof of concept. Biomaterials 2006;27(3):315–23.
118. Saini S, Wick TM. Effect of low oxygen tension on tissue-engineered cartilage construct development in the concentric cylinder bioreactor. Tissue Eng 2004;10(5–6):825–32.
119. Detamore MS, Athanasiou KA. Use of a rotating bioreactor toward tissue engineering the temporomandibular joint disc. Tissue Eng 2005;11(7–8):1188–97.
120. Seidel JO, Pei M, Gray ML, Langer R, Freed LE, Vunjak-Novakovic G. Long-term culture of tissue engineered cartilage in a perfused chamber with mechanical stimulation. Biorheology 2004;41(3–4):445–58.

Section V

The Future

29

The Future of Musculoskeletal Tissue Regeneration: A Clinical Perspective

Anna V. Cuomo[1] and Jay R. Lieberman[2]

Abstract: Over the past decade significant advances have occurred with our understanding of the molecular pathways related to the repair for hard and soft tissues of the musculoskeletal system. It is essential that this information be translated from the bench to the bedside to create novel treatment regimens that advance the care of patients. The purpose of this chapter is to elucidate therapeutic regimens that may be developed in the future. Over the next two to 10 years there will be an intense focus on developing targeted delivery of bioactive substances that employ minimally invasive surgical techniques. Treatments in the remote future will require knowledge related to the host biologic potential, disease risk stratification and prevention strategies for the musculoskeletal patient. A case study is presented to explore the potential clinical future.

Keywords: Tissue regeneration, gene therapy, pharmocogenomics, orthopaedic genome, molecular diagnostics, future.

29.1. Introduction – Hurdles from the Bench to Bedside

The purpose of this chapter is to define the essential issues that will enable critical advances in molecular medicine to be translated from the bench to bedside. While the immediate future holds great promise for novel surgical interventions, a paradigm shift in clinical care will become available that will make surgical intervention less necessary. In order for this paradigm shift to occur, an increased knowledge of the pathophysiology of diseases such as osteoarthritis and the natural history of hard and soft tissue repair will be imperative. This information will determine the basis of musculoskeletal health care in the future.

[1]Department of Orthopaedic Surgery, David Geffen School of Medicine at UCLA, Los Angeles, CA

[2]Director, New England Musculoskeletal Institute, Professor and Chairman, Department of Orthopaedic Surgery, University of Connecticut Health Center, Farmington, CT

From: *Orthopedic Biology and Medicine: Musculoskeletal Tissue Regeneration, Biological Materials and Methods*
Edited by W. S. Pietrzak © Humana Press, Totowa, NJ

29.2. The Keys to Musculoskeletal Regeneration: Cells, Signals and Matrices

The disparate structures and functions of various musculoskeletal tissues, such as bone, cartilage, muscle, tendon, ligament and meniscus, are united by their common elements: cells, signals and matrices. Ultimately, all three elements are required for tissue regeneration. In the following section clinically relevant questions for each of these elements are identified and their potential influences on treatment regimens are discussed.

29.2.1 Cells: How do We Identify, Harvest, and Stimulate Cell Precursors?

Stem cells have been a central focus in tissue engineering due to their capability for self-renewal, plasticity, expansion and possible immune privileged status. Musculoskeletal progenitors, also called adult stem cells (ASCs), include mesenchymal stem cells (MSCs) [1], mesoangioblasts [2], endothelial progenitor cells [3], and mesoderm adult progenitors [4]. However, their phenotypes remain elusive, thereby limiting their harvest, expansion, and optimization for tissue regeneration. Once ASCs are better characterized, and their lineages defined, specific stem cells can be harvested with higher yield and less morbidity for a variety of clinical applications.

Exactly where ASCs reside within mature tissue remains speculative. They are potentially dependent on environmental cues to retain their 'stemness' and a 'stem cell niche' has been an area of active research. For instance, the homing mechanism of transiently circulating hematopoietic stem cells to bone marrow, as well as the migration of stem cells into specific anatomic sites within tissue, has been more clearly delineated in the past three decades [5]. Other stem cells are likely to have similar mechanisms and understanding these pathways will lead to improved tissue regeneration techniques.

In the laboratory ASCs have been harvested from skin, fat, muscle, liver, brain, peripheral nerve, bone marrow, peripheral blood and vascular tissue. Sources such as skin, nerve and brain pose obvious cosmetic or functional donor site morbidity and, thus, are poor donor sites. Although the feasibility of harvesting autogenous adult stem cells from adipose tissue has spurred considerable clinical interest [6], bone marrow continues to be the major source of musculoskeletal cell precursors in the clinical setting. Bone marrow has several important limitations. Donor site pain is a significant source of morbidity and the quantity and quality of bone marrow can be variable. Furthermore, the concentration of progenitor cells under ideal conditions is still relatively low. A recent study suggests a concentration of one osteoprogenitor per 10^4 to 10^6 nucleated cells in an average donor. Assuming minimal dilution with peripheral blood to yield an average of 20 million nucleated cells per cubic centimeter, this number extrapolates to 500 stem cells per cubic centimeter of fresh marrow aspirate [7]. The same study also found that a threshold of 1,000 progenitors per cubic centimeter was necessary to stimulate bone healing in human tibial nonunions treated with a percutaneous injection of concentrated bone marrow aspirate. The results suggest that a minimum number of progenitor cells are necessary to promote healing, but this may be influenced by the biologic potential of the host and the size of the defect. In addition, identifying carriers that support or enhance healing is critical.

Efforts to better characterize stem cells are underway. Microarray analysis of various culture expanded stem cells has identified 260 genes that are upregulated approximately three-fold in various stem cells. The majority of these genes, presumably identifying a cell's 'stemness,' govern yet unidentified cellular functions and phenotypes [8]. Stem cell phenotypes have been particularly difficult to study, since isolation *in vitro* has been shown to alter their surface markers. Since cell-specific surface markers are vital to providing a mechanism to tag, harvest, quantify and monitor ASCs, the recent discovery of the MSC-specific surface protein CD105 is an exciting step forward in this area of research [9]. The ability to isolate and concentrate MSCs without *ex vivo* expansion has the potential to revolutionize clinical applications with same-day procedures for bone, tendon, muscle and nerve regeneration. However, it is also possible that stem cell harvest will become unnecessary. Recent research suggests that committed cells can dedifferentiate "backwards" to become stem cells by changing intracellular regulators. *In vitro* studies with synthetic factors such as reversine [10], a 2,6-disubstitued purine similar in structure to naturally occurring cyclin-dependent kinase inhibitors, has spurred both *in vitro* and *in vivo* dedifferentiation of fibroblasts. Therefore, it is possible that the number of progenitors within tissue may simply be the number of committed cells available for dedifferentiation.

The potential clinical impact of ASC research is profound. The appropriate stem cell concentration required to heal a tissue defect could be calculated based on the defect size and tissue bed characteristics. Bone marrow aspirate could be harvested and concentrated to the appropriate concentration and volume. Or, the nucleated cells from a small tissue sample, such as peripheral blood, could be dedifferentiated to an appropriate precursor before re-implantation for *ex vivo* therapies. Minimally invasive techniques could be developed to implant matrices seeded with stem cells that can promote the regeneration of bone, cartilage, ligament or meniscus. In theory these therapies could be directed at early stage disease. Treatment of early knee osteoarthritis could have a profound effect on quality of life and health care costs, since it has been projected that the number of primary (first-time) total knees will increase to 3.48 million by the year 2030 [11].

Although ASCs have clinical potential, it is embryonic cells that may revolutionize the tissue engineering strategies for the musculoskeletal system. Research with these cells is limited at this time, but they clearly possess an immune privileged status and the plasticity to become a variety of progenitors depending on the signals received from the local environment [12]. As such, surgeons are interested in tissue engineering strategies that combine embryonic stem cells with matrices for off-the-shelf products. An understanding of the biological behavior of these cells is essential to create new treatment paradigms for tissue repair.

29.2.2. Signals: The Orthopaedic Genome, Pharmacogenomics and Targeted Therapies

Many therapies that alter cell signaling by targeting extracellular proteins have been developed. These include a multitude of growth factors, inflammatory cytokines and cell receptors. One of the most studied is bone morphogenetic protein (BMP). Urist first characterized BMP as an extract from demineralized bone matrix (DBM) in the 1960s and, since then, recombinant human

BMPs have been utilized for creating osseous fusions and reconstructions of bone defects [13]. Other recombinant proteins have recently been FDA-approved and are available to clinicians to augment naturally occurring pathways. Insulin-like growth factor-1 and its recombinant form (rhIGF-1) can be used to increase the longitudinal growth of bone in children deficient in these proteins [14]. Recombinant human platelet-derived growth factor is used as a topical agent to enhance healing of chronic pressure ulcers [15]. Also, erythropoietin, which increases hematopoeitic precursors, can be given systemically to decrease the need for perioperative transfusions in orthopaedic patients [16].

Although recombinant proteins show great promise, there are three major problems with their clinical applications at this time. First, supraphysiologic doses at frequent dosing intervals are required to be effective. For instance, there are only nanogram amounts of BMP in the human body, but the milligram doses are necessary to induce spinal fusion or heal an open tibia fracture [17-18]. Second, the effects can be systemic and may not specifically target the pathologic tissues. For instance, rhIGF-1 also disrupts the insulin-glucagon endocrine system and can adversely lead to hypoglycemia [19]. Third, extracellular cytokines are still relatively "upstream" signals and can produce heterogeneous effects. For example, PDGF has been shown to both enhance and inhibit bone regeneration in various *in vivo* models. Although poorly understood, this is likely attributable to local competing signals and the character of the recipient tissue bed [20–21]. These three major drawbacks have led to a greater interest in therapies that directly alter intracellular events. The direct effect on protein expression can result in a prolonged therapeutic effect that is highly specific to a cell phenotype, thereby providing a 'tailored therapy.'

However, understanding intra- and extracellular signaling is still in its infancy. There is an increasing appreciation of the complexity of these pathways with redundant or overlapping feedback loops. For instance, there are 16 known types of BMP that can form homo- or heterodimers, each with variable affinity to several extracellular receptors: type I, IIa, and IIb. Receptor activation initiates three intracellular pathways with Smads, MAPK and protein kinase-C, and their downstream signals may antagonize each other and produce variable effects [22–23]. As a result the potential outcomes can be difficult to predict. Thus, efforts have focused on identifying the key signals in these pathways that may serve as therapeutic targets. Innovative techniques, such as quantitative-PCR and reporter gene assays, are critical to these efforts.

Other novel technologies, such as gene microchip arrays, provide powerful tools for studying multiple genes at once. Microchip arrays are capable of defining relative gene expression of approximately 50,000 oligonucleotide probes on a single chip with high accuracy. The probes are used to identify regions of a gene and the microchips can be designed to study a particular subset of genes, such as the 'orthopaedic genome [24].' This is a broad subset of the 40,000 genes identified by the Human Genome Project that are involved in the genesis and maintenance of the musculoskeletal system. It includes gene families coding for connective tissue matrix molecules, the factors controlling skeletal development, bone and cartilage metabolism and the intracellular and extracellular signaling pathways involved in the autocrine, paracrine and endocrine control of the musculoskeletal function and repair. Inflammation and other indirect processes also affect many of these pathways (Table 29.1).

Table 29.1 Orthopaedic genome related proteins

Protein	Function	Associated disease
Extracellular		
PTHrP	Chondrocyte proliferation	Jansen metaphyseal chondrodysplasia, enchondromatosis
BMPs	Embryologic and bone growth factor	
Noggin	BMP antagonist	Multiple synostosis syndrome
Hedgehog family	Chondrocyte proliferation	Brachydactyly type A1
GDF5	BMP antagonist	Brachydactyly type A2
RANK ligand	Osteoclast stimulation	Lytic lesions in multiple myloma
Osteoprotegrin	Osteoclast inhibition	Heredetary hyperphosphatasia
Wnt	Osteoblast differentiation	Tetra-amelia
Sclerosin	Wnt antagonist	Sclerosteosis
IGF-II	Growth hormone	Beckwith-Wiedemann syndrome
NGF	Survival and maintenance of sensory neurons	Congenital insensitivity to pain
Transmembrane		
BMP-IR	BMP receptor	Fibrodysplsia ossificans progressiva
LRP5	Wnt coreceptor	Osteoporosis-pseudoglioma syndrome
Collagen I	Bone matrix	Osteogenesis imperfecta
Collagen 2a1	Bone matrix	Kniest's dysplasia
Collagen 10a1	Cartilage matrix	Metaphyseal chondrodysplasia
Fibrillin	Connective tissue matrix	Marfan's diseaase
Intracellular		
SMADS	TGF-b related transcription factor	Juvenile polyposis
Runx	BMP related transcription factor	Cleidocranial dysplasia
b-catenin	Wnt related transcription factor	Embyologic joint fusion
Inflammatory		
IL-1	Stimulates cellular immunity and bone resorption	
COX2	Mechanotransduction signaling and skeletal repair	
TNF-alpha	Acute systemic inflammation and bone resporption	

Gene microchip arrays could also serve as a screening mechanism to characterize a patient's biochemistry profile and host potential. One major drawback, however, is that proteins, not genes, are responsible for the biologic activity of cells. Since there are at least 300 different posttranslational modifications, protein microchip arrays will be a necessary adjunct to provide comprehensive biochemistry profiles [25].

Another interesting and clinically useful subset of genetics is the study of single nucleotide polymorphisms (SNPs). These are DNA sequence variations unique to an individual that occur when a single nucleotide (A, T, Cor G) in the genome sequence is altered. There are an estimated 10 million SNPs in each human genome that serve to alter gene expression and protein conformation to a degree that makes each organism unique. Many SNPs have been linked to various risk factors for certain diseases, and there is a strong consensus that more SNPs will be linked with a variety of conditions to help stratify patients into risk categories for both the development of a condition and the susceptibility to a specific treatment. Pharmacogenomics, or how an individual's genetic inheritance affects the body's response to drugs, is particularly exciting since it offers therapies tailored to an individual's biochemical profile. For example, polymorphisms of the liver enzyme P450 are responsible for poor responses to codeine as a pain medication in up to 10 percent of the population [26]. Screening for this polymorphism allows a patient's pain management to be tailored prior to surgery. The use of SNP screening and pharmacogenomics may also serve an indispensable role in the application of tissue engineering, since the host environment plays a critical role in supporting new tissue. For example, the host genome could be screened for vasculogenesis or inflammatory potential that may lead to assimilation or rejection of the engineered tissue. To improve the therapeutic benefit, the engineered tissue could be individually tailored to optimize vasculogenesis or to decrease the risk of rejection for that patient.

As we discover more potential cell-specific therapeutic targets, therapeutic delivery remains a challenge. Therefore, there is great interest in developing gene therapy to enhance tissue repair and regeneration [27–28]. The goal could be to replace a defective gene, such as dystrophin, or may serve to overexpress a normal gene, such as BMP, insulin-like growth factor or vascular endothelial growth factor. Gene therapy may also interfere with expression of another gene by indirect effects on transcription factors or directly by binding to mRNA or intracellular proteins. Finally, of great interest to oncologists, it may act as a cell suicide signal and induce apoptosis [29–30].

The obstacles associated with developing gene therapy for tissue regeneration are safety and cost. Potential problems associated with the inflammatory response to adenoviral vectors and safety concerns about retroviral oncogenicty will require further study. The type of gene therapy that will be most useful will be determined by the duration of protein expression that is needed and whether an *ex vivo* or *in vivo* approach can be used. Therefore, a variety of vectors are likely to have clinical utility.

Vector mediated cell-specificity can be achieved in different ways. Viruses can be directed to cell-specific surface markers for entry into the 'tagged' cells. Also, the vector can contain a target gene with a promoter that is specific to a cell phenotype. For instance, hypertrophic chondrocytes are the only known cells to produce Type X collagen. A vector containing the target gene with a promotor for Type X collagen will restrict expression of the target gene to hypertrophic chondrocytes, even though other cell populations may also carry the vector. The use of an appropriate promotor also provides control over the quantity and duration of gene expression. Systemic use of an antibiotic such as tetracycline can initiate gene expression in cells carrying a vector with a tetracycline promoter [31]. Importantly, gene expression can also be terminated when the exogenous signal is stopped. Once the sequence of events in tissue regeneration are better understood, a clinician may be able to noninvasively orchestrate these signals with great precision and recapitulate the necessary events for appropriate tissue regeneration.

Safety of gene therapy is an important consideration that has limited its clinical utility. There is valid concern over triggering oncologic processes, such as leukemia, as a result of nonspecific infection of hematopoietic stem cells with retroviral vectors [32]. Preventative therapies requiring long-term gene expression and systemic therapies with extensive exposure generate the greatest concern for obvious reasons. As new cell-specific markers are identified, such as the CD105 marker for MSCs [9], cell-specific targeting would eliminate many of these safety concerns and open the door for future clinical applications of gene therapy.

The future of musculoskeletal regeneration depends on both the understanding of normal intracellular signaling and influential role of the host environment. Microchip arrays, pharmacogenomics and gene therapy all promise an exciting future for discovering therapeutic targets and providing individually tailored therapies. Since these tools form the bridge between the benchtop and the bedside, they offer a powerful thrust into the future.

29.2.3. Matrices: Tailoring Form and Function

The function of cells and signals are organized by the surrounding extracellular matrix. A matrix provides one or more of the following: mechanical support, physical form, transmission of mechanical signals and/or influence over the delivery of chemical signals to the resident or migratory cells. In general, engineered matrices will fail *in vivo* if there is discrepancy between the biologic and mechanical properties of the graft and the surrounding host tissue. Unfortunately, providing all the requisite properties is a difficult task. For this reason, many clinically available matrices designed to support tissue regeneration are less than ideal.

A certain matrix may provide adequate strength initially, but then fail from poor tissue ingrowth and eventual material fatigue. Alternately, matrices may provide excellent inductive and conductive signals, but ultimately fail without additional mechanical support. As an example, one of the few FDA-approved bone graft substitutes is recombinant human BMP-2 (rhBMP-2) on an absorbable collagen sponge (InFUSE ®) that does not provide any mechanical stability until bone has formed [33]. Similarly, demineralized bone matrices (DBM) are osteoconductive scaffolds that provide minimal or no osteoinductive activity, and surgeons must use these matrices in appropriate anatomic environments [34–35]. There are a number of other commercially available matrices, such as allograft cortical and cancellous chips and synthetic ceramics that can be used as bone graft substitutes. However, the biologic activities of these materials are variable and there are concerns related to their incorporation and eventual resorption, limiting their clinical utility.

A mechanically stable and bioactive substance would dramatically change the practice of reconstructive fields, such as orthopaedic, plastic and oromaxillofacial surgery. Percutaneous procedures with injectable, bioactive and resorbable cements could replace invasive treatments of acute fractures, chronic nonunions, and critical-sized bone defects. Management of soft tissue defects that also require mechanical strength, such as rotator cuff patches, anterior cruciate ligament (ACL) reconstruction, and cartilage or meniscal repair could likewise be performed with minimally invasive procedures and incur little functional loss during recovery.

For this reason there has been considerable research in nanotechnology, which considers the biomaterial properties such as chemistry, charge, wettability, and surface roughness. These determine the extracellular protein interactions and mediate cell interactions at the tissue/matrix interface, which are critical for biocompatibility and longevity of the implant. *In vitro* research of surface morphology has suggested the importance of nanometer roughness. Up to four times the calcium-mineral deposition occurs when osteoblasts were cultured for 28 days in the presence of ceramics with grain sizes below 100 nm, compared with conventional alumina surfaces [36]. Even greater osteoblast performance has been reported in grain sizes below 60 nm. This has been correlated to osteoblast interactions with vitronectin, which shares a linear dimension of approximately 60 nm [37]. Multiple techniques are now being explored, such as e-beam lithography, polymer demixing, chemical etching, cast-mold techniques and spin casting to fine-tune surface characteristic for optimal biologic interactions [38]. In addition, three-dimensional (3D) printers can construct 3D organic-inorganic composite matrices with a defined internal architecture. These have also demonstrated osteoblast ingrowth and proliferation *in vivo* [39].

Other novel techniques in the field of nanotechnology include local delivery of pharmaceuticals or gene therapy in polymer nanospheres embedded within carriers. This could control the timing and concentration of inductive signals for improved cell ingrowth, expansion and/or differentiation. Currently available matrices, such as absorbable collagen sponge, provide only minimal retention of signal proteins, which can be problematic. Recombinant BMPs, for example, have a half-life of 0.8 to 15.3 minutes when injected systemically into rats, depending on the initial dose. However, rhBMP-2 within an absorbable collagen sponge results in a mean residence of four to fivedays, and up to 4 percent retention of the growth factor at two weeks *in vivo* [40]. Yet supra-physiologic doses are still needed to achieve adequate bone formation. Not only does this make treatment more expensive, but dissipation of the signal may result in poor bone fusion. Thus, future matrices with embedded pharmaceuticals or nanospheres with the potential for timed release of growth factors would be a substantial development.

Certainly, the potential for developing sophisticated matrices is growing. However, tailoring the properties of matrices to encourage ingrowth of viable tissue requires a basic understanding of the cells and signals involved in regeneration. As these areas are better understood, the ability to provide an appropriate matrix will only be limited by the technology required in their construction.

29.2.4. Cells, Signals and Matrices: The Keys to Primary Care?

Advances in each of these three active areas of research– cells, signals and matrices – will undoubtedly result in the ability to provide systemic or local delivery of targeted therapy for rapid tissue regeneration with little functional loss. The controlled expansion and differentiation of stem cells, guided by timed delivery of the appropriate growth signals within a suitable implant, is no longer science fiction, but an emerging reality. Eventually, large segmental bone defects secondary to trauma or tumors could be healed and soft tissues in functionally sensitive areas, such as rotator cuffs and menisci, could be repaired. Is it possible, then, that an entire organ could be engineered? Would joint arthroplasty come to mean joint replacement with a newly grown autologous shoulder, hip or knee? Will there be a role for metal, ceramic or plastic implants at all?

While this is not impossible, the utility of engineered whole tissue autografts will be limited in the future. Parallel advances in diagnostics and cell biology will ultimately lead to earlier disease recognition, opening the door for improved primary care of musculoskeletal diseases. The end-stage diseases we see today, such as large chronic rotator cuff tears, severe arthropathy and osteoporotic fractures, may become as rare as polio is today. Therapeutics will likely be directed at reversing pathologic cytokine production or bolstering appropriate protein production to maintain or improve musculoskeletal health in a primary care setting.

29.3. Characterizing the Future Musculoskeletal Patient

29.3.1. Molecular Diagnostics: Refining Risk Stratification

The host environment is an extremely important consideration in the application of tissue engineering. There is a growing awareness of predisposing factors to musculoskeletal diseases and these same factors may determine the efficacy of specific therapies *in vivo*. Understanding patient phenotypes, therefore, will be a critical component to developing treatment algorithms.

Patient screening will become a critical tool for musculoskeletal health providers. Osteoporosis, for example, is predisposed by environmental factors such as poor nutrition and exercise. It is also caused by defects in the collagen 1a1 and 1a2 genes [41]. A few factors alone, however, are unlikely to account for the widespread prevalence and variance of osteoporosis [42]. In fact twin and family studies in idiopathic osteoporosis suggest that genetic factors may account for 50 to 80 percent of the interindividual variation of bone mineral density [43–47].

A major discovery has been the variations of the Wnt coreceptor, LPR5, that are linked to normal variability of bone mineral density within the general population. As recently as 2001, loss-of-function mutations in LPR5 were discovered to cause autosomal-dominant osteoporosis pseudoglioma syndrome [48]. This rare disease occurs in children with very low bone mass, but no other identifiable defects in collagen synthesis, anabolic and catabolic hormones, calcium homeostasis, endochondral growth or bone turnover [49]. Subsequent studies of the LPR5 gene sequence in various populations led to the identification of several SNPs which may either be directly responsible for subtle variations in protein kinetics, or may simply be linked to nearby genetic variations [50]. Regardless, differences between phenotypes can be predicted by identifying SNP for a disease that affects millions each year.

Other screening factors for orthopaedic diseases have been identified. Osteolysis and implant loosening have recently been linked to variations in the TNF gene promoter, IL-1 gene family, and frizzled-related protein 3 [51–52]. Increased or decreased expression of these factors in an individual with osteoarthritis may influence a clinician's decision to recommend a total joint arthroplasty. Other performance biomarkers such as urine metal ion levels [53], serum cytokines [54], and lymphocyte response [55] could be used to monitor patients postsurgically. Recognizing implant failure earlier may allow for novel interventions to prevent catastrophic events and provide faster feedback for implant design assessment.

Identifying multiple risk factors is increasingly simple. As discussed earlier, microchip arrays are currently capable of holding up to 50,000 probes, and their number and accuracy continues to improve. In fact, the exponential growth of such biotechnology is reminiscent of the growth of informatics as recognized by of Moore's Law. In 1965 Gordon E. Moore, the co-founder of Intel, published his empirical observation that the complexity of integrated circuits, with respect to minimum component cost, doubles every 24 months [56]. This trend has continued to present day with 65 nm chips replacing the 500 nm chips from only a decade ago. As biotechnology and bioinformatics become increasingly linked, the potential for defining a patient's unique genetic blueprint and interpreting their predisposition to various diseases is truly profound. The increasing availability of such patient information also raises concern over privacy and health-related ethical issues.

29.3.2. Issues in Primary Care: Taking Heed from the Osteoporosis Model

Improved medical knowledge and technology does not necessarily enable patients to lead healthier lives. Osteoporosis is responsible for approximately 1.5 million fragility fractures annually within the United States [57]. After one fragility fracture, there is a 1.5 to 9.5-fold increase in risk for future fractures, yet it is reported that 40 to 70 percent of patients treated for a fragility fracture did not believe they had osteoporosis [58]. Furthermore, patients are often not compliant with medical regimens [59]. Advice to eat a healthy diet and partake in moderate exercise is frequently ignored, and newly available treatments with bisphosphonates or denosumab are not initiated. Therefore, patient education and motivation will likely be just as important as developing sophisticated therapeutics if they are ever to yield any benefit.

29.3.3. New Ethical Considerations: Are We Ready?

Genetic testing demands responsible management of potentially harmful information. The mental burden of a lethal or debilitating disease – without effective treatment – on patients, their families and caregivers can be extremely detrimental. Also, knowledge of predisposing factors can influence medical insurance providers and render patients without adequate medical coverage. Fortunately, this has been an active area of public debate. Topics such as genetic discrimination, implications of genomic research on policy and balancing intellectual property rights with the need for research continues to be addressed by the National Human Genome Research Institute at the National Institute of Health. There is no doubt that genetics will enhance primary care. However the dilemmas inherent to such powerful knowledge will need to be recognized and resolved as a society over time.

29.3.4. The Musculoskeletal Patient in 2020

The following case study is a hypothetical assessment of a patient adapted from the "Shattuck Lecture – Medical and Societal Consequences of the Human Genome Project: by F.S. Collins [60]."

A 50-year-old female suffers from severe degenerative osteoarthritis of her right knee with significant cartilage and bone loss, and her treatment algorithm is initiated (Fig. 29.1). After a thorough history and physical examination, her genetic and proteomic profile is scanned from her medical identification microchip. It shows she has an osteoporosis risk of 6.3, an osteoarthritis risk index of 4.2 and an "arthroplasty loosening index" of 3.5, which are based on the relative expression of genes known to be involved in bone turnover, cartilage degradation and prosthetic loosening. After factoring in other factors, such as her age, weight and activity level, it is recommended that she undergo a total knee arthroplasty. The implant surface will be treated with a matrix that encourages osteoblast ingrowth and also harbors viral particles

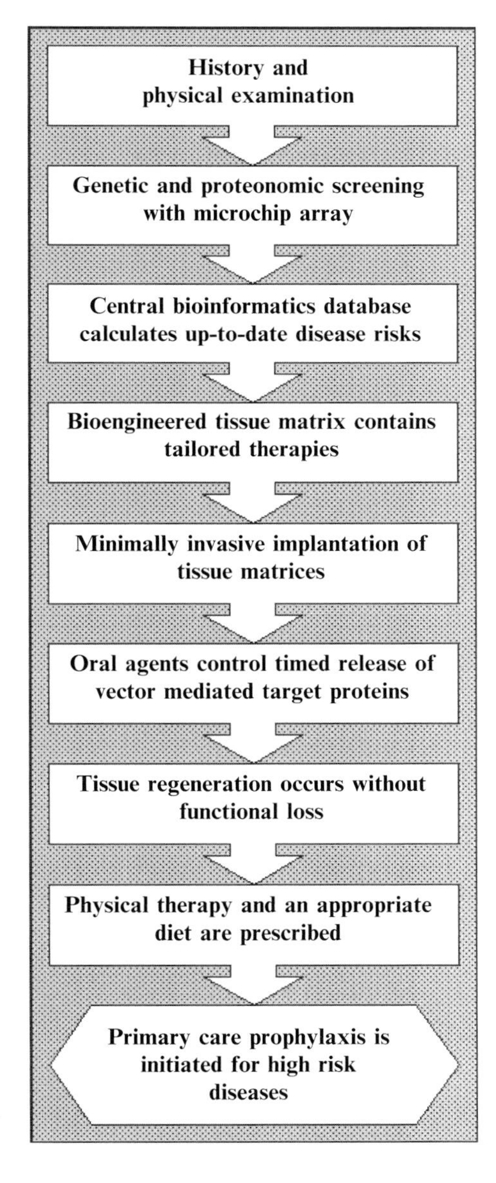

Fig. 29.1 Future musculoskeletal regeneration treatment algorithm

encoding proteins designed to block transcription factors involved in pathologic osteolysis. Expression of therapeutic genes can be controlled by an oral agent. She undergoes surgery and, prior to leaving the hospital, she is well informed by a medical education team regarding her risk factors for various diseases and what preventative therapies are available.

Several years later during her routine follow-up, she describes a recent twisting injury to her 'good' knee while skiing and her work-up reveals a torn ACL and meniscus, with a chronic full-thickness loss of medial compartment cartilage and subchondral bone. She is advised that total joint reconstruction now has better success rates with tissue engineering and she is scheduled for a minimally invasive implantation of hyaline cartilage. On the day of the procedure, off-the-shelf ACL and hyaline cartilage matrices that have been seeded with embryonic stem cells are selected. The ACL matrix contains fibers with enough tensile strength to allow immediate mobilization of the knee. The bioactive fibers are engineered so they are replaced by *de novo* ligament at different rates to maintain tensile strength during ligament regeneration. The hyaline cartilage matrix contains nanospheres that release bioactive factors when they experience a critical shear threshold. This helps to stimulate assimilation of the graft into the surrounding cartilage and bone. Finally, during her minimally invasive implantation, her meniscus is repaired with fibrin glue containing small viral particles encoding for several dedifferentiation and proliferative factors to initiate *de novo* mensical repair. One week later she is functionally well, and is able to continue her walking exercises that are part of her disease prevention plan. She also begins systemic oral therapy for osteoporosis prevention, based on her age-related risk factors and biochemical profiles.

References

1. Bianco P, Gehron Robey P. Marrow stromal stem cells. J Clin Invest. 2000 Jun;105(12):1663–8.
2. Tagliafico E, Brunelli S, Bergamaschi A, De Angelis L, Scardigli R, Galli D, Battini R, Bianco P, Ferrari S, Cossu G, Ferrari S. TGFbeta/BMP activate the smooth muscle/bone differentiation programs in mesoangioblasts. J Cell Sci. 2004 Sep 1;117(Pt 19):4377–88.
3. Kawamoto A, Gwon HC, Iwaguro H, Yamaguchi JI, Uchida S, Masuda H, Silver M, Ma H, Kearney M, Isner JM, Asahara T. Therapeutic potential of ex vivo expanded endothelial progenitor cells for myocardial ischemia. Circulation. 2001 Feb 6;103(5):634–7.
4. Jiang Y, Jahagirdar BN, Reinhardt RL, Schwartz RE, Keene CD, Ortiz-Gonzalez XR, Reyes M, Lenvik T, Lund T, Blackstad M, Du J, Aldrich S, Lisberg A, Low WC, Largaespada DA, Verfaillie CM. Pluripotency of mesenchymal stem cells derived from adult marrow. Nature. 2002 Jul 4;418(6893):41–9. Epub 2002 Jun 20.
5. Nilsson SK, Simmons PJ. Transplantable stem cells: home to specific niches. Curr Opin Hematol. 2004 Mar;11(2):102–6. Review.
6. Dragoo JL, Lieberman JR, Lee RS, Deugarte DA, Lee Y, Zuk PA, Hedrick MH, Benhaim P. Tissue-engineered bone from BMP-2-transduced stem cells derived from human fat. Plast Reconstr Surg. 2005 May;115(6):1665–73.
7. Hernigou P, Poignard A, Beaujean F, Rouard H. Percutaneous autologous bone-marrow grafting for nonunions. Influence of the number and concentration of progenitor cells. J Bone Joint Surg Am. 2005 Jul;87(7):1430–7.
8. Ramalho-Santos M, Yoon S, Matsuzaki Y, Mulligan RC, Melton DA. "Stemness": transcriptional profiling of embryonic and adult stem cells. Science. 2002 Oct 18;298(5593):597–600.

9. Aslan H, Zilberman Y, Kandel L, Liebergall M, Oskouian RJ, Gazit D, Gazit Z. Osteogenic differentiation of noncultured immunoisolated bone marrow-derived CD105+ cells. Stem Cells. 2006 Jul;24(7):1728–37.
10. Anastasia L, Sampaolesi M, Papini N, Oleari D, Lamorte G, Tringali C, Monti E, Galli D, Tettamanti G, Cossu G, Venerando B. Reversine-treated fibroblasts acquire myogenic competence in vitro and in regenerating skeletal muscle. Cell Death Differ. 2006 May 26.
11. Kurtz SM, Lau E, Mowat F, Ong K, Halpern, MT. The Future Burden of Hip and Knee Revisions: U.S. Projections from 2005 to 2030. AAOS 2006 Annual Meeting: Paper 403. Presented March 24, 2006. Electronic publication: *http://www.aaos.org/education/*anmeet/anmt2006/podium/podium.cfm?* Pevent=403* (accessed Dec 20, 2006).
12. Gan Q, Yoshida T, McDonald OG, Owens GK. Epigenetic Mechanisms Contribute to Pluripotency and Cell Lineage Determination of Embryonic Stem Cells. Stem Cells. 2006 Oct 5. (Electronic publication ahead of print)
13. Urist MR, Mikulski A, Lietze A. Solubilized and insolubilized bone morphogenetic protein. Proc Natl Acad Sci U S A. 1979 Apr;76(4):1828–32.
14. Shaw NJ, Fraser NC, Rose S, Crabtree NJ, Boivin CM. Bone density and body composition in children with growth hormone insensitivity syndrome receiving recombinant IGF-I. Clin Endocrinol (Oxf). 2003 Oct;59(4):487–91.
15. Steed DL. Clinical evaluation of recombinant human platelet-derived growth factor for the treatment of lower extremity ulcers. Plast Reconstr Surg. 2006 Jun;117 (7 Suppl):143S–149S.
16. Spivak JL, Ferris DK, Fisher J, Noga SJ, Isaacs M, Connor E, Hankins WD. Cell cycle-specific behavior of erythropoietin. Exp Hematol. 1996 Feb;24(2):141–50.
17. Boden SD, Kang J, Sandhu H, Heller JG. Use of recombinant human bone morphogenetic protein-2 to achieve posterolateral lumbar spine fusion in humans: a prospective, randomized clinical pilot trial: 2002 Volvo Award in clinical studies. Spine. 2002 Dec 1;27(23):2662–73.
18. Govender S, Csimma C, Genant HK, Valentin-Opran A, Amit Y, Arbel R, Aro H, Atar D, Bishay M, Borner MG, Chiron P, Choong P, Cinats J, Courtenay B, Feibel R, Geulette B, Gravel C, Haas N, Raschke M, Hammacher E, van der Velde D, Hardy P, Holt M, Josten C, Ketterl RL, Lindeque B, Lob G, Mathevon H, McCoy G, Marsh D, Miller R, Munting E, Oevre S, Nordsletten L, Patel A, Pohl A, Rennie W, Reynders P, Rommens PM, Rondia J, Rossouw WC, Daneel PJ, Ruff S, Ruter A, Santavirta S, Schildhauer TA, Gekle C, Schnettler R, Segal D, Seiler H, Snowdowne RB, Stapert J, Taglang G, Verdonk R, Vogels L, Weckbach A, Wentzensen A, Wisniewski T; BMP-2 Evaluation in Surgery for Tibial Trauma (BESTT) Study Group. Recombinant human bone morphogenetic protein-2 for treatment of open tibial fractures: a prospective, controlled, randomized study of four hundred and fifty patients. J Bone Joint Surg Am. 2002 Dec;84-A(12):2123–34.
19. Sherwin RS, Borg WP, Boulware SD. Metabolic effects of insulin-like growth factor-1 in normal humans. Horm Res 1994;41 (suppl 2): 97–102.
20. Nevins M, Giannobile WV, McGuire MK, Kao RT, Mellonig JT, Hinrichs JE, McAllister BS, Murphy KS, McClain PK, Nevins ML, Paquette DW, Han TJ, Reddy MS, Lavin PT, Genco RJ, Lynch SE. Platelet-derived growth factor stimulates bone fill and rate of attachment level gain: results of a large multicenter randomized controlled trial. J Periodontol. 2005 Dec;76(12):2330–2.
21. Ranly DM, McMillan J, Keller T, Lohmann CH, Meunch T, Cochran DL, Schwartz Z, Boyan BD. Platelet-derived growth factor inhibits demineralized bone matrix-induced intramuscular cartilage and bone formation. A study of immunocompromised mice. J Bone Joint Surg Am. 2005 Sep;87(9):2052–64.
22. Gallea S, Lallemand F, Atfi A, Rawadi G, Ramez V, Spinella-Jaegle S, Kawai S, Faucheu C, Huet L, Baron R, Roman-Roman S. Activation of mitogen-activated protein kinase cascades is involved in regulation of bone morphogenetic protein-2-induced osteoblast differentiation in pluripotent C2C12 cells. Bone. 2001 May;28(5):491–8.

23. Dudley AT, Godin RE, Robertson EJ Interaction between FGF and BMP signaling pathways regulates development of metanephric mesenchyme. Genes Dev. 1999 Jun 15;13(12):1601–13.
24. Puzas JE, O'Keefe RJ, Lieberman JR. The orthopaedic genome: what does the future hold and are we ready? J Bone Joint Surg Am. 2002 Jan;84-A(1):133–41.
25. Melton L: Protein arrays: Proteomics in multiplex. Nature 2004; 429: 101–107.
26. Gardiner SJ, Begg EJ. Pharmacogenetics, drug-metabolizing enzymes, and clinical practice. Pharmacol Rev. 2006 Sep;58(3):521–90.
27. Baltzer AW, Lieberman JR. Regional gene therapy to enhance bone repair. Gene Ther. 2004 Feb;11(4):344–50. Review.
28. Lieberman JR, Ghivizzani SC, Evans CH. Gene transfer approaches to the healing of bone and cartilage. Mol Ther. 2002 Aug;6(2):141–7. Review.
29. O'Keefe DS, Uchida A, Bacich DJ, Watt FB, Martorana A, Molloy PL, Heston WD. Prostate-specific suicide gene therapy using the prostate-specific membrane antigen promoter and enhancer. Prostate. 2000 Oct 1;45(2):149–57.
30. Li X, Zhang J, Gao H, Vieth E, Bae KH, Zhang YP, Lee SJ, Raikwar S, Gardner TA, Hutchins GD, VanderPutten D, Kao C, Jeng MH. Transcriptional targeting modalities in breast cancer gene therapy using adenovirus vectors controlled by alpha-lactalbumin promoter. Mol Cancer Ther. 2005 Dec;4(12):1850–9.
31. Nakagawa S, Massie B, Hawley RG. Tetracycline-regulatable adenovirus vectors: pharmacologic properties and clinical potential. Eur J Pharm Sci. 2001 Apr;13(1):53–60. Review.
32. Check E. Cancer risk prompts US to curb gene therapy. Nature. 2003 Mar 6;422(6927):7.
33. Minamide A, Kawakami M, Hashizume H, Sakata R, Tamaki T. Evaluation of carriers of bone morphogenetic protein for spinal fusion.. Spine. 2001 Apr 15;26(8):933–9.
34. Peterson B, Whang PG, Iglesias R, Wang JC, Lieberman JR. Osteoinductivity of commercially available demineralized bone matrix. Preparations in a spine fusion model. J Bone Joint Surg Am. 2004 Oct;86-A(10):2243–50.
35. Oakes DA, Lee CC, Lieberman JR. An evaluation of human demineralized bone matrices in a rat femoral defect model. Clin Orthop Relat Res. 2003 Aug;(413):281–90.
36. Webster TJ, Ergun C, Doremus RH, Siegel RW, Bizios R. Enhanced functions of osteoblasts on nanophase ceramics. Biomaterials. 2000 Sep;21(17):1803–10.
37. Webster TJ, Schadler LS, Siegel RW, Bizios R. Mechanisms of enhanced osteoblast adhesion on nanophase alumina involve vitronectin. Tissue Eng. 2001 Jun;7(3):291–301.
38. J.B. Thomas, N.A. Peppas, M. Sato, and T.J. Webster. Nanotechnology and Biomaterials in *CRC Nanomaterials Handbook*, Y. Gogotsi ed. CRC Press, Boca Raton, 2005.
39. Manjubala I, Woesz A, Pilz C, Rumpler M, Fratzl-Zelman N, Roschger P, Stampfl J, Fratzl P. Biomimetic mineral-organic composite scaffolds with controlled internal architecture. J Mater Sci Mater Med. 2005 Dec;16(12):1111–9.
40. Friess W, Uludag H, Foskett S, Biron R, Sargeant C. Characterization of absorbable collagen sponges as recombinant human bone morphogenetic protein-2 carriers. Int J Pharm, 1999;185: 51–60.
41. Mann V, Ralston SH. Meta-analysis of COL1A1 Sp1 polymorphism in relation to bone mineral density and osteoporotic fracture. Bone. 2003 Jun;32(6):711–7.
42. Liu YJ, Shen H, Xiao P, Xiong DH, Li LH, Recker RR, Deng HW. Molecular genetic studies of gene identification for osteoporosis: a 2004 update. J Bone Miner Res. 2006 Oct;21(10):1511–35.
43. Duncan EL, Cardon LR, Sinsheimer JS, Wass JA, Brown MA. Site and gender specificity of inheritance of bone mineral density. J Bone Miner Res. 2003 Aug;18(8):1531–8.

44. Pocock NA, Eisman JA, Mazess RB, Sambrook PN, Yeates MG, Freund J. Bone mineral density in Australia compared with the United States. J Bone Miner Res. 1988 Dec;3(6):601–4.
45. Arden NK, Baker J, Hogg C, Baan K, Spector TD. The heritability of bone mineral density, ultrasound of the calcaneus and hip axis length: a study of postmenopausal twins. J Bone Miner Res. 1996 Apr;11(4):530–4.
46. Garnero P, Arden NK, Griffiths G, Delmas PD, Spector TD. Genetic influence on bone turnover in postmenopausal twins. J Clin Endocrinol Metab. 1996 Jan;81(1):140–6.
47. MacInnis RJ, Cassar C, Nowson CA, Paton LM, Flicker L, Hopper JL, Larkins RG, Wark JD. Determinants of bone density in 30- to 65-year-old women: a co-twin study. J Bone Miner Res. 2003 Sep;18(9):1650–6.
48. Gong Y, Slee RB, Fukai N, Rawadi G, Roman-Roman S, Reginato AM, Wang H, Cundy T, Glorieux FH, Lev D, Zacharin M, Oexle K, Marcelino J, Suwairi W, Heeger S, Sabatakos G, Apte S, Adkins WN, Allgrove J, Arslan-Kirchner M, Batch JA, Beighton P, Black GC, Boles RG, Boon LM, Borrone C, Brunner HG, Carle GF, Dallapiccola B, De Paepe A, Floege B, Halfhide ML, Hall B, Hennekam RC, Hirose T, Jans A, Juppner H, Kim CA, Keppler-Noreuil K, Kohlschuetter A, LaCombe D, Lambert M, Lemyre E, Letteboer T, Peltonen L, Ramesar RS, Romanengo M, Somer H, Steichen-Gersdorf E, Steinmann B, Sullivan B, Superti-Furga A, Swoboda W, van den Boogaard MJ, Van Hul W, Vikkula M, Votruba M, Zabel B, Garcia T, Baron R, Olsen BR, Warman ML; Osteoporosis-Pseudoglioma Syndrome Collaborative Group. LDL receptor-related protein 5 (LRP5) affects bone accrual and eye development. Cell. 2001 Nov 16;107(4):513–23.
49. Gong Y, Vikkula M, Boon L, Liu J, Beighton P, Ramesar R, Peltonen L, Somer H, Hirose T, Dallapiccola B, De Paepe A, Swoboda W, Zabel B, Superti-Furga A, Steinmann B, Brunner HG, Jans A, Boles RG, Adkins W, van den Boogaard MJ, Olsen BR, Warman ML. Osteoporosis-pseudoglioma syndrome, a disorder affecting skeletal strength and vision, is assigned to chromosome region 11q12–13. Am J Hum Genet. 1996 Jul;59(1):146–51.
50. Koay MA, Woon PY, Zhang Y, Miles LJ, Duncan EL, Ralston SH, Compston JE, Cooper C, Keen R, Langdahl BL, MacLelland A, O'Riordan J, Pols HA, Reid DM, Uitterlinden AG, Wass JA, Brown MA. Influence of LRP5 polymorphisms on normal variation in BMD. J Bone Miner Res. 2004 Oct;19(10):1619–27.
51. Wilkinson JM, Wilson AG, Stockley I, Scott IR, Macdonald DA, Hamer AJ, Duff GW, Eastell R. Variation in the TNF gene promoter and risk of osteolysis after total hip arthroplasty. J Bone Miner Res. 2003 Nov;18(11):1995–2001.
52. Hausler KD, Horwood NJ, Chuman Y, Fisher JL, Ellis J, Martin TJ, Rubin JS, Gillespie MT. J Bone Miner Res. Secreted frizzled-related protein-1 inhibits RANKL-dependent osteoclast formation. 2004 Nov;19(11):1873–81.
53. Skipor AK, Campbell PA, Patterson LM, Anstutz HC, Schmalzried TP, Jacobs JJ. Serum and urine metal levels in patients with metal-on-metal surface arthroplasty. J Mater Sci Mater Med. 2002 Dec;13(12):1227–34.
54. Granchi D, Verri E, Ciapetti G, Stea S, Savarino L, Sudanese A, Mieti M, Rotini R, Dallari D, Zinghi G, Montanaro L. Bone-resorbing cytokines in serum of patients with aseptic loosening of hip prostheses. J Bone Joint Surg Br. 1998 Sep;80(5):912–7.
55. Hallab NJ, Anderson S, Stafford T, Glant T, Jacobs JJ. Lymphocyte responses in patients with total hip arthroplasty. J Orthop Res. 2005 Mar;23(2):384–91.
56. Moore, G. Cramming more components onto integrated circuits. Electronics Magazine 19 April 1965.
57. Boden SD, Einhorn TA, Morgan TS, Tosi LL, Weinstein JN. An AOA Critical Issue. The Future of the Orthopaedic Surgeon–Proceduralist or Keeper of the Musculoskeletal System? J Bone Joint Surg Am, Dec 2005; 87: 2812–2821.

58. Chevalley T, Hoffmeyer P, Bonjour JP, Rizzoli R. An osteoporosis clinical pathway for the medical management of patients with low-trauma fracture. Osteoporos Int. 2002;13(6):450–5.
59. Adami S, Isaia G, Luisetto G, Minisola S, Sinigaglia L, Gentilella R, Agnusdei D, Iori N, Nuti R; on behalf of ICARO Study Group. Fracture incidence and characterization in patients on osteoporosis treatment: the ICARO study. J Bone Miner Res. 2006 Oct;21(10):1565–70.
60. Collins FS. Shattuck lecture–medical and societal consequences of the Human Genome Project. N Engl J Med. 1999 Jul 1;341(1):28–37.

Index

R